WITHDRAWN

PRINCIPLES OF

Urology

An Introductory Textbook to the
Diseases of the Urogenital Tract

MEREDITH F. CAMPBELL, M.S., M.D., F.A.C.S.

*Emeritus Professor of Urology, New York University.
Consulting Urologist to Bellevue Hospital, New York;
to Variety Childrens Hospital, Miami, and to St. Francis
Hospital, Miami Beach, Florida; Lecturer in Urology,
University of Miami School of Medicine.*

W. B. SAUNDERS COMPANY

Philadelphia & London

1957

Each one of us, however old, is still an undergraduate in the school of experience. When a man thinks he has graduated, he becomes a public menace.
       —John Chalmers Da Costa, M.D.

Preface

THE TWOFOLD purpose of this book is suggested by its title: for the instruction of the student in the broad fundamentals of Urology, and to serve as a practical guide for the physician who is not a urologic specialist, as he encounters urologic problems. This is not intended to be a complete reference textbook nor an armchair urology. The conceit implied by its writing is founded on an experience of thirty-five years in the teaching of Urology to both undergraduate and graduate students of medicine.

Somewhat of an innovation but sound pedagogy, a brief consideration of urologic semantics is followed by a short syllabus of the more frequently employed urologic terms; many are doubtless new to the undergraduate student, yet are certain to be important tools in his clinical career. On the assumption that the upper class student has been away from the dissecting room for at least one and usually two years, and the practicing physician has left the benches much longer, a brief review of the more important aspects of urogenital tract anatomy and physiology are included as an introductory refresher. Urologic symptoms and their potential significance as indications for special urologic examination are discussed, while the pathogenesis, clinical aspects, diagnosis and treatment of the more common urologic diseases are considered adequately, it is hoped, to the needs of active daily general practice either in the office or at the bedside. It is not expected that the urologically untrained physician will undertake the more highly technical procedures which occasionally are here mentioned but he should at least know what they are and why and how they are employed.

Special effort has been made to instruct the reader in the requisites of physical and laboratory examination and diagnostic study up to the point of cystoscopic investigation or major urosurgical therapy. Minor urologic office procedures such as meatotomy and the passage of catheters and sounds are illustrated; properly every practitioner should be com-

petent in their use. Unlikely theories, contentious points, and descriptions
of major operative procedures are omitted.

A useful and stimulating inclusion in a book of this type is a chapter
of questions with page references to the answers. This will be helpful to
the student reviewing his medical school course in Urology and later,
perhaps, in preparation for state and other board examinations.

Some illustrations shown here have also been used in my CLINICAL
PEDIATRIC UROLOGY (1951), and three-volume UROLOGY (1954),
but since both of these were published by W. B. Saunders Company no
special notation or credit has been made except when the original was
other than mine.

I am grateful to my colleagues and special associates of past years,
many of whom have aided immeasurably in the scrupulous collection
with me of data concerning all phases of urogenital tract pathology as
observed in 51,291 autopsies, and of personal operating room records at
hospitals with which I have been associated. I am indebted to the pub-
lisher who, as always, has been most cooperative, generous and artistic.

MEREDITH F. CAMPBELL

Miami, Florida
March, 1957

Contents

Contents   xv

CHAPTER 1 *Introduction to Urology*

Definition and Scope. Urology is that branch of medical science concerned with the urinary organs in both sexes, and the genital apparatus in the male. Diseases of the female reproductive tract are in the province of Gynecology. During the past twenty years the adrenals have become included in the field of Urology, a thoroughly logical incorporation for both embryologic and clinical reasons (cf. Chapter 13).

Urology is here considered on the basis of the various urosystemic mechanisms such as obstruction, infection, calculous disease, tumors, neuromuscular disease and so forth, as distinguished from the teaching of Urology as a collection of pigeonholed anatomic entities such as diseases of the kidneys, diseases of the ureter, and diseases of the bladder, for example. Thus, either organic or neurogenic obstruction may cause urinary stasis or urinary constipation which favors the development and perpetuation of urinary infection (cf. Chapter 7). Obstruction and/or infection account for at least 90 per cent of the urologic problems in infants and children and for an even higher incidence of urologic lesions in older patients. In the young most obstruction is congenital in association with anomalous development (Chapter 6). Continuing, either obstruction or infection or both are the principal etiologic considerations in the formation of most urinary calculi. Furthermore, it is generally accepted that chronic bacterial irritation (infection) is a frequent etiologic factor in the development of cancer, particularly of the urinary organs.

Thus a clear understanding of the fundamentals of uropathy as it results from these various mechanisms will enormously clarify for the physician the pathogenesis of the usual conditions clinically encountered in the urogenital apparatus and comparably simplify both accurate diagnosis and the selection of rational treatment. In keeping with the purpose of this book little space is devoted to the highly technical details of

1

cystoscopy, pyelography, and special instrumentation, but an effort has been made to describe succinctly the methods and means of physical, laboratory, and even some radiographic examinations which the upper class medical student or nonurologist practitioner should be able to make himself or, at least, closely supervise. This arrangement of presentation has proved the most logical and effective; without clear appreciation of the initial discussion and somewhat didactic review of the basics in Urology, the remainder of the book can be little more than a quasi urologic almanac for which it is not intended. For greatest practical facility, the Index is somewhat more meticulous and extensive than usual. The nonurologist who finds himself completely in the dark on a urologic clinical problem may, by noting the symptoms and learning their more usual causes as given in Chapter 2, be enabled to establish the probable diagnosis with reasonable accuracy.

SEMANTICS AND WORD USAGE IN UROLOGY

The medical student's instruction in acceptable composition and speaking has usually terminated with his course in college Freshman English (or other mother tongue). While no special attention is generally devoted to it in medical school, it is nevertheless most desirable that the student be properly indoctrinated in the use of scientific terminologies for speaking and writing and especially to discourage his employment of clinical jargon or slang which, unfortunately, is all too readily and impressively acquired by the medical neophyte. Equally unfortunate is the fact that the sloppy jargon and slang expressions so avidly gained in his professional formative years are more than likely to become part and parcel of his subsequent career as a depreciating detriment.

Limitation of space sharply restricts the discussion of semantics and word usage in Urology; only a few of the more common errors can be cited but a sensitive ear will detect many others.

Except in statistical and impersonal clinical recording, the unfortunate person with disease is not a case but a patient. Properly one does not take a history from a case but from a patient. A patient, not a case, is operated upon. Similarly and particularly in the history, the patient should be referred to as a man or a woman and not as a male or a female, but the sick one may be a male infant or a female child. A patient has symptoms, not symptomatology.

Kidneys, bladders and other organs are not spoken of or recorded as negative, but as normal if they are; yet the examination, not the structures, may be negative. An organ such as the ureter does not show pathology but rather a pathologic condition; pathology is the science of disease.

In speaking of or recording a roentgenographic examination it is an *x-ray film* that is examined not an x-ray plate—yet, originally, fifty years ago they were glass plates! The roentgenologist is a physician expert in roentgenology and not a mere photographer. The preliminary x-ray exposure may be a *plain* or *scout* film. In urography, either retrograde or excretory, the radiopaque solution employed is a *medium* (media, plural) and is not a dye. Indigo carmine, methylene blue and phenolsulfonphthalein are *dyes*. What is too commonly referred to as *intravenous urography* should properly be designated as *excretory urography;* the medium may be injected intravenously, subcutaneously, intramuscularly and, as in present-day cholangiography, a medium to be taken by mouth may be discovered.

Note the difference between the frequently and commonly incorrectly and interchangeably used terms *dilation* and *dilatation.* One dilates a urethral or ureteral stricture with a dilating instrument (dilation), but instrumental dilatation is not carried out. Dilatation is an abnormal quantitative increase in the caliber of the lumen of a hollow structure or viscus such as the bowel or heart, and in the urinary apparatus results from obstruction, inflammation, infection or neurogenic paresis whether in the bladder, ureter or kidney pelvis. Dilatation of the ureter is known as *ureterectasis;* dilatation of the kidney pelvis is designated as *pyelectasis.*

The plural of *diverticulum* (L.) is diverticula and not as so often written or spoken, diverticuli or diverticulae. Today the term *orchiectomy* (removal of the testicle) is preferred to orchidectomy and many choose the use of *cryptorchism* (condition of improperly descended testis) to cryptorchidism, or *hermaphrodism* rather than hermaphroditism. A man is not a prostatic; he is a patient with hyperplasia, hypertrophy, adenoma, inflammation or other disease of the prostate. A patient does not have a neisserian disease, he has gonorrhea. A *tubercular* lesion is a nodular one (e.g., tubercular syphilides) and does not necessarily have anything to do with tuberculosis. A *tuberculous* lesion, on the other hand, is caused by Mycobacterium tuberculosis.

One of the most frequent examples of spoken jargonese is the use of the word *cystoscope* as a verb which it is not but, rather, a noun. Its use may be enlarged; it is recognized that word usage makes the language. Yet, properly, one does not cystoscope a patient any more than one lithotomizes or "T and A's" a patient, or one microscopes a slide or an astronomer telescopes the sky. *Cystoscopy* is performed, or a patient is subjected to cystoscopy, or a cystoscope is passed or introduced, or a cystoscopic examination is made. Similarly, a patient is not sounded; rather, *sounds* are passed or a urethral stricture is dilated with sounds. A patient is *prepared* for operation, not "prepped." He is *operated upon*, not operated on nor operated. Etymologically, operate means to work but no conscientious surgeon "works" his patients. The frequently erroneously employed term *fulgurate* means the destruction of a lesion by unipolar current or by sparking. It is impossible to use this current under water as in cystoscopic surgery which requires a bipolar current; properly, such electrodestruction of tissue should be designated as *electrocoagulation.*

The citations in the last few paragraphs by no means exhaust urologic jargon nor are they hypercritically presented, for in the literary compositions of many of our best scientific writers and even more so in the "scientific" produce of the "popular" nonscientist authors, semantic lint pickers can find much for technical criticism.

SYLLABUS OF COMMON UROLOGIC TERMS

It is likely that as the student progresses in this book, he will find many words which are as completely new to him as are the conditions or the procedures they denote. Since these words are certain to become helpful tools in his clinical speaking and recording, the more frequently employed, useful or confusing are here listed with the Latin (L.) or Greek (Gr.) derivations, irregular plural forms, and often with examples of their derivative application. A few prefixes and suffixes the student should know are also given.

ORGANS

KIDNEY(S)	(L. ren; Gr. nephros) e.g., renal; nephritis, nephrosis.
PELVIS(ES)	(L. pelvis, "basin"; Gr. pyelos) e.g., pyelitis, pyelotomy.
URETER(S)	(Gr. ureter) e.g., ureteral (adj.).
BLADDER(S)	(L. vesica; Gr. kystos) e.g., vesical; cystitis.
PROSTATE(S)	(Gr. prostates (pro, before; statos, standing); literally, to stand in front of the bladder; e.g., prostatitis, prostatectomy.
SEMINAL VESICLE(S)	(L. seminalis); adjective: vesicular (note difference from vesical).
URETHRA(S)	(Gr. urethra) e.g., urethritis.
PENIS(ISES)	(L. penis) e.g., penile (adj.).
SCROTUM(TA)	(L. scrotum ("bag")) e.g., scrotal (adj.).
TESTICLE(S)	(L. testiculus; Gr. orchis) e.g., testicular; orchiectomy.
EPIDIDYMIS(IDES)	(Gr. epididymis) e.g., epididymal.
VAS DEFERENS	(L. vas deferens); plural: vasa deferentia.

PREFIXES

A-
AN-   Without or not; used chiefly with words of Greek origin, e.g.:

abacterial:	Devoid of bacteria (often a virus infection).
agenesis:	Defective development or absence of parts.
aplasia:	Incomplete or defective development of tissue.
anemia:	Blood deficient in quantity or quality.
anuria:	Total suppression of urinary secretion by kidney.

AZO-   denoting the presence of the -N:N- group:

azotemia:	Presence of urea or other nitrogenous bodies in excess in the blood.

DYS-   (Gr. dys); difficult, painful, bad, disordered, etc.:

dysuria:	Difficult or painful urination.
dystrophy:	Faulty or defective nutrition.

HYDRO-   (Gr. hydōr); some relation to water or to hydrogen:

hydronephrosis:	An abnormal collection of urine in the kidney pelvis causing pelvic distention and atrophy of the organ (lit. water disease of the kidney).

HYPER-   (Gr. hyper); over, above, beyond, excessive:

hyperplasia:	Abnormal multiplication or increase in number of normal cells in normal arrangement in tissue.
hypertrophy:	Morbid enlargement or overgrowth of an organ or part due to an increase in size of its constituent cells.

HYPO-	(Gr. hypo); under, lack of, deficiency, less than the ordinary or norm:
	hypochloremia: Lowering of chloride content in the blood.
	hypogenesis: Defective growth or development.
MACRO-	(Gr. makros); large or long; combining form meaning abnormally large in size or length:
	macropenis: Abnormally large penis.
MEGA-; MEGALO-	(Gr. megas, megalou); great, huge, enormous.
	megacolon: Giant colon; Hirschsprung's disease due to enlargement and hypertrophy of colon.
	megalo-ureter: Enlargement of the ureter.
MICRO-	(Gr. mikros); abnormally small:
	micropenis: Diminutive penis.
NEO-	(Gr. neos); combining form meaning new:
	ureteroneocystostomy: Reimplantation of the ureter into a new site in the bladder.
OLIGO-	(Gr. oligos); small, little, deficient, scanty, few:
	oliguria: Deficient secretion of urine.
	oligospermia: Few spermatozoa in semen.
PARA-	(Gr. para, par); faulty or disordered condition, abnormal; also beside:
	pararenal: Beside the kidney; also associated in a subsiding or accessory capacity (parasympathetic) or closely resembling the true form (paratyphoid).
PERI-	(Gr. peri); anat.: around, enclosing, surrounding a part:
	perirenal: Around the kidney.
	perivesical: Around the bladder.
PNEUMO-	(Gr. pneuma, pneumatos); air, wind; also soul, spirit. (pneumōn); lung:
	pneumocystogram: A roentgenogram made after injecting air into the bladder.
	pneumaturia: Air in the urine.
POLY-	(Gr. polys); many, much, more than normal or usual number:
	polyuria: Passage of abnormally large amount of urine.
	polydactyl: Extra fingers.
PRE-	(L. prae); before (in front of or in time):
	prevesical: In front of the bladder.
	pre-adolescent: The period preceding adolescence.
PRO-	(L. pro; Gr. pro); before or in front of, priority in point of time, for, in behalf of:
	pronephros: The primordial kidney.
PSEUDO-	(Gr. pseudēs); false or spurious:
	pseudohermaphrodism: Spurious hermaphrodism; the gonads of one sex but abnormalities of the external genitalia, or existing secondary sex characteristics cause doubt as to true sex.
RETRO-	(L. retro); back, backward or located behind:
	retroperitoneal: Behind the peritoneum.
	retropubic: Behind the pubis.
SUB-	(L. sub); under, near, almost, moderately, or in an inferior degree:
	subvesical: Under the bladder.
	subnormal: Less than normal.
SUPRA-	(L. supra); above or over, chiefly in position:
	suprarenal: Hormonal gland above the kidney (adrenal).

TRANS-   (L. trans); across, over, through, beyond:
                    transurethral: Performed through the urethra, e.g., re-
                                            section of the prostate.
URO-   (Gr. ouron, urine); relation to urine, urinary tract, or urination:
                    urolithiasis: The disease condition in association with
                                            urinary stone.
                    urology: Literally, the science of the urine.

SUFFIXES

-ALGIA   (Gr. algos, pain); a painful condition:
                    nephralgia: Painful or aching kidney.
                    orchalgia: Painful testicle.
-CELE   (Gr. kēlē); hernia, tumor, or swelling:
                    hydrocele: A collection of fluid in the tunica vaginalis of the
                                            testicle or along the spermatic cord.
                    cystocele: A hernial protrusion of the bladder.
-ECTASIS   (Gr. ekstasis); distention, or dilatation of:
                    ureterectasis: Dilatation of the ureter.
                    pyelectasis: Dilatation of the kidney pelvis.
-ECTOMY   (Gr. ektomē); surgically, to remove or to cut out.
                    nephrectomy: Removal of the kidney.
                    cystectomy: Removal of the bladder.
-EMIA   (Gr. haima); blood; pertaining to the condition of the blood:
                    uremia: "Urea" in the blood.
                    hyperemia: Excess blood in any part of the body.
-PATHY   (Gr. pathos); a disease, suffering, affliction, or feeling:
                    nephropathy: Kidney disease.
                    apathy: Literally, no feeling.
-PEXY   (L. pexia; Gr. pexis); a fixing or making fast of a part:
                    orchiopexy: The operation of fixing an undescended testicle in the
                                            scrotum.
                    nephropexy   Making fast of a kidney, usually in a high position.
PLASIA   (Gr. plasis); a molding, development or formation:
                    hypoplasia: Defective or incomplete development.
-PLASTY   (Gr. plastos); formed; surg.: Plastic surgery applied to a specified body
                                            part.
                    urethroplasty: Operative repair of a wound or defect of the urethra.
-RRHEA   (Gr. rhoia); flow, discharge:
                    gonorrhea: Discharge due to gonococcus infection.
-SIS   (Gr. sis); a termination or ending of words of Greek origin denoting state
                    or condition and with a combining vowel usually appears as: -asis, -esis,
                    -iasis, -osis.
-OSIS   (L. osis; Gr. osis); a disease, state, process, or morbid condition as nephro-
                    sis; a physiologic increase or formation:
                    hydronephrosis: Water disease of the kidney.
-GRAM   (Gr. gram, graph); a radiographic picture of a hollow viscus:
                    cystogram: Cystography of the bladder.
-GRAPHY   (Gr. graphein, to write); a radiographic picture made after injection of a
                    viscus with a (opaque) medium; rarely air is the medium.
                    pyelography: Pyelogram of the renal pelvis.
-OMA   (Gr. ōma); a morbid affection of some part, usually a tumor.
                    nephroma: A tumor of the kidney.
-OSTOMY*   (Gr. stoma, a mouth); to establish permanent opening (drainage):
                    pyelostomy;   Drainage of kidney pelvis.
                    cystostomy;   Drainage of the bladder.
-OTOMY*   (Gr. tomē); a cutting; cut into, to cut:
                    cystotomy;   Opening the bladder.

-URIA   (Gr. ouron); urine; pertaining to the condition of the urine, especially an abnormal or diseased condition caused by the presence of a (specified) substance:

pyuria:	Pus in the urine.
hematuria:	Blood in the urine.

DEFINITIONS

ABERRANT	Wandering or deviating from the usual or normal course.
ACHALASIA	Failure to relax on the part of a bodily opening; in Urology, chiefly at the bladder neck.
ADRENERGIC	Activated or transmitted by epinephrine (adrenalin); a term applied to those fibers which liberate sympathin at a synapse when a nerve impulse passes, i.e., the sympathetic fibers.
ADRENOLYTIC	Inhibiting the action of the adrenergic nerves; inhibiting the response to epinephrine.
ANDROGEN	Any substance which possesses masculinizing activities, such as the testis hormone.
ANOMALY	Marked deviation from the normal standard.
CALYCECTOMY	Excision of a renal calyx.
CASTRATION	Removal of both testes (or ovaries).
CHILDHOOD	Period from second birthday until puberty.
CONGENITAL	Present at birth.
CORDOTOMY	Neurosurgical division of the sensory tracts in the spinal cord without injury of the motor tracts; performed for relief of intractable pain.
CYSTOSCOPE	An electrically lighted instrument for examining the bladder interior.
ECTOPY (IA, IC)	Displacement or malposition, especially if congenital.
ENCOPRESIS	Incontinence of stools, a habit analogous to enuresis.
ENURESIS	Involuntary discharge of the urine.
GONADOTROPIC	Having special affinity for or influence on the gonads.
INFANCY	Period from sixth week after birth until the second birthday.
NEONATAL	The first six weeks after birth.
NOCTURIA	Frequent urination at night.
RHIZOTOMY	Surgical division of the roots of the spinal nerves for pain or paralysis.
SYNDROME	A complex or set of symptoms which, occurring together, reflect a morbid state or disease.

* Thus one performs cystotomy to open the bladder to remove a foreign body or a stone (the latter sometimes designated as cystolithotomy); cystostomy is performed to establish prolonged or permanent bladder drainage as in inoperable carcinoma of the prostate.

CHAPTER 2   *Urologic Symptoms and Their Interpretation*

UROLOGIC ailments are usually manifested by a more or less characteristic variety and sequence of symptoms which, systematically elicited from the patient, by themselves at once generally suggest the probable diagnosis. However, as the focus of these clinical stories becomes more and more concentrated, the diagnostic possibilities sometimes may be inversely expanded and confusing. Painless hematuria in a child most often results from nephritis or urinary infection but in an adult renal neoplasm, stone, urinary infection, tuberculosis of the kidney is the order of causative incidence and, rarely, hematuria follows the ingestion of a drug such as methenamine or salol (salicylic acid and phenol) to cite a few of the more than half hundred potential causes of blood in the urine.

    The prime purpose of careful history taking and comprehensive examination is the same in every patient: to make the correct diagnosis and institute proper treatment. Constantly it must be kept in mind that urologic disease is fundamentally the same in patients of all ages; only the patients and their age-group reactions to identical uropathy differ. After the age of seven years, the clinical picture in children resembles that in adults. A child is not just a small adult but shows pronounced anatomic, physiologic, pathologic, and immunologic differences from older patients in whom identical etiologic factors generally cause strikingly different manifestations. The pronounced lability of the metabolism in the young and the gravity of its derangement by urinary infection or by urinary toxemia, for example, is often so frightening as to cause the underlying urologic disease to be overlooked or, too commonly, not even thought of. Gastrointestinal disturbances of urotoxic origin are present in over half of all patients with chronic prostatic obstruction, the usual

8

diagnosis in these cases being chronic gastrointestinal indigestion, biliousness, liver disease, or even gastric ulcer; the faulty digestion being eventually evident by constipation, diarrhea, anemia, malaise, undue fatigability, failure to gain or, more likely, loss of weight. Similarly, neurologic, cardiovascular, or febrile disturbances are commonly seen in urinary toxemia and regardless of its underlying cause (obstruction, infection and the like).

In both the historic and investigative survey, the patient must be considered as a whole rather than just a lot of bone and tissue surrounding a diseased urogenital tract. Unless this broad view is maintained, serious disease and, perhaps even more important, a disease of other organs or other body systems may be overlooked. In many conditions and especially urinary infection, the primary focus or condition lies outside the urologic apparatus and invades it via the blood stream, lymphatics, or even by direct extension. Common examples are hematogenous renal infection, (1) of the diffuse focal suppurative type from an acute pharyngitis or dental infection, or (2) the renal carbuncle from a paronychia or a skin abscess or (3) renal tuberculosis from tuberculous lungs. An appendiceal abscess may invade the bladder, or gonorrheal urethritis may give rise to gonorrheal arthritis. Although an experienced urologist can often venture a correct diagnosis after taking a surprisingly short history, such brevity is decidedly to be frowned upon, and investigative short cuts are more than likely to lead to serious diagnostic error. In short, it is the physician's moral duty to obtain a comprehensive, though not necessarily verbose history, and to give the patient a thorough physical examination and as much urologic study as the doctor is reliably trained and equipped to make. Certain symptoms, and especially when they persist, are indications for complete urologic examination which properly should be entrusted to a qualified urologist for the highly technical procedures such as cystoscopy, retrograde pyelography and the interpretation of the findings. Advisedly the urologist should have charge of or at least actively assist in the urologic treatment.

UROLOGIC SYMPTOMS AND THEIR INTERPRETATION

Pyuria, pain and hematuria are the commonest symptoms in urologic disease and together constitute the symptomatic cardinal triad of urinary tract inflammation which is generally caused by infection. Other symptoms suggesting uropathy include disturbances of urination, disturbances of digestion, or injury. These and their collateral clinical manifestations are now discussed.

Pyuria (Gr. πύον, pus; ὂ υρον, urine), *pus in the urine.* This is the commonest symptom of urinary or juxta-urinary tract infection but this reciprocal relationship is not absolute. Figure 1 schematically shows the usual direct and indirect causes of pyuria. In some cases of mild anaerobic bacteriuria and in some viral (abacterial) infections the urinary leukocyte count is normal: not over 5 per high power field of fresh aseptically collected and freshly shaken urine. *Abacterial pyuria* has also been ascribed

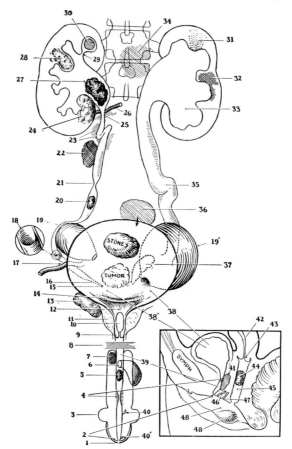

FIGURE 1. Direct and indirect causes of pyuria.

1. stenosis of prepuce
2. stenosis of urethral meatus, etc.
3. paraphimosis
4. urethral stricture
5. urethral stone
6. urethral diverticulum
7. periurethritis; periurethral abscess
8. cowperitis; chronic external sphinctero-spasm
9. congenital valves of posterior urethra
10. hypertrophy of verumontanum; verumontanitis; enlarged utricle or utricular diverticulum
11. prostatitis; prostatic abscess
12. contracted bladder neck; median bar
13. periprostatitis or pelvic suppuration
14. mucosal fold at bladder outlet; trigonal curtain
15. stricture of ureteral meatus; ureterocele
16. ureterovesical junction stricture
17. vascular obstruction of lower ureter
18. congenital ureteral valves
19. ureteral obstruction by diverticulum compression
19'. diverticulum
20. ureteral stone
21. ureteral stricture
22. periureteritis; periureteral phlegmon or abscess
23. ureteral kink, periureteral fibrous bands
24. renal tumor
25. ureteropelvic junction stricture
26. aberrant vessel (obstruction of upper ureter)
27. pelvic stone
28. renal tuberculosis
29. stricture of calyceal outlet
30. calyceal stone
31. pyelonephritis
32. pyonephrosis
33. "pyelitis"; infected hydronephrosis
34. perirenal suppuration invading urinary tract; spinal disease (Pott's, etc.)
35. hydro-ureter

to (1) syphilis because it so often disappears with antiluetic treatment, and (2) toxins originating in an extra-urinary bacterial focus.

Sterile pyuria is rare, the chief causes being (1) trauma caused by instruments or calculi, (2) chemical inflammations, (3) infection that has disappeared but an irritant agent remains and, in infancy and childhood, (4) extreme dehydration and (5) exsiccosis. In the newborn, pyuria occurs more often in males.

The *amount of pus* in the urine is no indicator of the nature or gravity of existing uropathy. Urologists constantly encounter patients with far-advanced hydronephrosis, especially in the young, whose urine is crystal clear and microscopically shows little or no pus although many casts, albuminuria and other harbingers of nephritis may be present. Similarly, a mild low-grade pyuria may be overlooked by the patient for months or years and ultimately be discovered by urinalysis prompted by the examination for a suspected nonurologic condition.

On the other hand, urine grossly cloudy or discolored by pus, blood, desquamated epithelial debris, or precipitated urinary salts is certain to startle most people who, according to intelligence, will consult a reputable physician, or the corner druggist.

The microscopic urinalysis in pyuria is described on page 42, and the multiple glass test for pyuric shreds is considered in Chapter 8.

Pain. Unquestionably pain along the course of the urogenital tract is the *urologic* symptom which more than any other makes the majority of patients want to find out what *may be wrong* and to seek relief. The character of the pain will largely depend upon its cause. For example, the congestive or edematous swelling of the acutely inflamed renal parenchyma or the hydronephrotic distention increases the renal capsular tension to produce a variety of pains—dull aching if the process is mild or acute throbbing if severe. In general, *renal pain* is most severe in the isolateral costovertebral angle, but by *renorenal reflex* through spinal centers (sixth dorsal to first lumbar) may appear in the normal contralateral organ. Urologic pain, especially renal, generally reflects the acuteness or severity of the lesion; too often disease severe enough to threaten life exists painlessly and only the appearance of hematuria, urinary frequency or other symptoms causes diagnostic urologic study to be made. The sudden cessation of severe pain may not mean clinical improvement or spontaneous relief of obstruction but rather that the obstructed organ may have ruptured or, in torsion of the spermatic cord for example, the testicle has become gangrenous. Adults and children, except with language

---

FIGURE 1. Direct and indirect causes of pyuria (*continued*).

36. pericystic abscess rupturing into bladder
37. seminal vesiculitis
38. neuromuscular vesical disease
38'. cystitis
39. urethritis
40. folliculitis (Littré)
40'. folliculitis (Morgagni)
41. periurethritis; periurethral abscess
42. endometritis
43. cervicitis
44. foreign body in vagina
45. vaginitis; hydrocolpos; fusion of labia minora
46. skenitis
47. folliculitis of introitus
48. bartholinitis

barrier, may be expected to describe and localize their pain. *Infants with acute pain* usually emit a sharp distinctive cry, contract the face, become irritable, and may even try to localize the pain with their hands. In any event, the infant's reaction indicates he does not want to be handled or moved.

Renal and Ureteral Colic. Most upper urinary tract colic designated as renal is actually ureteral and consequent to acute obstruction of the ureter and is generally caused by the passage of stone or blood clot. True renal colic occurs when the pelvic outlet of the kidney is effectively blocked. These colics are a smooth muscle spastic reaction to distention and usually are sharp, stabbing, excruciating, often cause sweating, prostration, shock, and collapse. Such severe reno-ureteral pain originating in the retrorenal region of the back or in the upper outer loin generally radiates down the course of the ureter towards the bladder. By *reference through the genitocrural nerve* from its irritated cord center, pain is commonly felt in the testis in the male, in the ovary in the female, and frequently in both sexes radiates to the bladder outlet and urethra to cause urinary frequency or pain. As I can personally attest, only Dietl's classic description of renal colic can begin to transmit to a reader never thus afflicted the exquisite pain and suffering ureteral colic engenders.

The *viscerosensory reflex* (ilio-inguinal), which so regularly appears under these clinical circumstances, offers a confirmatory diagnostic test that the abdominal pain is of ureteral origin and not from disease of the appendix, gallbladder, fallopian tube, or other intraperitoneal viscus (Fig. 2). In this reflex there is variable hyperesthesia of the skin over the iso-lateral upper inner thigh, roughly an area bounded by the lower border of Poupart's ligament, medially by the adductor muscle, and laterally by the sartorius muscle. When this area is coarsely pinched it causes severe cutaneous pain and sharp exaggeration of testicular retraction upwards (subinguinal syndrome of renal colic). Comparable coarse pinching of the contralateral area elicits no pain, causes only the usual cremasteric contraction and correlates the simple test which almost always is of practical differential value.

Other radiation and distribution of pain in reno-ureteral colic is governed by the spinal connections of the renal nerves, chiefly the tenth dorsal to first lumbar segments. By the passage of *pain stimuli through the vagus* (celiac ganglion) to the medulla oblongata, nausea, vomiting, diarrhea, and other gastrointestinal symptoms appear while in the circulatory system *vasomotor reactions* are likely to cause sweating, fainting, and even collapse. *Intraspinal overflow* in acute renal pain may produce pain reference to the other side of the body including the kidney (reno-renal), to the isolateral chest, shoulder, or even to the knee, as well as protective *visceromotor reflex* rigidity of the abdominal muscles and elevation of the testicle through cremasteric contraction consequent to genito-crural nerve stimulation.

Even with lesser pains originating in the ureter or in the lower urinary channels, nerve reference may cause pain in the tip of the last rib (tenth dorsal nerve), over the posterior iliac spine (eleventh dorsal nerve), or even the soles of the feet (third sacral). Reflexly through the inferior hemorrhoidal nerve, *vesico-urethral disturbances may cause pruritus ani*. Chronic ureteral obstruction and, notably, stricture may reflexly cause abdominal pain; especially is this so in right-sided disease when the diagnosis of appendicitis is almost always made and the organ needlessly removed. It should be a standing rule in every hospital that *no operation for chronic appendicitis should be permitted until the patient has had at least a satisfactory excretory urographic study* to make sure the urinary tract is normal and, practically, that it is free of ureteral stone or stricture. In most cases removal of the stone or adequate cystoscopic dilation of the stricture may be expected to cause the "chronic appendicitis" to disappear. Inversely, and of *diagnostic consideration in acute appendicitis*, sensory transference of these same pathways frequently induces urologic manifestations and symptoms such as pain in the costovertebral angle, loin, ovary, testicle, suprapubic area, groin, penis, sometimes with urinary frequency, burning, hesitancy, and by direct contact of the acutely inflamed appendix with the ureteral or bladder wall, gross hematuria and even pyuria. Pain in the renal area or the loin is sometimes caused by inflammatory or arthritic changes in the lumbar spine (Fig. 3).

Bladder pain is usually localized to the viscus and of itself is seldom diagnostic. Mild pain may induce only slight frequency of urination.

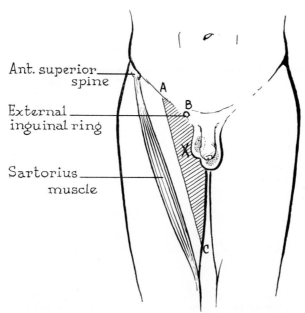

Ant. superior spine

External inguinal ring

Sartorius muscle

FIGURE 2.   Viscerosensory (subinguinal) syndrome of reno-ureteral colic. Coarse pinching of skin over shaded area causes acute pain in contrast to "normal" pain on pinching uninvolved contralateral side. X indicates usual point of maximum hyperesthesia within skin triangle ABC. Note elevation of right testis by reflex cremasteric contraction.

Great frequency of urination, tenesmus and strangury are often present in acute cystitis and acute prostatitis or with foreign bodies or vesical calculi, these symptoms often being referred to the tip of the penis, the perineum, or rectum. The pain of vesical overdistention is extreme and sometimes rhythmically recurrent. In a conscious patient with a painless greatly overdistended bladder, make sure that he does not have tabes dorsalis, or a spinal cord otherwise seriously damaged by traumatic injury or degenerative disease. In the ulceration of the bladder in the late stages of spinal disease, the anesthesia consequent to spinal cord or peripheral nerve disease may prove a blessing.

Urethral pain customarily results from acute inflammation or foreign body in the canal with burning, dysuria, and strangury, aggravated by urination and accompanied by terminal urinary spasm (tenesmus). Deep urethral pain is commonly referred to the perineum, frenum, or to the external meatus. Occasionally upper urinary pain tract is referred to the urethra, especially with vesical foreign bodies and stone.

Genital Tract Pain. Pain originating in the external genitalia may be due to penile lesions, testicle (trauma, orchitis, abscess), epididymitis, torsion of the spermatic cord or of the testicular appendix, varicocele, tumor, hydrocele, abscess or trauma. It is generally severest at the point of most acute disease from which it may radiate to the inguinal cord, groin, loin, back or to the epigastrium. Referred testicular pain in acute ureteral disease is well known.

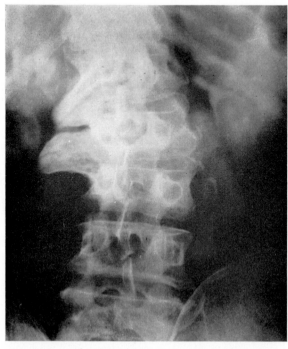

FIGURE 3. Pain in right renal area consequent to upper lumbar vertebral productive arthritis. Normal right upper urinary tract.

Headache is a variety of pain or discomfort, is often a manifestation of urinary toxemia in chronic nephritis especially in hypertensive disease, and may be accompanied by tinnitus and/or vertigo.

In summary, the chief causes of urologic pain are listed according to anatomy:

1. *Kidney:* abnormal mobility, ectopia, horseshoe formation, fused, pronounced hypoplasia, hydronephrosis, calculus, tumor, pyelonephritis, pyonephrosis, solitary abscess, perirenal tumor, cyst or abscess.
2. *Ureter:* obstruction by stricture, stone, tumor, kink, valve, diverticulum; compression by (a) aberrant vessel, (b) fibrous bands, (c) peri-ureteral masses.
3. *Bladder:* stone, foreign body, tumor, ureterocele, retention (neuromuscular, contracted outlet, benign or malignant prostatic tumor).
4. *Urethra:* stricture, meatal stenosis, stone, tumor, valve, diverticulum, hypertrophic verumontanum.
5. *Scrotum and Contents:* tumor, trauma, torsion of spermatic cord or testicular appendages, inflammation, abscess, cyst of scrotum or its contents.
6. *Adrenal:* tumor or abscess.
7. Infection and inflammation of these structures not otherwise indicated.

Hematuria. The sudden appearance of blood in the urine is always of serious import and, except in acute nephritis, neither time nor effort should be lost in determining fully the source and nature of the bleeding. The most likely causes of hematuria are shown in Figure 4. If possible, watch the patient while he voids to see if the blood comes at first (initial hematuria), at the end of urination (terminal hematuria), or if the blood is well mixed with the urine throughout the voiding.

Unfortunately even today physicians often fail to appreciate the potential significance of blood in the urine and thereby needlessly doom the life they should have saved. Hematuria in an infant or child is most likely to mean acute nephritis, pyelonephritis or other acute infection, or tumor, in this order in contrast to the order in adults: tumor, infection, stone, trauma, and tuberculosis. One condition, congenital stenosis of the external meatus with ulceration, is a frequent cause of hematuria in young boys. Often it splotches the clothing with blood stains to draw the parent's attention to the condition (see Section on Anomalies).

In addition to the local causes of hematuria there are many systemic and other conditions which may be responsible: in infancy especially— hemorrhagic disease of the newborn, uric acid infarction, hereditary telangiectasis and, in children and adults, acute bacterial endocarditis (renal infarction), acute rheumatic fever, measles, severe renal passive congestion, renal papillitis, renal and vesical angioma and varices, hypothrombinemia, aplastic anemia, purpura, hemophilia, leukemia, scurvy, bilharzia, trauma, sepsis, appendicitis, physical exercise, hemoglobinuria from exposure to cold; drug poisoning and idiosyncrasies as with methylene blue, sodium salicylate, salol, phenol, turpentine, sulfonamides, Dicumarol, allergy to unboiled milk, tetanus antitoxin, fish, shell food. Hereditary or familial hematuria has been reported with several fatalities following circumcision in hemorrhagic disease of the newborn, suggesting the low threshold for blood loss through the kidney circulation. *Blood casts* reflect intraparenchymal renal bleeding. In highly acid urine the blood turns brown but remains reddish or red in alkaline urine. Bloody-looking urine may be due to the ingestion of beets (anthocyanin), a consideration of particular diagnostic concern in children in whom the condition is most common.

Disturbances of Urination. These are present in half of all cases of urologic disease and reflect inflammation—congestive or bacterial—at or near the bladder outlet (trigone, prostate, posterior urethra, meatus, glans, or prepuce) but directly or reflexly may result from upper urinary tract or rectal disease.

Frequency of Urination. Two thirds of all cases of urinary tract inflammation or infection and nearly all cases of obstruction at the bladder outlet or peripherally are accompanied by urinary frequency. It may also be caused by highly alkaline or acid urine, or pronounced crystalluria (oxalate, phosphate, uric acid). Frequent urination is normal in infancy

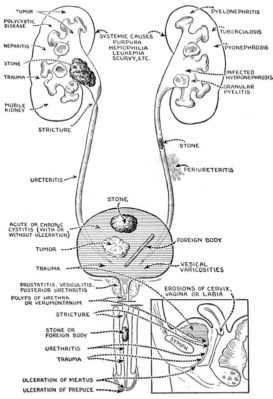

FIGURE 4.   Usual causes of hematuria. Systemic, allergic, toxic and other unusual causes of hematuria are enumerated in the text.

but by two years the child should hold his urine for at least two hours. The normal urinary schedule for 24 hours in children follows: 3 to 6 months, 20 times; 6 to 12 months, 16 times; 1 to 2 years, 12 times; 2 to 3 years, 10 times; 3 to 4 years, 9 times; by 12 years the schedule and output are essentially those of adults: 4 to 6 times, none at night, with 1200 to 1500 cc. output.

A large vesical residuum correspondingly reduces the functional or net capacity of the bladder and frequency is a prominent symptom. Anatomic diminution of the bladder capacity by inflammation (spasm), or sclerotic contracture also causes urinary frequency.

Urgency is the hurried call to urinate ("When you've got to go, you've got to go!"). It results from an intensification of the same factors as cause frequency and in advanced degree there may be incontinence.

Tenesmus is the extremely painful spasm occurring at the end of urination and results from even greater intensity of the same conditions which cause frequency and urgency. The tense squeezing of the inflamed tissues at or near the vesical outlet may cause *terminal hematuria,* the blood being mechanically squeezed from the congested inflamed tissues. Tenesmus is especially severe in vesical or prostatic urethral stone, in foreign body in the bladder, or in vesical neck ulceration.

Strangury is due to the same causes as tenesmus; the patient voids drop by drop with extreme pain, burning or scalding. It signifies intense inflammation at or near the vesical neck.

Vesical *spasm* may result from the same causes as tenesmus or may be due to the passage of highly concentrated acid urine, bladder stone, appendicitis, vulvitis, acute perivesical inflammation or even reflexly in acute hip-joint disease.

Burning on urination is generally caused by intense urethral or vesical inflammation.

Hesitancy is initial dysuria. It may be a nervous inhibition but, persisting, usually reflects obstruction at the vesical outlet or peripherally. The trigonal muscle hypertrophies in its attempt to open the bladder outlet obstructed by contracture or prostatic hyperplasia which, by the same token, interferes with usual bladder neck closing to cause *terminal dribbling.* Yet dribbling after the completion of urination may result from ballooning or diverticulum of the urethra behind a stricture; the pocketed urine slowly dribbles away after voluntary urination is finished.

Polyuria. This is abnormal frequency and volume output of urination, is physiologic in cold weather, with a large fluid intake, during a high emotional or excitement state such as an examination (academic or physical), in some cases of sclerotic nephritis, diabetes insipidus, diabetes mellitus, and often in the postconvulsive state. *Diabetes insipidus* occurs once in about 60,000 persons; there is extreme thirst (polydypsia), and low specific gravity of the urine (1.001 to 1.005). Its cause is unknown but it has been frequently associated etiologically with cerebral concussions, falls on the head, chronic hydrocephalus, brain tumors, luetic meningitis and, notably, disease or functional deficiency of the posterior pituitary lobe.

Nocturia is suggestive of bladder-neck obstruction but there may be stone or foreign bodies in the viscus or the polyuria of nephritis. *Nycturia* is a variety of nocturia in which the patient passes more urine at night than in the daytime, and it is generally the result of advanced sclerotic nephritis.

Dysuria is difficult urination and is seen particularly in infravesical obstruction, pronounced inflammation of the deep urethra (e.g., severe prostatitis), neuromuscular or chronic inflammatory vesical atony or, psychologically, when one tries to urinate in the presence of others.

In *initial* dysuria, there is difficulty in starting the stream after which it flows freely, and in *total* dysuria the difficulty persists throughout the struggling act.

Urinary Retention.   This may be incomplete or complete. Complete urinary retention may be (a) acute, or (b) chronic.

Acute urinary retention results from any condition which completely blocks the outflow of urine. This may be caused by a stone jammed in the bladder outlet or urethra, or the sudden edematous swelling of a urethral stricture, enlarged prostate or other pre-existing blockage following (1) instrumentation, (2) exposure to cold, (3) overindulgence in alcohol or sexual excitement, or (4) external trauma.

Chronic urinary retention may be caused by any condition obstructing the outflow of urine including in addition to stone, prostatism, stricture, or neuromuscular vesical disease. The more frequent causes of the latter are spina bifida, spinal cord tumor, central or peripheral neuritis from syphilis, trauma, primary anemia, poliomyelitis, and so forth.

In *chronic complete vesical retention* the urine overflows by dribbling —paradoxical or pseudo-incontinence. In children this overflow commonly and erroneously causes the diagnosis of enuresis to be made.

Anuria is the arrest of output of urine, either (1) from renal failure (secretory type), or (2) from upper urinary tract blockage (excretory type). Anuria normally occurs for the first twenty-four hours in a third of all newborn infants but after that time it is of grave import in a patient of any age. Neonatal anuria is believed to result from failure of the bladder to initiate the emptying reflex or from sphincterospasm, and will disappear with a copious fluid intake. *In true anuria, there is no urine in the bladder.*

Etiologically, anuria requires bilateral defection of two kidneys or is unilateral in solitary kidney and may be classified as:

(1) PRERENAL.   This is concerned with factors operating before the blood reaches the kidney and includes hypotension, thrombosis of the renal vessels, thyroid deficiency, hepatic disease, neurogenic reflex as in cystoscopy or other instrumentation, dehydration by vomiting, with urinary sepsis, diarrhea, shock or excessive perspiration, all of which are combated by circulatory replacement with whole blood, plasma or isotonic glucose-saline solution.

(2) RENAL. These causes are directly operative in the kidney itself and include severe degeneration, bilateral renal inflammation, bismuth or bichloride of mercury poisoning, tumor, polycystic disease, shock, suppuration, reflex mechanism, histamine or allergic factors. Renal anuria may also be caused by blockage of the renal tubules with sulfonamide crystals, by hemoglobin crystals in mismatched transfusions, by myoglobin and hemoglobin in crush syndrome and extensive burns, together with associated tubular degeneration, sometimes designated as the lower nephron-nephrosis syndrome.

(3) POSTRENAL. These factors interfere with the drainage of urine formed by the kidney and are chiefly bilateral ureteral blockage by calculi or unilateral in solitary kidney.

(4) ARENAL. Congenital absence of the kidneys is excessively rare and is found only in nonviable monsters, but the unwitting removal of a solitary kidney has sometimes occurred, or an inadequate kidney may remain after nephrectomy on the opposite side.

Diagnosis of anuria is made by the discovery that no urine is entering the bladder and this should be firmly established by catheterization.

Treatment of anuria demands prompt ureteral catheterization to identify or relieve the obstructing factors. Copious fluid is given, chiefly intravenous physiologic saline and 5 per cent glucose or $\frac{1}{6}$ molar sodium-r-lactate solution for systemic alkalinization and the combat of acidosis. In mismatched transfusions, the crush syndrome, and hemoglobinuric anuria due to severe extensive burns, employ 2.5 per cent sodium sulfate given slowly intravenously, 15 cc. per kilogram of body weight (Olson and Necheles, 1947); the success of this treatment depends upon the re-establishment of upper urinary tract drainage by ureteral catheter.

If ureteral catheterization is inadequate to establish free renal drainage in these cases, employ nephrostomy, ureterostomy, or other procedure as necessary. The final definitive surgery to correct the obstructive factor is performed later when the acute crisis has passed and the condition of the patient warrants.

Only sufficient fluid is given to maintain fluid balance in anuria—that is, the fluid intake equals the fluid loss by skin, lungs, bowel or vomiting. For an average size adult, this will be about 1000 cc. per day; more than this may soon drown the patient by pulmonary edema and anasarca. Extraction of toxic metabolites from the circulation may, in desperate cases, call for gastrointestinal lavage, peritoneal irrigation or, if available, the use of the artificial kidney. The artificial kidney can selectively remove metabolites and electrolytes from the body in about six hours; correction of acid-base balance by cation replacement may be necessary.

With obstruction eliminated, the renal function may be expected to resume after six to nine days and if life can be preserved this long with free urinary drainage operating, most kidneys will revive and resume function.

In *metallic renal poisoning*, by mercury or bismuth in particular, administer BAL (0.3 cc. of 10 per cent solution in oil of 2, 3-dimercaptopropanol) intramuscularly every four hours for several days if necessary. Renal decapsulation is seldom if ever of value. Therapeutic sweating does no good and only further weakens the patient.

Incontinence of Urine. True incontinence is usually the result of neuromuscular disease consequent to congenital neural defects (spina bifida, meningocele, etc.), injury of the spinal cord by inflammation or infection (syphilis, poliomyelitis, transverse myelitis), tumor, trauma as in fractured spine or, rarely, surgical procedures as occasionally with transurethral or perineal prostatectomy. It may also follow other perineal operations which involve severance of the pudic nerves, or as a result of grave surgical disturbance or disruption of the pudendal plexus; true or false (overflow) incontinence occurs in more than a third of patients undergoing radical rectosigmoidectomy. Enuresis of childhood is generally not a true incontinence but rather a manifestation of ill-formed habits. Inflammation at or near the vesical outlet may cause such pronounced urinary frequency and spasm as to simulate incontinence but the sharp distinction must be made.

Temperature. Fever of unexplained origin in a patient of any age always demands a careful urinalysis. Although fever of urologic origin is usually the result of infection, in Wilms' tumor in children fever may be the only symptom for some time. With acute obstruction of an infected urinary tract, the temperature usually rises abruptly and high with premonitory chills, headache, hyperirritability, sweating, and gastrointestinal upsets with anorexia, nausea, vomiting, diarrhea, malaise and/or acidosis. Drenching sweats with a picket-fence type of temperature suggest suppuration which may be renal carbuncle or perinephric abscess.

Palpable Mass. A palpable mass along the urogenital tract is a frequent symptom. It may result from urinary retention, as in hydronephrosis, distended bladder, or from fluid distention as in hydrocele, may be due to a neoplasm, cystic disease of the kidney, mesonephric or urogenous cyst development. A palpable solid abdominal mass in a child should always be considered malignant until proved otherwise, and this is a good rule to follow when the patient is an adult.

Pneumaturia is the passage of gas in the urine and at once suggests a uro-enteric fistula, the most common being of the vesicorectal or congenital urethrorectal varieties, and is especially disturbing when feces pass with the air and urine. Rarely, gas is passed from the bladder when diabetic urine is infected with a gas-producing organism.

Infection elsewhere in the body may be of prime etiologic importance in renal or perirenal infection, especially in Staphylococcus aureus renal carbuncle or perirenal abscess. The most frequent extra-urogenital focal infections encountered are acute pharyngitis, tonsillitis, otitis media, pneumonitis, gastroenteritis, boils, osteomyelitis, infected wounds and paronychiae. Such data should be included in the history.

Edema is seldom a symptom of urologic disease although it is common enough in parenchymatous nephritis and other forms of Bright's disease. Here the swelling first involves one or both eyelids, there is puffiness of the face, lips, hands, and fingers, and later ankles, legs and feet. In edema of cardiac decompensation and circulatory failure, the swelling appears first in the ankles, feet, and legs and later in the scrotum, penis, lower abdomen and, when true anasarca is present, within the abdomen as free fluid.

Injury of the urinary tract should be included in the history, noting especially the character, site of impact, and nature of the trauma, the duration and type of pain produced, hematuria, and urinary disturbances such as dysuria and retention, or even loss of sensation as it occurs in spinal fracture and crushing of the spinal cord.

Reflex and neurotoxic disturbances are often so pronounced as to overshadow or completely obscure the symptoms of urinary infection, especially in children. Gastrointestinal disturbances with faulty nutrition are prominent in at least half of all cases of severe chronic uropathy, notably infection and/or obstruction. The symptoms may be indigestion, biliousness, constipation, diarrhea, anemia, malaise, easy fatigability, loss of weight or failure to gain—all of which call for at least a careful urinalysis and sharp clinical consideration.

Uremia. This may be described as a symptomatic phenomenon caused by the toxemia of renal failure. Its most usual manifestations are nausea, vomiting, vesical disturbances, headache, pronounced irritability, nervousness and, terminally, convulsions and coma.

Renal injury giving rise to uremia may be due to infection, obstruction, "medical" nephritis, bilateral or solitary atrophic, hypoplastic, polycystic or multicystic kidney disease, crush injury of the muscles (crush syndrome), circulatory failure, or any of the causes of anuria (q.v.). The precise cause of uremia is unknown; it is not as once thought simply the result of urea retention in the blood. Some phases of uremia simulate those in phenol poisoning, and there is actually increase in the blood phenols, probably associated with the retention of by-products or end-products of metabolism. The *chief systemic symptoms* are due to salt and water loss while the neurologic manifestations are those of choline and trimethylamine excess. The terminal picture is that of acidosis.

Yet renal insufficiency in uremia may be reversible in some situations with corresponding extension of the patient's life. Reversible causes of renal insufficiency include congestive heart failure (improved by digitalization); reduction of edema and hypertension; prompt treatment of bacterial endocarditis, pyelonephritis, systemic infections, dehydration, hyponatremia, alkalosis, hypercalcemia, anemia, renal depletion or acute glomerular nephritis. To the active remedial measures must be added rest and a high protein diet.

The uremia of obstructive uropathy is largely due to dehydration, hypocalcemia, vitamin deprivation, anemia and inorganic acidosis, correction of which brings about improvement even though the blood nitrogen level may stay high. Thus with a high nonprotein nitrogen blood level and a normal carbon dioxide combining power, preparation for definitive surgical treatment requires only free drainage—by catheter or otherwise—to reduce the intertubular hydrostatic pressure sufficient to restore the filtration pressure relations and the excretion of nitrogen (ammonia). Following the establishment of free urinary drainage, recovery is enhanced by the combat of acidosis with intravenous administration of 100 cc. of ⅙ molar sodium-r-lactate solution for each volume per cent the carbon dioxide combining power is below 60 per cent.

Two main types of uremia are encountered: (1) the acute or convulsive, and (2) the chronic or retentive.

1. Acute Uremia. Usually there is a prodromal period when suddenly the acute manifestations appear. The etiology is any condition causing sudden severe renal injury. Acute nephritis is perhaps the most common cause in children as it often is in older patients, but in the last group its occurrence is frequently a flare-up of chronic nephritis or acute urinary obstruction; mercury poisoning or crush injury are rare causes. In the prodromal period there are headaches, muscle twitchings, increased nervous tension, nausea, vomiting, and sometimes diarrhea with bloody stools. The manifestations are believed to be the result of excess chloride retention in the body and the enteric irritation of ammonium carbonate which, as a decomposition product of urea, is vicariously eliminated by the stomach and bowel. Persistent hiccup is nearly always present and, with advancing dehydration, the oral mucosa is red and dry, a uremic breath and ulcerative stomatitis are the rule, and the parched red tongue usually becomes brown and boardy. With the acute onset of uremia, there are usually epileptiform or eclamptic convulsions which may be continuous or intermittent, or sudden acute mania with stertorous breathing due to cerebral edema.

Sudden blindness (amaurosis) without ophthalmic or eye-ground changes, and dyspnea (paroxysmal, continuous or intermittent Cheyne-Stokes type) are due to acidosis, appear late, and portend death. Terminally, a peculiar whitish urea frost may appear on the skin and with acute or gradually occurring coma, spells the end. Few recover from the terminal stage of uremia and then only with such heroic therapeutic measures as the artificial kidney.

Chronic Uremia. This is the more usual variety of uremia and may be the late result of severe persistent urinary retention, chronic hyperparathyroidism with renal calcinosis, hypertensive pyelonephritis, subacute bacterial endocarditis, chronic nephritis of "salt-losing" (chiefly sodium) type, intoxication with irradiated sterols, or other conditions producing progressive renal injury. The course of the disease may be weeks or months. The symptoms usually seen in increasing severity are: lethargy, dullness, anorexia, malaise, loss of energy and appetite, chronic indigestion, and biliousness, obstinate constipation or debility, toxic diarrhea with nausea and vomiting. The sallow skin of the failing patient becomes scaly, harsh, hypersensitive and, late, deeply pigmented. Co-existing manifestations are a glossiness of the eyes, loss of weight, insomnia, headache—especially occipital—with commonly altered personality. Muscular twitching, dry, red buccal membranes with dysphagia (difficult swallowing), brownish dry boardy tongue, urinous breath, hiccup, and hemorrhagic manifestations (petechiae, ecchymosis, mucosal bleeding, melena, hemoptysis, hematuria) are likely to appear. Most of these patients with chronic uremia fall easy prey to terminal pneumonia. *Terminal convulsions do not occur in chronic uremia.*

Latent Uremia. This is the usual picture in chronic obstructive uropathy involving the entire functioning renal parenchyma as in bilateral ureteral obstruction—calculous anuria, chronic urinary obstruction, or inadequate renal function of any cause. Terminally, the clinical picture resembles that of acute uremia but without convulsions.

Diagnosis of uremia is suggested by the clinical manifestations which have been described and is confirmed by demonstration of the underlying cause, a high blood nitrogen level (urea, nonprotein nitrogen, uric acid, creatinine) and a startlingly low carbon dioxide combining power, even to zero.

While the *prognosis* in uremia due to obstructive uropathy is normally guarded when the blockage is relieved, it is far more hopeful than in the usual uremia of nephritis which is regularly hopeless.

Treatment of Uremia. This is based on the etiology and may be summarized as follows:

1. Administer the fluid intake to three fourths of the normal average for the age or weight of the patient.
2. Correct electrolyte imbalance or deficiency as guided by frequent determinations of the diagnostic serum levels.
3. Correct acidosis by oral sodium and chloride feeding together with intravenous ⅙ molar sodium-r-lactate solution (p. 22).
4. If there is suggestion of tetany, clinically or by serum calcium determination, give calcium chloride or calcium gluconate.
5. Give high protein intake 1.0 to 2.0 gm. per kilogram body weight by mouth, as amino acids intravenously, or as blood serum albumin (plasma), together with carbohydrates, especially glucose, to furnish calories.
6. Combat hypoproteinemia and malnutrition by continuous intravenous blood plasma (serum albumin) when patient cannot take or assimilate food by mouth.
7. Give continuous whole blood transfusions if hemoglobin falls below 70 per cent (10.0 gm. per cent).
8. Administer sedation as necessary.
9. Effect cardiac digitalization as indicated, employing the drug least likely to cause nausea or vomiting.
10. Withhold any food, drug, or laxative, or enema irritating to the gastrointestinal tract.
11. Administer aluminum salts (gels) by mouth to retard the absorption of phosphates from the intestinal tract and thus, in turn, diminish the appearance of hypocalcemia.

12. Reduce blood nitrogenous retention by
    a, exsanguination transfusion
    b, continuous gastrointestinal lavage
    c, use of the artificial kidney.

Coma and convulsions due to cerebral edema, especially in the young, are combated by the intravenous injection of hypertonic saline solution (30 per cent), 40 cc. to a five year old child and 100 to 150 cc. to an adult. As an alternative, 20 per cent glucose in 1 per cent magnesium sulfate may be given on the dosage basis of 0.2 cc. per kilogram body weight. This will usually stop the convulsions in fifteen minutes; an oxygen tent or oxygen by nasal tube will give cardiac relief.

Low or deficient blood sodium (hyponatremia) is a frequent complication in urologic patients whether the uropathy is chronic obstructive, chronic pyelonephritis, or other condition, especially cardiac complications. The cardiac group in particular have probably been on a low salt diet or have been given a mercurial diuretic. Yet in the treatment in all major urologic diseases and notably after obstruction is relieved, diuresis is generally promoted. But in many of these patients tubular damage prevents their normal retention of sodium which becomes lost from the body. Most of these patients eat poorly so have a low salt intake for that reason alone. Variable adrenal deficiency or failure may also result in salt loss. Evidence of hyponatremia is given by (1) the presence of azotemia without severe renal damage; (2) a large output of urine associated with a rising nonprotein blood nitrogen; (3) dehydration and a dry boardy tongue despite an adequate fluid intake; (4) undue or disproportionate muscular weakness; (5) pronounced anorexia and general debility. With recognition of the condition of hyponatremia, the administration of sodium chloride is the treatment, both as intravenous physiologic saline and sodium lactate solution and orally as sodium chloride tablets. Small doses of adrenal cortical extract may be beneficial in some patients who respond slowly to salt administration alone.

CHAPTER 3   *The Clinical History and Urologic Examination*

The History. Despite present-day instrumental and accessory investigative aids such as roentgenography, the careful taking of a complete history and a thorough physical examination and urinalysis are fundamental in the diagnostic study of urologic disease. The story of an infant's problem must be obtained from the parents, guardian or nurse, but after three or four years of age young patients can usually speak for themselves and may even tell a truer and more helpful story than the nervous, defensive or inadequate mother, trying to obscure her own shortcomings and neglect of the child.

The taking of the history logically falls into three divisions: (1) chief complaint—the patient's own word of what symptoms he has—their duration, sequence, rate of development and appearance; (2) the previous history in some cases should include the more important childhood diseases such as measles, scarlet fever, or mumps which may give a clue; chronic respiratory or urinary infections are often of direct bearing on the present condition; (3) family history is of concern as regards possible blood relationship of parents in whom mental defects and genetic anomalies are reasonably frequent fruits of cousin intermarriage. Other family history should include notes regarding exposure to active tuberculosis, especially open pulmonary with cavitation and coughing, and hypertension, syphilis, adrenal or Bright's disease, the last often being the diagnosis given to unrecognized congenital polycystic renal disease in the ancestors. Include all such data as clinical mileposts.

Present History. The historical data of chief concern in urologic disease should, if possible, be systematically acquired, the physician shaping his questions to the revelations of the patient's answers. The following

25

résumé indicates the more important historical data, both negative and positive answers being important.

1. *Pyuria*

Time, nature of onset and recurrences
Duration and nature of course
Character—initial, total (throughout), or terminal with urination
Bacteria, present or not
Associated pain, stone, injury, exposure or infection
Associated gastrointestinal or neurologic disturbances

2. *Disturbances of urination*

Frequency
  Character and time of onset and recurrences
  Duration and degree
  Periodicity—constant, intermittent, diuria, nocturia
  Nycturia (passing more urine at night than in daytime)
Enuresis
  Duration, events preceding onset
  Night wetting
  Day wetting
  Sociologic factors—home training, neurotic mother or nurse, other children in family, punishments, institutional life, and so forth
  Past treatment
Dysuria
  Duration and character of onset and recurrences
Character of disturbance
  Constant, intermittent, tenesmus, urgency, hesitancy, change in stream (small, divided, lack of force, dribbling), crying on urination
Relation to
  Other urologic symptoms, instrumentation or known infections elsewhere in the body
Retention
  Character of onset and recurrences
  Degree, periodicity
  Relation to neurologic symptoms, injury to urethra or bladder, urethral stricture, instrumentation and acute infections elsewhere in the body

3. *Pain*

Location
Character—sharp, dull, mild, severe, constant, periodic
Cry—character, duration, relation to other symptoms
Radiation
Duration of present and past attacks
Relation to urination, vomiting and so forth
Relation to urinalysis—before, during, or after pain

4. *Hematuria*

Time and duration of onset and recurrences
Character—clots, initial, during or terminal to voiding
Degree of bleeding
Relation to injury, pain, stone, exposure or known infection elsewhere in the body

5. *Fever*

Chills
Character and duration of onset and recurrences

	Relation to urologic symptoms
	Relation to pyuria
	Associated gastrointestinal and neurologic symptoms

6. *Abdominal tumor*   Location, duration, consistency
Movable or fixed
Size—constant, variable, disappearing, factors altering, associated symptoms

7. *Injury*   Character, duration, point of impact
Urinary symptoms before and after
Pain, hematuria, fever, masses, effect of movement and position

8. *Stone passage or crystalluria*   Time and character of onset, duration
Pain—location, radiation, duration
Hematuria
Pyuria
Recurrence

9. *Genital lesions*   Malformations
    Interference with normal function
    Symptoms produced
Phimosis, balanitis, urethritis, vaginitis
Epididymitis, orchitis
    Location, duration, character of onset
    Pain, radiation, crying and so forth
    Relation to infection elsewhere
    Relation to other urologic disease
    Relation to trauma or straining (torsion of spermatic cord)
Hydrocele
    Duration, character
    Relation to infection or trauma
    Size—constant, increasing or variable
Varicocele
    Side involved, character, rapidity of size increase
    Relation to abdominal tumor and to abdominal cutaneous vascular dilatations or varices
Testicular tumor
    Side, duration, character, rapidity of enlargement
    Pain, metastasis, loss of weight

10. *Pneumaturia*   Duration, coexistent fecaluria

It is seldom necessary to interrogate concerning every symptomatic subdivision here given; the fruitfulness of the interrogations and the economy of time will be largely dependent upon the clinician's experience.

GENERAL EXAMINATION

A careful complete physical examination should precede instrumental urologic investigation.

Inspection. The patient should be undressed sufficiently so that all external parts of the body can be satisfactorily observed. *Bagginess* under the eyes usually reflects nephritis (Bright's disease or obstructive urinary tract injury) but may mean myxedema. *Edema* of cardiac failure is evident first in the feet and legs, but in advanced disease scrotal or even penile edema may be present. Normally *edema appears when the body fluid excess increases the lymph volume by 10 per cent.* Edema of the lower extremities may also result from lymph blockage (filariasis, carcinomatous lymphatic metastases, lymphatic leukemia, avitaminosis—especially A, B complex, and C). When a bed patient is receiving too much fluid intravenously, engorgement of the external jugular veins may be seen, the jugular engorgement also being observed in anoxemia and myocardial failure.

Not only should the examiner inspect the buccal membranes which, in uremia, are red and dry or even boardy, but he should also touch and feel the tongue.

Virchow's supraclavicular node (also known as the *sign of Troisier*) is sometimes seen or felt on the left side, this being a frequent site of metastasis from prostatic or gastric carcinoma. *Continuous hiccuping* in urologic disease usually means uremia; the diaphragm reflex contraction is generally triggered by the toxemia of grave disease, peritonitis, or pleurisy.

Gynecomastia designates enlargement of the male breast. The breast enlargement may be unilateral or bilateral; the breast substance is composed of proliferated connective tissue and ducts but no true acini, histologically resembling the breast tissue of an adolescent girl. Secretion, if present, is albuminous or mucinous, not lacteal.

While it is hypothesized that gynecomastia results from pubertal androgen-estrogen imbalance in the male, neither hormonal assays nor clinical observations are supportive of this. Thus it is found that gynecomastia may be induced by the administration to males of androgens (methyltestosterone but not testosterone), chorionic gonadotrophin (stimulates adrenal and/or testis to induce their hormone output), adrenal cortical extracts, desoxycorticosterone acetate (replacement therapy in Addison's disease); it has developed in pituitary, testicular, thyroid and adrenal endocrinopathy. Klinefelder, Reifenstein and Albright have hypothesized that a normal "x" hormone secreted by the testis is inhibitory to mammary growth and lack of this "x" hormone permits testosterone to stimulate breast growth without opposition. Yet, this hypothesized hormone has not been demonstrated. In any event, prepubertal and senile gynecomastia usually disappears spontaneously and requires no direct treatment, when it can be established in males of all ages that the condition does not reflect local neoplasia or endocrinologic tumor. It has also been observed to occur in pulmonary disease (bronchiectasis, bronchogenic carcinoma, tuberculosis, emphysema), hepatic disease (carcinoma, cirrhosis, hepatitis), spinal cord disease (paraplegia, transverse myelitis), renal disease (chronic pyelonephritis, glomerulonephritis), lymphoblastomas (including mycosis fungoides and leukemia), and severe malnutrition. Surgical relief is rarely necessary but is locally corrective.

Inspection may further disclose a renal or vesical swelling (tumor), hydrocele, varicocele, hypospadias, epispadias, vesical exstrophy, hypogen-italism, balanitis, periurethral abscess, scrotal fistulae (granulation tissue about the orifice of the discharging sinus) or inguinal adenitis. The adenitis may result from infection in the toe, foot or leg, penile or labial skin. In genital infection the nodes tend to be hardened and small, or "shotty" while as a rule in extragenital lesions the nodes are extremely enlarged and fluctuant. The last type, and especially with ulceration, should make one suspect lymphogranuloma venereum (Frei test positive), or granuloma inguinale (demonstrate Donovan bodies).

In *hernia* the cough impulse is usually much better seen than felt. The undressed patient, standing, coughs at command with his head turned to one side while the examiner, seated in front, watches the external inguinal ring area for impulse bulging.

When the differential diagnosis rests between hydrocele and hernia, if the examiner can get his fingers above the mass, it is not a hernia (see Chapter 8). A hydrocele of the cord will descend if downward traction is put on the testicle. In acute epididymitis not only is the enlarged tender organ palpable, but with acute vas deferentitis there is pain at the external inguinal ring.

The *prepuce* should be widely retracted exposing the coronal sulcus and frenum, with special attention not to overlook a stenosed pinhole meatus, ulcerative meatitis, preputial edema or calculi, gonorrheal or other urethral discharge, neoplasm, chancre, chancroid, or lymphogranu-loma inguinale (tropical bubo). A phimotic prepuce may require dorsal slit to permit its full retraction. Having retracted the prepuce, always replace it to its normal position lest paraphimosis develops (Fig. 167).

An abnormally small or *stenosed external urethral meatus* should be recognized. The glans penis is compressed transversely from before back-wards between the thumb and first finger; this causes the meatus to gape open. Even more certain, grasp the glans on each side of the meatus with the thumb and first finger of each hand and actively spread the opening. Stenosis should be promptly corrected by meatotomy in males and ure-thral dilation in the female. The meatus of the hypospadiac urethra is almost always smaller than normal and sometimes only pinhole size (see Stenosis of the Meatus, Chapters 6 and 8).

Lymphogranuloma may involve the genitalia, perineum, rectum or buttocks and cause intestinal symptoms in white patients but apparently Negroes are relatively exempt. It begins as a herpetic lesion with sec-ondary inguinal and iliac node spread and subsequent granulomatous formation; the Frei test is positive.

Posteriorly above the intergluteal groove, look for meningocele, pressure on which in a young infant causes bulging of the fontanel. Poor leg development or paralysis usually reflects lumbosacral spinal mal-formation (spina bifida, meningocele, myelocele, meningomyelocele, etc.) in children, and spinal injury or cord disease (syphilis, tumor) in adults. In true spina bifida there is a depression over the upper central sacrum posteriorly and the depressed area is generally covered with a coarse hairy growth.

Pilonidal cyst may form as the result of incomplete closure of the neural groove, opening in the midline near the coccyx. If drainage from its sinus is impaired, the cyst mass fills with inflammatory debris and becomes extremely painful.

Palpation. By touch one determines the rate and quality of the pulse, and the characteristics of palpable lymph glands, splenic, hepatic, renal, and other intra-abdominal enlargements or masses. *Masses* of urogenital tract origin are predominantly due to urinary obstruction, cyst formation or neoplasm. Abdominal masses in children are chiefly renal or vesical, and these show variation in size as a hydronephrosis or distended bladder is evacuated. The loin mass may be solitary or polycystic disease of the kidneys or a mesonephric cyst which may cause dystocia, while a suprapubic mass may be a urachal cyst or occasionally an ectopic kidney, often hydronephrotic. Rarely, a thickened tuberculous or over-distended ureter can be palpated.

Just before abdominal examination the bladder should be emptied, by catheterization if necessary. In abdominal palpation, properly one uses the sensitive flat flexor surface of the warmed hand and fingers and not just the finger tips, the patient being supine on the table and comfortable with arms relaxed at the sides. Sometimes abdominal relaxation can be encouraged by a slight flexing of the knees, a pillow placed under the knees, deep breathing through the open mouth, dropping the lower jaw, or even by engaging the patient in conversation. Boisterous uncooperative infants and young children can often be most satisfactorily examined by laying them face down.

It is usually best to begin palpation on the opposite side from the site of pain, watching the patient's face for pain reaction. A tumor or tenderness in the upper loin generally means renal or perirenal involvement while a fixed mass is probably perinephritis, chronic pyelonephritis, or neoplasm. A tense hydronephrosis may simulate neoplasm and, in children especially, any solid abdominal tumor should be considered malignant until proved otherwise. A mass which will move in a plane from the right hypochondrium to the left iliac fossa but not in a plane at right angles to this, is almost certainly a *mesonephric* cyst.

On the right side a tumor whose lower border is crossed by the hepatic flexure is almost always renal while an enlarging left renal tumor reaching the anterior abdominal wall pushes all viscera ahead of it, hence there is no colonic tympany over the growth. In differentiating hydronephrosis and hydrops of the gallbladder, the examiner's left hand is placed under the supine patient while the right hand is placed over the abdominal right upper quadrant. The left hand gently exerts pressure upward by which in hydronephrosis, the right hand will be lifted upwards by the renal mass, but will be unaffected by a large gallbladder.

Renal Palpation. This may be performed by ballottement or by manual compression (Fig. 5).

Ballottement. In a child renal palpation is most satisfactorily performed by ballottement and this is true in general when the patient is an adult. As shown in Figure 5 the fingers of the hand below the loin are used to throw the kidney against the more or less stationary hand compressing the loin anteriorly. With the patient comfortably flat on his back and the arms at his side, the knees slightly flexed and the abdomen relaxed, the fingers of the examining hand on the abdomen are placed external to the rectus muscle just below the free border of the ribs. As the patient breathes in and out, firmer pressure is made with the fingers in front and, when they are down as much as seems possible, at the moment of abdominal relaxation immediately after the deepest inspiration, the kidney is sharply thrown forwards by the fingers of the hand under the loin behind. A low or large kidney will be thrown against the fingers of the anterior hand and if the organ is tender pain will be felt. By this method, many kidneys will be palpated which cannot be felt by the usual and much more uncomfortable bimanual procedure. In infants one-handed manual compression as well as ballottement is often practicable, only the thumb being used in front and one or two fingers behind the loin.

Bimanual palpation by the usual technique consists of a gradual

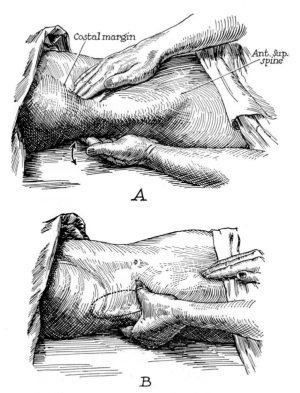

FIGURE 5. Renal palpation. *A*, by ballottement; the kidney is gently thrown upwards by the under hand. *B*, by manual compression with one hand as shown here (infants) or bimanually as in *A*.

approximation of the fingers of the hand over the loin in front and those of the hand under the loin behind, gently bringing the fingers of these two hands closer together in the renal region as the patient breathes and, finally, when he takes a deep breath on command, a quick attempt is made to feel the kidney.

In *renal palpation for nephroptosis* the patient stands chiefly on the leg opposite the organ to be examined, the other leg being slightly flexed and the body bent a little forward. As the patient breathes deeply, the examiner attempts to get a hand above the kidney and another below it for orientation and then, if possible, to trap the kidney between the two hands brought together above from in front and from behind and above the organ. Often palpation of the kidney, spleen, and liver is more satisfactorily accomplished with the patient lying on his side in which position the organ falls forward.

Pain caused by fist percussion or thumping over the posterior loin (Murphy sign) is suggestive of renal or perirenal disease but is an uncomfortable procedure and rarely used by urologists. Palpation of the lower abdomen properly should not be undertaken until the patient has emptied his bladder or has been catheterized. An empty bladder cannot be felt. The *distended bladder* is usually palpated as a symmetrically rounded mass just above the symphysis and may extend to the umbilicus or even higher. In chronic vesical distention, the mass may feel lobular, with or without diverticula, may fall to one side, or even extend into a scrotal hernia. By bimanual examination (rectal finger and counterpressing suprapubic hand) under anesthesia, larger infiltrating bladder tumors may be felt and especially for evidence of lateral pelvic tumor extension (see Chapter 12). In the same manner, a bladder stone may be palpable.

Palpation of the penis is essential in tumor ulceration, both epithelioma and chancre being hard and indurated. There may be hard, cord-like, thrombosis of the dorsal penile vein. Palpation along the urethra and especially with an instrument within the canal will disclose localized areas of periurethritis, stricture, indurated or cystic nodules.

Palpation of the inguinal region, scrotal contents, and the *rectal examination* should be mastered by every clinician. In this rather limited area, extremely difficult problems in differential diagnosis arise, including indirect and direct inguinal hernia, femoral hernia; improperly descended testes, inflammation or tumor of the testicle, epididymis, or tunical coverings; inflammation, tumor, cyst or torsion of the spermatic cord.

Examination should begin with the patient standing and the area fully exposed, his pants dropped down or taken off, and his shirt raised above the nipples. A lax or weak lower abdominal musculature—Malgaigne's bulgings—predisposes to hernia. The *external inguinal ring* is located in the average adult about ½ inch (1.5 cm.) above and external to the spine of the pubis which, in turn, is located by following the pubic crest laterally. The *internal inguinal ring* lies a half inch above the midpoint of Poupart's ligament. Thus oriented, the examiner watches the external ring for bulging on coughing; this is likely to be more prominent in direct hernias.

If no striking irregular bulging is seen when the patient coughs, palpate the inguinal opening. In the male this is done by evaginating the scrotum upward with the little finger, beginning first just above the testis and with the flat side of the fingernail against the cord which will guide the finger directly to the external inguinal ring. The normal ring orifice is slightly triangular with the base located mesially below while with hernia, round enlargement of the orifice, sometimes to great size, may be encountered and on coughing the expanse of impulse is felt.

In females, the counterpart of the inguinal canal in the male is the canal of Nuck which contains the outer end of the round ligament, and occasionally hernia descends through the canal. Here one palpates for cough impulse just below the external inguinal ring and with two or three fingers.

If a mass is found above the external inguinal ring, and one can palpate above and around it, it is not a hernia. When it cannot be palpated around, grasp the sac between the thumb and forefinger and pull it down, then have the patient cough. If there is no impulse, the hernia is probably irreducible. To test its reducibility, the patient flexes the iso-lateral thigh and rotates it inwards. Gentle traction is meanwhile exerted on the hernial sac with one hand while the thumb and first finger of the other hand attempt to compress the contents of the sac mass and work them back into the abdomen. When this is successful, in omental hernias the first part goes easy enough but adhesions may keep the last part of the hernial contents from reaching the abdomen. In intestinal hernia on the other hand, the first part of the reduction goes with difficulty and the last part goes easy; a final gurgle announces successful reduction.

Direct Hernia. These pass through Hesselbach's triangle* medial to the deep epigastric artery. Direct hernia is generally acquired through excessive physical exertion as in straining or undue lifting and is rarely seen before the fifth decade. On digital examination the finger introduces directly into the abdomen rather than obliquely and outwards as in indirect inguinal hernia. Occasionally in direct hernia the pulsating epigastric artery can be felt laterally to the inguinal hernia.

Femoral hernia occurs chiefly in women, the hernial path being beneath Poupart's ligament, through the cribriform fascia of the femoral canal, and then passing externally upwards. It is seldom of urologic interest except when hydrocele of the canal of Nuck may develop in a woman or an ectopic testicle may localize there in a man. The bulge is below and slightly lateral to Poupart's ligament at the upper and outer sides of Scarpa's triangle. It always develops lateral to the pubic spine. When the hernial mass extends upwards over Poupart's ligament, it is usually strangulated.

* Bordered by Poupart's ligament below, lateral border of rectus muscle sheath medially, and deep epigastric vessels laterally.

Rarely, psoas or perinephric abscess points at the femoral ring as may massive abdominal ascites.

The *scrotal skin* is normally free over the scrotal contents and if adherent, look for underlying disease, usually inflammation. Sebaceous cysts, usually multiple and like wens in the scalp, are commonly found in the scrotal skin of older men.

By gently feeling, one distinguishes the separate structures within the scrotum—the testicle, epididymis (palpating its head, body and tail, Fig. 35), and the cordlike, slate-pencil size vas deferens which leaves the tail of the epididymis below to pass up the cord mesially and behind to the external inguinal ring to which point the entire cord should be carefully palpated. Normally the adult spermatic cord is about as large around as one's little finger and feels somewhat soft and pliable like a drapery pull cord. In the scrotum will be normally felt many stringlike longitudinal structures which are chiefly cremasteric muscle bundles.

By scrotal palpation the size, position, number and consistency of the testicles are noted, whether hydrocele, spermatocele, epididymal or spermatic cord cysts, hematocele or tumor are present; whether the vas deferens is normal or is beaded as in chronic nontuberculous infection or as it frequently is in tuberculous disease. In nontuberculous nongonorrheal epididymitis the organ is enlarged, lumpy, indurated, often somewhat tender, and in tuberculous epididymitis there are likely in addition to be tuberculous scrotal fistulae.

Mumps and syphilis are the two chief causes of *orchitis;* in the former the acutely swollen gland is often accompanied by mild collateral epididymitis, but in luetic orchitis the gland is smooth, hard, relatively painless, and freely movable, the so-called billiard-ball testis, thus differing from other varieties of orchitis or epididymitis which anchor the organ down to adjacent structures by scar. The Wassermann test is positive.

Hydrocele swellings occur anterior to and, for the most part, above the testis. The translucency test is applied; grasp the hydrocele mass by the neck of the scrotum and put a light behind it, preferably in a dark room but lacking this, use a rolled-up heavy paper or a mailing tube will do to look through. Clear hydrocele illuminates with a pinkish or reddish tinge or color; in hematocele, tumor, neoplasm, or thickening or calcification of the tunica vaginalis, transillumination is absent. Spermatocele cysts lie above the testis, may transilluminate well; on aspiration the fluid looks like barley water and will be found teeming with spermatozoa.

Tumors of the testicle and scrotal contents demand special and prompt recognition. *Do not squeeze any testicular mass*, especially if it feels slightly heavier than normal; this could spread tumor cells (or tubercle bacilli) into the circulation. A neoplastic mass will not transilluminate; Papanicolaou stain of cells from aspirated fluid may give a positive clue, as may a positive Aschheim-Zondek test for prolan A in the urine (see Chapter 12). Some intrascrotal tumors do not elaborate prolan A. Chorioepithelioma (choriocarcinoma), the most malignant testicular tumor, elaborates a high excess of estrogens to cause pronounced gynecomastia and feminization changes.

Palpate and inspect the perineum for ectopic testis, Cowper's, peri-urethral or ischiorectal inflammation or abscess, urinary extravasation or perineal fistula.

Rectal Examination. "If you don't put your finger in it, you put your foot in it!" This study should be performed as part of every complete physical examination regardless of the age and sex of the patient. The proper technique of rectal examination is learned by few clinicians; the educated finger is indispensable for exploration of the anus and lower 4 inches of rectum. In fairness to their patients, all clinicians and especially urologists should have a rectal examination performed on themselves and have a soft rubber catheter and a steel sound passed that they may learn first hand the patient's reaction, discomfort and viewpoint. Certainly this lesson would make for gentler and more considerate examinations.

Our autopsy studies in 19,000 infants and children showed that about one in 3000 had either (1) imperforate anus, (2) patent anus, with rectal atresia at a higher level, or (3) a normal anus and rectum but atresia just above the rectal segment, or (4) imperfect anus and rectum with a blind-ending rectosigmoid pouch 3 to 4 inches above the anal level. Ten per cent of all newborn children have an abnormally tight anal ring, a tight fissured rectal sphincter or anorectal bands, while other conditions such as fissures, condylomas, rectal prolapse, skin tags or loss of muscle tone are not infrequently present. Fortunately, the anorectal dilation coincident to the rectal examination often cures the lesser rectal obstructions and lesions in the newborn and young children.

Preliminary inspection of the anus and perianal area may reveal pruritus ani, rectal prolapse, external hemorrhoids, prolapsed internal hemorrhoids, anal fissure, fistula or fistula-in-ano. If pruritus ani is found, make skin scrapings and look for fungi; examine the urine for sugar, and the stool for thread worms, especially in the young.

In *performing rectal examination* first have the patient empty the bladder completely lest a distended bladder may erroneously suggest an enlarged prostate! The *position of the patient* for the examination is the next important consideration, and this will largely depend on whether he is ambulatory or bedridden. The ambulatory patient may be examined in the *knee-chest* or *knee-elbow* position which is satisfactory for the examiner but most awkward and uncomfortable for the patient.

Standing Position. A simpler and more comfortable position for the patient and one I routinely employ is to have him stand with both feet planted firmly on the floor, legs separated, the body bent forwards at right angle at the hips and the hands resting on a table or chair. The patient then points his heels outwards (pigeon-toed) to spread the buttocks and the examination begins.

If the patient, young or old, is in bed, the examination is satisfactorily and comfortably performed with him turned on his side in the Sims' position with the upper leg flexed upward and the under leg extended.

If the patient is bedridden and must be examined lying flat on his back, his knee on the side of the examiner is flexed upward. The examining hand is passed under the drawn-up leg and in some instances even a bimanual examination can be made. If the patient is sunken deeply in the bed, put a pillow under the buttocks to facilitate the examination.

The index finger is the examining finger used in adults and older children while the little finger is used in infants and young children whose anal ring would be needlessly traumatized by the larger finger. *The examining finger protected by rubber glove or finger cot should be generously lubricated by surgical jelly or white petrolatum.* This is most important, for most of the discomfort or real pain produced by rectal examination results from lack of lubrication with needless friction between the dry rubber glove or finger cot and the sensitive dry rectal tissues, in addition to the painful pulling of unlubricated perirectal and anal hairs caught up in the process.

First separate the buttocks widely to expose clearly the anal opening and be sure the finger goes in the rectum and not, in the female, in the vagina. For the study one uses which ever hand he customarily employs for delicate examination or efforts. If one makes the examination with the left index finger, the buttocks about the anus are widely separated with the thumb and fingers of the right hand (Fig. 6).

Now tell the patient what you are going to do, warn him when you start to introduce the examining finger, and try to get him to relax by taking several deep breaths or by bearing down as in moving the bowels.

Rather than bluntly, coarsely, and crudely trying to quickly spear the anal canal as is so commonly done at rectal examinations, the well-lubricated finger should first be gently rested against the external sphincter (Fig. 6). Remember the anus is closed by a most sensitive irritable ring which readily responds to roughness and haste with pain and spasm. As the anus relaxes in response to increased digital pressure, the finger is carefully and gently introduced with a slight twisting motion (Fig. 6). Don't hurry! Go slow! Take your time! And be gentle, *gentle*, GENTLE!

At first the finger is directed forward and upward until the internal sphincter is passed, then backward into the rectal ampulla.

In performing the rectal examination, one notes the anal tonus, anorectal lesions (ulcerations, cryptitis, hypertrophied papillae, perirectal abscess, fistula opening), the size, shape and texture of the prostate gland and seminal vesicles. The examiner notes also the condition of the rectal walls, palpates the hollow of the sacrum and coccyx, and the pouch of Douglas. Internal hemorrhoids, unless thrombosed, cannot be identified by digital rectal examination.

A hyperspastic sphincter remaining tight despite the patient's effort to relax, is suggestive of fistula-in-ano; the examination causes exquisite pain. Should this occur look for the cutaneous tag of the "signal pile" which "watches" over the fissure. A dilated relaxed rectal sphincter suggests spinal cord disease, reflects the tonus of the vesical outlet, and when accompanied by a relaxed ballooned rectum, is almost pathognomonic of disease of the lumbosacral nervous system.

One should scarcely confuse constipated stool in the rectum or the feeling of the cervix with neoplasm although a hard curved cervical pessary might strongly suggest malignancy, but the observation will disappear with removal of the pessary. If palpable *rectal carcinoma* exists, determine if it encircles the bowel, if it is ulcerated, fixed, cauliflower, pedunculated, and can the finger get above it. Occasionally *rectal polyps* can be hooked down by the examining finger and seen. A *rectal stricture* feels like a hole in a diaphragm, firm and sclerotic, or is soft "like a hole in Swiss cheese." Induration or *abscess of Cowper's glands* is palpated between the index finger in the rectum and the thumb outside on the perineum over the gland (Fig. 6). *Ischiorectal abscesses* are similarly palpated, being indurated and tender. Examine the mucocutaneous junction at the anus and the immediate surrounding skin for the orifice of a fistula-in-ano. If the fistulous tract is high, it may feel like a cord or a pencil under the movable overlying rectal mucosa.

Palpation of the Prostate. The prostate of a five-year-old boy feels flat and triangular with the apex just within the anal sphincter. It is usually difficult to outline the normal prostate in males younger than four years of age; when the organ is inflamed, no great difficulty is apt

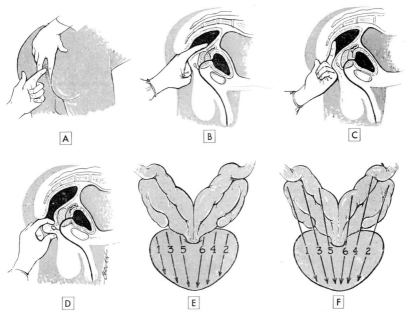

FIGURE 6. Rectal examination. *A*, introduction of protected well lubricated finger. *B*, palpation of prostate and seminal vesicles, lateral view. *C*, palpation of anterior surface of sacrum and coccyx. *D*, palpation of Cowper's gland. *E*, massage of prostate for specimen collection or treatment; order of "strokes" is indicated gradually working toward the center (verumontanum). *F*, massage of seminal vesicles and prostate.

to be encountered in digital examination of the organ. As a rule, the prostate of a three year old boy feels about the size of one's little finger nail. In the young the normal seminal vesicles are not palpable, but congested or otherwise diseased, they may be felt especially in boys practicing habitual masturbation. In *prostatic abscess* or *sarcoma*, there is variably great enlargement; not infrequently a soft sarcoma and fluctuant prostatic abscess feel strikingly alike, or the neoplastic gland may be enlarged, nodular, and firm.

In an adult male, the *prostate* is about the size and shape of a chestnut; 2.5 to 3.0 cm. wide; 2.5 cm. in the long diameter, and 2.0 cm. thick at the heaviest point posteriorly. By rectum one can feel the prostatic lateral lobes and the anatomic apex or posterior lobe. *One cannot feel the median or anterior lobes!* Also felt are the seminal vesicles, one on each side, at the bladder base; these may be palpable if diseased or indurated.

To the examining finger the normal adult prostate feels strikingly like an orange, firm, smoothly elastic, but neither hard nor soft. The anatomic apex of the gland fuses forward with the soft membranous urethra between the layers of the triangular ligament (urogenital trigone) within the confines of which are also, one on each side, Cowper's bulbo-urethral glands (Fig. 6). These are palpable only when inflamed.

The abnormalities of the prostate and its contiguous structures as detected by rectal examination are given under the various headings: Acute prostatitis, prostatic abscess, hyperplasia, carcinoma, sarcoma, and so forth (see Index).

Prostatic fluid is obtained by stripping down the gland with long, firm strokes as suggested by Figure 6. Digital expression will not begin to deliver nearly as much seminal fluid as will physiologic seminal ejaculation. Usually both the prostate and seminal vesicles are stripped down for this examination (q.v.).

Palpation of the Seminal Vesicles. The vesicles are high up from the anal level and a long finger is advantageous but is not a necessity especially if the patient is hyperflexed forward at the hips and bimanual palpation is used: One finger in the rectum and the other hand above the spine of the isolateral pubis pushing inward towards the examining finger. In this manner most seminal vesicles can be felt. When inflamed, they are variably enlarged, tender, indurated, and may be fixed and lumpy, especially with tuberculosis, or stony hard with tumor spread upward from prostatic carcinoma.

Seminal vesicle fluid is obtained by stripping down the gland, beginning at the tip of the organ and expressing the secretion with two or three downward digital strokes in the direction of the vesicle on each side (Fig. 6 *F*).

Vaginal examination and palpation of the urinary tract in the female are separately and briefly considered in Chapter 13.

Percussion. Vesical distention is recognizable by percussion which should begin high and progress downward toward the pelvis. In a five-year-old child, 3 ounces of urine distends the bladder 1 inch above the symphysis pubis as does 6 ounces of urine in an average size adult. The note of a distended bladder is flat in contrast to the tympanitic note of the abdomen just above, or the colon over a renal tumor, for example.

Auscultation is employed in estimating the blood pressure, the diastolic pressure usually being about half the systolic. During the first year of life the systolic pressure rises to 90 to 100 mm. Hg where it remains approximately the same until the tenth year, when it increases to 115 to 120 mm. Hg at fifteen years, and 130 to 135 mm. Hg at thirty years.

UROLOGIC EXAMINATION

The indications for urologic examination are:
1. Pyuria
    (a) acute, persistent
    (b) chronic
2. Disturbances of urination—dysuria, frequency, urgency, etc.
3. Hematuria (except acute nephritis)
4. Abdominal pain
5. Abdominal tumor
6. Anomaly of the external genitalia
7. Urogenital injury
8. Spinal cord injury and disease
9. Enuresis
10. Renal insufficiency
11. Renal retarded growth
12. Hypertensive vascular disease

The precise diagnosis of urologic disease demands adequately comprehensive examination in which the practitioner who initially sees the patient must be expected to fulfill a most important role. An acceptable routine of procedure in the investigation of a patient with urologic disease may be outlined as follows:

1. A thorough history taking.
2. Careful physical examination, especially with palpation of the urinary and reproductive tracts. Rectal examination. Blood pressure observations.
3. Examination of the urine which in females should always be obtained by catheterization (see text): specific gravity, albumin, sugar, pus, blood, casts, bacteria (stain and culture).
4. Complete blood count, often with blood typing.
5. Residual urine estimation.
6. Two hour phenolsulfonphthalein excretion test: intravenous injection preferred to intramuscular.
7. Blood chemistry: nonprotein nitrogen or urea nitrogen; CO_2 determination; other studies as indicated, e.g., chloride, sodium, sugar, serum albumin and globulin; serum calcium and phosphorus, creatinine, and so forth.
8. Plain x-ray of urinary tract for calculi and spinal defects.
9. Excretory urographic examination.

10. Cystogram if excretory cystogram (9) is not satisfactory or to demonstrate vesico-ureteral reflux; urethrograms occasionally.

11. Cystourethroscopy (general anesthesia in about 50 per cent):

    (a) Observation of bladder wall, outlet, posterior urethra, anterior urethra.

    (b) Ureteral catheterization—bilateral unless contraindicated.

    (c) Divided renal function test (indigo carmine or phenolsulfonphthalein intravenously).

    (d) Divided renal specimen collection for urea, pus, blood and bacteria.

    (e) Retrograde pyelography and ureterography—preferably bilateral.

In the urologic investigation the nonurologist may be expected to carry out procedures 1 to 10 with helpful interest to himself and benefit to the patient. Procedures 11-a to 11-e may advisedly be delegated to a qualified urologist, not only for the technical study but for help, advice and guidance in the treatment of the patient.

The history taking and physical examination are assumed to have been accomplished. In the laboratory examination, the following studies should be carried out *seriatim:*

URINALYSIS

This is the keystone of urologic diagnosis. Unless the urine specimen is properly collected the whole structure of further study is likely to be erroneous and, if the examination of the improperly collected specimen is accepted as reported by the laboratory, is utterly unfair to the patient whose life may be hopelessly jeopardized.

First, the urine specimen should be freshly collected; stale specimens have no place in the diagnostic study. When infection is suspected or known to be part of the clinical picture in a female of any age, only a catheterized specimen is worth examining. Moreover, as a matter of precision, only a properly collected urine specimen should be examined in any urologic case.

Only aseptically collected fresh uncentrifuged urine specimens merit serious study.

Collection of the Urine. Unless a "clean catch" specimen can be obtained from the male, employ aseptic catheterization. In collecting the "clean catch" specimen, the prepuce is widely retracted, the glans and separated meatus are thoroughly washed with antiseptic solution such as oxy-cyanide or bichloride of mercury 1:500; lacking these, use green soap. The patient voids a few cubic centimeters of urine free, and then a sterile beaker or other sterile collecting receptacle is introduced into the voiding stream; the specimen thus obtained is utilized for routine analysis, culture, and/or Gram stain of sediment from a centrifuged portion.

In the female of any age, the specimen for urinalysis and for culture should be taken only by catheter. No amount of scrubbing of the labia and introitus will cleanse well enough to avoid bacterial and cellular contamination by these areas in the voiding process. Examination of casually collected specimens is undoubtedly the greatest fundamental error commonly made in urologic investigation by inadequately trained urologists and by most general practitioners!

Catheterization in the male is simple to perform. First, the separated meatus and environs are thoroughly cleansed with a mercurial or green soap solution. A sterile soft rubber catheter or, in a boy, the Campbell 8 F. male miniature metal catheter (Fig. 7) is then passed with aseptic precautions to the bladder and after a few cubic centimeters of urine have run out free, subsequent urine flow is collected in a sterile receptacle.

In the female, the introitus is similarly exposed and cleansed and the catheter is passed through the urethra under vision. For this a soft rubber catheter is satisfactory; *glass catheters should never be used.* For catheterization of females of all ages, the Campbell miniature metal catheters are unsurpassed (Fig. 7).

Unless the physician will employ aseptic catheterization for the collection of urine as just described, further investigation will proceed on false sands, to wit: many patients have been diagnosed as having urogenital tuberculosis because in the examination of a specimen voided through a long prepuce, acid-fast smegma bacilli, not recognized as such, were found. Many patients of all ages and of both sexes have been referred for urologic examination because of persistent pyuria, yet whose

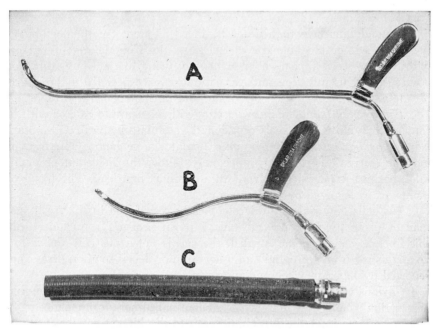

FIGURE 7. Campbell miniature (8 F.) stainless steel catheters. *A*, male catheter. *B*, female catheter with fin handle to facilitate instrumentation. This catheter is routinely used for both female adults and children. *C*, rubber tubing with male Luer connection fitting to facilitate collection of catheter specimen or irrigation of the bladder. (Courtesy of Journal of Urology.)

aseptically collected specimens were analytically normal and sterile, and whose "pyuria" was due to a long tight prepuce, vaginitis or just local filth.

The *urine in the neonatal period* is scant (15 to 150 cc. a day) and highly concentrated but the specific gravity is low because the glomerular and tubular filtration function is low at this period. Other constituents which would be considered abnormal in an older patient include a strongly acid reaction, albumin, sometimes sugar, and urate crystals, mucus, casts, uric acid, or uric acid crystals, and epithelial, red and white blood cells.

After the neonatal period, the urine constituency becomes more what we are accustomed to find in adults, of which *to the urologist the sugar, urea, pus, blood and bacterial content are of prime concern.*

Color and Appearance of the Urine. Although the rudiments of urinalysis are known to the second or third year medical student, some features of this study are of special interest in the diagnosis of urologic disease. The *clarity* of the urine will vary with its crystalline (urate, carbonate, phosphate, etc.), its cellular (white, red, epithelial), and mucous content. Fresh *hematuria* appears bright red, while old blood is mahogany color or "smoky." *Anthocyanin* in the urine after the ingestion of beets gives it a bright red color which must be distinguished from hematuria, a problem encountered chiefly in children. Urates are stained pink by *uro-erythrin*—a blood derivative—and settle out in the urine as red "brick dust."

Hemoglobinuria is manifested by blood pigment (methemoglobin) in the urine without red blood corpuscles, results from laking of red cells within the vessels, appears as a mahogany urine like old hematuria, and occurs in serious infection and parasitic disease, especially malaria, from nitrate absorption, ingestion of poison, and mismatched transfusions.

Paroxysmal hemoglobinuria occurs with exposure to cold or with late congenital syphilis, and may occasionally simulate hematuria. Similarly, *hematoporphyrinuria* may simulate hematuria or hemoglobinuria, and may be congenital. Its appearance may follow the ingestion of phenol, salol, barbituric acid derivatives, sulfanilamide, and lead. The blood pigments are recognized by spectroscopy.

Pus cells (pyuria) are microscopically recognized in the fresh specimen of urine by their polymorphic ("pawn broker's") nucleus; unless this nucleus can be demonstrated, the cell is not a pus cell and is to be distinguished from epithelial and other cellular debris so often erroneously reported by laboratory technicians as pus.

Chylous urine is milky suggesting pyuria and results from lymphatic obstruction usually due to filariasis, abdominal tumor, or other mechanical blockage. Sometimes the lymphatic path to the kidney can be urographically demonstrated by *pyelolymphatic backflow* (Fig. 21). **Lipuria** (oil or fat globules in the urine) is rare except in an occasional case of advanced diabetes mellitus.

Odor of the Urine. In colon bacillus infection this is of a dead mouse quality and in Proteus infections, it is fishy or of dead fish. Ammoniacal urine denotes decomposition of urea by bacterial "urea-splitters." The peculiar aromatic odor of the urine which appears after eating asparagus is due to its hippuric acid content.

Reaction of the Urine. Normally this is *acid* because of diacid phosphate and sodium phosphate. *Alkalinity* is derived chiefly from the earthy carbonates. With increased respiratory activity in the morning, carbon dioxide is eliminated through the lungs, hence less acid is excreted in the urine as acid sodium phosphate and the urine at this time may be neutral or alkaline, a phenomenon known as the *alkaline tide.*

Normally the *urine titer* ranges between pH 6.0 and pH 7.5, and is conveniently estimated with nitrazine paper (Squibb) and its color chart; the greater the urinary acidity the more mustard yellow the paper turns, and the more alkaline, the bluer the paper gets. Potentiometer and pH titration are unnecessary for practical urinalysis.

The normal **specific gravity** ranges between 1.002 and 1.030 reading, as high as 1.060 being recorded in low fluid intake and dehydration. A *fixed specific gravity* suggests renal damage or congenital renal deficiency and demands further study. (See Concentration Test, page 46.)

Total Output of Urine. Normally the urine output from a five year old child ranges between 500 and 700 cc. in twenty-four hours, and in an adult 800 to 1500 cc. In *polyuria* (unusually large fluid intake, diabetes insipidus, diabetes mellitus, chronic nephritis, brain tumor, parathyroid tumor, postepileptic and postasthmatic states) enormous quantities of urine are passed. *Polydipsia* (excessive thirst) and great frequency of urination are the chief symptoms.

Albuminuria. To the urologist the degree of albuminuria is of secondary importance; every patient with hematuria or relatively acute urinary infection will show albuminuria as will nearly every patient with an indwelling drainage tube (indwelling catheter, cystostomy, ureterostomy, pyelostomy, nephrostomy, for example). Under these conditions, albuminuria is neither abnormal nor of grave concern. Albuminuria is common (1) after a heavy protein intake, (2) in the newborn, (3) with fever, and (4), in the orthostatic variety, albumin is passed only when the patient is in the upright position. The reason for the last phenomenon is at present unknown, being variously ascribed to a large pulse pressure or to lumbospinal anomalies which interfere with the renal circulation when the patient is in the upright position. When all the usual laboratory studies are normal in early life except the lordotic albuminuria, there is no evidence that nephritis will appear in later life.

Bence Jones proteinuria is usually associated with multiple myeloma, leukemia, lymphosarcoma, and occurs occasionally in nephritis or carcinoma. The protein is precipitated from the serum at 40° to 60° C. (104° to 140° F.) and disappears after heating to 65° to 66° C. (150° F.).

Glycosuria. The presence of sugar (glucose) in the urine is of special import to the urologist when localized suppuration is suspected in or about the urinary tract and especially in perinephric abscess. In diabetes mellitus there is special susceptibility to Staphylococcus aureus infection—urinary or otherwise.

The important normal chemical constituents of the urine are given in Table 1.

Microscopic Examination of the Urine. First and foremost the specimen should be properly collected to avoid contamination; it should be fresh to avoid cellular disintegration and it should be uncentrifuged so that a constant factor in all cell counts is maintained. Microscopically the *pus cell* is recognized as slightly larger than the red blood cell, contains neutrophilic granules as well as granular degeneration debris and the nucleus may appear as a bilobed or trilobed body or as two or three separate small nuclear bodies which are sharply brought out in relief if a little dilute acetic acid is run under the cover glass. By distinction the epithelial cell is larger than the pus cell and has a large round nucleus. Cell structures are well preserved in acid urine but in alkaline urine degenerate to an amorphic slimy mass.

Normally the combined output of epithelial and blood cells in the urine of a male is 300,000 to 500,000 cells in twelve hours, or less than one cell per cubic millimeter, the upper normal limit being 600,000 in the male and a million in the female. In short, an occasional leukocyte and red blood cell in the urine is normal.

These occasional *red blood cells in the urine* are physiologically increased by vigorous exercise, exposure to cold or may be profuse with urinary tract infection, obstruction (congestion), tumor, nephritis, calculous disease, or trauma. *Hematuria* may also be caused by a wide variety of other conditions as indicated in Figure 4. In the fresh specimen red blood cells show no crenation but this rapidly occurs in standing specimens. The addition of a drop of dilute methylene blue to the speci-

TABLE 1.   COMPOSITION OF A NORMAL URINE

(Volume—24 hours—1500 cc.)

CONSTITUENT	ABSOLUTE WEIGHT GRAMS	APPROXIMATE PERCENTAGE
Water	1440.00	96.0
Solids	60.0	4.0
Urea	35.0	2.33
Uric acid	0.75	0.05
Hippuric acid	0.7	0.05
Oxalic acid	0.015	0.001
Aromatic oxyacids	0.06	0.004
Creatinine	1.0	0.07
Thiocyanic acid (as KSCN)	0.15	0.01
Indican	0.01	0.001
Ammonia	0.65	0.04
Sodium chloride	16.5	1.1
Phosphoric acid	2.5	0.15
Total sulfuric acid	2.5	0.15
Silicic acid	0.45	0.03
Potassium (K_2O)	2.5	0.15
Sodium (Na_2O)	5.0	0.3
Calcium (CaO)	0.25	0.015
Magnesium (MgO)	0.30	0.02
Iron	0.005	0.0004

men before microscopic examination brings out the erythrocytes in sharp contrast because of their failure to absorb the dye.

Casts are molds of the renal tubules, their type depending upon their genesis. Hyaline casts are formed from coagulated albumin, granular casts from degenerated tubular epithelium; pus, blood and epithelial casts are conglomerate masses of these cells bound together in a transparent matrix. *Pus casts are always pathognomonic of pyelonephritis.*

Urine Culture. This demands aseptic collection of the specimen as previously described earlier in this chapter. Culture and gram-stained smears of centrifuged specimen sediment do not always agree, in our experience the culture being the more reliable. For immediate information as to the probable nature of the invading bacteria in an acute severe urinary infection, examination of the gram-stained urine sediment is most valuable to enable prompt administration of a drug or antibiotic whose therapeutic spectrum includes the type organisms observed. Thus one would not prescribe penicillin for a gram-negative bacillary infection which might well be a colon bacillus (see Chapter 7 on Infections). The fresh aseptically collected urine is centrifuged at 2500 revolutions per minute for fifteen minutes after which the supernatant fluid is poured off and, using a fine pipet, the sediment is taken up, smeared on a slide, dried, and fixed by heat and stained by Gram's method.* The examination for tubercle bacilli is similarly performed, the Ziehl-Neelsen stain being used instead of Gram's technique.

It is axiomatic that *the identification of the bacterial invader(s) is essential to the choice of rational therapy.*

TESTS OF RENAL FUNCTION

These are of two types, (1) the excretory, which tells us what the kidneys can do now, and (2) the retention, which tells us what the kidneys have been doing in the recent past. The normal physiologic activity of the renal unit is (a) glomerular filtration, (b) tubular absorption, (c) tubular excretion; the various tests thereof are discussed in Chapter 4. They are but briefly reviewed here.

TESTS OF RENAL EXCRETION

Phenolsulfonphthalein Test. This determines the ability of the renal tubules to excrete the dye and normally, when the intravenous route of administration is employed, to the extent of at least 25 per cent dye return during the first fifteen minutes after injection. Prior to the test injection** it is customary to give the patient two glasses of water that the

---

* A rapid Gram-stain technique: Cover the fixed preparation for thirty seconds with a 2 per cent solution of crystal violet in methyl alcohol; (2) wash with water; (3) apply Gram's iodine solution for thirty seconds; (4) wash with alcohol until purple color ceases to come away; (5) apply contrast stain such as 1 per cent aqueous safranine; (6) wash in water, dry thoroughly, and examine under the oil immersion objective lens.

** While the decubital vein is usually used for making the injection in adults and older children, in infants and in young children one must often use one of the superficial veins of the lower arm, wrist, back of hand, foot, scalp or, occasionally, the external jugular vein or even the anterior fontanel when it is open.

resulting polyuria may call into activity all of the functioning tubular secretory ability for the dye since this gives a truer estimation of the total secretory capacity. The collected specimens will be amber if the urine is acid, and magenta-red if alkaline. To ensure the full alkalinity before making the test readings against known standards, alkali such as a few drops of 10 per cent sodium hydroxide is added to each test specimen.

Intravenous Route. One cubic centimeter of standard (0.6 mg.) phenolsulfonphthalein solution is given intravenously and specimens are collected at fifteen-minute intervals, the normal excretion being 25 to 40 per cent the first fifteen minutes, 15 to 18 per cent the second, 8 to 10 per cent the third, and 4 to 5 per cent the last fifteen minutes; about 5 per cent is secreted during the following hour, a total excretion of 75 to 90 per cent in two hours.

Intramuscular Route. When this method is employed, 1 cc. of dye is given into the muscle (usually deltoid or buttocks) and a ten-minute delay for absorption is allowed. Total voided specimens at 30, 60, 90, and 120 minutes are collected. Normally 40 to 60 per cent of the dye is excreted the first hour and 10 to 25 per cent the second for a total output of 60 to 85 per cent in two hours. Because of the uncertainty of dye absorption (edema, faulty circulation, and so forth) following intramuscular injection the intravenous test is preferred.

Indigo carmine, a deep bluish dye, is given intravenously during cystoscopic examination as a comparative test of renal function, the intensity of the dye output being the criterion. It is not an accurate quantitative test, but for practical purposes it may be accepted that a kidney which will put out a good or deep indigo carmine excretion will probably support life. The test is given both intramuscularly and intravenously; the last is the usual and preferred method.

Dilution Test. A criterion of good renal function is the ability of the kidneys to secrete a large amount of water at low specific gravity (1.001 to 1.002) in half an hour. Five hundred to 1000 cc. of fluid is given in the morning. The patient stays in bed and no food is taken until the test is completed. Voided specimens are collected every half hour for four hours and the specific gravity readings are made.

Concentration Test. The capacity of the kidneys to concentrate urinary crystalloids is reflected in the specific gravity of the urine. Renal injury which prevents the organ from concentrating the urine also renders it unable to put out urine more dilute than 1.008 to 1.010; this is known as *fixation of specific gravity*. High fixation indicates low fluid intake and except in diabetes insipidus and a very large fluid intake, a low fixation denotes serious renal disease. The test as usually carried out is as follows: At the evening meal the patient takes a considerable amount of protein. The night's urine is discarded. The next morning's urine is saved. The patient stays in bed for one hour after awakening when a second sample is separately collected. The patient arises, moves about and another specimen is taken in an hour. When the renal function is unimpaired, the specific gravity of at least one sample will be between 1.022

and 1.032. In severe impairment, the specific gravity may be down to 1.008 or 1.010, and with moderate injury, between 1.010 and 1.020. Other criteria include: (1) variation of specific gravity in the different specimens, (2) maximal specific gravity in any one specimen, (3) total night output, (4) the urea, sodium chloride, and total nitrogen output in any particular specimen, and the total output in all specimens.

Interpretation. Normally there should be a variation in specific gravity of at least eight to ten points between the highest and the lowest, the night specimen being small in amount and with a specific gravity of 1.020 or higher in the morning. Renal injury is evident by inability to vary widely the specific gravity; the range might not be over one or two points. In nephritis the night specimen will be larger in amount and have a lower specific gravity.

Other tests than these and of greater refinement are generally too complex for any but hospital procedure. These include the urea, inulin, hippuran, and para-aminohippurate clearance tests and are briefly described in Chapter 4 under Physiology of the Kidney.

TESTS OF RENAL RETENTION

These indicate what work the kidney has recently been doing, whether secreting waste metabolites or, injured, retaining them. If one kidney is badly diseased but its mate is sound, the blood constituency will usually remain normal. On a theoretic basis, Homer W. Smith states that the total renal function must be reduced to 30 per cent of its normal value in order to raise the blood urea from 21 to 36 mg. per cent. In renal disease grave enough to cause retention of waste metabolites, examination of the blood will show increase in nitrogen elements—the urea, nonprotein nitrogen; disturbances of acid-base and electrolyte balance, changes in blood minerals, and the development of lipemia. Increase in blood creatinine rarely occurs until the nitrogen levels are at least twice normal, i.e., the urea is 30 mg. per cent, or the nonprotein nitrogen 50 to 55 mg. per cent, a damage of considerable magnitude since the urea quotient is seldom elevated until two thirds to three fourths of the renal units have ceased functioning.

The normal blood and other chemistry values in the human are given in Table 2.

REACTION OF BODY FLUIDS

This is normally neutral (pH 7.4) but with increased metabolic activity the production of acid exceeds that of base. In conditions such as dehydration, edema, acidosis, and alkalosis there is pronounced water and metabolite disturbance with alteration in the relation between the *intracellular* and *extracellular* fluids. Sodium chloride and sodium bicarbonate components are changed, potassium is lost chiefly from the muscles, or is replaced by sodium in the tissues. Thus in *acidosis* intracellular sodium is primarily reduced but the muscle potassium remains normal or but only slightly increased while in *alkalosis* there is potassium loss from the

TABLE 2. NORMAL BLOOD AND OTHER CHEMISTRY VALUES

	INFANTS AND CHILDREN	ADULTS	
Nonprotein nitrogen	25–30	15–40	mg. per 100 cc.
Urea nitrogen	7–15	9–17	" " " "
Uric acid	3–4	2–4	" " " "
Creatinine	1–2	1–2	" " " "
Total plasma protein			
Albumin	6.5–7.5	6–8	per cent
Globulin	4–5	1.3–3.2	" "
Fibrinogen	.2–.5	.2–.6	" "
Chlorides			
Whole blood	450–500	500–550	mg. per 100 cc.
Plasma	500–520	570–620	" " " "
Sodium	300–350	315–333	" " " "
Calcium (serum)	10–12	9–11	" " " "
Potassium	15–20	15.5–19.7	" " " "
Phosphorus (serum)	4–5	2.5–4.5	" " " "
Phosphate activity			
Acid	0–0.5	1.5–3.5	units (King)
Alkaline	1.0–2.0	1.0–3.5	" "
Sugar	80–120	80–120	mg. per 100 cc.
Cholesterol (whole blood)	140–170	140–250	" " " "
Acetone bodies	5–8	6–9	" " " "
Lactic acid	10–15	10–15	" " " "
Carbon dioxide combining power	45–60	53–65	volumes per cent
Urea clearance			
Standard	40–65 or 75–120	57 per cent average normal function	
Maximum	60–95 or 80–125	75 per cent average normal function	
Prothrombin time (Quick)	12–16	12–14	seconds
Ascorbic acid (vitamin C)	1.5	0.5–1.5	mg. per 100 cc. average

muscle and intracellular replacement of the potassium deficit by sodium. The serum carbonate component varies directly with the intracellular sodium but inversely with muscle potassium, so that in serum alkalosis there is potassium and chloride deficiency and in acidosis there is sodium deficiency.

Thus, in serum alkalosis with potassium deficiency, treatment with sodium salts alone is inadequate and potassium should be added to the solution.

The *acid excess* is eliminated in the urine largely as acid phosphates ($N_aH_2PO_4$) and in the expiration as carbon dioxide (CO_2). Thus through this normal renal mechanism tissue neutrality is maintained. As excess acid (chiefly aceto-acetic) ions are formed in the blood in all acute and some chronic diseases, their neutralization causes a diminution of the basic carbonate in the blood with a relative or absolute diminution or reduction of sodium. The acid increase may result from hyperproduction of acid in the tissues or a failure of the process by which acid is normally eliminated from the body and commonly in the form of ammonia salt. The basic carbonate component in the blood is estimated as the carbon dioxide combining power of the plasma—normally 45 to 60 volumes per cent in an adult, 50 to 65 volumes per cent in children—and is an index of the gravity of the toxemia. The fundamentals of treatment are (1) combat of dehydration and (2) restoration of normal electrolyte balance by the administration of electrolytic fluid usually containing glucose.

Acidosis. This develops as the basic carbonate level of the blood is lowered, either by increased acid ion production or by excess loss through disease of carbonate and basic minerals, sodium and potassium. The potential causes of acidosis are numerous and in every case in some way are connected with renal injury interfering with the normal electrolyte maintenance and control by the kidney (see Physiology). Acidosis is especially frequent in children, particularly the young ones, is generally evidenced by pronounced gastrointestinal upset with vomiting, diarrhea, starvation, anal or other acute infections; ingestion of acids or acid-producing salts such as ammonium chloride; and in severe fever produces a picture of its own which may even overshadow that of the initial underlying disease, and especially is this so in acute renal infection in the young.

The onset of acidosis is usually noted as marked irritability, malaise, weakness, apathy, loss of appetite, nausea and vomiting with, later, dehydration, loss of conjunctival luster, dry, bright red buccal and oral mucous membranes and tongue. Hyperpnea (rapid breathing) and often delirium develops with, later, true air hunger and coma, all of this being the usual picture in the clinical course of grave uremia, the manifestations of which are largely due to its acidotic component.

The *diagnosis* of acidosis is made by recognition of the signs, symptoms, and clinical course as just outlined, and a lowered carbon dioxide combining power of the blood plasma is its confirmation. Commonly the carbon dioxide combining power will be reduced to the twenties but I have seen it as low as 7 volumes per cent in a young girl with massive suppuration of a solitary kidney. As treatment succeeds, the carbon dioxide combining power estimation may be expected to increase to the normal 55 to 65 volumes per cent.

Treatment. Acidosis is serious in patients of all ages and demands immediate treatment, the objective being to restore the normal blood electrolyte balance. The immediate intravenous administration of 5 per cent glucose in normal saline, Ringer's or $\frac{1}{6}$ molar sodium-r-lactate solution is urgent. The glucose supplies calories and fluids to combat ketosis, the saline solution will assist the kidney in regulating electrolyte balance through retention of necessary electrolytes and the sodium-r-lactate solution augments the alkaline reserve by metabolism of the lactate ions to release the sodium ions which are deficient in acidosis. One cubic centimeter of $\frac{1}{6}$ molar sodium-r-lactate solution per kilogram body weight will increase the plasma bicarbonate by 0.54 volume carbon dioxide combining power per cent.

Alkalosis occurs less frequently than acidosis and results from an increase of basic ions in the blood plasma. This increase of base results from (1) loss of hydrochloric acid (anions) by protracted vomiting, acidosis or diarrhea, (2) excessive administration of alkalies, especially sodium bicarbonate (rare) or, as I have thrice observed, (3) from the intravenous injection of too much glucose. Alkalosis is seldom of renal origin but may be when diminished fluid intake sufficiently reduces the renal excretion of excess sodium bicarbonate.

Symptoms are like those of acidosis except the breathing is shallow and apneic (irregularly slow). As the disease advances and this is particularly notable in children, there develop tetany, muscular twitchings, carpopedal spasm, Trousseau's* and Chvostek's** signs, convulsions and, terminally, coma. The observation of these symptoms and the clinical course together with the finding of a high carbon dioxide combining power in the blood plasma level establishes the diagnosis. The highest level I have encountered was 89 carbon dioxide volumes per cent in a patient with persistent vomiting induced by a renal carbuncle.

Treatment of alkalosis must be prompt and energetic with the intensive administration of the electrolytes used in combating acidosis plus the administration of potassium because, as stated earlier, in alkalosis there is potassium loss from the muscles and intracellular replacement of the potassium deficit by sodium. The large fluid intake, chiefly intravenously, combats the dehydration and accelerates sodium bicarbonate elimination through the increased kidney function. The combined use of normal saline and Ringer's solutions will enable the kidney to adjust the electrolyte retention and restore normal biochemical balance. The employment of Darrow's solution (sodium chloride 4.4 gm., potassium chloride 2.7 gm. and sodium bicarbonate 4.0 gm., per liter) is recommended for the treatment of both acidosis and alkalosis, and in the treatment of diarrhea in infants (alkalosis) has alone reduced the mortality from the usual 25 to 35 per cent level to less than 5 per cent. As the patient improves, the previously high carbon dioxide combining power of the blood plasma will descend to normal levels.

METHODS OF FLUID ADMINISTRATION

Water is preferably given by mouth, but the administration of fluids containing electrolytes, glucose, or amino acids, for example, is best achieved *intravenously* though in the infant this often means cutting down on the vein. When it proves impossible to get a needle into a vein, employ *hypodermoclysis* through a 20 gauge hypodermic needle placed in the breast or upper inner thigh. *Hyaluronidase* (1.0 mg. per 25 cc. electrolyte solution) is often co-administered with the hypodermoclysis solution and will stimulate tenfold the absorption of the fluid from the subcutane-

---

* Trousseau's sign. A muscular spasm on pressure over large detached arteries or nerves; seen in tetany, tache cerebral and thrombosis of the extremities in visceral cancer.

** Chvostek's sign. A spasm of the facial muscles resulting from tapping of the muscles or branches of the facial nerve; seen in calcium tetany.

ous tissues or muscles. Hyaluronidase is a mucolytic enzyme which acts on and depolymerizes the mucopolysaccharide hyaluronic acid existing in the ground substance of connective tissue and which normally restrains fluid diffusion and absorption in the tissues.

Rectal administration of fluids may be employed in some cooperative patients if they can retain a small (14 to 20 F.) two or four eye catheter in the rectum. Normal or half-normal saline (0.5 to 0.9 per cent NaCl) is given, at a rate of not over 50 drops a minute. Unfortunately, glucose and other nutrients are insignificantly absorbed by the rectum. The greater the hydration, the greater and more rapid will be the fluid absorption. This method should be remembered for the emergency when facilities for more rapid methods of fluid administration are not at hand.

UROGRAPHY

This is roentgenography applied to Urology, a further anatomic identification being used to designate which part of the urinary tract is thus shown. A urogram is a generic term indicating any x-ray of the urinary tract *in toto* or only a separate portion. A *plain urogram* is one made without the injection of contrast medium or air into the tract; this is also known as a preliminary or *"scout"* film. Urographic demonstration of the renal pelvis is a *pyelogram;* of the ureter, a *ureterogram;* of the bladder, a *cystogram;* of the urethra, a *urethrogram;* of the seminal vesicles a *vesiculogram.* When the upper urinary tract is radiographically outlined by radiopaque medium injected through a ureteral catheter, it is known as a *retrograde* pyelogram, ureterogram, and so forth, and when delineated by medium excreted by the kidneys following its intravenous, subcutaneous, or intramuscular injection, it is known as an *excretory* pyelogram. It is an *intravenous pyelogram* only when the medium is thus given. A urogram made while the patient is voiding radiopaque medium is a *voiding cystogram,* or voiding cystourethrogram.

Urographic Media. There are now available several nontoxic intravenously injectible urographic media made radiopaque by firmly bound iodine in content varying approximately from 35 to 70 per cent. These include Skiodan, Neo-iopax, Diodrast, Urokon, Hypaque, Hippuran; directions and contraindications for their use accompany the commercial package. Today the higher concentrations, 50 to 70 per cent, are being increasingly used for greater urographic clarity but also with greater risks. Unfortunately some patients are iodine sensitive and some serious, as well as a few fatal, reactions have resulted from the use of most of these media. For this reason a 1 cc. test ampule is sold with each large ampule; a drop or two is injected intradermally to form a bleb and is observed for twenty minutes. If a pronounced allergic skin reaction occurs, it is best judgment to forego the excretory urographic study and perform retrograde pyelography instead, prophylactically administering an antihistaminic substance such as Benadryl (25 to 50 mg.) or chlor-trimeton (Chlorprophenpyridamine Maleate) 5–10 mg. intramuscularly or subcutaneously a few minutes before the retrograde pyelographic injection is made.

Without urography we can hardly make a precise anatomic diagnosis of surgical disease of the upper urinary tract. The diagnostic films should be made with the greatest precision and care; radiographically poor films may not only be misleading but should be discarded and re-examination carried out. Certainly one should not be guilty of jeopardizing a patient's life through culpable diagnostic reliance on urograms which are neither satisfactory nor definitive. This consideration is much more likely to arise with excretory urography than with retrograde injection of contrast medium. Yet even in retrograde urography, unsatisfactory or indeterminate urograms occur with distressing frequency, the incidence varying largely according to the ability of the x-ray technician, the pre-examination preparation of the patient, the elimination of intestinal gas and fecal shadows, and the technique of the instrumenteur who is more likely to underinject than overinject the ureter(s) and pelvis(es). The inadequately injected urogram is commonly misleading by failing to demonstrate the true extent of hydronephrosis, or an early tumor, polycystic disease, rarely tuberculosis or ureteropelvic obstructions, for example, and which would be clearly demonstrated in urograms of a patient whose upper urinary tract is adequately injected.

The vital importance of these frequent technical errors is stressed here because many practicing physicians untrained in urographic interpretation are today, by necessity or choice, undertaking the reading of urograms showing disease which, if not properly recognized and promptly treated, generally by major urosurgery, spells the patient's doom. Thus in the early days of excretory urography—and the situation is not yet entirely rectified—many normal kidneys were removed, largely by general surgeons and general practitioners, because the intravenous pyelogram showed a "good" kidney on one side but no renal shadow on the other. Therefore it was deduced that the kidney failing to show a pelvic shadow must be seriously diseased or dead and should be removed. Both urologists and roentgenologists know by experience that this occurs frequently enough as a urographic freak and for inexplicable reasons. Yet often in the patient whose normal kidney was erroneously removed, the pyelographic shadow on the opposite side thought to be the "good" one, was actually pathologic because the shadow demonstrated there denoted unrecognized asymptomatic obstruction at the pelvic outlet or in the ureter which caused retention of the excreted medium in the kidney, while the normal kidney secreted well and emptied itself rapidly and prematurely. Because the chances for diagnostic error are great, and by virtue of considerable experience and observation, I no longer perform upper tract urosurgery on the basis of excretory urographic findings alone but employ definitive bilateral retrograde pyelo-ureterography except when the ureter is impassable by tuberculosis, tumor, stone or other obstruction. In this circumstance, one must of necessity be guided solely by the excretory urographic data and chromomeatoscopy (q.v.).

Preparation of the Patient for Urography. Every roentgenologist has his own pet routine and so instructs the patient. The main items in these routines of preparation are (a) night preceding examination: (1) laxative (castor oil or licorice powder, 1 oz.); (2) no food or fluid after six in the evening; (b) morning of examination: (1) cleansing enema; (2) no breakfast; (3) no fluids.

In my practice no preparation is employed, since I have found that freedom from gas is largely a matter of chance, that no meal should be omitted because the longer the interval from the last meal, the more gas there will be in the bowel. In short, I prefer to "take the patient right off the street." Children especially should be spared purging, "enemas, until the return is clear," and starvation; certainly there is nothing better designed than starvation to encourage intestinal gas formation and distention. The rectum should be cleared of feces with a low enema if lower spinal defects are properly to be demonstrated but a preliminary or scout film will show whether fecal or gas shadows are likely to prevent a satisfactory examination, and if they are present, a mild laxative is given and the examination is postponed until the next day or such time as the scout film shows a satisfactory urographic study can be made.

Do not use parasympathomimetic drugs (pitressin, acetylcholine, pituitrin, etc.) to stimulate the bowel to rid itself of gas as these drugs also induce contraction and variable spasm of the renal pelvis and ureter (see Physiology).

Requisites of a Good Film. A satisfactory initial plain or scout film (urogram) should show in detail the spine and transverse processes to the tip of the coccyx, the eleventh and twelfth ribs, the bony pelvis including the prostatic area, the soft structures, the renal and lower hepatic borders, and psoas muscle outlines (Fig. 8). In infants the renal and psoas muscle outlines may not be clearly shown but the liver shadow will be. A hazy indistinct renal shadow on an otherwise clear film may mean hydronephrosis, pyonephrosis, tumor, or renal hypoplasia. Unilateral obliteration of the psoas muscle shadow always suggests perinephric abscess but it may also occur in perinephritis without abscess, other retroperitoneal inflammation especially retrocecal appendicitis, or the psoas shadow may be beclouded by intestinal gas.

Indications for Excretory Urography. These are:

1. When visualization of the upper urinary tract in its normal physiologic status is desired (Fig. 9).

2. As a preliminary examination prior to complete urologic investigation, the usual indications for which are summarized in Chapter 2.

3. In genital anomalies, to avoid cystoscopy, the upper urinary tract being anomalous in about one in three of these cases.

Contraindications to Excretory Urography. These are recognized by some as:

1. Marked renal insufficiency (uremia, or impending uremia). While I have never seen ill effects from excretory urography in the azotemic patient, when the renal function is low the procedure is a waste of time

and material because the output of the contrast medium is negligible or zero and no urographic shadows are cast. It is a good working rule that the method will be fruitless when the blood urea is over 25 mg. per cent, or the nonprotein nitrogen level is 50 mg. per cent or higher.

Hypersensitivity to the urographic medium to be used is also a contraindication to the method. Some patients who are only mildly sensitive may thus be examined when antihistaminic drugs such as Chlor-Trimeton or Benadryl are given first.

Limitations of Excretory Urography. These are:

1. Inability to administer the urographic medium, but this is rare. As a last resort an intramuscular, preferably pectoral, injection may be given but in several thousand urographic studies, I have employed the subcutaneous or intramuscular method but five times and in one of these a sterile abscess developed.

2. Faulty roentgen technique. This accounts for more unsatisfactory results than does abnormal renal function or other uropathy.

3. Confusion of gas and fecal shadows.

4. Polyuria, oliguria, or reflex suppression of urine.

5. Poor renal function: Here the "best" film may be made from four

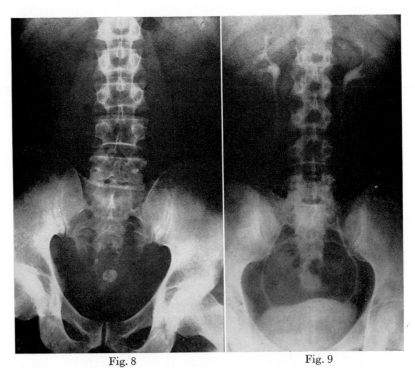

Fig. 8   Fig. 9

FIGURE 8.   Plain or scout urogram. The vertebral column is clearly shown from the eleventh ribs to the tip of the coccyx as are the lumbar transverse processes and the outlines of the kidneys and psoas muscles. The shadow of a small bladder stone is seen. In young children, especially under four years of age, these features are seldom so well shown.

FIGURE 9.   Normal excretory urogram. Renal pelvic, ureteral and vesical outlines are satisfactorily delineated.

to twenty-four hours and even up to three days after the injection, and notably in obstructive uropathy with hydronephrotic retention.

6. Partial or indefinite ureteral shadows.

7. Poor pelvic shadows, often seen in tuberculosis, tumor, or pronounced infection of the kidney.

8. Extremely important, the *inability properly to interpret urograms*. Maneuvers to obtain satisfactory urograms are chiefly:

1. Dehydration for twelve to eighteen hours; this increases the concentration of the excreted medium in the urinary tract, and is our greatest aid in achieving satisfactory urographic clarity. We do not employ the Trendelenburg position, nor the lower abdominal compression bag.

2. In infants gastric distention achieved by giving the child (a) his formula with which he swallows considerable air, or (b) a carbonated beverage, the gas from which balloons the stomach to make a wide clear field over the renal pelves and upper ureters. The shadow of the lower ureter is usually obliterated by the intestines and their contents pushed downwards by the distended stomach. Note: Food or drink is not given until just before injection of the medium is completed (Fig. 10).

3. Proper spacing of x-ray exposures. In infants the exposures should

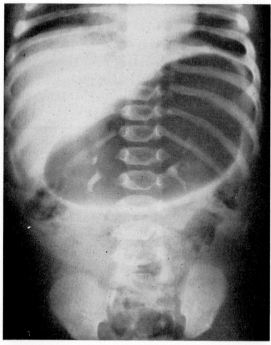

FIGURE 10. Visualization aid in excretory urography in infants (Matthei, 1950). Several ounces of formula or carbonated beverage are given immediately following the intravenous injection of urographic medium; with the liquid, considerable air is swallowed to balloon the stomach. This affords a clear gastric field to enable satisfactory visualization of the renal pelves and adjacent ureters. The shadows of the gas-filled bowels displaced downward usually obscure the ureteral urographic shadows.

be made at much shorter intervals than is the general practice; I take them three, six, nine, twelve, and fifteen minutes after injection with concurrent development of the films as the examination proceeds. In poor renal function or when obstruction, for example, is evident delayed urograms may be indicated. In adults and especially when the 50 and 70 per cent concentrations of medium are given, exposure at five, ten, fifteen, and twenty minutes are usually satisfactory but here, too, inspection of the films as they are being developed concurrent with the series may call for late or delayed exposures, even up to the next day.

Reactions to Excretory Urography. These are remarkably few. In my experience about one in three patients feels warm in the face as the intravenous injection is being made; one in five feels variably nauseated; one in ten vomits, and one in fifty shows cutaneous welts, and one in a hundred more severe allergic reactions with swelling of the lips and tongue, but these are readily controlled with epinephrine (5 to 10 minims of 1:1000 solution intramuscularly), or Benadryl (50 mg. by mouth). For immediate effect, use epinephrine. Mild reactions such as warmth of the face or nausea will usually stop promptly if the patient will take a few deep breaths. Vomiting calls for temporary cessation of the injection (without removing the needle from the vein) which can usually be resumed uneventfully in a few minutes.

Results in Excretory Urography. The method yields satisfactory diagnostic information in a third of all infants and in half of older children and adults. In an additional 10 per cent of all patients the findings are "suggestive" although neither conclusive nor diagnostically reliable. Despite the failures, the method is highly valuable especially when its revelations, or even its very failure, point up the necessity for complete cystoscopic and retrograde pyelographic study.

AORTOGRAPHY

Lumbar aortography is the injection directly into the aorta of excretory urographic medium (70 per cent strength) to outline the renal arterial supply especially (1) when hypoplasia (Goldblatt kidney) exists, (2) when the question of renal resectability* enters the picture and (3) to distinguish between cysts and solid tumors. In solid tumors, especially neoplasm, there is "puddling" or pooling of the opaque medium in the neoplastic mass giving it an irregular fuzzy granular shadow (Fig. 245); in renal cystic disease, the field of the avascular fluid mass is clear and is surrounded by the arterialized parenchyma.

* Here the decision may rest between (1) conservative resection when the blood supply of the remaining renal segment is good (and if so, what vessels to preserve), or (2) performing nephrectomy because the arterial supply is demonstrably inadequate. Enthusiasts to the contrary, aortography (renal angiography) is still a dangerous procedure; the reported toll of those killed or injured by this method is nearly 100 to date and is constantly increasing in the world's radiologic literature. I know of three deaths this past year in one Miami hospital alone.

CYSTOGRAPHY

This is the radiographic delineation of the bladder when it is filled with a radiopaque medium or with air. Today excretory cystography as part of excretory pyelography has largely replaced the cystogram made by injection of opaque medium through a catheter. Cystography may be used in patients of all ages; my youngest was three days old.

Media. Although many still use 5 or 10 per cent sterile sodium iodide solution as the radiopaque medium, it is frightfully irritating to the bladder urothelium and he who does not believe this should put a few drops of the solution in his eyes! The preferred contrast medium is 5 to 15 per cent solution of any of the media employed in excretory urography. The bladder is filled enough so the patient just feels the fullness and urographic exposures are made in the anterior-posterior, oblique, and lateral positions, the last so as not to overlook a diverticulum of the bladder floor or trigone. Stereoscopic exposures are best. After this the bladder is usually emptied by voiding, during which an x-ray exposure is made (*voiding cystogram*). This will show the action and any morphologic abnormality of the empty-ing mechanism as well as a contracted or dilated bladder outlet, urethral valves, hypertrophic verumontanum, diverticulum, stricture or other gross pathologic alteration of the urethra. When the voiding is completed, an immediate final urogram will indicate the approximate vesical residuum, retention in a diverticulum, or in a dilated upper urinary tract.

When air is injected into the bladder instead of radiopaque medium, the resulting urogram is a *pneumocystogram* and is of particular value in demonstrating vesical diverticulum, tumor, and relatively non-opaque stone or foreign body (Fig. 236). About fifty cases of fatal air embolism due to pneumocystography have been reported.

A normal cystogram is shown in Figure 11.

Abnormal cystograms are recognized by:

1. Irregularity, indentation, or bulging of the bladder wall.

2. Vesico-ureteral reflux.

3. Changes about the vesical neck as in prostatic obstruction, con-tracture or paralysis.

4. Filling defects of the vesical outline as in trauma (often with extravasation!), tumor, extracystic growths, or masses (Fig. 267).

Items 1 to 3 are generally the result of infection, obstruction (Fig. 42), diverticulum (Fig. 98), ureterocele (Fig. 86), or neuromuscular disease (Figs. 203–206). Cystitis when hyperacute or of long duration commonly produces a fuzzy or moth-eaten cystographic outline with which, because of inflammatory injury of the ureterovesical junction valve mechanism, vesico-ureteral reflux also may be present (Figs. 12, 42).

Reflux may also be caused by myogenic obstruction as with vesical neck contracture, posterior urethral valves, urethral stricture, or neuro-genic as in spastic neuromuscular vesical disease with spasm of the vesical outlet or of the external urethral sphincter. This obstruction may cause sufficient intracystic back pressure to pull open, injure, or destroy the ureterovesical valve mechanism and thus, by reflux when lower

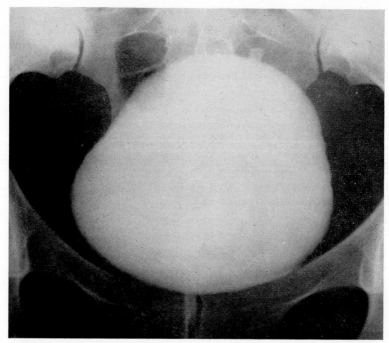

FIGURE 11.   Normal cystogram. The vesical outline is smooth; the vesical outlet is crescentic without leakage into the adjacent deep urethra and there is no vesico-ureteral reflux.

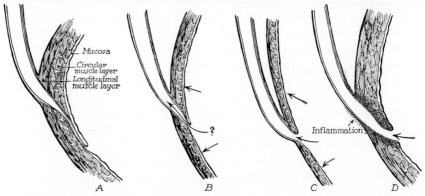

FIGURE 12.   Mechanics of the ureterovesical valve and vesico-ureteral reflux. *A*, normal relationships. The obliquity of the course of the ureter through the bladder wall and the mucosal valve leaflet elongated from above downward is shown. *B*, the effect of moderate vesical distention on the function of the ureterovesical valve. The obliquity of the intramural ureter is diminished and the valve leaflet is foreshortened. These changes may or may not result in reflux. *C*, with marked vesical distention the bladder wall becomes greatly thinned, the obliquity of the intramural ureter is reduced and the mucosal valve flap is pulled away permitting reflux to occur (after Gruber). *D*, ureteral reflux induced by inflammatory infiltration of mucosal valve leaflet and of intramural portion of duct which is thus converted into a rigid tube. This commonly occurs in prolonged urinary infection but may also be present temporarily in acute cystitis.

urinary tract infection exists, the upper tract and especially the kidneys become seriously infected (Fig. 42).

Vesico-ureteral reflux may cause renal pain on voiding and can be demonstrated only by urography. In a cystographic study of 722 consecutive child patients, an eighth (12 per cent) showed vesico-ureteral reflux, bilaterally in half of these and in two thirds of those with bilateral reflux the entire upper urinary tract was outlined, sometimes revealing supravesical anomalies, ureteral reduplication being the most common. *Reflux was not observed in any unanesthetized child with a normal bladder.* By vesical overdistention under anesthesia, reflux sometimes occurs as the protecting overhanging mucosal meatal valve-leaflet is drawn upwards as the bladder is overdistended to leave the ureteral orifice unprotected and the intramural ureter shortened and dilated (Fig. 12).

Delayed cystography has demonstrated that normally with physiologic bladder filling the periodic opening of the ureterovesical valve permits the influx or regurgitation of some of the vesical contents into the ureter. The occurrence of this normal natural phenomenon has led some observers to attach great importance to the demonstration of a variably filled upper urinary tract thirty minutes after filling the bladder by catheter with a radiopaque medium. These observers have failed to distinguish a normal regurgitation from pathologic reflux, the latter occurring promptly with cystographic filling of an unanesthetized patient and occurring only when demonstrable disease is present.

URETHROGRAPHY

Urethrography outlines the urethral canal by x-ray following injection of contrast medium. The method is of particular diagnostic value when obstruction (especially stricture, stone, tumor) diverticulum, rupture, or neuromuscular paralytic relaxation of the bladder neck or external

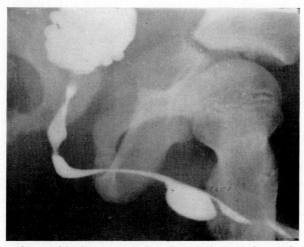

FIGURE 13.   Urethrographic demonstration of diverticulum of the urethra proximal to stenosis of external urethral meatus.

sphincter exists and is of special interest in the young with congenital stenosis of the external meatus (Fig. 13). The best exposure is taken with the patient on the side with legs in exaggerated bicycle-riding position, the under leg drawn up on the abdomen, and the upper leg extended far back and the x-ray tube focused on the perineum.

PERIRENAL PNEUMOGRAPHY

The injection of air into, and its dispersion within, the retroperitoneal space will usually outline the kidney and adrenal, unilaterally if the injection is so made, and bilaterally if a presacral injection is performed.

In *unilateral direct perirenal pneumography* the air injection is usually best made with the patient sitting on the edge of a table, the feet resting firmly on a chair or stool in front, and the body bent forward with the elbows resting on the knees. In an adult of average size the site of injection is three to four finger breadths lateral to the vertebral midline and two finger breadths below the border of the last rib. The skin and the tract of the injecting needle down to the perirenal area is first anesthetized by local infiltration with 1 per cent procaine solution. An 18 or 20 gauge spinal tap needle with beveled point is then carefully introduced, usually about 5 cm. and until the "click" of its passage through the perirenal fascia is felt. Withdraw the stylet and test for bleeding by syringe suction. If the needle is introduced too deeply and is in the kidney, the outer end will move up and down with respiration with the body wall as the fulcrum.

If all seems well and the needle is not in the kidney, *slowly* inject 400 to 500 cc. of filtered air, stopping if the patient shows shock or has extreme isolateral shoulder pain (diaphragmatic reflex and reference). When the air injection is completed, withdraw the needle, apply collodion, and let the patient lie down. Subsequent x-ray exposures are made at one, four, eight, twelve, and twenty-four hours. When the injection technique and radiologic examination have been successful, the films will show the kidney and adrenal clearly outlined (Fig. 296) unless perinephric or periadrenal inflammation or sclerosis prevent the desired infiltration of the injected air.

Bilateral retroperitoneal pneumography is analogously performed by the injection of about 500 cc. of air through a spinal puncture needle introduced (under local anesthesia) into the space between the posterior rectal and anterior sacral walls. For this injection the patient is on his side, in knee-chest or in lithotomy position. With a gloved finger in the rectum for orientation and as a guide, the 18 or 20 gauge blunt beveled needle is introduced in the midline just in front of the coccyx and directed backward to follow the anterior sacral wall upward for about 2 inches. Following its injection the air infiltrates upward retroperitoneally on each side to radiographically outline the kidneys and adrenals. In children proportionately smaller quantities of air are injected and because of the relative paucity of retroperitoneal fat, the gaseous infiltration and, by the same token, the success of the examination, are generally less satisfactory than in adults.

INSTRUMENTAL EXAMINATION

A general practitioner without special urologic training should possess and be able to use properly certain urethral catheters and steel sounds.

Catheters. The various types it would be well to have in the office are shown in Figure 14. For general use boilable soft rubber (latex) catheters with two eyes (Robinson type), even sizes 10 to 20 F.* being preferable to the usual Nélaton's ("drug store") single or velvet eye catheter and especially for indwelling catheter drainage. Woven silk catheters with a modified natural curve should also be on hand and in even sizes 10 to 18 F. These are ruined by boiling and autoclaving and, after first washing and cleansing well with soap and water, should be sterilized by soaking them in a solution of oxycyanide of mercury 1:500 for at least four hours.

The Campbell (8 F.) stainless steel urethral catheter for young males conforms to the outline of the deep prostatic urethra and is passed in the same way as sounds (Fig. 7). The Campbell curved miniature modified-S metal catheter is invaluable for its purpose in the catheterization of females of all ages, even though it was initially designed for use in infants and young girls (Fig. 7). The metal catheters are sterilized by boiling. *No catheter should be introduced except under clear vision* and this applies particularly to catheterization in the female.

Glass catheters are mentioned only to be condemned.

Sounds. Preferably these are made of noncorrosive (stainless) steel and should be smooth with a curved tip conforming to the natural curva-

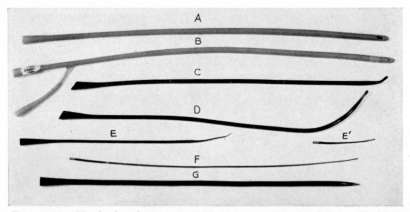

FIGURE 14.　Urethral catheters. *A*, Robinson types, two-eye latex used chiefly in males, a shorter one being made for women. *B*, balloon catheter (balloon uninflated; inflation shown in Figure 55); *C*, Coudé-tip silk catheter; *D*, modified natural curve woven silk catheter. *E*, miniature woven silk catheter with long filiform for infants and children (Hutchins); *G*, Phillips' follower catheter with screw tip filiforms: *F* (long) and *E'* (short).

* French scale 1 F. equals ⅓ mm., e.g., 30 F. equals 30 mm. circumference or approximately 10 mm. diameter.

ture of the deep male urethra (Fig. 15). They are readily sterilized by boiling. The practitioner would do well to have a set of these sounds in even sizes 10 to 30 F. Sounds are employed chiefly to dilate the urethra either preparatory to passing another instrument such as the cystoscope, or therapeutically to dilate a stricture or other dilatable obstruction.

The Campbell miniature stainless steel sounds are especially designed for young boys and are put up in sets 8 to 22 F. caliber (Sklar, Long Island City, New York).

Straight sounds are used chiefly for dilating the female urethra. While the small or tight urethra may be adequately dilated with the male type Van Buren sound, in therapeutic dilation of urethral stricture in the adult female large caliber instruments are needed and sizes 30, 32, 34 and 36 F. are recommended.

Filiform tipped woven catheters of the Phillips whip type are occasionally needed in emergency for relief of acute obstruction due to stricture or other soft tissue urethral blockage (Fig. 14); sizes 10, 14 and 18 F. are adequate for most problems of this type. They must be soaked in a sterilizing solution as woven silk catheters are and must not be boiled.

Cystoscopes, urethroscopes, ureteral catheters, other ureteral instruments, and retrograde pyelographic technique are not discussed here; it is assumed the urologically untrained practitioner will not attempt their use but will obtain the services of a qualified urologist.

URETHRAL INSTRUMENTATION

Urethral catheterization must be an aseptic procedure. The instruments to be introduced are sterilized and the hands of the instrumenteur must be rigidly cleaned (if sterile gloves are not worn), and must be *gentle!*

Catheterization in the Male. First, the prepuce must be widely retracted and, together with the glans and the separated meatus, it is thoroughly washed with green soap solution, 70 per cent alcohol, or an antiseptic solution such as oxycyanide (my preference) or bichloride of mercury 1:1000. With the patient lying comfortably and relaxed on his back on a table, bed or couch, the cleansed penis is held at right angles

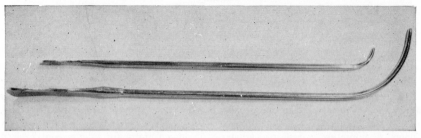

FIGURE 15. Campbell miniature sound. Designed to conform to the curvature of the deep urethra in infant and young males. These instruments, manufactured in even sizes (6 F. to 22 F., Sklar) are of stainless steel and may be employed equally well for urethral dilation in female children. Comparison of size and curve with adult size Van Buren sound.

to the body and the *well-lubricated* tip of the catheter is gently introduced into the canal. Be sure to use a good surgical lubricant such as K-Y, J & J, or Lubafax brands; sterile oil will do if nothing else is available, but never Vaseline. The catheter is gently passed—rotating it slightly back and forth helps to ease it along—until it meets the involuntary resistance of the external sphincter muscle within the layers of the urogenital trigone which is anchored above on each side to the under surface of the pubic arch. Usually the catheter will pass right on into the bladder but often enough by reflex sphincter spasm the catheter or other instrument may be held up at the triangular ligament. If, at this point, the patient's attention can be distracted by asking him to take a deep breath or to attempt urinating, the sphincterospastic contraction will usually relax and the catheter will slide into the posterior urethra and bladder.

Catheterization in the Female. In females of any age, the labia are first thoroughly washed with one of the antiseptic solutions (except alcohol) indicated in the preceding paragraph. The labia are then separated as widely as possible and the introitus, clitoric area, and especially the external urethral meatus are thoroughly cleansed with the antiseptic solution. Still keeping the labia widely apart, the meatus is identified and the catheter with a well lubricated tip is ever so gently introduced directly to the bladder. In order to avoid contamination of specimens by urethral detritus caught in the eyes of the instrument, a few centimeters of urine are allowed to flow out before collection of the specimen proper is begun. Usually the specimen is subjected to complete routine urinalysis, bacteriologic culture, and a study of stained centrifuged sediment.

Passage of Sounds and Rigid Instruments. Having thoroughly cleansed the penis as indicated under catheterization of the male, begin the passing of the sound (or cystoscope) with the instrument in the line of the groin, rotating the outer end of the sound medially to the midabdominal line when its tip has reached the bulbomembranous junction (Fig. 16). The outer end of the instrument is then made to describe an arc

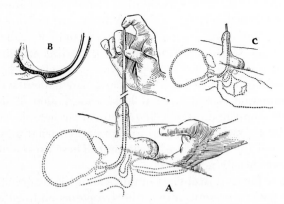

FIGURE 16. Passage of sounds. *A*, with index finger in the perineum to guide the instrument into the membranous urethra; *B*, the tip of the instrument is caught in a pouch of the urethral floor at the bulbomembranous junction; *C*, finger in rectum to help overcome difficulty in *B*.

downward so that eventually the shaft lies between and parallel with the thighs. Coincident with the downward sweep of the shaft, downward pressure is exerted by the other hand over the pubis to relax the suspensory ligament of the penis, this maneuver alone often causing the sound to fall into the deep urethra and bladder of its own weight.

In the passage of the rigid instrument, always keep its tip against the urethral roof—the surgical guide. If the downward sweep of the instrument is begun before the tip is at the triangular ligament, the beak will be forced upwards to form a pocket on the urethral roof (Fig. 16). If the urethral roof is not adhered to and the instrument has been pushed too far downwards before the external sweep of its outer end is begun, the tip may pocket in the deep bulbous urethra (Fig. 16). If there is difficulty introducing the tip of the instrument into the membranous urethra or vesical outlet, a guiding two fingers placed externally and perineally over the bulbous segment and scrotum or a guiding finger in the rectum may be used to elevate the beak into the proper location (Fig. 16).

By referring to the outline on page 39 showing an acceptable routine of procedure in the diagnostic investigation of a patient with urologic symptoms or known urologic disease it will be noted that a great part of the study can and should be done by the patient's nonurologist physician, these procedures being indicated in items 1 to 10. At this point the services of a qualified urologist should be engaged not only for the cystoscopic and technical instrumental studies but for an interpretation of these findings and assistance in rational treatment based on the diagnosis. In this sequence of investigation it is at this point that the urologist may actively enter the picture. The help he may be expected to give, the essentials of the technical urologic examination, and the fundamentals of therapy as based on the demonstrated uropathy are discussed in the next few paragraphs.

CYSTOSCOPY

Cystoscopy is the visual examination of the bladder interior and is at once a science learned only by study and an art acquired by long years of practice. An extensive discussion of cystoscopy and its collateral studies, notably retrograde pyelography, and urethral, vesical, and ureteral instrumental treatment is beyond the purpose and scope of this book. The nonurologist physician entrusted with the care of a patient who needs cystoscopic examination should have at least some notion of the procedure, its indications, contraindications, requisites of acceptable technique, the scope of the investigative study and interpretation, what may be expected to be found, and the rationale of treatment. These aspects of cystoscopic examination are briefly given here.

Indications for Cystoscopy. Complete urologic examination is called for when the patient presents any of the symptoms outlined on page 39 in Chapter 3; often two or even more indications may coexist. In addition, cystoscopy is employed (1) to treat lesions of the bladder, its outlet, or of the ureter (e.g., ureteral dilation); (2) to take biopsy specimens of suspicious lesions for histologic examination; (3) for re-examination to determine therapeutic success or, in some instances, (4) to learn why medical treatment has failed.

Contraindications to Cystoscopy. The principal ones are:

1. Acute urinary infection (except in persistent hyperacute renal infection).

2. Acute gonorrheal urethritis.

3. Pronounced renal insufficiency which may be expected to improve with proper treatment, free drainage, etc.; cystoscopy can later be performed under more favorable and safer circumstances.

4. Marked debility, extreme emaciation (rarely).

5. Hopeless urologic condition or grave extra-urogenital tract disease.

6. The absolute: Ignorance or incompetence on the part of the instrumenteur. Age is no contraindication; I have satisfactorily carried out complete urologic examination in newborn males; in one instance the findings indicated the emergency of nephrectomy for renal thrombosis which the child had and the operation at twelve days of age was successful.

The *cystoscope* used more often than any other is the Brown-Buerger model or some modification of it (Fig. 17). This electrically illuminated instrument carries a telescope with an optical system containing eighteen coated lenses corrected for visual interpretation so that the cystoscopist sees objects and structures right side up. Most cystoscopic assemblies have

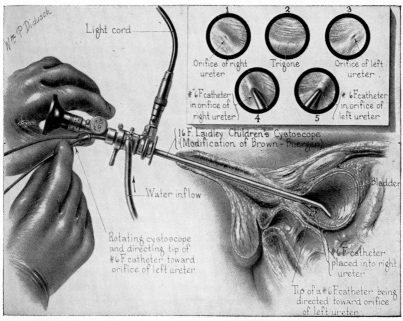

FIGURE 17. Brown-Buerger type double catheterizing cystoscope (Laidley 16 F. model, courtesy American Cystoscope Makers, Inc.). An observation telescope also fits this sheath.

a telescope solely for observation studies and a smaller catheterizing telescopic element which usually will accommodate two 5 or 6 F. ureteral catheters or a single larger one (7 or 8 F.) for ureteral dilation, or the use of cystoscopic cutting or grasping instruments (Fig. 18). Miniature cystoscopes equally useful are also available (Fig. 19).

Assured that the instrument is functioning properly and that the light burns, the cystoscope is introduced into the bladder as previously described for the passage of a sound. With the instrument in place, the bladder is

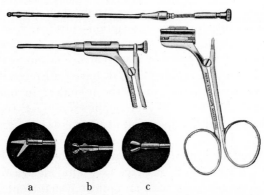

a   b   c

FIGURE 18. Cystoscopic operating instruments. These are made in a large size for adults and a miniature (7 F.) size for children. The last is used with Campbell cystoscope shown in Figure 19. *A*, scissors; *B*, rongeurs; *C*, grasping forceps. (American Cystoscope Makers, Inc.)

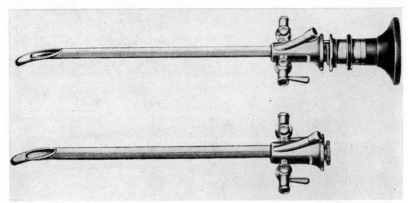

FIGURE 19. Campbell miniature (17 F.) cysto-urethroscope designed for urologic examination, ureteral dilation and transurethral surgical procedures such as removal of foreign bodies, electro-excision of tissue especially at the bladder neck and ureteral meatotomy. This instrument will accommodate a 9 F. or "small" 10 F. Garceau ureteral catheter comfortably, enables simultaneous catheterization of four or five ureters, and is used by the author more often than any single miniature instrument. *A*, assembled 17 F. instrument. *B*, 19 F. sheath. In later models an expanding obturator is provided. Employment of this instrument in infant males demands its introduction through an external urethrostomy opening and often so in young boys. Under no circumstances should the passage of this or any other instrument be permitted to cause preventable urethral trauma. (Courtesy American Cystoscope Makers, Inc.)

irrigated free of purulent, epithelial, crystalline or other debris, and the light is lit. Clean irrigating fluid is run in and the bladder interior including the outlet and deep urethra are thoroughly studied, chiefly as to the presence of inflammation: where, what type, and how severe. With pronounced inflammation around one or both ureteral orifices, infection of the isolateral kidney must be suspected. Hypertrophy of the trigone reflects obstruction, usually at the bladder neck. This, in turn, demands special study of the vesical outlet for contracture, adenomatous prostatic hyperplasia, middle lobe enlargement, hypertrophy of the verumontanum, or congenital valves of the prostatic urethra. A lax or atonic vesical outlet usually signifies paretic neuromuscular vesical disease such as is seen in tabes and is often found in the later stages of spinal fracture. Other common conditions and lesions to look for include ureterocele, ureteral stenosis, prolapsed ureter, prolapsed ureteral mucosa, vesical diverticulum, or varicose veins of the bladder floor.

Having completed the observation study catheterization of the ureters is then performed, gently passing the tip of the small catheter well into the kidney pelvis on each side (Fig. 17). Ureteral catheterization permits separated urine specimens to be taken from each kidney, and following the intravenous injection of indigo carmine, a blue dye, to observe the comparative renal function. Having collected the separated ureteral specimens to be examined for their comparative urea, pus, blood and bacterial content including culture, bilateral retrograde pyelography is performed.

RETROGRADE PYELOGRAPHY

Indications for Retrograde Pyelography. This is the radiologic determination of the anatomic conformation of the upper urinary tract as it lends itself to the interpretation of disease. It may be employed in patients of any age: I have performed it bilaterally in a five-pound premature infant with persistent acute urinary infection since birth—an urgent indication—and in many others less than a week old, and in still many more less than a month old.

Contraindications for Retrograde Pyelography. These are:

1. When the diagnosis can be made without it; occasionally excretory urography is satisfactory but usually is not a thoroughly reliable guide for surgery.

2. When the data obtained by retrograde urography will be of no value as in hopeless cases.

3. In the extremely ill, with rare exceptions.

4. Inexperience with the method or inadequate radiographic facilities.

Bilateral pyelography should be employed when (1) excretory urograms are unsatisfactory or have not been made, (2) the total renal function is good, and (3) the information potentially to be gained by it warrants the examination. I employ it almost routinely and have observed no disquieting sequelae attributable to the procedure.

Care must be observed to avoid pelvic overdistention as reflected by

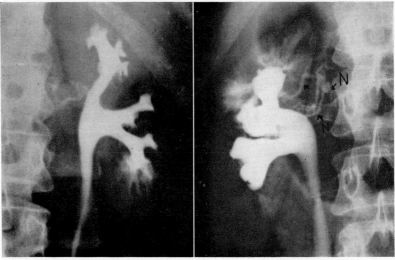

Fig. 20   Fig. 21

FIGURE 20.   Varieties of pelvic backflow. Pyelovenous backflow. Limited pyelovenous backflow in inverted crescent formation conforming to the parenchymal arcuate veins.

FIGURE 21.   Pyelolymphatic backflow. The course of the lymphatics is sharply outlined as well as the intermediate lymph nodes (N).

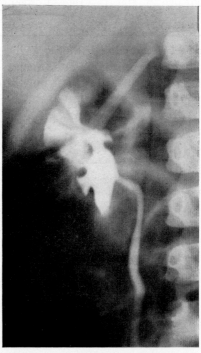

FIGURE 22.   Pyeloparenchymal backflow. Interstitial backflow which urographically appears as a brush or tuft formation extending from the papillary tip into the parenchyma. There is massive backflow extension of medium into the parenchyma, in this case the site of leakage apparently being the outer limb of the superior calyx.

abdominal or renal pain and for this reason *retrograde pyelography should not be performed on an unconscious patient.* The radiopaque medium used for excretory urography is also employed for retrograde pyelography in full strength (35 per cent) in infants and in half strength (17.5 per cent) in adults.

In performing retrograde pyelography, the average amount of medium injected on each side in an infant is 2 to 3 cc.; in a ten year old child 5 to 6 cc., and in an adult 8 to 15 cc., according to facility and absence of distention or pain. With pelvic overdistention pyelovenous (Fig. 20), pyelolymphatic (Fig. 21), or pyeloparenchymal (Fig. 22) back-flow may occur. Underfilling may also lead to diagnostic misinterpretation and especially in estimating the degree of hydronephrotic distention, ureteral or ureteropelvic obstruction, or the recognition of renal tumor, infection, and other pyelographically demonstrable lesions. Stereoscopic urograms are of greater diagnostic value than single exposures. Having performed retrograde pyelography, ureterograms are then made by continuing injection of the retrograde medium as the catheters are being withdrawn down the ureters. Satisfactory ureterograms may be expected to give considerable additional information as to the upper tract uropathy and are usually as diagnostically important as the pyelogram.

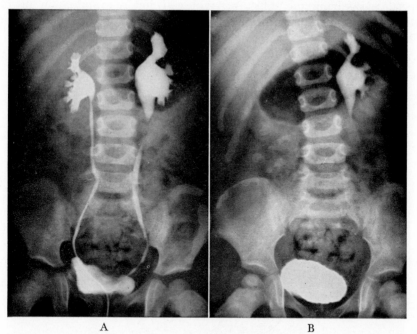

A   B

FIGURE 23.   Delayed or "trap" film in urographic exposure, which should routinely be made five to ten minutes following the pyelographic injection and withdrawal of the ureteral catheter to demonstrate pelvic and/or ureteral retention above the point of blockage. *A*, stricture of upper left ureter in a three-year-old boy. *B*, trap film taken ten minutes after *A* showing that the right upper urinary tract has completely emptied itself as has the left ureter below the stricture. Such retention is diagnostic of obstruction.

Delayed or *trap films* are then taken five minutes after withdrawal of the catheters in infants and young children, and after ten minutes in older children and adults. Failure of complete emptying of the upper tract in this time and particularly of the renal pelvis indicates variable urinary stasis and may well be the most important clue or finding in the entire examination, especially when chronic urinary infection or a persistent localized pain is under investigation (Fig. 23).

Pyelographic interpretation is fundamentally dependent upon knowledge of the usual and bizarre variations of the normal renal pelvis, and this is gained only by extensive experience in the study of urograms. Even with this background, errors are occasionally made. Normal pyelograms may show strikingly different outlines and a wide latitude of interpretation is often required because of physiologic changes in the caliber and shape of the normal urinary tract during peristaltic diastole and systole (Fig. 39). Segmental ureteral systolic contractions and diastolic dilatations often suggest changes due to obstruction so that the study of serial urograms should be made. Changes in the pelvic and minor calyceal outlines sometimes mean much in the urographic differential diagnosis and generally afford the critical clue (Fig. 24). Incomplete urographic filling, the movement of the patient, faulty roentgenography, or anomalous development may seem to offer diagnostically difficult problems but the expert, recognizing the difficulty, will call for re-examination of the patient rather than jeopardize him with a hazardous urographic interpretation.

Examples of the normal pyelogram are shown in Figures 9, 40; gross

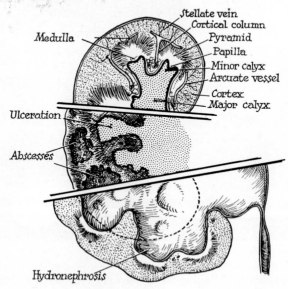

FIGURE 24.   Pyelographic diagnostic criteria in infections and hydronephrosis. Renal changes of urographic diagnostic importance. The urographic changes in renal and perirenal tumors are indicated in Figures 242 and 243.

alterations and pathologic changes urographically demonstrated are shown in other urograms distributed throughout this book.

Reactions to Urologic Examination. It is expected that following cystoscopic examination there will be transitory urethral and vesical irritation the first two or three times the patient urinates; there may be terminal hematuria. A small dose of codeine or aspirin will usually relieve this distress and a hot sitz bath* affords prompt relief. With a generous water intake before cystoscopy, gentle instrumentation, asepsis, careful pyelographic injection, rest, and a large fluid intake after examination with, when indicated, antibacterial therapy, complications are rare and seldom important. Complications or reactions occur chiefly when urinary stasis of obstruction or neuromuscular disease exists. Cystoscopic examination provokes reactions in fewer infants and children than in adults, comparatively. For this reason fear of instrumental reaction in the young should never be recognized as the sole contraindication to complete urologic examination when a cogent indication exists.

* This simple and effective means of getting localized heat to the pelvis should be known to every physician. The patient runs water into the bath tub to the depth of 6 or 8 inches at a comfortable temperature. He gets into the tub, sits upright with legs extended, the water level being approximately at the crests of the ilia. Hot water is now run into the tub to the point of tolerance by the patient—usually 108° to 110° F. by bath thermometer —and in this the patient sits for six to ten minutes. A drenching sweat or Turkish bath effect is to be avoided. To avoid catching cold, it is advised that the bath, when taken once a day, be the last thing done at night just before getting into bed. As the urinary frequency and pelvic distress ameliorate, the number and duration of the sitz baths are reduced.

CHAPTER 4 *Applied Anatomy and Physiology of the Urogenital Tract*

INTRODUCTION

THE GROSS anatomy of the urogenital organs as well as their relation to each other in continuity and to their surrounding structures are shown in Figures 25 and 31. Much can happen to the urine in its formation, transmission, and evacuation and, as in obstruction for example, to the involved organs themselves. In short, the clinical effects of alteration in secretion, transportation and/or expulsion of urine account for at least nine tenths of urologic problems. Though far from a complete enumeration, common examples of renal secretory problems are the *polyuria* of diabetes insipidus, diabetes mellitus, or sclerotic nephritis; the *oliguria* of dehydration, shock, acute glomerular nephritis of measles or scarlet fever, or the *anuria* in mismatched blood transfusions, grave renal parenchymal injury by bichloride of mercury poisoning, renal thrombosis, or total upper urinary tract obstruction as it occurs in calculous disease. Transmission difficulties are exemplified by stricture, calculus, neoplastic obstruction, or neuromuscular dysfunction; the proximal tract above the point of transmission interference shows characteristic back-pressure damage (see Chapter 5). The same obstructive factors when present in the lower urinary tract are concerned in faulty urinary evacuation whether the lesion be an enlarged prostate, a tight meatal or preputial orifice or a tabetic bladder.

THE KIDNEY

The kidneys normally are retroperitoneally situated, one on each side of the lumbodorsal spine, with the hilum at approximately the level of the transverse process of the first lumbar vertebra (Fig. 25). The upper renal poles are slightly closer than the lower, the left upper pole being at the level of the eleventh rib posteriorly and on the right, one half to one vertebra width lower. This lower position of the right kidney is relatively more pronounced in children in whom it is thought by many to be a contributing factor in the high incidence of renal infection on the right side, through the mechanism of predisposing urinary stasis produced by ureteral angulation.

On the average, the length of the kidney is twice the width and three times the thickness of the organ, varying at different ages from 4 to 5 cm. long at birth to 10 to 12 cm. long in the adult. The average kidney weight at birth is 23 gm. each, and 125 gm. in adults, with a combined renal weight to body weight ratio of 1:140 in infants to 1:170 in adults. The ratio of cortex to medulla is 1:5 in infants and 1:2 in adults. At birth the kidney is numerically a finished product, its postnatal growth being due to elongation and widening of the tubules, especially the convoluted, and the doubling in size of the glomeruli. The cortical surface of the kidney is lobulated (fetal lobulation indicating pyramidal boundaries) until about the fifth year and in about 5 per cent of all people this persists into adulthood but is of no clinical concern.

Normally its blood supply enters the kidney and the pelvis joins the

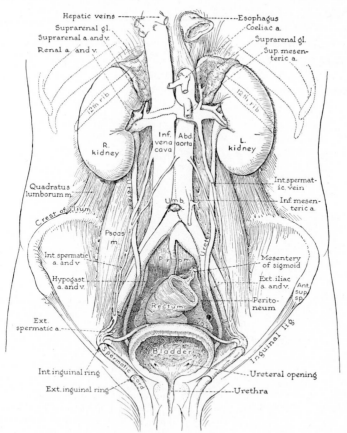

FIGURE 25. The upper urinary tract and its topographical relations. (Jones-Shepard).

ureter at the notched hilum. Dense roentgen shadows just laterally to the area between the second and third transverse lumbar processes suggest renal pelvic calculi.

The firm fibrous renal capsule which encloses the parenchyma extends into the hilum and sinus, and its stretching by edematous swelling in renal trauma, acute inflammation or infection causes pain. The three main components of the kidney are shown in Figure 26: the cortex, medulla, and pelvis.

The reddish brown *cortex* engulfs the bases of the bluish tinged medullary pyramids between which it extends to the pelvis to form the columns of Bertin (Fig. 26). The medulla is comprised of thirty to forty inversely conical grouped pyramids whose bases are in contact with the cortex, and whose papillae (apices) enter the pelvis to help form the minor calyces. In the upper and lower segments of the kidney, four to seven pyramids unite to form a papilla, while in the renal midsection only two to three pyramids thus join, a total of eight to ten papillae (minor calyces) projecting into the pelvis, this being an average number but subject to great numerical alteration.

The *nephron is the renal unit* and, as shown in Figure 27, begins in the glomerular Bowman's capsule found only in the cortex and cortico-medullary zone and most numerous towards the cortical periphery. It is estimated that normally each kidney has about two million glomeruli, although count estimates as high as 4,500,000 have been made (Traut). Figure 27 indicates the changing caliber and course of a typical tubule as it conducts urine through the tortuous first convoluted tubule, the

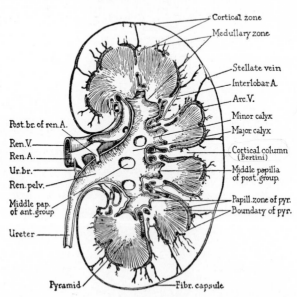

FIGURE 26. The kidney. Cross section. Schema of gross renal architecture (after Broedel). The character of minor calyx (cupping) formation by intrapelvic projection of the papillae of the pyramids is noteworthy. Because of the nature of renal function, the vascular supply is disproportionately large.

straight descending loop of Henle, reversing direction to the cortex as the ascending loop of Henle, again becoming tortuous (second convoluted tubule) and thence to unite with other collecting tubules to drain into the renal papilla in the minor calyces.

It is believed by many that tuberculous renal infection characteristically begins near the papillae because tubercle bacilli which have passed the glomerular barrier are held up at the constricted apex of the loop.

In the *interstitial* (connective) *tissue*, which separates the tubules from one another and comprises the renal reticulum, passes the arterial, venous, lymphatic and nerve supply of the kidney—a fact of vast importance in the distribution, localization, and pathogenesis of renal infection (see Chapter 7 and Fig. 143). The usual lesion in "pyelitis" is an interstitial suppurative nephritis.

Since the lymphatics and blood supply of the pelvic walls freely communicate with those of the parenchyma, and the orifices of the tubules of the medullary papillae open in the minor calyces, "pyelitis" is most unlikely to exist without associated infection of the parenchyma and vice versa, a consideration of utmost practical interest in the problem of renal infection in patients of all ages (cf. Chapter 7).

Although the pelvis is usually situated half in and half out of the kidney, it may be entirely intrarenal or extrarenal. In hydronephrosis the extrarenal pelvis becomes much larger but the intrarenal hydronephrosis

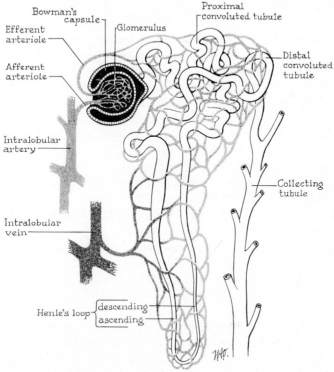

FIGURE 27. The nephron or renal unit. Course of the renal tubules. Lymphatics (not shown here; see Fig. 143) accompany the arteriovenous circulation in the interstitial tissues between the tubules.

more rapidly compresses the parenchyma and, unrelieved, irreversibly damages the organ. Most often the normal renal pelvis has three major calyces but occasionally only two, composed of the union of groups of two to four minor calyces. Urographically demonstrated changes in the minor calyces are of prime diagnostic importance especially in infection, hydronephrosis, cystic and neoplastic renal disease (see Urography, Chapter 3).

Blood Supply. Every minute blood equal to twice the weight of the kidney passes through its arteries and veins, disproportionately large because of the vital function of the organ. Before entering the kidney, nutrient vessels from the renal artery are given off to the adrenal and perirenal fat; bacterial embolism through these vessels explains many cases of adrenal or perinephric abscess (Fig. 153). The renal arteries— one or two in number but anomalous vessels up to ten have been encountered—subdivide within the kidney into interlobar, arcuate, and interlobular arteries and eventually terminate by afferent arterioles in the glomerular tuft. Ninety-nine per cent of the blood reaching the arcuate arteries ultimately passes through the glomeruli (Huber). From the glomeruli the "cleared" blood passes by efferent arterial capillaries between the renal tubules as nutrients, the arteriolae rectae, and eventually to the venous collection (Fig. 27). Thus bacteria which may fail to lodge in the afferent or in the glomerular capillary system may be held up on the efferent side to incite metastatic infection (interstitial suppurative nephritis Fig. 144).

Because the renal arterial supply is a terminal circulation (end arteries), the anatomy is conducive to embolism, infarction, or thrombosis, the extent of involvement depending upon the size of the involved main vessel and likely to be comparatively small, if cortical, and massive, if deep medullary (Fig. 153). The renal veins may be multiple and anomalous especially on the left side (90%; Anson). The clinical aspects of aberrant vascular obstruction are discussed in Chapter 6.

Renal lymphatics course through the kidney in the interstitial spaces and surround the blood vessels and tubules. The subcapsular lymphatics and those of the perirenal fat comprise a superficial system while those of the parenchyma are the *deep* system and anastomose both with the superficial lymphatics and the four to six large trunks at the hilum which pass to the lateral aortic glands. The superficial and perinephric lymphatics empty into the superior aortic nodes.

Nerves. These are both sympathetic and parasympathetic. The renal *sympathetic nerves* of greatest clinical importance arise from the tenth dorsal to second lumbar levels although there are connections as high up as the sixth dorsal. These fibers contain vasoconstricting and vasodilating elements.

The *parasympathetic* supply arises from the vagus nerve through the celiac ganglion which explains many reflex (medulla) manifestations in acute renal disease: nausea, vomiting, salivation, as in renal colic. Entering the kidney the fibers are widely distributed, largely following the vascular distribution proper. Capsular distention causes pain. Arterial denervation by stripping the nerves from the renal arteries does not interfere with renal secretion, nor is calycopelvic peristalsis disturbed.

Relation of the Kidney to Surrounding Structures. The kidney is surrounded by a loosely fitting fatty capsule which, until the eighth year, is extremely scant and in infants and emaciated children may be scarcely discernible. In the obese adult the perirenal fat may be extremely voluminous. The *anterior* or *subperitoneal* layer of this fatty perirenal capsule is thin so that anterior renal cortical lesions, especially traumatic or suppurative, are commonly manifested by pronounced peritoneal irritation and, simulating an "acute abdomen," have caused many needless laparotomies to be performed (Fig. 28). The value of these operations because of this misdiagnosis lies in the possibility that the underlying and obviously unsuspected renal suppuration will be discovered. Mesially, the perirenal fat surrounds the aorta and vena cava and extends into the hilum to surround the pelvis and calyces (Fig. 29).

Laterally and posteriorly, the perirenal fat is relatively abundant. This fatty capsule is enclosed and guided by the perirenal *fascia of Gerota* which is open below; it extends downwards to be continuous with the sub-

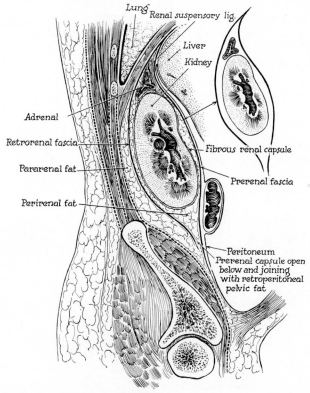

FIGURE 28. Perirenal fascia; longitudinal section showing localization and routes of spread of perirenal suppuration. Fused above at the diaphragm, the anterior and posterior sheaths pass downward enclosing the kidney and its perirenal fat. The last, due to lack of fascial fusion below, is continuous with the fat of the pelvis. Because of this, pelvic infections may subsequently become clinically manifest as perinephric abscess or vice versa.

peritoneal fat of the iliac area to which perirenal infection may extend to simulate psoas or appendiceal abscess. The anterior layer of Gerota's fascia is continuous in front of the spine with that of the other side, and fuses laterally and above with the posterior layer to enclose perirenal fat, kidney, its vessels, nerves and ureter (Figs. 28, 29).

The *pararenal* fat, usually scant, surrounds the posterior layer of Gerota's fascia. These fatty capsules are well supplied with lymphatic and blood vessels, which may be primarily involved by bacterial metastasis.

The kidney is *held in position* (1) by its vascular pedicle, (2) by the perirenal fascia which, in turn, is anchored above to the diaphragmatic aponeurosis, (3) by peritoneal attachments, (4) by the pressure of the intra-abdominal contents and, to some extent, (5) by the shape of the organ as it fits into the lumbar gutter which is narrower below. In nephroptosis, loss of perirenal fat is doubtless the usual explanation, the condition being most common in skinny, nervous, adult women.

The *surgical relations* of the kidney posteriorly are the lower portion of the diaphragm, quadratus lumborum, transversalis, and psoas muscles upon which it lies, and the twelfth thoracic, iliohypogastric and ilio-inguinal nerves which pass between the organ and the quadratus muscle and, slightly lower, the genitocrural and femoral nerves. These intimate relationships account for pain reference to the lower abdomen, genitalia, hip, thigh, or even the knee, especially in severe renal or acute perirenal infection. Similarly there is often protective reflex spasm of the quadratus and erector spinae muscles causing a rigid posterior loin and stiff back with, usually, scoliosis toward the side of the acute lesion (Fig. 158). Yet *tenderness in the costovertebral angle*—the area at the junction of the last rib and outer border of the erector spinae muscles—is the most commonly encountered finding, reflecting underlying renal or perirenal disease of which it may be considered a pathognomonic sign.

Above, the *adrenal* caps the kidney and each of these organs may be

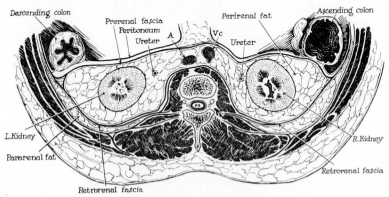

FIGURE 29.   Perirenal fascia; transverse section. It is noteworthy that the anterior fascial sheath passes from side to side in front of the ureters, great vessels, and vertebral column, and fuses laterally with the posterior fascial sheath. The last in turn is attached medially to the vertebral column. Separation of the perirenal and the pararenal fat by the posterior fascial sheath is indicated.

reciprocally involved by inflammatory or neoplastic lesions of the other. On the right, the liver, descending or second portion of the duodenum, and the hepatic colonic flexure overlie the kidney, while on the left a portion of the stomach, the jejunal and the splenic colon flexures overlie the kidney. Generally, in tumor or other renal enlargement, the colon is in front of the kidney, passing towards the inner side of a right renal mass, and the outer side of a growth on the left.

THE URETER

The ureter transports urine from the kidney to the bladder, is subject to several anomalous, obstructive, and inflammatory conditions which of themselves are of vital importance, particularly as the kidney above is secondarily involved.

The ureter begins in the infundibulum of the pelvis (the ureteropelvic junction) and in passing downward to its oblique termination in the ureteral orifice at the upper outer angle of the vesical trigone, shows three distinct areas of normal physiologic narrowing (Fig. 30). The first narrowing is at the uretero-pelvic junction, the second is at the point of crossing the iliac vessels, and the third is at the ureterovesical junction. The upper or abdominal portion of the ureter is clinically divided into (1)

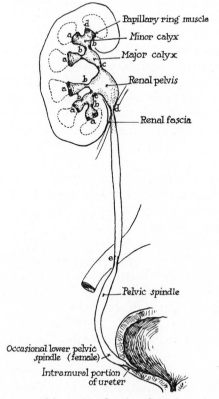

FIGURE 30.   The ureter and its course showing the points of normal narrowing.

a lumbar segment (ureteropelvic junction to iliac crest), (2) an iliac division (iliac crest to the iliosacral crossing), and (3) pelvic part (remainder to the bladder). The relative dilatations of the duct between (d) and (e) (Fig. 30) and (e) and the bladder are known respectively as the *lumbar* and *pelvic spindles*. Recognition of these normal narrowings and spindles is imperative for correct interpretation of ureterograms. In humans of all ages, the length of the ureter is about half that of the trunk. The normal diameter of the ureter lumen in the newborn is 1.0 to 1.3 mm. and in an adult 3.0 to 4.0 mm.

The ureter has three coats: (1) an inner mucosal layer covered with transitional epithelium, (2) a middle muscular (an inner and outer longitudinal layer with a much thicker circular layer between), and (3) an outer fibrous layer. The last is surrounded by an areolar layer containing blood vessels and lymphatics. Layers (1) and (2) are separated by a submucosal areola containing blood vessels, nerves and lymphatics.

Shortly before entering the bladder wall, the muscular coat of the ureter becomes chiefly a thick tube of longitudinal muscle known as Waldeyer's sheath, continuous with the trigone and distinctly separate from the bladder wall musculature proper. Normally the ureter enters the bladder obliquely for a distance of 5.0 mm. in an infant and 20.0 to 25.0 mm. in an adult, thus forming an oblique valve arrangement with a thin overhanging ureteral meatal lip to prevent backflow of urine from the bladder to the ureter (see Physiology of the Ureter). *There is no sphincter at the ureterovesical junction!* The oblique entrance of the ureters explains the ureterovesical valve mechanism: the anterior ureteral wall is longer than the posterior and there is slight redundancy of the vesical mucosa on the sides and roof of the orifice (Fig. 12, Gruber). By compression the intracystic pressure normally squeezes the intramural ureter together and closes the valve mechanism which periodically is opened by the peristaltic ejaculation of urine from the ureter.

Inflammatory changes frequently convert the intramural ureter to a stiffened (indurated) tube and thus destroy the valve action as may vesical dilatation or overdistention as occurs in peripheral obstruction. Unless the obstruction is relieved, vesico-ureteral reflux tends to become permanent, as is so often seen in some forms of neuromuscular vesical disease (Fig. 12 and Chapter 9).

Vesico-ureteral regurgitation is to be distinguished from *reflux* and is favored by any condition which causes marked vesical irritation and may occur in a normal bladder whose emptying is interfered with, and reflex detrusor contraction results.

The arterial blood supply of the abdominal ureter is from the renal and spermatic (or ovarian) vessels; the pelvic ureter is supplied by the superior vesical and inferior hemorrhoidals. The venous return parallels the arteries.

The *lymphatics* are: (1) longitudinal in the submucosa and the periureteral areola, and extend from the bladder, prostate, seminal vesicles, uterus, and tubes to the kidney and its fatty capsules; (2) *segmental drainage* occurs in three divisions to the retroperitoneal, lumbar, and pelvic glands. These lymphatics are of special importance in the ascending dissemination of infection, whether directly or by the lymphohematogenous route (see Chapter 7).

Applied Anatomy. Progressing downwards from the kidney, the abdominal ureter lies on the psoas muscle and is covered over by and attached to the posterior peritoneum. On the right the appendix and cecum overlie the ureter; diseases of each of these structures may simulate diseases of the others. Ureteral inflammation from underlying acute appendicitis often causes blood and pus in the urine. Scarcely less often do we find appendectomy being performed for "chronic appendicitis" (whatever that is!) when the true lesion is ureteral, chiefly stricture. Moral: No operation should be performed for "chronic appendicitis" without having at least a satisfactory excretory urographic study performed first, making sure that the urinary tract is normal. Occasionally, acute ureteral obstruction by ureteral or renal pelvic stone causes needless appendectomy for "acute appendicitis."

The pelvic ureter on each side as it approaches the bladder in the male is crossed by the vas deferens and enters the bladder beneath the seminal vesicle. Rarely is the ureter compressed by the vas deferens but inflammatory lesions in this area are not infrequent and may lead to ureter stricture formation. In the female the ureter, after passing through the base of the broad ligament and just before it enters the base of the bladder, is crossed by the uterine artery. By anomalous development vascular obstruction of the ureter at the point of crossing may occur, as I have seen in four children, and a few cases in adults have been reported by others.

THE BLADDER

The bladder is a muscular bag comprised of three sets of muscles: detrusor, trigone and "internal sphincter" (Fig. 25). It is lined by transitional epithelium and is surrounded by loose areolar tissue. Blood and lymph vessels and nerves course in the loose submucosal areola. Excepting the trigone, the bladder musculature—the detrusor urinae, designed to empty the bladder—is essentially a solid wall of interlacing concentrically contracting muscle fibers. An inner and outer longitudinal, and a circular middle coat are usually described by anatomists.

The *trigone*, although incorporated in the bladder base, is anatomically separated from the bladder wall proper having been derived from wolffian ducts and Waldeyer's sheath, the last spreading out over the trigone and continuing on each side to the bladder outlet as Bell's muscle which, together with the internal longitudinal muscle layer of the posterior urethra, fuse to pass forward beyond the verumontanum. Contraction of this muscle bundle group depresses the inferior segment of the vesical outlet to initiate urination (see Physiology of Urination). Yet the physiologic anatomy of the bladder outlet is still in doubt. The orifice is not surrounded by a true circular sphincter. Most present day studies indicate the "internal sphincter" represents a thickening and concentration of the longitudinal muscle bundles of the bladder detrusor which continue to the posterior urethra and in both sexes. As Emmett has observed, when the anatomy and mechanics of the "internal sphincter" have been satisfactorily settled, the full details of the mechanism of voluntary urination and urinary control will become known.

It is notable that the bladder in infancy and early childhood is an abdominal organ; definitive descent begins about the fourth year so that by puberty the viscus is pelvic, and by the twentieth year is in its adult position on the pelvic floor. The bladder is held in position at four fixed points: (1) the urachal attachment, (2) the vesical outlet, and (3, 4) the ureteral junctions. Yet the chief support is the pelvic floor. Anteriorly, the pubovesical space of Retzius and the lateral perivesical spaces are filled with fibrofatty, highly vascular, areolar tissue.

The normal bladder capacity at birth is 20 to 50 cc., by the end of the first year is four times greater, and in adulthood varies from 300 to 600 cc.

Blood Supply of the Bladder.   This is bilateral from branches of the anterior division of the internal iliac arteries and, in the female, from the vaginal and uterine branches. The veins, rather than accompanying the arteries, form a freely anastomosing perivesical plexus draining downward to the prostato-vesical plexus, and from there to the hypogastric or internal iliac veins. Any venous compressing factor such as constipation with sigmoidal and rectal distention by feces or, so commonly, pregnancy is likely to cause intense vesical congestion and thereby predispose to infection.

Lymphatics.   These are in rich plexuses in the submucosa, muscularis and subperitoneal tissues but have not been demonstrated in the bladder mucosa. Continuity of the vesical and ureteral lymphatics has been shown, a matter of clinical importance in the ascending spread of urinary infection. The vesical lymphatics drain to the external iliac nodes and glands at the aortic bifurcation while those of the bladder base, prostate, seminal vesicles, and rectum drain, in addition, to the hypogastric nodes.

THE GENITALIA AND SPERMATIC TRACT

The Male Urethra.   The external sphincter muscle within the urogenital triangle divides the male urethra into an anterior or penile segment (*pendulous* portion from meatus to penoscrotal junction and *bulbous* from this junction to the external layer of the triangular ligament), and a posterior or deep segment—*membranous* between the layers of the triangular ligament and *prostatic* as the urethra traverses this gland to the bladder outlet (Fig. 31). The part externally adjacent to the triangular ligament is sometimes called the *bulbomembranous* urethra, all of these terms being convenient for descriptive anatomic localization of lesions. The anatomic divisions of the urethra, their average normal caliber, the normal points of urethral narrowing, and the S-shape urethral curvature are shown in Figure 32. The male urethra in the newborn averages about 6 cm. in length, at ten years of age 10 or 11 cm., and in the normal adult 15 to 20 cm.

Between the normal narrowings are the dilated portions of the canal: the fossa navicularis, the bulbous and the prostatic—*deepened at the expense of the urethral floor.* The *roof* (surgical wall of Guyon) and the posterior segment are fixed—a matter of great moment in the passage of rigid instruments to the bladder; the instrumenteur tries to keep the tip of the instrument hugging the urethral roof until the bladder is reached.

The anterior urethra and its innumerable mucous glands are lined with columnar epithelium on which gonococci grow luxuriantly. Transitional epithelium lines the posterior urethra as well as the upper urinary channels. Most strictures of the membranous and prostatic urethra are traumatic, while the severest gonorrheal strictures are found in the deep bulbous and the bulbomembranous urethra.

The structure of the prostatic urethra is shown in Figure 31, the *verumontanum* sits in the midline and into it open the utricle (vagina masculina, a müllerian derivative) and the ejaculatory ducts of the seminal vesicles. Laterally to the verumontanum are fifteen to twenty openings of the prostatic ducts.

The *external urethral sphincter*, a wide band of striated muscle and part of the compressor urethrae, encircles the prostatic apex and membranous urethra to control (via the pudic nerves) voluntary urination. Some fibers from the external sphincter pass to join the levator ani muscles so that, in the act of urination, levator contraction reduces the angle of the prostatic urethra and distinctly aids in starting the stream.

The *membranous urethra* between the layers of the triangular ligament and the *external meatus* are normally the narrowest portions of the urethra, while the bulbous segment is the widest and extremely vascular.

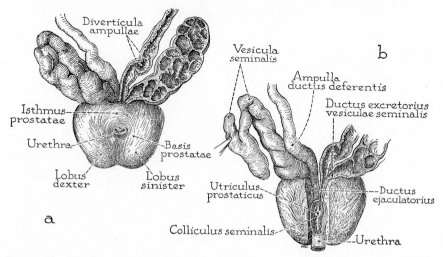

FIGURE 31.   The lower urinary tract and reproductive organs in the male. (Anson—Maddock after Spalteholz.)

The bulbomembranous glands of Cowper, one on each side, are located between the layers of the triangular ligaments just anterior to the bulbo-membranous junction, and may become foci of infection or abscess, especially gonococcic (Fig. 6). Numerous small mucous glands (of Littre) found in the anterior urethra and larger glands (of Morgagni) located in the upper urethral wall may tenaciously harbor infection, especially gonorrheal, or abscess may later be followed by stricture.

The Penis. The three erectal tissue components of the penis (corpora cavernosa and the corpus spongiosum) and their relation to each other are shown in Figure 33. These bodies are bound together by dense fascia (Buck's), the boundaries of which control the spread of phlegmons. The corpora cavernosa are anchored to the ischiopubic rami, and passing between them below is the corpus spongiosum which begins in the urethral bulb and external layer of the triangular ligament. The entire organ is fixed to the pubis at its root by the suspensory ligament. The size of the penis perhaps bears less constant relation to the body development than any other organ and functionally one "cannot tell the depth of the well by the length of the pump handle." The thin delicate, lax, elastic penile skin favors enormous inflammatory edema on comparatively slight traumatic insult, and hematoma increases rapidly and widespread.

The *blood supply* is from the internal pudic artery, the deep branches supplying the erectile tissue, and an artery to the bulb supplies the corpus spongiosum. The dorsal penile veins and the prostatic plexus are the venous drainage. Because of this unusually rich vascular supply penile wounds generally heal kindly even when the organ is severely crushed or nearly severed. Conservative therapy is favored.

The penile *lymphatics* are arranged in a superficial and a deep series.

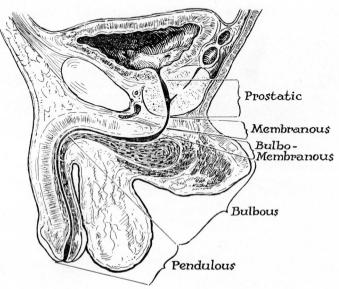

FIGURE 32.   Anatomic divisions of the male urethra.

Those of the skin and prepuce drain into the inguinal nodes superficial to Poupart's ligament and then to the external iliac glands. Those of the glans penis drain to the intra-abdominal (in and above the crural nodes); one chain enters the inguinal canal and runs behind the spermatic cord. Thus because of the bilateral lymphatic anastomosis at the base of the penis, bilateral or contralateral inguinal adenitis may exist and direct extension to the iliac nodes may occur. Submucosal lymphatics of the urethra and bladder, by experimental evidence, interconnect with those of the upper urinary tract (Chapter 7) and may be a *modus operandi* of retrograde spread of infection.

The penile *nerve supply* is the internal pudendal nerves, the hypogastric and the pelvic plexuses. The sympathetics supply the erectile corpora, and the vagal elements the cutaneous structures.

The Scrotum. This structure encloses the testes, epididymides, lower part of the vasa deferentes and the spermatic cords. The scrotal skin is lax, thin, redundant, elastic and wrinkled, and amply supplied with sebaceous glands. Because of these characteristics, wide extension of cellulitis, hematoma or edema is favored. The scrotum readily distends to accommodate large hernia, hydrocele or testicular tumors. Only with extreme distention or inflammatory thrombosis does scrotal skin gangrene occur.

In the deeper layer of the scrotal skin is the dartos fascia which joins the penile fascia above and the perineal fascia below (Fig. 34). Thus the dartos fascia guides the extension of scrotal inflammatory, suppurative or phlegmonous processes as (1) they leave the scrotum, or (2) approach it from penile or perineal lesions (periurethral phlegmon, urinary extra-

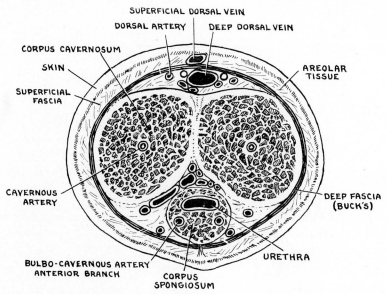

FIGURE 33. Cross section of the penis showing relation of the corpora cavernosa to the urethra surrounded by the corpus spongiosum.

vasation). When penile suppuration or extravasation breaks through Buck's fascia, Colles' fascia becomes the restraining envelope within which the phlegmon may extend to the anterior abdominal wall, scrotum and perineum. The two scrotal compartments are separated by the median raphe and nearly always keep a scrotal suppuration on its own side.

The *testicle* is anchored to the lower scrotal pole by the *gubernaculum*. Tapping of hydrocele should always be performed in the anterior upper scrotal segment to avoid injury to the cord or large superficial veins. The *scrotal blood supply* is from the superficial branches of the internal pudic arteries and the external pudic branches of the femoral artery. The venous return accompanies the arterial supply. The scrotal *nerves* are derived from the superficial perineal branches of the internal pudic and the internal branch of the small sciatic nerve. The ilio-inguinal nerve supplies the anterior upper scrotum. In neuromuscular disease originating below the second lumbar level, disturbance of the cutaneous branches of these nerves is often diagnostic.

The Prostate.   The prostate is a glandulomuscular organ which surrounds the urethra at the bladder outlet and is enclosed in a fibrous capsule (Fig. 31). The adult prostate is about the size and shape of a horse chestnut with apex forwards. The bulk of the gland is placed laterally to the urethra (lateral lobes); these are joined above by a thin commissure of glandular substance—the anterior lobe—and medially just below the vesical outlet is the glandular group of the median lobe. The posterior lobe constitutes the anatomic apex of the prostate, as rectally palpated. On the floor of the prostatic urethra are the verumontanum and the ejaculatory ducts (Fig. 31). The prostate is supplied by the arterial branches of the inferior vesical from the middle hemorrhoidal vessels. The venous

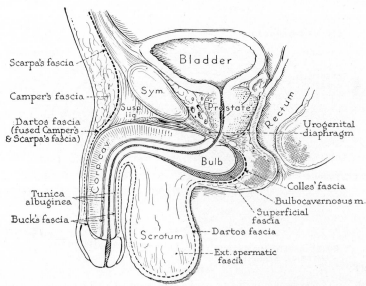

FIGURE 34.   Scrotal and perineal fasciae. These are of great importance in both directing and limiting the spread of periurethral phlegmons (extravasation) (Jones-Shepard).

return is by the prostatovesical plexus emptying into the internal iliac veins. In pelvic fracture, vesical rupture, laceration of the prostatic urethra and other grave injury in this area, hemorrhage into the perivesical and periprostatic spaces may be profuse and even fatal (Figs. 215, 216).

The prostatic *lymphatic drainage* is (1) to the lower lumbar nodes through the presacral glands, (2) to the iliac glands via the perivesical lymphatics, and (3) to the hypogastric chain. The prostatic *nerves* are from the hypogastric plexus.

In adults diseases associated with the prostate are chiefly ancient venereal or the hyperplastic or neoplastic obstruction of declining years; inflammation and obstructive prostatic disease is not uncommon in young boys.

The Testicle. The testis is enclosed in a dense fibrous capsule, the tunica albuginea (Fig. 35). The testicle is held in position by (1) the gubernaculum which passes from its lower pole to the bottom of the scrotum, (2) the mesorchium or testicular mesentery which, when absent or ill-joined, permits axial rotation or torsion of the spermatic cord (testicle), a condition frequent enough in young boys but seldom seen after the age of fifteen years (Chapter 8). As shown in Figure 36, the testis is composed of numerous spermatic tubules which conduct spermatozoa from the spermatogenic cells lining these ducts (Fig. 36*B*). These tubules are imbedded in and separated by a reticulum in which are the interstitial cells of Leydig (Fig. 36*B*), which elaborate androgenic hormone influencing sexual characteristics, development, and activity.

The bulk of the testicular parenchyma is divided into tubulous lobules by fibrous septa which converge at the hilum (body of Highmore). There the 600 or so testicular tubules join to form the *tubuli recti*, 15 to 20 in number, which then unite to form the *vasa efferentia* (Fig. 35). These ducts in turn unite in the globus major (head) of the epididymis to become the *canal of the epididymis* which comprises the bulk of this structure, and eventually becomes the vas deferens at the lower pole or globus

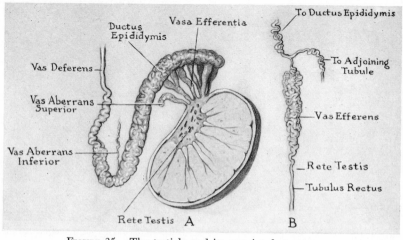

FIGURE 35.   The testicle and its associated structures.

minor (tail) of the epididymis. A small inflammatory process in the epididymis may readily seal off the spermatic ducts to produce isolateral sterility. This lesion may occur in boys as well as in adult males.

The *tunica vaginalis* is a remnant of the peritoneal prolongation preceding testicular descent (Fig. 105). The parietal layer lines the scrotal cavity, the visceral layer covers most of the epididymis and overlies the dense tunica albuginea of the testicle. The endothelial lining of the tunica vaginalis secretes a variable amount of fluid (normally 3 to 5 cc.) which fills the space between and separates the parietal and visceral walls of the tunica vaginalis. Although the processus vaginalis is usually open at birth, it is closed by the first month in nine tenths of infants. Failing to close, congenital hydrocele and often hernia result. Inflammatory epididymitis or orchitis or traumatic irritation of the tunica vaginalis with excessive exudation of serum causes clinical hydrocele (Fig. 178).

The *blood supply* of the testicle and epididymis is the spermatic artery directly from the abdominal aorta. An accessory artery of the vas deferens supplies this structure. The venous return joins to form the pampiniform plexus which, in turn, empties into the spermatic vein leading to the vena cava on the right and renal vein on the left. The longer blood column on the left with its increased hydrostatic pressure is believed to be a frequent cause of varicocele (Fig. 187). In right varicocele, situs inversus or abdominal (renal?) tumor must be ruled out.

The testicular *nerves* from the aortic and renal plexus (tenth dorsal segment) accompany the spermatic artery. Because of the intimate connection of the spermatic, aortic and solar plexuses, a sickening abdominal pain is commonly caused by testicular trauma or an acute epididymal lesion.

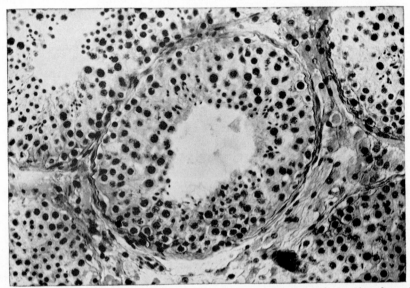

Figure 36A.   Normal testicle: histology. Microscopic appearance of a section through a normal adult testicle, illustrating the spermatogenic cycle.

The Spermatic Cord.   This is composed of a dense sheath having (1) an external fibrous layer (intercolumnar fascia) from the aponeurosis of the external oblique muscle and (2) cremasteric fascia containing thin cremaster muscle fibers and originating in the transversalis abdominal fascia. The sheath of the spermatic cord is closed everywhere except at the pelvic opening (Bogros' space) through which pericystic phlegmons or suppurations may penetrate and extend down the cord, usually to cause vascular thrombosis and resulting testicular gangrene. Within the sheath of the cord run (1) the *vas deferens* from the tail of the epididymis to the inguinal canal and thence retroperitoneally to the dilated ampulla of the vas before it empties into the seminal vesicle, (2) the artery of the testicle and the artery of the epididymis. The venous return is by the

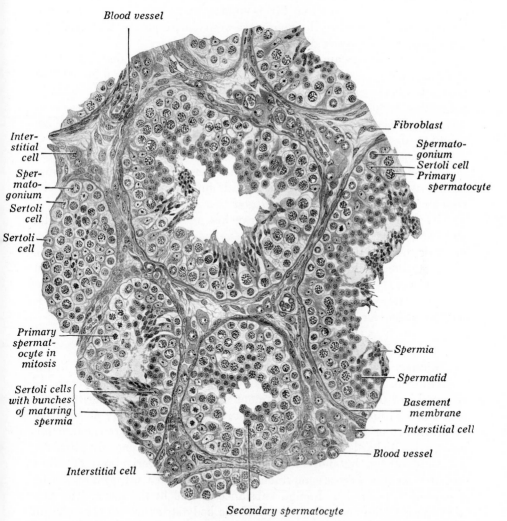

FIGURE 36*B*.   Human testis (from operation). The transections of the tubules show various stages of spermatogenesis. 170 ×.

pampiniform plexus which, when engorged and varicosed, is clinically recognized as varicocele (Fig. 187). The plexus ultimately opens into the vena cava on the right and renal vein on the left.

On physical examination the *vas deferens* is recognized in the adult as a slate pencil size (3 to 5 mm.), firm tubular structure located mesio-posteriorly in the cord. The vas which is composed largely of longitudinal muscle fibers becomes enlarged when inflamed, and especially in tuberculosis may become nodular or beaded.

The *seminal vesicles*, one on each side, are monotubular structures which function as spermatic reservoirs situated above the prostate between the bladder floor and the rectum. They are joined medially by the iso-lateral vas deferens near the entrance of the duct of the seminal vesicles into the prostate (Fig. 31). The muscular wall of the seminal vesicles— a circular and a longitudinal layer—upon sympathetic stimulation contracts to expel semen. In the young the vesicles are poorly developed and are palpable only when diseased.

The intimate relationship of the seminal vesicles to the floor of the bladder, trigone, prostate, posterior urethra and rectum explains why in vesiculitis there may be urinary frequency, dysuria, urgency, occasionally hematuria, rectal tenesmus or painful defecation. In acute seminal vesiculitis and prostatitis the patient often complains of the feeling of a "hot potato in the rectum."

The *ejaculatory ducts* of the vesicles open through the verumontanum into the posterior urethra from which ascending infection may cause vesiculitis, especially in gonorrhea. With inflammatory occlusion of the vesicles and their ducts, isolateral sterility results.

The vesicles are supplied by branches of the inferior hemorrhoidal and inferior vesical arteries and the venous return is via the vesico-prostatic plexus. The nerve supply is from the pelvic plexus and the lymphatics drain into the internal iliac nodes. The dense fibrous fascia of Denonvilliers separates the seminal vesicles and prostate from the rectum; only in advanced suppurative or neoplastic disease of these structures is the fascial barrier broken through and the rectum invaded.

PHYSIOLOGY OF THE UROGENITAL ORGANS

Kidney.   "The kidney plays an indispensable and major part in the regulation of the composition of body fluids to preserve that degree of constancy of the internal environment which is essential to health. Cessation of its function causes death as surely if not as quickly as stoppage of the heart or respiration." This capsule summary of renal function written by Richards in 1929 has been expanded to volumes by physiologists and others, but not more succinctly stated. Derivations of every structure in the body are represented in the excreted nitrogenous waste, water, salts, as well as foreign substances found in the urine. The kidneys preserve the normal alkalinity of the body structures so necessary to the maintenance of the many physicochemical reactions constantly taking place. In pronounced renal disease, the severe ionic disturbances of the blood and other body tissues are clinically recognized as acidosis or alkalosis. This is especially pronounced in children who, with their high metabolic rates, display rapid and pronounced alteration in the hydrogen ion (pH) concentration of the blood, the degree of which may be readily and accurately determined by blood CO_2 combining power estimation.

While the elimination of useless protein waste products—chiefly urea, creatinine, and uric acid—via the kidney is popularly recognized, it is less well appreciated that the kidney also secretes valuable body fluid components when they are in excess, and retains them when they are quantitatively below normal in the body. This is of greatest importance as concerns the salt and fluid factors by which the kidney maintains the osmotic pressure and proper electrolyte content of the circulating plasma and the interstitial fluid. Obviously, an understanding of the fundamentals of renal function is of utmost importance in the proper treatment of urologic disease, requiring as it so often does the correction of fluid and electrolyte disturbances by diet, liquids, and ionic chemotherapy.

Urine is formed in the kidney by secretion, this function being dependent upon: (1) the chemical composition of the blood, (2) the rate of blood flow through the kidney, (3) the volume of blood flow through the kidney, and (4) the blood pressure.

Other factors influencing renal secretion are (a) loss of body fluids through other channels (skin, lungs, intestines), (b) psychic factors in which excitement and nervous tension stimulates the cardiac rate and output with greater blood flow through the kidneys, and (c) neurogenic factors, chiefly polyuria, as in some brain injuries or tumors, skull fractures, diabetes insipidus. Yet the kidney will function normally with its nerve supply completely severed.

Briefly, the mechanism of urine formation consists of glomerular filtration, tubular reabsorption and tubular secretion.

Glomerular Filtration. An ultrafiltrate of the blood plasma is expressed through the interstices of the endothelial membrane of the glomerular capillary tuft (Fig. 27), the impelling hydrostatic force being the blood pressure; a pressure head of 35 mm. is sufficient to drive the fluid through the pores of the capillary membrane. This ultrafiltrate, iso-alkaline with the plasma, contains all the constituents of the plasma except lipids; the excreted protein is but a trace. According to Smith (1951), in the average normal man 132 ml. (cc.) of blood plasma are filtered through the glomerular pores each minute, a volume of about fifty gallons in a day or approximately one drop per glomerulus. So great is the glomerular filtration activity that the entire volume of circulating blood with both its waste and valuable constituents is filtered through the glomeruli every twenty-seven minutes (Pitts, 1954).

Tubular Reabsorption. The enormous filtration volume output of the glomeruli is reduced nearly 200 times by tubular absorption, the useful ionic salt components being retained as necessary to maintain normal electrolyte equilibrium. Thus, as Pitts has computed it, in the fifty gallons (about 190 liters) of blood plasma circulating in a day through the glomeruli, there are (1) a pound of sodium bicarbonate, (2) 2.7 pounds of sodium chloride, (3) a half pound of glucose, (4) a quarter pound of amino acid, and 4.0 gm. of vitamin C together with lesser amounts of other substances valuable to the body including, in most instances, re-absorption of the traces of protein in the glomerular filtrate. These amounts just given are not the total body content of these substances but the total amount, by recirculation, the kidney is exposed to in a day as contained in the 3.5 liters of blood circulating throughout the kidneys every 27 minutes in a man weighing 70 kilograms.

Tubular absorption takes place by several methods—at least four and probably more:

1. *Passive absorption by diffusion*, e.g., the withdrawal of water and some urea (up to 60% of the filtrable urea) as the filtrate passes through the tubules. Yet unless a generous fluid intake is maintained, an increased back diffusion of urea into the blood stream occurs—a consideration of great moment in much of urologic therapy.

2. By the phenomenon of *active transport mechanism* in which, by energy expenditure, a substance is moved from a medium of low concentration to one of higher concentration. Thus glucose, phosphate, sulfate, vitamin C, and amino acids are reabsorbed by the tubules. Under abnormal loading a point is reached beyond which the tubule cannot absorb (for glucose, 375 mg. per minute). This is denoted as the maximal tubular absorption capacity Tm, the initial of the substance under consideration being added as Tm_{in} for inulin, or Tm_g for glucose. Amounts of glucose above this figure filtrated by the glomeruli will pass unaltered into the final urine output, e.g., as in transient alimentary glycosuria.

3. Apparently there is no maximal tubular absorption capacity for the sodium chloride and bicarbonate ions as well as the major ions in the plasma and extracellular fluid, only the concentration in the filtrate reaching them determining how much will be reabsorbed by the tubules.

Normally a hormone of the adrenal cortex controls the fine mechanism of ion reabsorption but in the physicochemical osmotic disturbance induced by hypoproteinemia, for example, water and salt retention are likely to be evidenced by edema.

4. About 80 per cent of the glomerular water filtration is reabsorbed by the proximal segment of the renal convoluted tubule, the osmotic mechanism being dependent upon absorption of chloride, sodium bicarbonate, and glucose. The remaining 20 per cent or so of fluid is absorbed in the distal convoluted tubules under influence of pitressin, the pituitary antidiuretic hormone.

Despite the enormous amount of ionic substances passing through the glomeruli in a day, only relatively small amounts or even traces are found in the voided urine (Table 2).

Tubular Secretion.   By this mechanism the tubules rapidly eliminate from the plasma products undesirable at the time at least, and serve as an exchange process for the necessary elements in the tubular urine. Thus, carboxylic, sulfonic, and hippuric acids are eliminated as are the diagnostic dyes and chemicals phenolsulfonphthalein, Diodrast, Hippuran, para-aminohippuric acid, and so forth, and apparently chiefly in the proximal convoluted tubules. Evidence suggests that in the distal convoluted tubules hydrogen, potassium, and indirectly ammonium ions from the peritubular blood are exchanged for sodium ions in the tubular fluids and, indirectly, ammonium ions for sodium ions, thus building up the plasma bicarbonate base reserve (Fig. 37). *The acidosis of chronic renal disease reflects failure of this mechanism of ionic interchange and conservation.* Yet, the tubular cells cannot produce urine of greater acidity

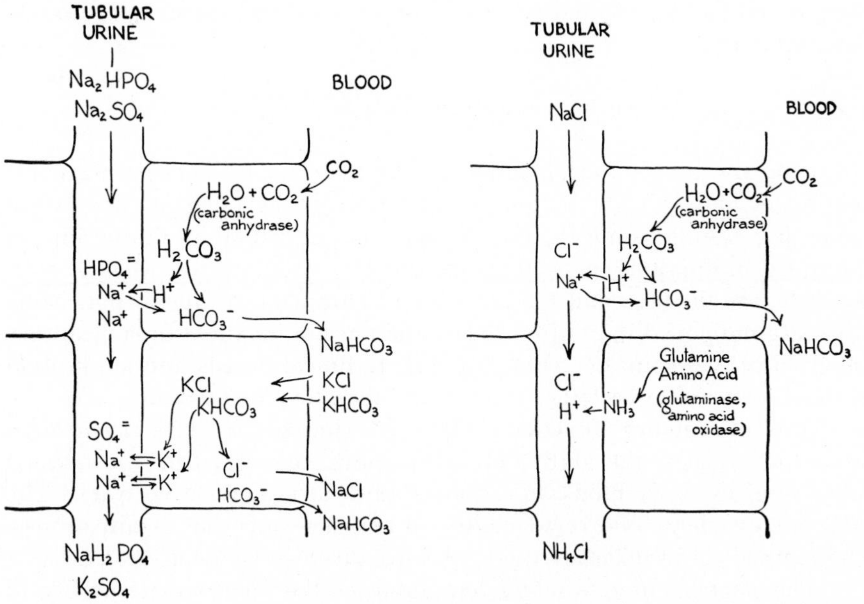

FIGURE 37.   Schematic representation of the tubular secretory mechanisms concerned with the regulation of acid-base and potassium-sodium balances. Presumably all of these mechanisms are localized in cells of the distal convoluted tubules. *Left:* Hydrogen-sodium and potassium-sodium exchange mechanisms. *Left upper:* Hydration of carbon dioxide to form carbonic acid is speeded by the enzyme, carbonic anhydrase. Hydrogen ions dissociated from carbonic acid are exchanged for sodium ions in the tubular urine. Sodium and bicarbonate ions are returned to the peritubular blood stream to build up the bicarbonate bound base reserves of the body. *Left lower:* Potassium ions are likewise exchanged for sodium ions in the tubular urine, permitting excretion of potassium and conservation of sodium. Some step in this exchange mechanism appears to be common to the one concerned with hydrogen ions, for the active transfer of hydrogen ions depresses potassium exchange, and the active transfer of potassium ions depresses hydrogen exchange. *Right:* The role of ammonia in acid-base regulation. Since the tubules are incapable of elaborating urine more acid than pH 4.5, they can exchange very little hydrogen for sodium if the acid formed is a strong acid, such as hydrochloric, rather than a weak acid, such as primary phosphate, shown on the left. However, if this acid is neutralized by ammonia as rapidly as it is formed, the exchange can go on. The ammonia is formed by the hydrolysis of glutamine and amino acids and diffuses rapidly into the tubular lumen if the reaction there is an acid one. (Pitts.)

than pH 4.5, the higher acidity encouraging the diffusion of ammonium ions from the cells to the urine to variably neutralize its high acidity. The *ammonia is formed* in the tubular cells by the deamination (oxidation) of amino acids and the hydrolysis of glutamine rather than as formerly thought by the hydrolysis of urea.

Applied Physiology.   The various commonly employed clinical tests of renal function as reflected in renal excretion (urea clearance test, phenolsulfonphthalein, indigo carmine, etc.) and renal retention (blood urea, nonprotein nitrogen, creatinine, etc.) are discussed in Chapter 3.

The *plasma clearance* of inulin is the only exact measurement of glomerular filtration, determining the number of cubic centimeters of plasma completely cleared of inulin in one minute time according to the formula

$$\text{Clearance of Inulin } (C_{in}) = \frac{U_{in} \times V}{P_{in}}$$

U_{in} being the inulin concentration in the urine in milligrams per cubic centimeter (ml.); V the volume or rate of urine excreted in cubic centimeter per minute, and P_{in} the plasma concentration in milligrams of inulin in milligrams per cubic centimeter. Similar, but slightly less accurate, are the urea and the creatinine clearance tests, the former being clinically employed most often today, the normal maximal urea clearance being 75 cc. per minute (Table 2). The technical details and application of these tests are to be found in clinical laboratory manuals.

Tests of Tubular Function.   Here the simplest is the *concentration* test which reflects the ability of the kidneys, in regulating the osmotic pressure of the body fluids, to excrete solutes in preference to water. The *dilution* test shows the renal ability to excrete water but retain solutes. The methods of performing these tests are given in Chapter 3.

The *phenolsulfonphthalein test* indicates the approximate ability of the tubules to excrete the dye. The crucial consideration is the total excretion in fifteen minutes (normal 25%) following intravenous injection, and a total of 65 to 85 per cent in two hours. When intramuscular injection is employed, the test is far less accurate because of variables in dye absorption from the site of injection (see Table 2).

Two accurate tests of tubular activity are the (a) *glucose absorptive capacity*, and (b) the *para-aminohippuric acid secreting capacity*.

As stated previously, the normal top limit of tubular absorption of glucose is 375 mg. per minute. By maintaining by intravenous infusion of glucose a blood plasma level of over 400 mg. per cent, the tubular "overflow" in the voided urine is estimated. By the synchronous injection of *inulin*, its filtration rate is also estimated, thus giving an estimate of glomerular and tubular activity.

When *para-aminohippuric acid* is injected some is secreted by the glomeruli as well as by the tubules to give an over-all estimate of total renal function.

Methods have also been devised for measuring the adequacy of the renal vascular supply and its circulation to determine the effective blood flow, a matter of clinical importance in the prognosis and management of advanced renal sclerosis, and of the Goldblatt type of renal disease with hypertension. Generalized or localized tubular ischemia consequent to vascular inadequacy (especially arteriosclerosis or obliteration) explains the hypertension; the inability of the tubules adequately to form ammonia and neutralize the acid explains the accompanying hyperchloremic acidosis.

Renal Function in Utero. Renal secretion begins about the fifth month of intra-uterine life, a function attested to by the following:

1. The finding of urine in the fetal bladder of five months (Englisch).

2. The frequently observed urination by the fetus at birth, especially in breech presentation.

3. Sodium benzoate given the mother appears in the fetal urine as hippuric acid, a change occurring in the fetal kidney.

4. Phlorhizin given the mother causes glycosuria in the fetus.

5. Methylene blue given the mother appears in the fetal urine at birth.

6. Diodrast injected into the human fetus at cesarean section showed this medium to be excreted by the kidney by the fourth to fifth month (Kjellberg and Rudhe, 1949).

7. Excretion of ferrocyanide by glomeruli and phenol red by the tubules in the mesonephros and metanephros of the fetal rabbit, cat, opossum, and pig (Homer Smith, 1949, personal communication).

As if this were not enough, attention is drawn to the striking similarity of amnionic fluid and urine, and the frequent finding of far-ad-

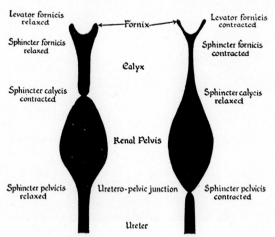

FIGURE 38. Mechanics of activity of the renal calyces in the transport of urine from the papillary collecting tubules. Collecting and emptying phases of calyx and true pelvis with cooperation of ureteropelvic junction. (Narath.)

vanced hydronephrosis and other pronounced obstructive uropathy in the fetus at six and seven months and often with total back-pressure renal destruction in the newborn fetus or infant.

Applied Physiology of the Renal Pelvis and Ureter.   Urine secreted by the kidney is propelled from the minor calyces to the bladder by ureteral peristalsis. This normally rhythmic, progressive, propulsive action is both a sympathetic and parasympathetic reaction to urinary distention of these channels but may also be myogenic as it will continue though the nerve supply of these ducts is completely severed from the central innervation centers.

The secreted urine as it enters the terminal collecting tubules (canaliculi) of the medullary papillae in the minor calyces is helped forward by the contraction of the musculi levatores fornicis (Narath) which temporarily elevate or shorten the papillae (Fig. 38). The urine passes, with closing and opening of calyceal sphincters, into the cavity of a minor calyx from which it is progressively impelled into the major calyx and pelvis, then across the pelvis and down the ureter to the bladder (Figs.

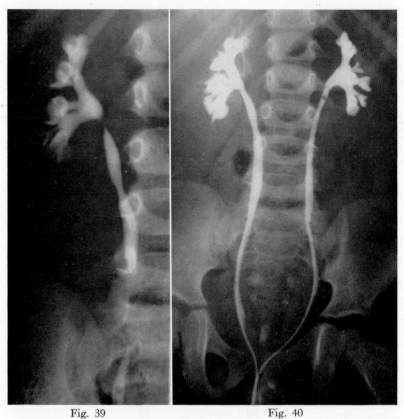

Fig. 39   Fig. 40

Figures 39 and 40.   Normal ureteropyelogram showing an "average" degree of variation in the shape and peristaltic outline.

39, 40). The *normal rate of peristaltic contraction* is every fifteen to forty seconds, depending mostly upon the rate and volume of urine secretion. With acute ureteral obstruction, the rate and force of peristaltic contracture is increased, even to the point of ureteral spasm recognized clinically as colic.

Substantial excretory urographic studies have shown that the renal pelvis never empties itself completely, always a few drops or even a cubic centimeter of urine remaining. Yet certain standards of normality are recognized: the pelvis of a small child should empty itself in two to two and a half minutes. A forceful peristaltic contraction will empty the pelvis in one and a half seconds (Narath). After normal urographic distention with a nonirritating medium, an older child's pelvis should empty in four to five minutes. Retention of medium after this time is significant and suggestive of (1) peripheral obstruction, (2) neuromuscular disease, and (3) chronic pelvic and peripelvic inflammation. In the adult, pelvic emptying usually occurs every three to five minutes and following pyelographic injection and removal of the ureteral catheter, the pelvis should be empty in five to six minutes, retention at ten minutes being pathologic (trap or delayed-emptying film, Fig. 23), and probably due to one of the causes just cited.

Ureteral peristalsis and contraction may be simulated by parasympathomimetic drugs such as prostigmine, acetylcholine derivatives, and pitressin, drugs which have sometimes been given to reduce intestinal gas and its conflicting shadows in the urographic film. Yet these drugs cause radiographically demonstrable contraction of the pelvic and ureteral outlines, often to a half reduction as I have shown (1941) and thus engender seriously erroneous urographic interpretation.

PHYSIOLOGY OF THE BLADDER

For better continuity of presentation, this is discussed under Neuromuscular Diseases of the Urinary Tract in Chapter 10.

PHYSIOLOGY OF THE GENITAL TRACT

Urethra.   The purpose of the urethra is to transport urine and, in addition in the male, semen. Following urination, the anterior urethra empties by collapse of the mucosal walls. In the absence of urethral or bladder neck obstruction the size and shape of the urinary stream will depend on the nozzle—the external urethral meatus, congenital stenosis of which is common in both sexes although more often recognized in the male and notably in young boys. The condition may cause advanced back-pressure injury of the entire proximal urinary tract in both sexes (Figs. 109, 110; also see 111). Moreover the condition, by producing urinary stasis, not only predisposes to urinary infection but intensifies and prolongs an existing one.

The function of the penis is both urinary and sexual.

The Male Reproductive Tract.   The testicle forms spermatozoa from the spermatogenic tissue and elaborates male sex hormone (androgen) in the interstitial cells of Leydig (Fig. 36*B*). The function of the remainder of the reproductive tract is to transport and deliver spermatozoa, formation of which normally begins at puberty. In improperly descended testes, the spermatogenic tissue commonly remains infantile, the developmental retardation setting in between the third and fourth year although many of these glands are hypoplastic from birth. In these cases the androgenic interstitial tissue may develop well but it is usually subnormal and sometimes with comparable secondary sexual characteristics and under development. It should be remembered that the adrenals elaborate two thirds of the androgenic hormone in the male, hence the precise degree of testicular interstitial cell hypofunction cannot always be accurately computed.

Castration before puberty checks development of the remainder of the reproductive apparatus; secondary sexual characteristics do not appear or are most elementary; facial and body hair is scant or absent, the pubic hair is of transverse female distribution. The epiphyses unite late while the bones grow longer and larger than normal with a tendency to a peculiar gigantism with long legs and trunk and a smallish head. This configuration together with abnormal distribution of fat over the buttocks, pubis, hips and breast, a high-pitched voice (laryngeal underdevelopment) may induce mental depression. In *eunuchoidism* bilateral testicular underdevelopment is accompanied by other endocrinopathy, especially pituitary (e.g., Fröhlich's syndrome, Fig. 191).

Erections may result from any local penile irritation such as phimosis in male infants and children while in adults sexual stimulation either erotic or physical is the usual inciting agent. Priapism is common in sickle cell anemia.

PHYSIOLOGY OF THE PROSTATE

The prostate in the male consists of two portions, the posterior lobe or anatomic apex in which carcinoma usually arises, and the remainder

TABLE 3.   CHEMICAL COMPOSITION OF FRACTIONS OF THE EJACULATE
(HUGGINS)

(Fructose arises chiefly from seminal vesicle; the other components are excreted chiefly or exclusively by the prostate)

COMPONENT	FRACTION OF EJACULATE	
	First	Last
Citrate, mg. per cent (Scherstén, 1936)	770	120
Calcium, mg. per cent (Scherstén, 1936)	52	20
Acid phosphatase units, 1 cc. (Gutman and Gutman, 1941)	2760	300
Fructose, mg. per cent (MacLeod and Hotchkiss, 1942)	157	377
Fibrinolysin, minutes per test (Huggins and McDonald, 1946)	120	288

or major portion in which benign hyperplasia arises but seldom carcinoma. There is no evidence that the prostate elaborates an endocrine hormone of its own although it is extremely sensitive to the pituitary hormone.

The prostatic secretion derived almost exclusively from the anterior lobe is energized by stimulation of the nervi erigentes. Immature or castrate animals do not have prostatic secretion. Curiously, intravenous injection of prostatic secretion causes a pronounced fall in blood pressure. The chemical composition of the prostatic secretion is shown in Table 3. Orchiectomy decreases prostatic secretion as do estrogens, while the administration of testosterone propionate stimulates it.

The Seminal Vesicle. This structure, contrary to some clinical opinion, is comparatively immune from infection despite major acute and severe infection of the adjacent and, in a measure, contiguous prostate. The presence of choline esters, phosphorus compounds and fructose characterizes the vesicular secretion from the numerous glands lining its walls. A streptokinase-like enzyme *fibrolysin* has been found to cause liquidification of the semisolidly ejaculated seminal fluid.

PHYSIOLOGY OF THE TESTICLE AND SCROTUM

As Moore has shown in a brilliant series of experiments, the scrotum acts as a testicular radiator in the confines of which the testicle matures and elaborates spermatozoa, the intrascrotal temperature being 2 to 4° F. lower than that of the abdomen. When the normal testes of rhesus monkeys are put in the abdomen, spermatogenesis ceases and degeneration of the spermatic tubules ensues. With replacement of the organs in the cooler scrotum, regeneration occurs and spermatogenesis returns. The testes are especially sensitive to x-radiation, most of the early radiologists having been sterilized unwittingly by exposure during routine radiographic practice.

The *chief function of the epididymis* is that of a satisfactory temporary residence for spermatids from the testis and which, in slowly passing through the tubule of the epididymis, become mature, active, fertile spermatozoa. Thus the spermatozoa in the upper epididymis near the rete testis are immature while those at the lower end or tail as they enter the vas deferens are fully active and mature. The time of residence in the epididymis depends largely upon the frequency of ejaculation.

Life of Spermatozoa. Clinical evidence indicates that, after insemination, spermatozoa may live up to 72 hours but more often only 24 to 36 hours. Outside the body at room temperature, motility persists from 20 to 24 hours, for less time at higher temperatures and, on ice, up to a week.

Under the stimulation of the testis hormone (testosterone), the epididymis, prostate, vas deferens, seminal vesicles, and Cowper's glands secrete the major portion of the seminal fluid; the contribution of the testis is chiefly spermatozoa with extremely small amounts of liquid secretion.

The benefit of administration of testosterone to elderly males and those suffering "declining youth" and alleged male climacteric is still *sub judice*, the claims of the hormone merchants notwithstanding. The administration of androgens is definitely contraindicated in carcinoma of the prostate. With deficient androgen elaboration by the testis, the administration of gonadotropins to stimulate interstitial tissue secretion of natural androgen is physiologically reasonable and preferred; the administration of thyroid gland may augment the "recovery."

CHAPTER 5

Urinary Obstruction

NINETY to 95 per cent of all urologic disturbances in patients of all ages are the result of obstruction and/or infection, urinary blockage and stasis being the fundamental predisposing etiology in nearly all cases of urinary tract infection (see Chapter 7). Nearly always in infants and children and not infrequently in adults the obstruction is congenital, generally as the result of anomalous development; too often congenital contracture of the bladder outlet, for example, is not recognized until the patient is 25, 35, or 45 years old. Prostatic obstruction of one variety or another occurs in at least half of all males over 50 years of age; one in seven men over 70 years of age develops carcinoma of the prostate.

By analogy, the urinary stasis or constipation caused either by obstruction or by atonic neuromuscular vesical disease resembles a stagnant millpond in which vegetation (bacteria) grows luxuriantly and in comparison to the clear clean swift running water of the unobstructed brook. Fundamentally this stagnation, called urinary stasis, is what happens in the obstructed urinary tract above the point of blockage.

In obstructive uropathy the effective urinary back pressure is the sum of (1) the renal excretory pressure and (2) the hydrostatic pressure of the urine. The last will vary with alterations of position of the person or of the total fluid mass weight which will change with the volume-capacity and tonicity of the urinary channels. The secretory pressure of the kidney is 35 mm. Hg and upward; the hydrostatic pressure will be largely influenced by the severity of the obstruction, in short, the amount of urinary residuum present. The back pressure is a measurable physical force just as is the pressure of the spinal fluid.

The vital consideration in obstructive uropathy is the back-pressure effect on the renal parenchyma with consequent diminution of its function. In unrelieved advanced destructive back-pressure injury, death from

TABLE 4. CONGENITAL AND ACQUIRED LESIONS PRODUCING URINARY
OBSTRUCTION: POTENTIAL CAUSES OF HYDRONEPHROSIS

I. URETHRA

a. *Congenital or acquired*
  Phimosis
  Meatal stenosis
  Meatal atresia
  Stricture
  Cysts
  Diverticulum
  Hypertrophied verumontanum
  Hydrocolpos

b. *Congenital*
  Posterior urethral valves
  Penile torsion
  Abnormal openings
    Epispadias
    Hypospadias

c. *Acquired*
  Polyps
  Trauma
  Calculi
  Tumor
  Extra-urinary masses, cysts, etc.

II. BLADDER

a. *Congenital or acquired*
  Contracture of vesical neck
  Hypertrophy of vesical neck
  Median bar
  Median lobe
  Hypertrophy of inter-ureteric ridge
  Diverticulum
  Neuromuscular disease
    1. Cord bladder
    2. Atonic bladder

b. *Congenital*
  Anomalies: Exstrophy, reduplicated,
    bipartate, etc.
  Trigonal curtain obstruction
  Ureterocele
  Hydrocolpos

c. *Acquired*
  Tumor
  Prostatic enlargement
  Prostatic neoplasm
  Calculi
  Foreign bodies
  Extravesical masses (sacral teratoma, anterior sacral
  meningocele, sacrococcygeal chordoma, hydrocol-
  pos, hematocolpos, etc.)
  Rectal distention by feces, appendiceal abscess, etc.

III. URETER

a. *Congenital*
  Stricture
  Stenosis
  Atony
  Spasm
  Cystic dilatation
  Kinks
  Angulations
  Diverticulum
  Herniation

b. *Congenital*
  Anomalies of number
  Anomalies of termination
  Valves and folds
  Ureterocele
  Vascular blockage
    1. Primary
    2. Secondary
  Torsion
  Retrocaval

c. *Acquired*
  Calculus
  Inflammation
    Ureteritis
    Peri-ureteritis
  Long-standing infection
  Blood clots
  Trauma
  Ligation
  Tumor
  Extra-ureteral masses, fibrous bands or enlarged glands
    which compress the ureter
  Fecal distention of rectum

TABLE 4. (*Continued*)

IV. PELVIS AND KIDNEY

a. *Congenital or acquired*
  Abnormal ureteral insertion
  Stricture at pelvic outlet

b. *Congenital*
  Renal anomalies of number, form, location, size, etc.
  Accessory renal vessels

c. *Acquired*
  Calculus
  Pelvic outlet blockage by intrarenal or extrarenal neoplasm
  Ptosis
  Trauma
  Infection, especially long-standing
  Aneurysm of renal artery (very large)
  Stress hypertrophy of pelvic and calyceal musculature

renal failure will result. The prime and immediate therapeutic objective in obstructive uropathy is the prompt establishment of free drainage by tube (urethral, ureteral, nephrostomy and so forth) in the acute emergency and later, when the condition of the patient permits, establishment of definitive permanent free drainage by plastic or other surgical methods.

In this chapter we are concerned primarily with the structural and functional alterations due to urinary obstruction as well as the attendant clinical manifestations. The most usual causes of urinary tract obstruction are shown in Figure 41 and Table 4. These are designated as (1) *mechanical* if anatomic, and (2) *dynamic* if consequent to neuromuscular disease of the urinary tract.

The nearer the obstruction is to the ureteropelvic junction (kidney), the more acute and earlier in appearance will be the symptoms of hydronephrosis and the more rapid the destructive process. When the pelvis is intrarenal, the back-pressure damage is greater and more rapid than in the extrarenal pelvis which, by accommodating dilatation, serves as a buffer mechanism to protect the parenchyma from the full brunt of the hydraulic compression. A consideration of the pathogenesis of hydronephrosis must include not only all urinary obstructive but inflammatory and neurogenous lesions as well. Often the obstructive conditions are congenital, especially in the young; so severe are some of these congenital lesions that they kill early and are not seen in adulthood. The usual encountered congenital or acquired lesions causing urinary obstruction are shown in Table 4.

PATHOLOGY IN URINARY OBSTRUCTION

With the onset of obstruction at any point along the urinary tract, congestion of the proximal tract occurs, often with diapedesis of red blood cells which is sometimes severe enough to be recognized as gross hematuria. Dilatation promptly ensues, its degree largely corresponding to the completeness of the obstruction. Blockage at the vesical outlet or peripherally causes bilateral back-pressure changes and damage (Fig. 42); supravesical bilateral ureteral obstruction is not at all rare, especially congenitally in children, and will bring about the same upper tract and renal changes as does prostatic hyperplasia or urethral stricture, for example.

In obstruction at the bladder neck or in the urethra, the bladder acts as an expansile cushion or protective buffer to spare the upper

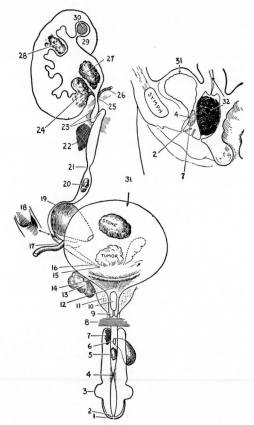

FIGURE 41. Commonest causes of urinary obstruction.

1, phimosis; stenosis of prepuce

2, stenosis of urethral meatus

3, paraphimosis

4, urethral stricture

5, urethral stone

6, urethral diverticulum

7, periurethral abscess

8, external sphincterospasm

9, congenital valves of the posterior urethra

10, hypertrophy of the verumontanum; diverticulum of utricle

11, prostatic abscess or growths

12, contracted bladder neck; median bar

13, periprostatic abscess

14, mucosal fold at bladder outlet; trigonal curtain

15, stricture of ureteral meatus; ureterocele

16, ureterovesical junction stricture

17, vascular obstruction of lower ureter

18, congenital ureteral valves

19, ureteral obstruction by compression by vesical diverticulum, fecal overdistention of rectosigmoid, pelvic cyst, etc.

20, ureteral stone

21, ureteral stricture

22, periureteritis or tumor

23, ureteral kink; periureteral fibrous bands

24, renal tumor

25, ureteropelvic junction stricture

26, aberrant vessel obstruction of upper ureter

27, pelvic stone

28, renal tuberculosis (secondary obstructive lesions consequent thereto)

29, stricture of calyceal outlet

30, calyceal stone

31, neuromuscular vesical disease

32, urethral compression by hematocolpometra or hydrocolpos urinary tract the full back-pressure effects. Its drainage impeded, to empty itself the bladder wall compensates by *work hypertrophy* which causes *trabeculation* as the first evidence of bladder injury by the obstruction. There is variable separation of the hypertrophic detrusor muscle bundles with evagination of the bladder mucosa between. A more advanced stage—recognized as cellule, then saccule formation—may develop and, finally, with massive blowout, a true diverticulum forms (Fig. 43).

Ultimately, as the obstruction persists or increases, the bladder reaches the point where it becomes decompensated and cannot empty itself. With the onset of decompensation, residual* urine makes its appearance and must be considered an approximate measurement of the degree of bladder wall decompensation. It should be recognized that a normal bladder full or overdistended for some time, and with its walls well stretched thereby, may show a small transient residual urine but this will disappear shortly. Moreover, in estimating the vesical residuum when the upper urinary tract is widely dilated, special effort must be made to perform the catheterization immediately after the patient has

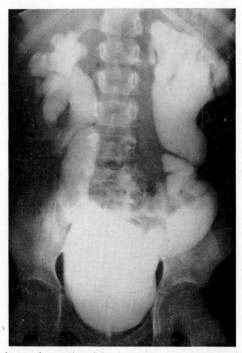

Figure 42. Urinary obstruction. Massive upper urinary tract dilatation due to congenital valves of the prostatic urethra in a six year old boy examined because of chronic pyuria. Grave renal destruction. Residuum 670 cc. Preliminary cystostomy drainage; six months later transurethral resection of the valves was limited (unilateral) by the poor condition of the patient, yet nineteen years later he appears healthy, is in college, but no urographic follow-up has been obtained.

* The residuum is determined by having the patient, preferably in his own privacy, empty his bladder as completely as possible. A catheter is then passed and the amount of urine obtained is the residuum.

emptied himself lest by downflow from the distended urinary reservoirs above, the bladder be variably filled and a false estimation of residuum be made. In such cases, it is often wise, after the initial voiding, to have the patient wait half a minute or so to allow further ureteral down-drainage, then try again to empty the bladder and catheterize at once to estimate the residuum. In advanced decompensation the residuum may be 20 or 30 oz. or more and in chronic complete retention with overflow incontinence, the bladder content is the residuum.

As the bladder dilates behind its obstructed outlet, the ureterovesical valve mechanism is physically altered so that it is no longer competent, but permits vesical contents to reflux into the ureter. Thus intracystic hydraulic pressure is directly transmitted to the ureters and renal pelves. Once the valve mechanism has given way, it stays impotent as long as the abnormal intracystic pressure persists (Figs. 12, 44).

The ureters similarly respond to urinary back pressure, first by increased rate and force of peristalsis but later, and especially with the advent of vesico-ureteral reflux, dilate and become decompensated. By lateral dilatation the ureters may become as large as the colon and by longitudinal dilatation, twice or more normal length (Fig. 42) with mul-

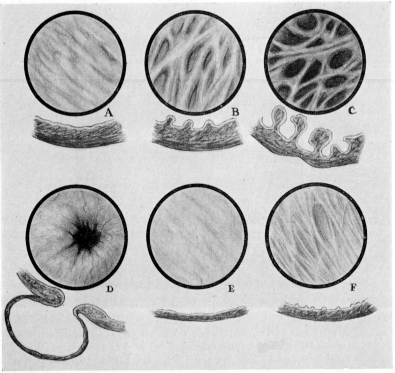

Figure 43. Bladder wall changes in infravesical obstruction. Cystoscopic appearance of changes in the bladder wall in infravesical obstruction. *A*, normal. *B*, early trabeculation. *C*, advanced trabeculation. *D*, diverticulum. *E*, late atony. *F*, fine trabeculation commonly seen in neuromuscular vesical disease. Trophic thinning of the bladder wall is indicated.

tiple curvatures and angulations, some of which may be true secondary kink obstructions. For this reason and as a therapeutic corollary, in establishing prolonged suprapubic cystostomy drainage, one must be certain the upper urinary tract is being completely relieved. This is readily determined by cystography when bilateral vesico-ureteral reflux exists, taking "trap" films ten minutes following bladder emptying after cystography and noting any retention of medium in the kidney pelves or upper ureters. Sometimes the cystographic reflux will not go above the point of secondary ureteral obstruction, but this is the clue that cystostomy alone is inadequate to give free renal drainage in the particular case. The point of secondary ureteral blockage usually can be identified and subsequently relieved surgically, employing interim nephrostomy drainage if indicated.

Frequently hypertrophy of the bladder wall prevents the uretero-vesical valve from giving way. Thus by compression of the intramural ureter, the hypertrophic bladder wall will cause ureteral blockage to increase the total urinary obstruction. In the ureterogram, this situation may be erroneously interpreted as a ureterovesical junction stricture; the etiologic distinction must be made.

To repeat: Urinary back pressure causes the greatest damage to the kidneys—truly vital organs. With increasing intrapelvic back pressure, the renal parenchyma is compressed between the hydraulic force inside and the dense fibrous renal capsule outside. The pressure thus exerted induces variable parenchymal atrophy, both by direct squeezing of the trapped nephron units and, equally important, by compression of their blood supply to cause tissue ischemia. This produces true atrophy of the secretory elements and, unrelieved, total destruction of the kidney (Fig.

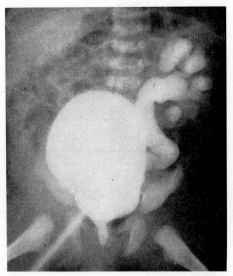

FIGURE 44.   Ureterovesical valve incompetence with reflux consequent to congenital valvular obstruction of the prostatic urethra in a newborn. Also note filling of the deep urethra proximal to the valves (Type I).

46). In the early stages, the back-pressure damage process is reversible but later becomes irreversible.

HYDRONEPHROSIS

This defines the changes in renal pelviocalyceal distention with urine and the associated parenchymal atrophy caused by urinary obstruction. Infected, the condition should be designated as *infected hydronephrosis* but when converted to a suppurative mass of little or no function, the condition is *pyonephrosis*. Let us here consider only uninfected hydronephrosis; the infected variety and its associated lesions are discussed in Chapter 7.

In *open* hydronephrosis, the usual variety clinically encountered, there is incomplete or intermittent obstruction, secretion of urine continues, and a massive hydronephrotic sac may develop (Fig. 45). In *closed* hydronephrosis the blockage is complete as with ureteral stone or accidental ligation of the ureter. Congenital ureteral stricture often causes large palpable hydronephrosis in infants and children. In some instances no anatomic lesion can be found to explain the pelviocalyceal dilatation which here must usually be attributed to neuromuscular disease—atonic or spastic. In *atonic hydronephrosis*, debilitation of the pelvic musculature may result from hydrostatic pressure and stagnation of the urinary fluid mass itself. Spasm of the ureteropelvic junction or even lower in the ureter is known to exist to produce obstruction exactly as it does at the vesical outlet.

The gross and histologic appearance of open and closed hydro-

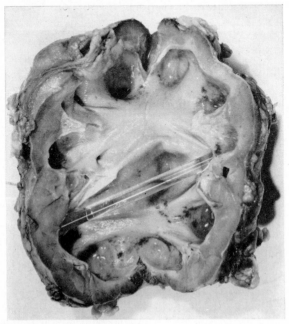

FIGURE 45. Hydronephrosis, advanced. Consequent to ureteropelvic junction stricture.

nephrosis is essentially the same except the open variety may become much larger and even enormous, sacs holding up to six liters having been encountered. In high obstruction the tissue changes occur more rapidly and are more pronounced than in lower blockage, calyceal dilatation occurring earliest in high obstruction and pelvic dilatation earliest in low blockage. In all cases of hydronephrosis, parenchymal congestion occurs with leukocytic infiltration in the renal pelvis and small hemorrhagic areas which explain the microscopic, mild or gross hematuria in many patients with hydronephrosis.

As the pelvic back pressure continues, the cortex and medulla (chiefly the pyramids) are further compressed as is the vascular parenchymal network, to cause tissue anemia and secondary atrophy with diminishing function. This *ischemia is the most important factor in the hydronephrotic damage.* The vessels, tubules and glomeruli farthest from the main arterial branches show the earliest and severest changes, later degenerate, function decreases, the parenchymal wall is weakened and, by vicious cycle, dilates still further to cause increased vascular compression.

Those islands of parenchyma whose blood supply is best maintained will be preserved longest, notably along the archings of the arcuate arteries and veins. No portion of the vascular tree is exempt. The fibrous renal capsule thickens, often becomes hyalinized, and generally strips easily from the hydronephrotic kidney. With relief of the obstruction, the kidney may return to relatively normal size, depending on the soundness of its blood supply which, when incompetent, leads to late *secondary hydronephrotic atrophy* and a shrunken, nonfunctioning, shrivelled kidney.

The severe arterial compression in advanced hydronephrosis may explain a variety of the Goldblatt renal mechanism in vascular hypertension so commonly seen in patients with either unilateral or bilateral involvement. Relief of the obstruction in most of these patients is followed by variable reduction in the blood pressure, sometimes to normal or thereabouts, unless generalized arteriosclerosis (and arteriolar sclerosis) exists. This mechanism of vascular compression in hydronephrosis has

TABLE 5. GROSS CHANGES IN PELVIC ARCHITECTURE: UROGRAPHIC INTERPRETATION

LOCATION	EARLY	LATER	ADVANCED*
Pelvis	Increase	Increase	Increase (round sac)
Major calyces	Broadening at base	Broadening throughout	Sacculation
Minor calyces	Flattening or clubbing	Obliterated	Obliterated
Papillae	Shortening	Shortening	Obliterated
Ureter	No change	Change in insertion angle	Elongated (usually not seen in urogram)

* All outlines are apt to be diffuse because of dilution of the urographic medium with residual urine in the pelvis.

been shown to explain some cases of "essential hypertension" in which obstructive uropathy had not been suspected, especially in the young.

The gross changes in the pelvic architecture are the basis of urographic interpretation (Table 5). With general pelvic dilatation, the earliest back-pressure changes occur in the minor calyces which become rounded and the cuppings blunted or obliterated, the normal cupping being caused by the projection of the papilla of a cluster of medullary pyramids into the tip of a minor calyx (Fig. 26). In progressive hydronephrosis, the minor calyces are flattened out and later disappear as such, the major calyces are dilated and rounded, and later they may even be obliterated and disappear, converting the kidney into a large lobulated multilocular fibrous shell filled with fluid (Fig. 46).

As hydronephrosis advances, the urea, sodium chloride and nitrogenous content of the pelvic urine are quantitatively reduced. Later the pelvic fluid becomes still more watery and contains albumin, leukocytes, epithelial debris, urinary crystals, or sodium chloride with little urea or uric acid. Terminally, in far-advanced hydronephrosis the pelvic fluid is only salt and water, sometimes with a trace of sugar, cholesterol, and with old or fresh blood (hematonephrosis). Following relief of obstruction and assuming the kidney can still function, voluminous compensatory polyuria occurs and the total urea and salt output may become greatly increased.

In rare instances the hydronephrosis is localized to one calyx. This

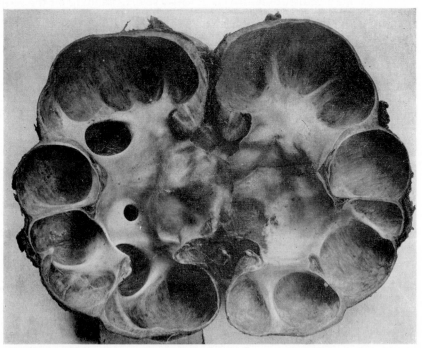

FIGURE 46. Hydronephrosis. Total renal destruction. Ureteropelvic junction stricture.

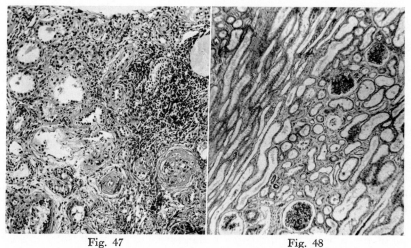

Fig. 47   Fig. 48

FIGURE 47.   Hydronephrosis. Glomerular atrophy, scarring and hyalinization. Tubular
injury, dilatation and degeneration.

FIGURE 48.   Hydronephrosis. Pronounced dilatation of tubules of the medulla.

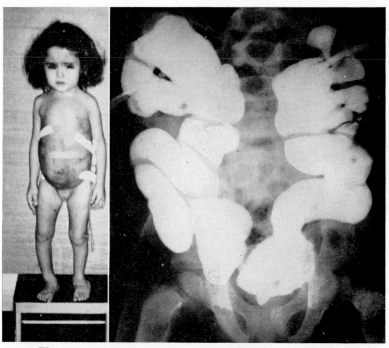

Fig. 49   Fig. 50

FIGURE 49.   Renal dwarfism (secondary renal hyperparathyroidism; osteitis fibrosa
cystica) due to congenital contracture of the bladder outlet with hopelessly advanced upper
tract back pressure damage in a five-year-old girl. Note the characteristic rachitic changes
which are most striking in the ankles and the unusually large squarish head.

FIGURE 50.   Cystogram in patient shown in Figure 49. Congenital contracture of the
vesical outlet with enormous dilatation of the upper urinary tract. The left kidney was
reduced to a thin functionless shell, while the right kidney showed slight but inadequate
function. Bilateral nephrostomy drainage was instituted with some clinical and renal
functional improvement. Subsequent death from renal failure.

111

is known as *hydrocalycosis* and is the result of sclerotic, calculus, stricture or other blockage of the calyceal outlet. Such hydrocalyces are often the site of stone deposit and because of their inadequate drainage and urinary stasis, serve as a persistent feeder of bacteria into the urinary tract to maintain generalized urinary infection. Conservatively, such hydrocalyces are resected to leave the healthy kidney segment (Figs. 228–230).

Fibrolipomatous perinephritis and *peripyelitis* occur in all long standing cases of hydronephrosis and frequently cause adhesions between the kidney and the peritoneum, and less often between the kidney and liver, diaphragm, spleen or intestines. In far-advanced disease the kidney may be nearly replaced with fibrolipomatous deposit.

Microscopic changes in the kidney in hydronephrosis are chiefly dilatation of the tubules, compression of the parenchyma with, later, atrophy of the glomeruli and convoluted tubules (Fig. 47). Terminally, progressive dilatation of the medullary collecting tubules ensues. Thus there is cortical atrophy with tubular dilatation in the medulla (Fig. 48). The terminal picture is chronic nephritis or nephrosclerosis and in children may induce the clinical picture of osteitis fibrosa cystica (secondary renal hyperparathyroidism), renal rickets, or renal dwarfism (Figs. 49–52).

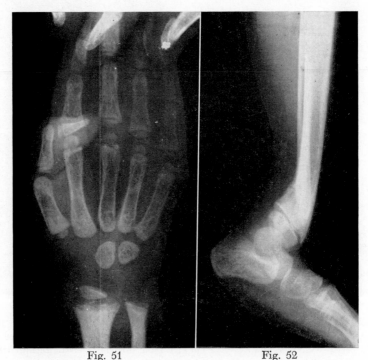

Fig. 51   Fig. 52

FIGURE 51.   Fibrocystic and rachitic changes in the bony structure of the hands in patient shown in Figure 49.

FIGURE 52.   The lower extremities in patient shown in Figure 49, showing deformity of the ankles and adjacent bony structures with fibrocystic changes.

In unilateral hydronephrosis *compensatory hypertrophy* of the sound kidney results from (1) increased vascularity coincident with increased burden, and (2) cellular hypertrophy. After the fourth or fifth year of childhood the renal cells do not multiply but simply enlarge, often to twice normal size. If the diseased kidney is not adequately treated or removed, variable toxic injury of the sounder kidney will occur and, if infected or otherwise gravely injured, renal failure and a uremic death may be anticipated.

Hydro-ureter. With continued obstruction infravesically, at the ureterovesical junction, or proximal, the entire ureter above the point of obstruction develops back-pressure changes. Obstruction at the uretero-vesical junction or peripherally first causes dilatation of the lower segment of the ureter, later the middle and upper portions dilate as does the renal pelvis. With ureteral obstruction above the ureterovesical junction, the proximal segment is dilated while the segment below remains normal. With complicating infection, the entire ureter commonly becomes enor-mously dilated.

Bladder. The progressive changes in the bladder consequent to vesical outlet or peripheral obstruction are shown in Figure 43. Concur-rent with the bladder wall hypertrophy there is hypertrophy of the trigone, the function of which is to open the vesical outlet. Trigonal hypertrophy is found with those obstructions involving the bladder neck (contracture, median bar, prostatic hyperplasia) but is not always present in valvular obstruction of the prostatic urethra, hypertrophy of the veru-montanum, or urethral stricture.

Following relief of chronic vesical retention, anatomic and func-tional restitution of the bladder wall generally ensues. This restitution will depend chiefly on (1) the duration of the obstruction, (2) the archi-tectural changes in the bladder wall, and (3) infection. With prolonged or severe vesical infection with intramural leukocytic infiltration and fibrosis, muscular degeneration and atrophy, its restitution following establishment of free drainage will be relative to the severity and dura-tion of these changes. Yet in some patients the bladder remains a large flabby, fibrosed atonic bag.

Urethra. Urethral obstruction leads to widespread dilatation which will vary according to the site and degree of blockage. In stenosis of the external urethral meatus—so common in infants and young boys—the entire urethra may be enormously dilated with only some narrowing where it passes through the membranous urethra (triangular ligament) which demarcates the anterior and posterior urethra. This dilatation is readily demonstrated urethrographically and may even show diverti-culum blowouts (Fig. 13). Similarly, urethral strictures and other ob-structions are recognized (Fig. 170). In addition to the urethral dila-tation and back-pressure uropathy, the bladder is likely to show collateral changes and even the upper urinary tract may become enormously dilated.

SYMPTOMS IN URINARY OBSTRUCTION

These may be none but in most cases there are pain, hematuria, urinary disturbances, and with infection there is likely to be fever, frequency and other alterations of urination.

Hydronephrosis itself may be asymptomatic but the advent of infection (to which the inadequate diagnosis of "pyelitis" is commonly given) generally causes fever and the manifestations of pyelonephritis—acute or chronic. The most frequent symptoms are pain, tumor caused by the mass itself, polyuria, hematuria, and pyuria, singly or in combination. Uremia appears in advanced bilateral hydronephrotic disease or in unilateral hydronephrosis when the renal mate is hopelessly diseased or is absent. In all obstructive uropathy, it is axiomatic that the clinical problem must be interpreted in terms of renal function, the chief therapeutic objective being the restitution and preservation of this function.

Pain in hydronephrosis may result from obstruction (stone, stricture, tumor, blood clots) which is often accompanied by infection. The pain may be sharp, dull, colicky, constant or intermittent. Small hydronephroses almost always cause more pain than large. The pain may radiate to the groin or genitalia to simulate ureteral stone colic. A low hydronephrotic kidney, especially on the right, may cause the erroneous diagnosis of "chronic appendicitis" to be made. Some patients find they can be relieved of the pain of hydronephrosis by manual compression over the mass, thereby forcing out some urine to lower the intrapelvic pressure and bring about temporary cessation or diminution of the distress.

Tumor. The commonest tumor of the abdomen in infants and children is hydronephrosis and generally in this age group develops on the basis of congenital obstruction. These enlargements in patients of all ages may cause displacement or compression of the stomach, bowel, and especially the colon, to produce constipation, dyspepsia, biliousness, and other alimentary disturbances. Massive hydronephrosis sometimes engenders dyspnea and respiratory or cardiac embarrassment by upward pressure of the mass on the diaphragm. Transient *polyuria* occurs with spontaneous relief of large hydronephroses. *Hematuria* occurs in about 15 per cent of all cases of hydronephrosis, usually results from congestion (parenchymal and pelvic) and may even be accompanied by clots and the ureteral colic induced by their passage. *Pyuria* occurs in sterile hydronephrosis but is nearly always the result of complicating infection, the usual clinical picture being inadequately diagnosed as "pyelitis." *Uremia* (1) occurs when hydronephrotic renal damage becomes grave, (2) is of poor prognosis, and (3) demands immediate relief of the obstruction and correction of blood electrolyte imbalance (q.v.).

Ureter. The symptoms of hydro-ureter are largely indistinguishable from those of hydronephrosis and the topical diagnosis is made by ureterography.

Bladder. Infravesical obstruction causes dysuria and urinary frequency which are aggravated by infection. Severe frequency suggests acute infection, a bladder stone, or a large residuum almost to the state of complete retention; chronic complete urinary retention with overflow or paradoxical incontinence gives rise to constant frequency (dribbling). In addition to the difficulty of urination, complicating infection may cause burning, strangury, tenesmus or terminal dribbling. When diverticulum complicates the vesical obstructive uropathy, the patient finds that if he waits a few seconds or a minute after emptying himself, he is able to pass a small or large amount more. This last urine represents emptying of the diverticulum and is often mucopurulent or foul. This symptom— the *pis en deux* or *miction en deux temps* of the French—must be differentiated from interrupted urination due to spasm or contracture of the vesical outlet, ureterocele, stone, or a tumor blocking this orifice.

Urethra. The symptoms of urethral obstruction are much like those

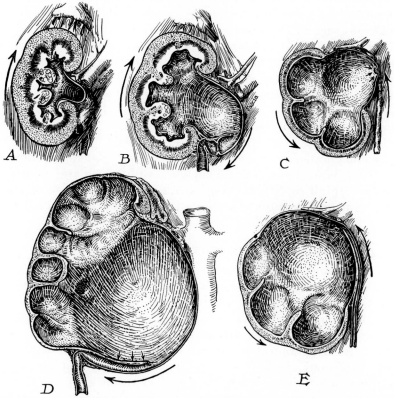

FIGURE 53. Development of hydronephrosis in a movable kidney. The periureteral fascia at the ureterovesical junction acts as a fulcrum to increase ureteral obstruction. Once begun, the process becomes a vicious cycle; the developing hydronephrosis causes increased renal sagging which, in turn, increases the obstruction. *A*, early clockwise rotation of kidney with beginning angulation of juxtapelvic ureter. *B*, increased obstruction with continued rotation. *C*, counterclockwise rotation and sagging of right kidney with elevation and often spur-valve formation at ureteropelvic junction. *D*, advanced clockwise rotation of right kidney with low spur-formation obstruction. *E*, same as *D*, but counterclockwise rotation.

of vesical outlet blockage just described. In both conditions bilateral renal back-pressure injury may progress to cause uremia, urotoxemia or urinary sepsis. Rupture of the distended urethra induces periurethral phlegmon or urinary extravasation.

A *tight phimotic orifice* causes ballooning of the prepuce with each voiding; ulceration of the underlying tissue may develop. Other symptoms are those of urethral blockage proper.

Diagnosis in all types of obstructive uropathy depends upon a complete urologic examination including cystourethroscopy and urography. The distended bladder may be palpable and disappear with catheterization. The progressive urographic changes are given in Table 5, and Figures 91 to 95 are illustrative. Some dilatation of the upper urinary tract will result from infection or atonic neuromuscular disease alone.

In hydronephrosis the ureteropelvic junction should be urographically demonstrated with special clarity to be sure there is no stricture, stone or vascular blockage at this point. As a rule, in large hydronephrosis, the pelvis rotates upwards and inwards towards the spine on an anterior-posterior horizontal axis, thus moving the ureteropelvic junction upward to make the angulation acute (spur-valve formation, Fig. 53). Similarly in ureterography, the results of obstructing stone, stricture, aberrant vessel(s), valves, and so forth will be recognized although their precise nature may be unknown until surgical exploration.

The *prognosis* in obstructive uropathy depends upon (1) the site, severity and duration of the blockage, (2) whether bilateral or unilateral, and (3) the promptness and thoroughness with which free drainage is established. In all cases relieved of obstruction, the prognosis should be guarded until sufficient time has elapsed to evaluate the renal rehabilitation.

TREATMENT IN URINARY OBSTRUCTION

The fundamentals of treatment in urinary obstruction are:
1. Immediate relief of retention and copious administration of fluids.
2. Establishment of the correct anatomic diagnosis.
3. Determination and improvement of renal function preparatory to
4. Definitive removal of the obstruction.

Thus in acute vesical retention prompt urethral catheterization is needed. In chronic vesical retention preliminary indwelling urethral catheterization may be necessary for a week or two to aid in renal stabilization before cystostomy is performed to give protracted free drainage. Similarly, an indwelling ureteral catheter is sometimes both life and kidney saving, awaiting sufficient recovery of the organ to warrant a nephrostomy for prolonged drainage. Repeated vesical or ureterorenal catheterization is advised against for, no matter how precise and careful the technique, one cannot avoid the introduction of bacteria into these congested debilitated fields with their minimal resistance to infection. Thus in 71 patients who died after vesical catheterization in the presence of large residual urine or chronic complete retention, Creevy found that in only five was death not caused by renal infection. Fortunately present-day antimicrobial therapy will do much to prevent and control instrumental infection but this does not permit laxity in aseptic technique nor poor surgical judgment.

A simple method for fixation of an indwelling nonballoon catheter is shown in Figure 54, and the use of the balloon catheter is illustrated in Figure 55. During the period of indwelling catheterization, it is well that the patient receive prophylactically a mild urinary antiseptic, for example a half gram of one of the newer sulfonamide preparations such as sulfa-soxazole (Gantrisin) four times a day. The catheter should be changed at least once a week and the method used for not over four weeks.

Vesical drainage by indwelling catheter may be prevented by inability to pass a catheter because of an obstruction, be contraindicated by intolerance of the urethra to the catheter and, frequently seen, complicating epididymitis and/or prostatitis. These conditions demand that cystostomy be employed at once for vesical drainage.

In any event, if prolonged drainage seems likely to be required, perform cystostomy; the Campbell *cystostomy trocar* permits rapid and simple suprapubic introduction of a balloon catheter into the bladder, it being the only instrument enabling introduction of a balloon retention tube (Figs. 56, 57).

With free bladder drainage established, copious fluid intake is given. There may be temporary oliguria but more often a compensatory polyuria

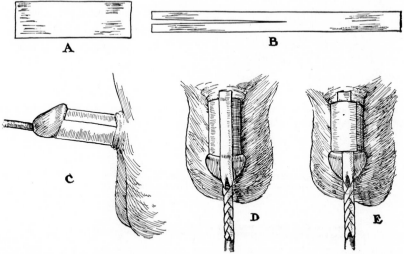

FIGURE 54. Method of fastening an indwelling catheter. *A, C,* small strips of adhesive tape are applied behind the glans from which the prepuce has been retracted. *B,* two tail strips of adhesive used to hold the catheter in place. As shown in *D,* one strip is applied on the dorsal and one on the ventral surface of the penis. *E,* application of a second strip of adhesive like *A* completes the technique. Today balloon catheters have largely replaced the usual type of urethral catheter for indwelling retention.

occurs with which the kidneys excrete a large amount of urine of low urea content, yet the total nitrogen output may be greater than normal. Care must be taken not to drown the patient with overhydration at this time. Ten glasses of fluid (2500 to 3000 cc.) by mouth or intramuscularly within twenty-four hours are usually sufficient, and in younger and smaller patients the fluid intake is correspondingly less. For variety and especially in children, fluids may be given as water, milk, glucose (1 to 2%), lemon, orange or limeades. Acidosis or alkalosis are treated as previously described in Chapter 2. Plasma protein deficiency is counteracted

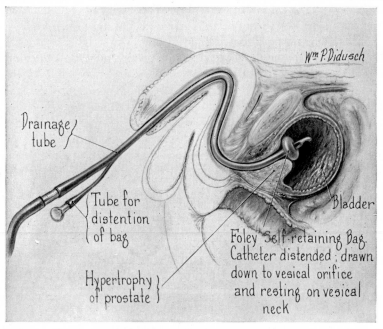

FIGURE 55.   Foley self-retaining urethral catheter with inflation bag. Sectional view showing the inflation bag distended, anchoring the catheter securely in the bladder. (Courtesy of American Cystoscope Makers, Inc.)

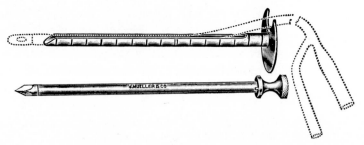

FIGURE 56.   Campbell cystostomy trocar for the introduction of balloon catheters. The obturator is tipped with a sharp stainless steel spearhead. With this trocar cystotomy has readily been performed in children as young as twenty-four hours of age. It has also been employed several times in establishing nephrostomy drainage.

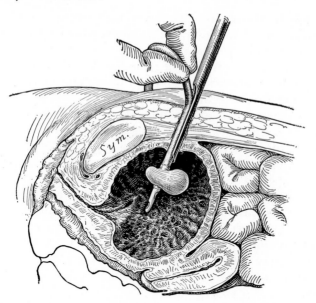

FIGURE 57. Suprapubic cystotomy employing the Campbell fenestrated trocar. As shown, the tube functions as a shoehorn or gorget along the groove of which the uninflated balloon catheter or other drainage tube is introduced into the bladder. Before withdrawing the trocar sheath, the balloon catheter should be inflated to prevent its accidental removal. The trocar is introduced into the well-distended bladder at a point about a third of the distance to the umbilicus and in a downward and forward direction judged to be toward the posterior border of the trigone. A small incision about 1 cm. long, made through the skin and the fascia of the rectus abdominus muscles, not only greatly facilitates the introduction of the instrument but minimizes trauma.

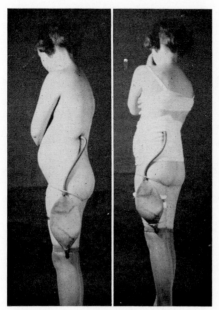

FIGURE 58. Nephrostomy. Method of maintaining nephrostomy tube drainage in an eight year-old patient. The nephrostomy tube drains into an 8-ounce rubber flounder bag.

by high protein intake or even the intravenous administration of whole
blood plasma or one of the amino-acid compounds of hydrolyzed casein
derivation (e.g., amogen).

When (1) the kidney is blocked off at the ureteropelvic junction and
is not spontaneously relieved or (2) when indwelling ureteropelvic catheterization is impossible because of impassable obstruction or is inadequate, perform nephrostomy and maintain this drainage until the blockage
can be relieved definitively and permanently. Do not attempt ureteropelvioplasty on the acutely inflamed edematous infected kidney as it is
poor surgical judgment and presaged to failure through faulty tissue
repair and postoperative sclerosis.

When full upper urinary tract drainage is not achieved by cystostomy, perform the necessary examination to determine the site and nature
of the blockage (page 39); the intrarenal back pressure will continue its
injurious activity until the pelvis is drained by nephrostomy or pyelostomy as necessary (Fig. 58). A convenient method of anchoring nephrostomy, ureterostomy, cystostomy or other drainage tubes is shown
in Figure 59.

Secondary ureteral obstructions, kinks, adhesions, and so forth, are
relieved by (1) ureterolysis (freeing of the ureter), especially at the
ureteropelvic junction, (2) resection of redundant ureter with oblique
end-to-end anastomosis, and (3) removal of stones or other conditions or
lesions which may obstruct. Ureteral dilation is seldom of value except
in low stricture and without secondary kink blockage. Other procedures
to relieve ureteral blockage include removal of aberrant vascular obstruction, plastic operation on the ureteropelvic junction or environs, nephros-

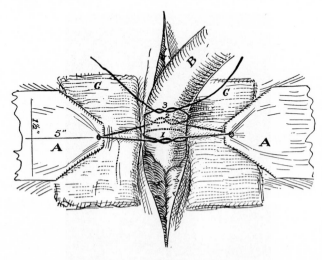

Figure 59. Drainage tube fixation. Author's method which can be employed for
holding tubes in any body cavity. *A*, adhesive skin-traction strips. *B*, drainage tube or
catheter tied in place by ligature. Knots 1, 2 and 3 are tied about the tube in the order
indicated; a small gauze dressing (*C*) is put beneath the traction ligatures.

tomy, renal resection (ureteroheminephrectomy), and often nephrectomy or ureteronephrectomy according to the demonstrated uropathy.

In sum, urinary back-pressure damage will be prevented or reduced only by complete eradication of all stasis producing conditions. To avoid needless reiteration here of the many obstructive lesions and their treatment, the reader is referred to Table 9 in Chapter 7.

CHAPTER 6 *Embryology and Anomalies of the Urogenital Tract**

INTRODUCTION

MORE THAN 10 per cent (10 to 14) of all humans are born with some urogenital anomaly. Excepting spina bifida occulta which 35 per cent of all people have and which is seldom clinically important, the urogenital anomalies comprise 35 to 40 per cent of all developmental mishaps. Some of the graver anomalies are never seen in adults because their bearers promptly die in infancy. The United States death registration in 1950 showed congenital malformations still to be the sixth most common cause of death in children one to four years of age: 15 per 100,000. It is obvious that in the absence of post-mortem examination only the more apparent malformations such as vesical exstrophy are recorded on the death certificate but these represent only a small portion of all urogenital tract developmental errors which will be discovered during life by adequate urologic investigation or after death by autopsy.

The influences and factors giving rise to anomalous development, in short, the causes, are unknown. No amount of unfavorable maternal impression can alter the chromosomal gene patterns of the primitive germinal union. Vitamin deficiency (riboflavin; Warkany), chemical substances (sterols and estrogens; Greene et al.), and virus infection, (especially eye opacities in children whose mothers had rubella (German measles) during the first trimester of pregnancy), have been advanced as possible causes. Many other agents thought to be unfavorable to normal fetal development have been cited with suggestive corroboration; these

* The reader interested in a detailed discussion of the Embryology and Anomalies of the Urogenital Tract is referred to Campbell's Clinical Pediatric Urology, Chapter III, W. B. Saunders Co., 1951.

include syphilis, x-rays, alcoholism, contraception, endocrine factors (infantilism, dwarfism, gigantism, cretinism), environment, heredity (Huntington's chorea, sickle cell anemia, gargoylism, Laurence-Moon-Biedl syndrome, and so forth), abnormal maturation of sex genes (hypospadias, pseudohermaphrodism), or of children born after a miscarriage, abortion, or premature birth. In a family with an antecedent background of congenital anomalies, it is not unusual to have spina bifida in one, vesical exstrophy in another, hypospadias in another, and cleft palate, for example, in still another. Dietary factors, parental age difference, illegitimacy, placenta previa, or rapid succession of pregnancies apparently are not acceptable as etiologic in anomalous development.

Murphy has probably made the best statistical study of the likelihood of occurrence of anomalies in siblings from a mother who, having given birth to a child with one or more congenital malformations, will have subsequent children with maldevelopments. It was found that anomalies occurred in 12.4 per cent (1 in 8) of families with another child subsequent to the deformed child; in about half (47 per cent) of the cases the malformations of two children in the same family were reduplicated and in 41 per cent the same anomaly had existed in distant relatives.

Whether they should have more children is a grave question of parents who have just given birth to a malformed child. The physician's advice is of vital concern here, not only in maintaining harmony, happiness and understanding in the family but in the possible relation and problem of subsequent children to society as a whole. On the basis of Murphy's findings, parents who have had a malformed child may well be advised: "Offspring presenting congenital malformations which are serious enough to warrant being recorded on death certificates are approximately twenty-four times as likely to occur in a family possessing a congenitally deformed child as in the population at large." However, clinical observation and statistical study suggest that this is not necessarily true with lesser malformations such as hypospadias for while we do occasionally encounter a family history of the condition in two or three generations, it is most unusual and in such cases the having of future children need not be interdicted. In sum: (a) when a congenital malformation has a genetic basis there is a greatly increased chance that subsequent brothers or sisters will also be malformed, but (b) when a congenital defect is due to factors that are not genetic, offspring subsequently conceived should be congenitally malformed only in the same frequency as is commonly observed in the general public.

Because of their associated embryologic development, the urinary and the genital tracts in each sex must be considered as one. The organs of the urinary and the genital tract (a) have a common origin from the intermediate cell mass, (b) primitive excretory ducts of the pronephros and metanephros are incorporated in the male genital organs, and (c) have a common relation with the primitive cloaca. As a corollary, when the genitalia show major malformation (hypospadias, vesical exstrophy, reduplicated uterus, uterus unicornis and so forth) there is a one in three chance that the upper urinary tract is also anomalous, ureteral reduplication being the most frequent finding. Conversely, with upper urinary tract malformations (renal hypoplasia, agenesis, horseshoe kidney formation for example) genital anomalies are common and in the female occur in two thirds of the cases. Urogenital anomalies are commonly multiple with collateral maldevelopment in each organ system as, for example, cryptorchism and isolateral renal agenesis or hypoplasia. An understanding of the fundamentals of embryology will make clear to the clinician the genesis and nature of the urogenital anomalies and are considered together in this chapter.

DEFINITION OF TERMS

Congenital means that the condition was present at birth.

Agenesis defines total absence of an organ or failure of a part to develop. It results from absence of primordial tissue from which the structure normally arises or from failure of the particular structure growth to be initiated, e.g., agenesis of the kidney or testes.

Aplasia means incomplete development of a structure resulting from (a) a slower than normal development ratio, or (b) retardation of normal progressive processes, or (c) arrest of the process already begun. This is observed in imperfect descent of the testis, ectopic ureteral orifice, or in abnormalities of renal size and position.

Hypoplasia designates incomplete or defective development and is usually used in describing organs which are smaller than normal size and consequent to imperfect formation of the structure such as hypoplastic kidney, testis, ureter or penis.

Paraplasia is structure formation away from normal development as exemplified in urethral or ureteral stenosis, renal fusion, or duplication of homologous sets of genital ducts.

It is axiomatic that an anomalous organ is more prone to disease than a normally formed one. For this reason, in Urology, a large portion of the clinical problems are derived from anomalous development and this is especially striking in infants and children. Many malformations of the upper urinary tract cause urinary obstruction which may produce symptoms of its own, predispose to urinary infection, or create an abnormal mass leading to erroneous diagnosis. At least 20 per cent of adults with upper urinary tract anomalies have had needless abdominal operations performed for symptoms caused by these malformations. This is especially notable in congenital ureteral blockage and particularly when congenital stricture or complicating stone erroneously leads to appendectomy for "chronic appendicitis."

EMBRYOLOGY OF THE KIDNEY

The development of the kidney is progressive through three separate structural stages: the pronephros, the mesonephros (wolffian body proper), and the metanephros which becomes the permanent kidney (Fig. 60, *A*).

The *pronephros* is an ontogenetic remnant of the excretory system in lower vertebrates, arises and develops independently cephalad on each side as six to ten pairs of tubules with a connecting duct called the *wolffian* or *primary excretory duct* which opens into the celomic cavity. The pronephros degenerates by the fourth week to leave only the woffian duct which rapidly grows to extend the length of the nephrogenic cord, and opens into the cloaca which is the dilated end of the cavity (Fig. 60, *B*).

The *mesonephros* appears just before the pronephros completely disappears. Derived from the mesoblastic intermediate cell mass, it consists of tubules which empty into the mesonephric (wolffian) duct, and appears first opposite the upper dorsal segments. When fully developed its caudal end is at the third lumbar level (Fig. 60). In its development, functioning glomeruli and collecting tubules appear. By the twelfth to fourteenth week, the mesonephros degenerates but a small portion of the collecting tubules persist in the adult female reproductive tract as the duct of Gartner, the epoophoron and paroophoron, and in the male as the ductuli efferentes, ductuli aberrantes, and paradidymis of the epididymis. Persistence of Gartner's duct explains ectopic ureteral opening into the vagina, cervix, or uterus.

The *metanephros* or true renal secretory anlage is composed of a secretory or glandular segment and a collecting or efferent drainage system; during mesonephric degeneration it appears caudally at the second and third sacral level as the nephrogenic cord (renal blastema). The renal vascular supply is established at this time and the collecting or drainage renal elements are formed by a posterior budding from the metanephric or wolffian duct when it turns sharply to enter the cloaca (Fig. 82). These ureteral buds grow cephalad to form the ureters, enter and become surrounded by the metanephrogenic blastema and, by division and subdivision of the upper end of the ureteral stalk, form the renal

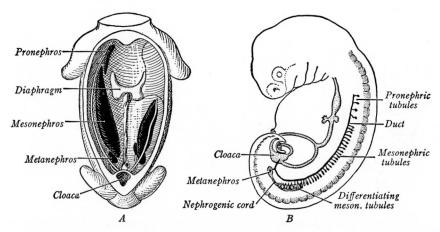

FIGURE 60.   Schematic indication of the location and relations of the three stages of development of the kidney in man. *A*, note the high thoracic origin of the pronephros, the abdominal site of the mesonephros and the extremely low initial location of the metanephros or permanent kidney. *B*, lateral schema of *A* (Arey).

pelvis, major and minor calyces, and dividing further, the renal collecting tubules.

By the fifth month the nephrogenic cap has been carried in with and surrounds the tips of the newly formed collecting tubules, enclosing the capillary tuft to form the glomerulus with its drainage tubule (nephron unit). Histocount estimations have variously placed the number of glomeruli in a kidney between 1,250,000 (Pitts) and 4,500,000 (Traut). With the union of the glomerular secretory unit and the end of the collecting tubule, the renal unit or reniculus (Fig. 68) is formed; failure of the glomerular and tubular structures to unite is believed to cause polycystic and some other varieties of cystic renal disease.

The *renal cortex* is derived from the metanephrogenic blastema, covers the bases of the medullary pyramids and imparts a surface lobulation phylogenetic of lower vertebrates and some mammals (ox, bear, bird). Usually this *fetal lobulation* is lost by the fifth year but in about 5 per cent of all individuals, persists into adulthood but without clinical importance. The primary renal columns of Bertin are formed as central extensions of the cortex between the papillae of the medullary pyramids. It is notable that there is true cellular multiplication in the kidney structure up to the fourth or fifth year but after that time in renal hypertrophy the kidney cells simply enlarge and do not regenerate or multiply as occurs in liver regeneration, for example.

The renal *fibrous capsule* is derived from mesoderm which surrounds the fetal kidney.

Ascent of the kidney from its primary low pelvic location begins about the seventh and eighth week, and the previously forward facing pelvis *rotates* medially (Fig. 61). Failure of these processes to occur explains renal ectopy and renal malrotation. Actually the kidney does not actively ascend but, rather, rapid spinal growth caudad occurs and away

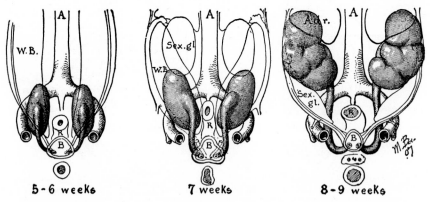

5-6 weeks   7 weeks   8-9 weeks

FIGURE 61.   Renal ascent and rotation during fetal life. The normal rotation of the kidney from facing forward to facing medially is shown. Fusion of either renal pole produces horseshoe kidney (compare Fig. 71). This fusion must occur by the seventh week. (Kelly-Burnham, courtesy Appleton Company.)

from the (pelvic) kidney, as it were. By the fifth month the upper pole of the kidney is at the level of the eleventh rib as found in normal adults (Fig. 25).

The *blood supply* of the kidney is established during the eighth or ninth week from the aorta and vena cava at the second lumbar level prior to which the nephrogenic blastema is supplied with vessels of more caudad origin which, by persisting, account for many cases of renal ectopy, the kidney being prevented from ascending by its initial vascular attachments which refuse to disappear. Normally the renal vessels enter at the pelvis (Fig. 62), but in a third of all individuals the arterial supply is multiple and in a far larger number the venous return is anomalous, especially on the left, considerations of vast moment to a surgeon operating upon a kidney (Fig. 63).

At birth the kidneys are disproportionately large and in a dehydrated emaciated newborn infant the comparatively huge renal masses may erroneously cause a diagnosis of polycystic disease, hydronephrosis, or tumor to be made.

The *adrenal gland* in early life is also disproportionately large, overlies and partially surrounds the kidney (see Chapt. 14).

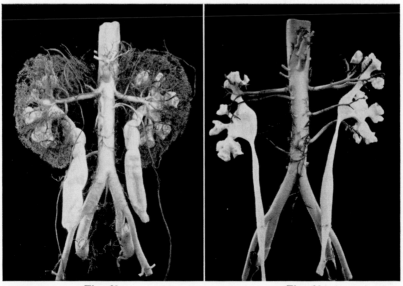

Fig. 62   Fig. 63

FIGURE 62. Normal renal blood supply. Corrosion specimen (late fetal life) showing the unusually rich vascularization of the organs (Morison). Note the normally large size of the ureters at this period.

FIGURE 63. Accessory renal vessels demonstrated by celluloid corrosion preparation. Full-term fetus. The renal pelves and ureters are shown in relationship to the main arterial distribution. On each side there are two accessory renal vessels above and one below, the lower one on the left being in proximity to the ureterovesical junction. The lowermost vessel on the left might well become a cause of ureteral obstruction by compressing the duct. (Morison.)

ANOMALIES OF KIDNEY

Congenital renal anomalies may be classified as

I. Anomalies of Number
  1. Bilateral agenesis
  2. Unilateral agenesis (solitary kidney)
  3. Supernumerary kidney

II. Anomalies of Volume and Structure
  1. Hypoplasia
  2. Congenital hypertrophy
  3. Solitary cystic disease
  4. Multilocular cystic disease
  5. Polycystic disease

III. Anomalies of Form
  1. Short, long, round, hour-glass or lobulated kidneys
  2. Horseshoe kidney
  3. Disc or doughnut kidney
  4. Sigmoid kidney or L-shaped kidney
  5. Lump kidney

IV. Anomalies of Location
  1. Simple ectopia
    a. unilateral
    b. bilateral
  2. Crossed ectopia with or without fusion
  3. Movable kidney

V. Anomalies of Rotation
  1. Incomplete
  2. Excessive

VI. Anomalies of the Pelvis
  1. Double kidney
    a. unilateral
    b. bilateral
    c. complete reduplication
    d. incomplete reduplication
  2. Pseudo-spider form
  3. Congenital hydronephrosis
  4. Extrarenal pelvis

VII. Anomalies of the Vessels
  1. Arterial
  2. Venous

I. Anomalies of Number

Bilateral renal agenesis occurs once in about 3000 (2721) autopsies*
and is incompatible with life, its duration at maximum being no longer

---

* In this chapter the average incidence of the anomaly is given as based on our study
of many reported series in the literature. Following this, in parentheses, is given the incidence in 51,880 autopsies in people of all ages as ascertained by minute protocol
abstraction and tabulation by myself and assistants at hospitals with which I have been

than that following bilateral nephrectomy, viz: ten to eleven days. Anomalies of other body systems are regularly found, many of which would eventually be fatal even if the patient had sound kidneys.*

Unilateral agenesis (congenital solitary kidney). This results from (1) failure of the renal bud to develop, (2) failure of the nephrogenic blastema to form, (3) both, or (4) failure of the vascular supply to form. The arrested development of the wolffian duct prevents formation of the isolateral primitive urogenital nucleus which accounts in turn not only for failure of the isolateral urinary tract to form but often of the isolateral genital apparatus as well.

Renal agenesis occurs once in about 600 persons (1:527; 1:391 in infants; 1:655 in adults). This occurs in each sex and on each side about

---

* With one urogenital maldevelopment, other anomalies commonly occur both elsewhere in the urinary tract and in other body systems. To emphasize this point and avoid subsequent repetition, the variety of the coexisting major anomalies observed in our autopsy series (51,880) is here given. Of course, not every case showing a urogenital tract anomaly had any of these other anomalies but the coincidence is high and clinically should ever be kept in mind.

The anomalies discussed in this chapter may be multiple, this likelihood being inversely proportional to their rarity. In the *gastrointestinal tract* were found maldevelopment of the bowel and particularly the lower segment, imperforate anus, atresia or stenosis of the rectum, urethrorectal fistula, patent cloaca, Meckel's and other intestinal diverticula, harelip, cleft palate, esophagus atresia, esophagotracheal fistula, situs inversus, congenitally small stoma, pyloric stenosis, duodenal or jejunal stenosis, incomplete rotation of the colon, rotation of the cecum, hepatic anomalies (absent, dwarf or cystic gallbladder), cavernous cholangitis, cystic pancreas, pancreatic tissue in the duodenum, hamartoma of the intestines; *cardiovascular anomalies:* patent ductus arteriosus, patent foramen ovale, mitral atresia, atresia of pulmonary artery, patent auricular septum, patent interventricular septum, anomalous coronary vessels, accessory coronary arteries, auricular hypertrophy, ventricular chamber dilated, cor loculare congenital heart, bicuspid aortic valve, congenital bicuspid valve, hypoplastic aorta, accessory aortic ostia, "congenital heart disease," cardiac hypoplasia, ventricular atresia, anomalous left carotid, accessory renal arteries, hypoplastic renal arteries, dextraposition of aorta; *skeletal anomalies:* clubfeet, clubhands, supernumerary digits, polydactilism, absent foot, leg, arm or hand, absent other bones, hemivertebrae, spina bifida, osteogenesis imperfecta, hyperplasia of mandible, syndactilism, talipes varus, rib fusion, hypertelorism, vestigial tail, vestigial auricle, atresia soft palate, agenesis of skeletal muscle, nonfusion of symphysis; *central nervous system:* hydrocephalus, anencephalus, mongolianism, meningocele, malformed brain, optic atrophy, meningomyelocele; *gynecologic anomalies:* double, unicorn, bicornuate, cystic, absent or infantile uterus, absent, infantile or double vagina, vaginorectal fistula, cystic ovary, parovarian cyst, absent cervix, malformation of uterus and tubes, persistance of Gartner's duct; *pulmonary anomalies:* absent, dwarf or anomalous lung, supernumerary lobe, absent fissures, diaphragmatic hernia, absent diaphragm, azygos lobe of the lung.

---

associated in the past (Bellevue, University, St. Vincent's, Willard Parker, Babies, New York Nursery & Childs in the city of New York, and the Mountainside Hospital in Montclair, N. J.). Of these 51,880 post-mortem examinations, 36.7 per cent (19,046) were in infants and children; 63.3 per cent (32,834) were sixteen years or older. Two thirds of the younger age group were less than six months of age and a little over half of all child patients (55.6 per cent) were males. Of the adults, nearly three fourths (71.9 per cent) were males while a third (32.2 per cent) were between forty-one and fifty-five years of age. This autopsy series is large enough accurately to reflect the average incidence of these urologic anomalies in the population at large. To these statistics from the dead house are added data from substantial series of personal clinical cases as well as selected citations.

equally.In one fourth of our autopsy cases the patient died of renal failure. In a few cases the only kidney has unwittingly been removed.

The solitary kidney itself is often hyperplastic and may be polycystic or ectopic. Accompanying anomalies in the pulmonary, gastrointestinal, cardiovascular and skeletal apparatus are frequent.

The *diagnosis* of congenital solitary kidney will be suggested by the excretory pyelogram which shows no renal shadow on one side and will be confirmed by complete urologic examination when an absent ureteral orifice or hemiatrophy of the trigone may be observed and only one kidney is demonstrable (Fig. 64).

The *treatment* of congenital solitary kidney is that of the existing disease and in all circumstances, since it is the only kidney, therapy must be conservative—whether surgical or nonsurgical. Many of these hopelessly incurable obstructed solitary kidneys can be treated only by permanent nephrostomy drainage; calculous anuria by blockage of the single ureter demands immediate ureterolithotomy.

Supernumerary Kidney. *Free.* This is probably the rarest renal anomaly, some 50 cases being reported; it was found in two of our autopsy series (1 in approximately 25,000). The *symptoms* of disease when present are those common to the particular type of involvement as in stone, hydronephrosis or infection in a normally formed kidney. The *diagnosis* is made by urography and *treatment* is removal of the diseased organ, assuming adequate renal tissue will remain.

Fused supernumerary kidney occurs once in about 4000 persons and must be considered as a reduplicated organ whose transverse separation is incomplete, the embryonic groove being that of the usual renal reduplication.

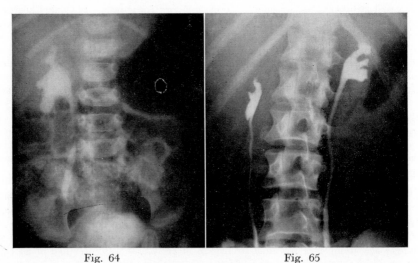

Fig. 64   Fig. 65

FIGURE 64.   Unilateral (left) renal agenesis suggested by excretory urography and later surgically confirmed.

FIGURE 65.   Bilateral renal hypoplasia in a five-year-old girl; the abnormality on the right is pronounced while that on the left is less so.

II. ANOMALIES OF VOLUME AND STRUCTURE

Renal Aplasia. Here the kidney is represented only by the faintest suggestion of renal development, there being no evidence of true kidney pelvis or vascular connection present and the "tubular" structures are most scant. When glomeruli are present, the condition should be classified as hypoplastic kidney (vide infra). The ureter is absent or without a lumen. The anomalous mass may cause pain by fibrotic compression of nerve endings or hypertension may exist on the basis of the Goldblatt renal ischemia mechanism (q.v.). Treatment is removal of the aplastic organ assuming a competent renal mate exists.

Renal hypoplasia occurs once in about 600 persons which is about the same incidence as renal agenesis (1:527) and results from failure of development of (1) the metanephrogenic blastema, (2) the metanephric duct, or (3) the blood supply. It is generally unilateral but may be bilateral and must be distinguished from secondary renal atrophy due to obstruction or infection. Characteristically, the organ, besides being smaller than normal and perhaps even only a little nubbin, shows poor development, often with rudimentary glomeruli and tubules, may be fibrofatty or cystic, and lies closer to the spine than normal (Fig. 65). The vascular supply and especially the arteries are smaller than normal, usually sclerotic, and account for the hypertensive vascular syndrome so often seen in these cases (Goldblatt kidney), and which generally is promptly cured by removal of the hypoplastic kidney. In a third of 112 cases of renal hypoplasia examined post mortem, death was due to renal failure.

The isolateral **adrenal gland** is hypoplastic or pathologic in 10 per cent of the cases while the **ureter** is hypoplastic in a third, strictured in 15 per cent, and occasionally entirely lacking.

Pain in the site of the hypoplastic organ is the usual symptom but hypertension may direct investigation to the urinary tract and here divided renal function tests and pyelography, particularly retrograde, may be expected to make the diagnosis. By urography, the pelvis is shown to be much smaller than normal, undeveloped, sometimes ampullatory or triangular, and occasionally of the unicalyceal or rabbit type (Fig. 65). Nephrectomy is the treatment.

Congenital hypertrophy of the kidney occurs as a compensatory embryologic mechanism in renal agenesis or hypoplasia. An acquired compensatory enlargement usually follows surgical removal of its mate. There is no treatment for renal hypertrophy nor is any desired.

Redundancy of the renal parenchyma usually appears as a double row of pyramids with a layer of cortex sandwiched between. The condition is of academic interest only.

Congenital renal cysts are rare (1:1600 in infants and children), are usually bilateral, occasionally produce an abdominal tumor with which there may be pain or, on occasion, hematuria. The condition is believed to be due to the same mechanism which causes polycystic renal disease (q.v.)—failure of union of the collecting tubules and the glomerular secreting unit, or by tubular obstruction.

Solitary cystic disease is quite different from polycystic disease or the cystic degeneration so commonly seen in sclerotic nephritis, or from dermoid cyst and hamartoma (q.v.). The cyst, more common at the lower pole, is thin walled, lined with serosa, and serous filled although blood and other debris may be present (Fig. 66). A cyst may (1) grow to enormous size, (2) compress the functioning parenchyma, (3) extend beyond the surface, or (4) by renal vascular damage cause hypertension. The cyst mass may compress the bowel. The diagnosis is made by urography which shows a localized and usually smoothly rounded or crescentic filling defect, or pelviocalyceal distortion caused by the cystic mass(es) (Fig. 66). Occasionally the cyst wall is calcified (Fig. 67). Cyst must be differentiated from malignant tumor. Renal angiography (aortography) may assist in the differential diagnosis, the avascular cyst area remaining clear while a tumor area is clouded with puddling of radiopaque medium in the neoplasm (Figs. 244 and 245). In most cases the cyst can be excised to preserve the good functioning renal parenchyma but when this is not worth saving, remove the kidney.

Congenital multilocular cysts may be considered as a collection of solitary cysts; doubtless the etiology is the same as in polycystic disease (q.v.) and the condition is rare. Pathologically the lesion must be differentiated from cystadenoma of the kidney and polycystic disease but the last is characteristically bilateral. The symptoms are those caused by pressure of the cystic mass on adjacent organs. The diagnosis is made by

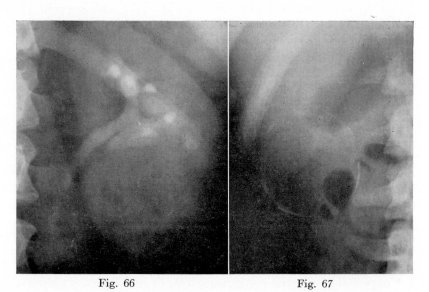

Fig. 66   Fig. 67

Figure 66. Solitary cyst of left lower renal pole causing upward compression and crescentic distortion of the inferior calyx. Surgical resection.

Figure 67. Calcified right renal cyst. Resected.

urography but often is erroneously that of renal tumor. When symptoms or the condition of the patient demands, nephrectomy is the treatment.

Congenital renal polycystic disease is recognized as a nodular cystic involvement, predominantly bilateral, and is to be distinguished from cystic renal degeneration so often seen in chronic nephritis (Fig. 68). About one in 265 infants are born with congenital renal polycystic disease but many of these die early so that the incidence in adults is approximately one in 300 (293). In cases apparently unilateral, only the demonstration of a renal mate free from cysts makes the diagnosis acceptable and this is most rare. As these congenital cysts enlarge, the intervening secretory parenchyma is seriously impaired and ultimately destroyed by compression. Large polycystic kidneys in the maternal pelvis or in the fetal abdomen may cause dystocia. In half of the cases the patients reach midlife before the diagnosis is made; as a general prognostic corollary, the later the diagnosis is made, the better the outlook.

Congenital hepatic cysts occur in about 5 per cent, splenic cysts in about 4 per cent, and pancreatic cysts in about 2 per cent of all cases of polycystic renal disease.

Congenital polycystic renal disease is one urologic condition which shows a striking *familial hereditary tendency* and has been traced through as many as five generations, the condition being a mendelian recessive.

The *etiology* of chronic polycystic disease is unknown. Hildebrandt's theory, one of the oldest, is still the most widely accepted and is based on the conception of failure of the nephrogenic blastemic elements (glomeruli) to unite with the wolffian derivatives—the renal tubules (Fig. 68). Blockage of the glomerular filtration by the nonunion results in cyst formation.

Polycystic kidneys may be enormous, ten to fifteen times normal size and extend from the diaphragm well down into the pelvis, gravely compressing and dislodging the abdominal viscera (Fig. 69). The cysts contain a watery yellow or brown fluid which may be colloid, mucoid, purulent or bloody but never urinous; cholesterol, leucine, cystine, uric acid, calcium oxalate or pus may be present. The cysts do not connect with the renal pelvis and seldom with each other. The compressed intercystic parenchyma shows interstitial nephritis to which the complicating lesions of infection, hydronephrosis or calculous disease may be added, greatly

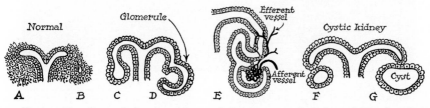

FIGURE 68. Congenital polycystic renal disease as attributed to glomerulo-tubular malunion. Formation of the glomerulus. *E*, ingrowth of the vascular tuft is indicated. *F*, *G*, schematically illustrate the prevailing theory of the etiology of renal polycystic disease, viz: failure of union between the excretory and the collecting elements of the renal units.

affecting the prognosis, and complicating treatment or rendering it entirely hopeless.

Symptoms. The clinical manifestations of nephritis are dominant but hematuria, pain, pyuria or tumor commonly occur. Compression of the abdominal viscera may produce pronounced gastrointestinal disturbances even to the point of obstipation. With advancing renal insufficiency, urotoxic gastrointestinal disturbances become pronounced. Much of the anemia results from nephrotoxic injury of the hemopoetic system (bone marrow) and therapeutically requires adequate whole-blood transfusion.

The *prognosis* is always bad; the earlier the diagnosis is made the poorer the prognosis and the shorter is the life expectancy. When recognized in childhood the patients are almost always dead within two years and commonly within three months but adults with the disease may live ten years or more after its discovery.

The *diagnosis* is suggested by palpation of the enlarged and usually nodular masses in the renal regions and especially when bilateral. On the basis of the urinalysis the diagnosis of chronic interstitial nephritis is usually made. The blood pressure may or may not be elevated. The diagnosis is confirmed by pyelography in which the retrograde is preferable to the excretory method. The pyelogram is characteristically bizarre, the more usual diagnostic changes being (a) shortening, obliteration, compression or elongation of the calyces with peculiar squared, oval or crescentic rounded outlines; (b) pelvic compression, distortion, displacement, obliteration or dilatation and (c) with infection, its superimposed changes (Fig. 70). While all of these changes are seldom found in a single pyelogram, many of them will be present and warrant the diagnosis of polycystic disease.

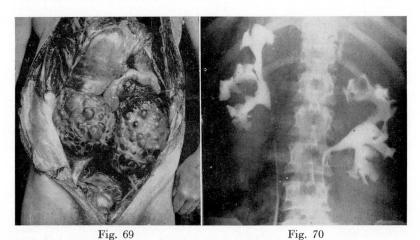

Fig. 69   Fig. 70

FIGURE 69.   Bilateral congenital polycystic renal disease as demonstrated post mortem in a 27-year-old woman.

FIGURE 70.   Congenital polycystic renal disease. Pyelograms show the usual bilaterality of the condition with the characteristic bizarre pelvic deformities caused by the cystic renal changes.

The *treatment* of uncomplicated polycystic disease is that of nephritis. The less surgical treatment is employed the longer the patient will live. Obstruction, infection, hematuria, stone or continued pain may require antimicrobial therapy and/or surgical intervention. Following nephrectomy, half of the patients will die during the immediate postoperative period; a third will die within the postoperative month. Cyst puncture may relieve pain in some cases but at best is a temporizing measure.

III. ANOMALIES OF FORM

Fetal lobulation of the kidney is normal up to the age of four or five years but in 5 per cent of all individuals persists throughout life. It is of no clinical concern.

Fusion of the kidney. This may be homolateral or contralateral. Reduplicated or double kidney is the common example of homolateral fusion and is discussed later in this chapter. Contralateral fusion is found once in about 400 persons and is generally of the horseshoe variety with fusion at the lower or upper poles but in some instances, of both poles giving rise to the doughnut, scutiform or disc kidney. The upper pole of one organ may be fused with the lower pole of its mate to produce an L-shaped or sigmoid kidney or the entire renal mass may be contra-

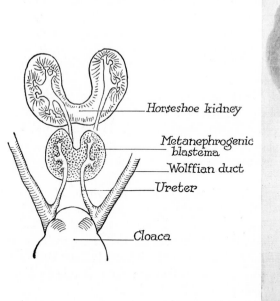
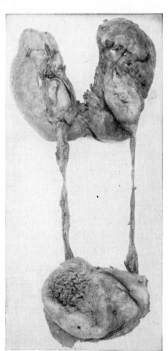

Fig. 71   Fig. 72

FIGURE 71. Horseshoe kidney. Schema indicating the embryologic etiology of horseshoe kidney formation. Lower polar fusion is here shown; superior polar fusion is most rare.

FIGURE 72. Horseshoe kidney. Resulting from fusion of the lower poles. The pelves face forward and the ureters arch over the renal isthmus.

laterally fused in one solid gnarled mass—the lump kidney—in which as in other forms of renal fusion the combined renal mass weight averages about equal to that of two normal kidneys. In renal fusion, the kidneys do not ordinarily reach their normal upper level but are held in the region of the fifth lumbar vertebra or below by early anomalous vascular attachments.

Horseshoe Kidney.   Here the two organs are fused across the midline, joined by an isthmus of solid parenchyma or only a dense band of fibrous tissue (Fig. 72), the fusion being at the lower pole in 90 per cent of the cases. In our autopsy study horseshoe kidney occurred in a ratio of 1:425, being observed nearly twice as frequently in children as in adults, an explanation being that many of these children died early of renal disease.

The horseshoe kidney formation results from fusion of the two nephrogenic blastemas, the fusion taking place at different periods but in any event earlier than the thirtieth day when the two renal masses in the pelvis are brought into contact by the developing umbilical arteries. When the fusion precedes the rotation by the eighth week, the ureters will be found leaving anteriorly and when the pelves face medially, the fusion follows rotation (Figs. 61, 71, 72).

Characteristically horseshoe kidneys lie closer to the spine and more obliquely than do normal kidneys, a point of urographic diagnostic importance (Fig. 73). The vascular supply is regularly anomalous.

Almost always the kidney and its isthmus lie anterior to the aorta and vena cava and the ureters pass anterior to the isthmus. Except for the malformation each renal half may be normal but one may be hypoplastic while the other is hyperplastic, cystic, polycystic, hydronephrotic or show other common renal lesions.

Because it is anomalous, the horseshoe kidney is especially prone to disease, chiefly hydronephrosis, infection and/or stone although neoplasm of one segment has frequently been found. The abnormal renal position favors urinary stasis which in turn predisposes to and perpetuates infection and particularly favors hydronephrosis and calculous disease.

The *symptoms* of horseshoe kidney disease are those of the complicating conditions—infection, hydronephrosis, stone, tumor and so forth, and are indistinguishable from these conditions in an unfused kidney. Pain around the umbilical area is often complained of as well as pain radiating to the lumbar region. Gastrointestinal disturbances may result from pressure or by reflex through the celiac ganglion. Meckel's diverticulum and lesions of the urachus must be ruled out.

The *diagnosis* in horseshoe kidney will nearly always be made by urography as a part of the urologic examination demanded by one or more of the presenting symptoms enumerated (Fig. 73). As ureterographically outlined, the curvature of each ureter conforms to the underlying renal mass over which it passes and usually curves upward and outward first, then in toward the spine.

When surgical disease involves only half of the horseshoe kidney, renal resection should be employed. Otherwise treatment is that of the local condition: removal of stone(s) by pyelotomy, eradication of obstruction by pelvio-ureteroplasty, or of infection by antimicrobial therapy, as necessary.

Lump, Clump or Cake Kidney. There is fusion of both kidneys into a solid, irregularly lobate mass of bizarre outline whose location is generally in the pelvis or just above. The vascular supply is derived from adjacent vessels, particularly the lower aorta, common iliac or hypogastric and usually enters the upper surface of the kidney. The ureters are short, anterior and enter the kidney abnormally (Fig. 74). As in horseshoe kidney the symptoms are those of complicating obstruction, infection, calculus, tumor or nephritis but lower abdominal pain may result from a dragging or pulling on the vascular supply by the mass weight of the ectopic kidney.

Diagnosis. Not infrequently the renal mass is diagnosed by abdominal palpation as neoplasm but it will be correctly recognized by bilateral retrograde pyelography which is preferred to excretory urography in these cases (Fig. 75). *Treatment* is that of the complicating disease, surgical interference being technically extremely difficult because of the

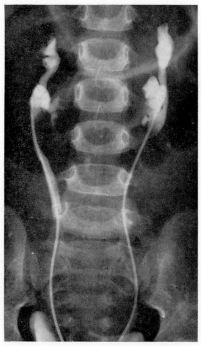

FIGURE 73. Horseshoe kidney disease in a three-year-old girl. The malrotated kidneys fused below are closer to the spine than normal. In a plain urogram the abnormal renal outlines may be noted, with the kidneys tilted toward each other at the lower or the upper pole and a breaking of the continuity of the psoas muscle outline by the transverse shadow of the renal isthmus.

location and vascular factors. Occasionally nephrostomy, pyelostomy or peritoneal marsupialization will give temporary relief.

IV. ANOMALIES OF LOCATION

Congenital Ectopic Kidneys. The organ is held in abnormal position by early formed anomalous vascular attachments, the length of the ureter corresponding to the position of the kidney. Both the renal vascular supply and the length of the ureter define the ectopia; in *acquired* renal ectopia the vascular supply and the ureteral length are normal but the anatomic renal supports (perirenal fascia, perirenal fat, adjacent abdominal organs) give way, and with the resulting ptosis the vascular supply accommodatingly lengthens and the ureter becomes secondarily curved or angulated. Most ectopic kidneys remain on their own side but about one in five cross over to join or at least lie near the renal mate.

Simple ectopia occurs about once in 100 persons but occasionally the ectopic kidney is solitary, an incidence of 1 in 2200 persons (our autopsy study showed once in 701). Pelvic dystopia is the most frequent site but the kidney may be sacro-iliac or as in two of our cases, thoracic.

Malrotation of an ectopic kidney is frequent, the pelvis usually facing forward but the adrenal remains in its normal position. Yet the kidney may be overrotated and face posteriorly or laterally. A deep

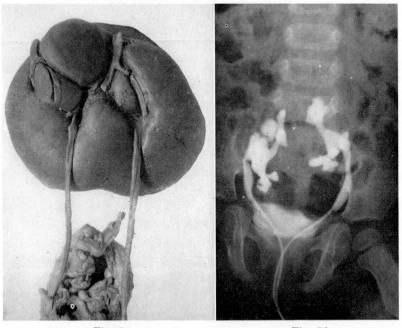

Fig. 74   Fig. 75

FIGURE 74.   Lump kidney showing the unusual anatomy with the anterior blood supply coming from above and the ureters leaving from below.

FIGURE 75.   Fused (lump) pelvic kidney in a two-year-old girl examined because of chronic pyuria. The organ was suprapubically palpable. Note shortness of the ureters.

pelvic kidney may compress the sigmoid or recto-sigmoid to produce constipation or obstipation, or to increase the difficulties of delivery.

The chief *clinical importance of renal ectopia* is concerned with (1) the high frequency of surgical diseases in these organs, especially infection and stone; (2) technical difficulties in surgical treatment, nephrectomy usually being the best procedure; (3) by producing pressure on nerves, blood vessels or neighboring organs, the dystopic kidney may cause lower abdominal symptoms such as pelvic neuralgia and, palpated, may lead to the incorrect diagnosis of neoplasm or disease of another organ such as cystic ovary. Other erroneous diagnoses made include appendicitis, iliocecal tumor or tuberculosis, sigmoidal tumor and mesenteric cysts.

The *diagnosis* of renal ectopy is at once established by urography which demonstrates the displaced kidney pelvis and abnormally short or long ureter, retrograde being preferable to excretory pyelography for this (Figs. 75, 76).

Crossed Ectopia. In the beginning, normal bilateral embryologic development occurs but early in renal ascent, one organ crosses the midline and fuses with its mate or lies adjacent (Fig. 77). In the crossing

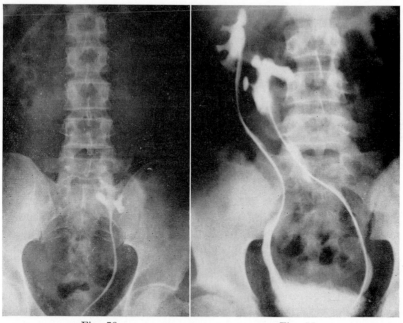

Fig. 76   Fig. 77

FIGURE 76.   Left ectopic kidney in upper pelvis of a forty year old man examined for hematuria proved to come from this organ. Antimicrobial therapy with no change in this kidney during fifteen years of subsequent observation.

FIGURE 77.   Crossed fused renal dystopia in an eight-year-old girl examined because of persistent pyuria and intermittent pain in the right loin; a normal appendix was removed during an acute attack of pain. The urogram portrays the characteristic pelvic misdirection in these cases.

over and fusion process a wide variety of renal formations may be achieved such as end-to-end, end-to-side, S- or L-shaped fusions. The condition is found at autopsy in one in about 2000 persons. The *symptoms* are those of the complicating disease as indicated under congenital renal ectopia and the *diagnosis* is made by urography (Fig. 77). The *treatment* of the ectopic unfused kidney is that of the complicating disease in a normally placed kidney, but in crossed ectopia with fusion the surgical difficulties are likely to be great, especially if resection is undertaken.

Abnormal Renal Mobility. This results chiefly from an unusually long vascular supply with the organ becoming engulfed by the peritoneum which together with the blood supply forms a long mesentery permitting the kidney free mobility in the peritoneal cavity. Under these conditions urinary stasis or obstruction is most likely to develop. Infection, stone or hydronephrosis are the anticipated end results and cause the *symptoms* to which the patient's attention is directed. The *diagnosis* is made by ureterography in which the freely movable kidney is demonstrated, with the patient in the upright, Trendelenburg, right and left lateral positions. Stereoscopic urograms will best show the character of accompanying malrotation. This condition must be distinguished from the mild or moderate nephroptosis frequently seen in nervous, frail women, especially spinsters, whose kidney has sagged largely from poor tissue support and lack of perirenal fat, and in whom ureteral obstruction is seldom demonstrable. For most patients of this type the diagnosis of "fallen kidney" is a curse for life and will only help to accentuate and accelerate their neurotic manifestations.

When pain can be attributed to the renal condition or there is urinary obstruction, high nephropexy rather than the wearing of a surgical belt is the *treatment*.

V. Anomalies of Rotation

Faulty Rotation. In the fourth week of renal life as the kidneys "ascend," mesial rotation begins and is completed by the eighth week (Fig. 61). The degrees of *malrotation* are (1) failure of, (2) incomplete, (3) reverse, or (4) excessive rotation. Malrotation is frequently observed in all varieties of renal malformation—the horseshoe, sigmoid, discoid and lump kidneys and in other forms of renal fusion. The condition is of clinical importance only when it is a factor in causing urinary stasis which in turn invites or perpetuates infection, stone formation or hydronephrosis. These complications produce the clinical symptoms. *Diagnosis* is made by pyelography in which stereoscopic urograms will best show the degree and nature of the malformation (Figs. 78, 79).

VI. Anomalies of the Pelvis

The renal pelvis is usually ampullate (85 per cent) with superior, medial and inferior major calyceal branchings which, in turn, subdivide into minor calyces (Fig. 26). Sometimes the median branch is missing. On the other hand pelvic branches up to six have been observed.

Double Kidney. This results from *reduplication* of the ureteral bud before it enters the nephrogenic blastema and is to be differentiated from the rare supernumerary kidneys in which two organs are formed on one side from separate blastemas (q.v.).

Double kidney is one of the commoner urinary tract anomalies, occurring in one in 152 persons in our autopsy series. In an examination of 4774 urograms Nordmark (1948) found 201 (4.2 per cent) cases of double pelvis. The condition has been observed twice as often in females as in males and more often on the right side.

In double kidney the ureter may be completely or incompletely reduplicated. Not infrequently in complete reduplication, the ureter from the upper pelvis opens ectopic in the urethra or elsewhere. Congenital ureteral stricture is one of the commonest co-existing anomalies observed

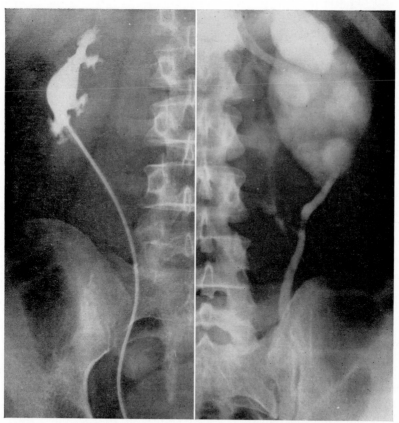

Fig. 78   Fig. 79

FIGURE 78. Congenital renal malrotation. Complete; cortex faces medially while ureter is carried laterally.

FIGURE 79. Congenital renal malrotation, ureteropelvic obstruction, advanced hydronephrosis and secondary stone formation (stone does not show in this pyelogram). Nephrectomy.

in renal reduplication and may occur in either or both of the separate ureters or ureteral branchings (Fig. 83). Often a small grooving or other embryologic evidence of the junction of the two renal segments is present and is a surgical guide in resection of the organ.

There are no *symptoms* of renal reduplication per se but because of the anomalous formation, the organ is far more prone to disease than a normally formed organ would be, infection and obstruction being of highest incidence and most often with involvement of the superior segment. The *diagnosis* is easily made by complete urologic examination in which the urograms will define the malformation (Fig. 83). In a study of 1102 children with persistent pyuria, I found 307 ureteropelvic anomalies, chiefly reduplication (26.9 per cent). When uncomplicated urinary infection exists, the treatment is antimicrobial therapy, but with surgical disease, heminephrectomy will usually conserve the sound half of the reduplicated organ although involvement of the entire kidney may demand nephrectomy.

Pseudospider pelvis describes a congenitally narrow, long, thin pelvis with calyces which urographically simulate the pyelogram of pelvic compression often seen in renal tumor.

Congenital hydronephrosis may result from practically every condition known to cause acquired hydronephrosis, the difference being that the etiologic factor was present during fetal life. The mechanism, pathogenesis, uropathy, symptoms, diagnosis and treatment of congenital hydronephrosis are essentially the same as in acquired hydronephrosis (see Chapter 5).

Congenital hydrocalycosis is the same etiologically and pathologically as the acquired variety (q.v.) except that it occurs in utero; many cases have been discovered in infancy and childhood.

Extrarenal pelves are a part of anomalous kidneys; the large pelvis is simply capped by renal parenchyma of various thickness and shape, often the major calyces entering the parenchyma more or less as separate tubes from the large extrarenal pelvis. The condition is important only when secondary infection, stone or other complications appear.

VII. Anomalies of the Vessels

Anomalies of the renal *arterial* blood supply occur in about 25 per cent of all individuals, are most variable and may be multiple, aberrant or as derivatives of the aorta, and are frequently of the ladder type (Figs. 63, 80). In a thousand autopsies in children under twelve years of age at the Boston Children's Hospital, thirty-eight cases of lower polar aberrant vessel blockage were found (White and Wyatt, 1942). In our autopsy study, renal arterial anomalies were recorded in 105 persons which is a much lower incidence than statistical studies of others have indicated. Unquestionably this reflects deficient observation or recording.

Renal vessels may be given off from the kidney pedicle, aorta, or vena cava and its branches, pass to the perinephric fat, diaphragm, adrenals, pancreas, and liver as well as to the renal poles. The *venous* return is characteristically far more anomalous than the arterial supply. The original renal blood supply is derived from the lower part of the aorta before the kidney ascends, and except for the final renal artery is normally lost as the kidney migrates upwards. Abnormally these vascular connections are retained, explaining not only the low attachments inducing renal ectopy but anomalous blood supply to a kidney in its normal position.

Most aberrant vessels pass to one or the other renal pole, are known as *polar vessels*, originate in or may communicate with relatively distant points of the aorta, vena cava or even adjacent branches of the great vessels. Lower polar vessels originating in the aorta, renal, or iliac arteries exist in about 6 per cent of all kidneys and are an important potential cause of urinary obstruction.

Anomalous renal vessels are of clinical importance as they may compress the ureter to cause obstruction or, at operation, may accidentally be lacerated to cause profuse hemorrhage.

There is still divergence of opinion as to whether the vascular obstruction is (1) *primary* or is (2) a *secondary* condition in which, through hydronephrosis with renal sagging or rotation, the ureter has been brought to lie snugly against the anomalous vessel which otherwise would be of no concern. All experienced urosurgeons know that either condition may be present.

Symptoms. The symptoms of vascular ureteral obstruction are those of the resultant hydronephrosis (see Chapter 5).

The *diagnosis* will be made by complete urologic examination instigated by the clinical manifestations and here urography is definitive. A transverse urographic filling defect is often demonstrable at the point where the vessel crosses the ureter and blots out the radiopaque medium (Fig. 81). Even more often, the dilated pelvis is urographically sharply

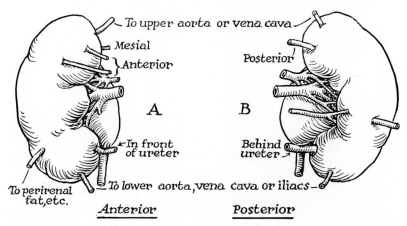

FIGURE 80. Aberrant vessels. Those which cross the ureter are potential causes of hydronephrosis but all are subject to laceration during mobilization of the kidney. Vessels of the deep pelvis in women, especially the uterines, may similarly compress the lower ureter.

cut off at the pelvic outlet and here the obstructing lesion may be a vascular blockage, congenital stricture, or peripelvio-ureteral sclerosis, the true nature of the condition being discovered only at operation. When the ureter is injected from below, the ureterogram generally stops abruptly at the point of vascular obstruction. When the pelvis has been filled, subsequent trap exposures may show retention as much as twenty-four hours later.

Treatment.   There is no medical treatment of vascular obstruction of the ureter, although intensive chemotherapy should be carried out to control or cure associated infection prior to the surgical attack. At operation the offending blood vessel or vessels are sometimes divided and the vascular obstruction is relieved. Yet nephrectomy must be performed in about half of these cases because of hopelessly advanced renal damage.

Aneurysm of the renal artery has been reported in about 125 cases. In some the condition resulted from trauma or from vasculitis, frequently of syphilitic origin. Symptomatically renal aneurysm causes pain in the side in half the patients, hematuria in a third, a palpable mass in a fourth, tenderness and hypertension in a fifth. With rupture of the aneurysm (*renal apoplexy*) profuse hemorrhage occurs, often with shock, and the development of a large perirenal hematoma. Moreover, the condition may cause a persistent pain in the renal region or even rapid death from hemorrhage. The *diagnosis* is suggested by a peculiar urographic filling defect of the pelvis or ureteropelvic blockage caused by compression by the aneurysm. Nephrectomy has given the best results with lowest mortality.

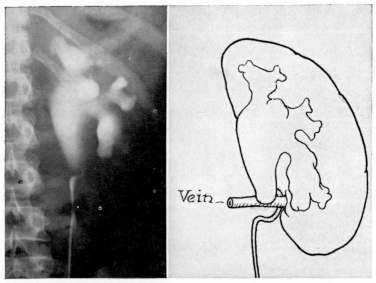

FIGURE 81.   Aberrant vascular obstruction in a six-year-old boy with pain in the left renal area and chronic pyuria. The upper ureter hooks over the vein. Treatment: division of the aberrant vein, ureteropelvioplasty for stricture at point of venous compression, and nephropexy.

EMBRYOLOGY OF THE URETER

As stated under Embryology of the Kidney, the ureter is derived as a budding from the wolffian duct (Fig. 82). In a four-week embryo (6 mm.) the cloaca is present as a dilated caudal segment from whose upper portion the allantois passes and into whose lower lateral portions the wolffian ducts open (Fig. 96). The anterior cloacal wall is composed only of ectoderm and entoderm designated as the *cloacal membrane*. Between the fifth and sixth week a frontal fold, the *urorectal septum*, passes downwards to separate the cloaca into a dorsorectal segment and a ventral *urogenital segment* (Figs. 82, 96). The ureteral buds spring from the urogenital segment (wolffian duct) to form ultimately the urinary collecting system as described under Embryology of the Kidney. The ureteral orifice is later carried upwards to the lateral angle of the trigone. Thus the wolffian duct also forms the posterior urethra, the vas deferens, epididymis, and, by budding, the seminal vesicles. This intimate embryologic relationship of ureter buds and wolffian derivatives explains certain unusual types of ureteral ectopic opening as in the seminal vesicles,

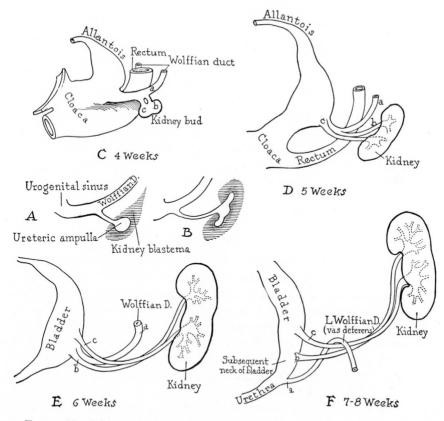

FIGURE 82. Schema of embryologic development of the kidney and wolffian duct. *A* and *B*, normal upper urinary tract. *C–F*, embryology of reduplicated kidney and ureter (after Kelly-Burnham).

in the vagina, cervix, or uterus (through persisting Gartner's duct, an early wolffian derivative).

ANOMALIES OF THE URETER

Ureteral anomalies are the most common major malformations of the upper urinary tract, and all are potentially obstructive. That they predispose to disease is well illustrated by the fact that in our autopsy studies the incidence of ureterorenal reduplication was one in 150 persons, but it occurred in 10 per cent of children clinically examined because of persistent pyuria. Most ureteral anomalies are dependent upon malformation of the ureteral bud and are in genesis by the third month of fetal life.

Ureteral anomalies may be classified as:

  I. Anomalies of Number
     1. Agenesis
     2. Duplication
     3. Triplication, and so forth
 II. Anomalies of Origin and Termination
     1. Ectopia
     2. Ureterocele
     3. Blind ending
     4. Ureteropelvic
     5. Postcaval ureter
     6. Herniation of ureter
III. Anomalies of Form, Caliber and Structure
     1. Aplasia
     2. Congenital stricture
     3. Congenital valves or folds
     4. Congenital dilatation without obstruction
     5. Congenital diverticula
     6. Spiral twists (torsion)
     7. Kinks
     8. Vascular blockage

I. Anomalies of Number

Bilateral ureteral agenesis is a part of bilateral renal agenesis, a phase of nonviable monster and is clinically unimportant.

Unilateral ureteral agenesis results from failure of the renal bud to develop and is almost always accompanied by renal agenesis or pronounced hypoplasia. The ureter may be present as a hypoplastic tube, a fine fibrous thread or even a short ureteral stump. Isolateral hemiatrophy of the trigone or a blind dimple at the normal site of ureteral opening may be present or a ureteral remnant may give rise to cyst formation simulating abdominal tumor.

Ureteral reduplication—so-called double ureter—may be incomplete or complete as previously discussed under renal reduplication (q.v.). The condition is found unilaterally six times as often as bilaterally and in one in five cases the bilateral involvement is mixed with complete reduplication on one side and incomplete division on the other (Fig. 83).

The embryologic explanation of ureteral reduplication is that two ureteral buds developed with fusion of the nephrogenic anlage (double kidney with or without fusion).

The embryologic *mechanism of the inversion relation* of the ureteral orifices and the corresponding pelves are indicated in Figure 82.

Ureteral reduplication presents no *symptoms* unless complicating obstruction and/or infection have developed or intervened. Stricture is the commonest obstruction and usually at the ureterovesical junction. The *diagnosis* of complete reduplication is made by cystoscopy when two ureteral orifices are discovered on the same side and confirmed by ureterography which will indicate the type and condition of the renal pelves.

In incomplete reduplication, urographic reflux from one injected branch of the ureter will usually outline the other ureteral segment and pelvis, especially if the injection is made as the catheter is being withdrawn (Fig. 83). Treatment is that of the underlying condition and in many of these cases when only half the kidney is involved ureterohemi-nephrectomy with removal of the diseased ureter and the renal segment it drains is curative (Fig. 84). When there is hopeless injury to the entire

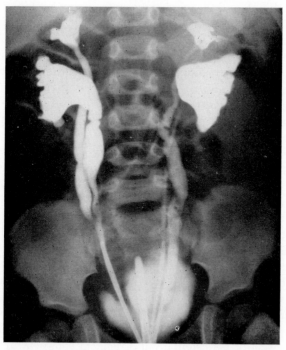

FIGURE 83. Ureteral reduplication in a two-year-old girl; complete on the left; incomplete on the right. At the point of junction of the ureteral segment from the right lower pelvis with that of the upper pelvis, there is a stricture which was later corrected by ureteroplasty.

organ, nephro-ureterectomy is the indication. Following surgical correction, the urine must be sterilized.

Ureteral triplication. A dozen cases of ureteral triplication have been reported; I have had two additional cases clinically and have seen such a case bilaterally at autopsy.

II. Anomalies of Origin and Termination

Ectopy. Here the ureteral orifice opens at some point other than the upper outer angle of the trigone. The condition is not unusual, occurs once in about 116 people and three times as often in females as in males. Yet all of the thirty-nine cases I have seen were in females and usually associated with ureteral reduplication, the ureter from the superior renal segment generally being the ectopic one although I have had several cases of bilateral ectopia and ectopia of both reduplicated ureters on one side and even one of all three ureters opening in the introitus.

The embryologic etiology is shown in Figure 82 where it will be observed that the ureteral buds arise from the ventral urogenital segment of the primitive cloaca into which the wolffian ducts also open. Shortly the ureteral orifices shift upwards on each side to open into the lateral angle of the trigone but anomalously they may fail to do this and the result is ureteral ectopy. In males the ectopic orifice is always within the external sphincter so that no incontinence results, while in females the opening is often beyond sphincteric control and incontinence results in at least half of the cases (Figs. 84, 85). As a rule in females, the ectopia is in the urethra or just adjacent to the external urethral meatus in the introitus, but it may open into a urethral diverticulum, or into the vagina, cervix or even in the uterus. Persistence of Gartner's duct explains the unusual ureteral ectopy in the vagina, cervix or uterus. Rarely the ureter opens into the rectum through faulty division of the cloaca by the urorectal septum.

In almost every case the orifice of the ectopic ureter is widely patent and in many will accept the miniature cystoscope. I have had six cases, however, in which the orifice was tightly stenosed and the ureter and renal pelvis above were massively dilated.

Symptoms of ectopic ureter are predominantly urinary disturbances and/or infection. There is variable urinary leakage in at least half the cases, sometimes not appearing early or even not until after childbirth. If the ectopic orifice is beyond the grasp of the internal sphincter, urinary dribbling is likely to occur but even with midurethral openings some of the patients stay dry. In young girls with ureteral ectopia, the diagnosis of and treatment for persistent enuresis is commonly maintained for many years. In these cases urinary infection occurs eventually and the *symptoms,* especially persistent pyuria, lead to complete urologic investigation and discovery of the anomaly. The *diagnosis* should always be suspected in any patient who has reasonably normal urinary control yet remains wet.

Treatment in ectopic ureter of an only kidney is generally trans-

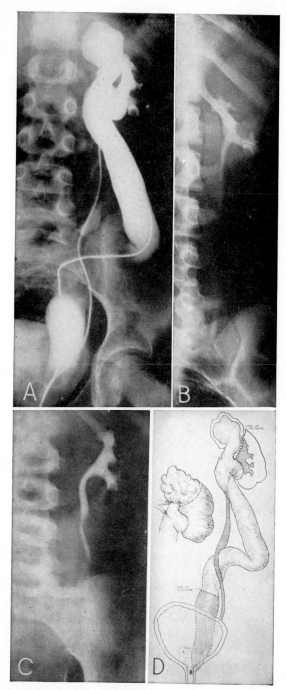

FIGURE 84.   Ectopic ureteral orifice in a five-year-old girl. A, reduplicated left ureters have been injected which disclosed a morphologically normal lower pelvis with a greatly dilated upper pelvis and ureter. Four weeks after ureteronephrectomy it was necessary to excise the remaining pyo-ureteral stump. (Bellevue Hospital.) B, urographic demonstration of the remaining left upper renal segment two months postoperative and C, sixteen years postoperative. Shortly before the last pyelographic examination, the girl went through pregnancy uneventfully. D, schema of the surgical anatomy showing the resected ureterorenal segment.

plantation to a new site in the bladder where sphincter control can be exercised. By a simple maneuver of endoscopically cutting the roof of the urethral ectopic ureter well back up into the bladder—1.5 to 2.0 cm.— the ureter will come to open into the bladder and continence will be restored (Fig. 85). When the ectopic ureteral segment drains the diseased half of the kidney, ureteroheminephrectomy is the indication but if the entire kidney is involved in the pathologic process, ureteronephrectomy should be performed removing the dilated, infected ureter to as near the ectopic orifice as possible. Ligation of the ectopic ureter should not be employed and especially when infection exists.

Ureterocele, commonly known also as intravesical cyst of the ureter, is a ballooning of the lower end of the ureter into the bladder cavity with involvement of all of the component layers of the ureteral wall, although the middle coat of muscle fibers and connective tissue is usually scant (Fig. 86). Ureterocele is not unusual, being observed in about 2 per cent of all routine cystoscopies although it was noted only in one of 3000 cases in our autopsy series. The condition is a frequent one in children; I reported a series of 100 instances of the lesion (1950) in the young and have since seen many more.

The *genesis* of ureterocele is dependent upon a small ureteral mu-

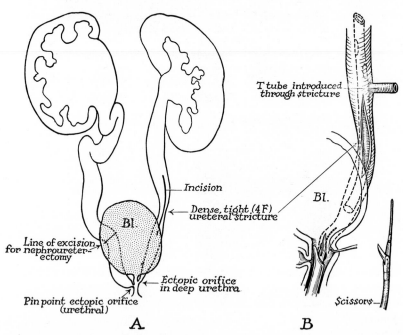

FIGURE 85. Bilateral ureteral ectopia in a three-year-old girl showing incision of ectopic ureteral roof on the left using Campbell miniature ureteral meatone scissors. This permitted the urine to collect in the bladder and cured the incontinence. The destroyed right upper urinary tract had to be removed and a tight congenital stricture of the lower ureter of the left "good" kidney was corrected by lineal incision and intubation.

cosal orifice which initially obstructs the urinary downflow as seen in Figure 87.

Ureterocele may be unilateral or bilateral (15 per cent), single or reduplicated, and accompanied by (1) dilatation of the ureter draining through the ureterocele, (2) isolateral ureteral reduplication or ureteral ectopia (in the urethra, diverticulum, etc.) or (3) prolapse through the urethra as I have observed in seven females. The condition involves each side about equally, and in one instance two ureteroceles were found on the same side. Curiously, the condition is observed four times as often in females as in males; in two-thirds of the cases the ureterocele drains the upper of reduplicated pelves, and in half the cases of ureterocele there are associated urologic or other anomalies.

The ureter above the ureterocele is almost always widely dilated. Prolapse of the ureterocele through the urethra may suggest inversion of the bladder and from which it must be distinguished. In the male the ureterocele may block the vesical outlet in ball-valve formation but it

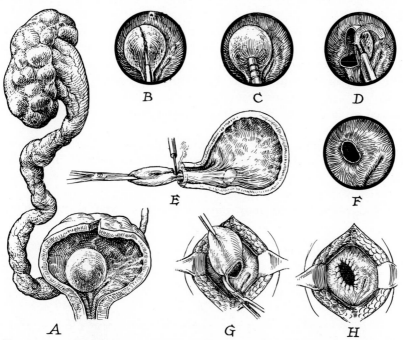

FIGURE 86.   Ureterocele. *A*, appearance of a small ureterocele which drains a greatly dilated ureter and kidney pelvis. *B*, cystoscopic division of the ureterocele by an electrode. *C*, cystoscopic dilation of the ureteral orifice by the pasasge of a large bougie, a method which is rarely effective. *D*, transurethral resection or removal of the crown of the ureterocele leaving a wide open ureteral orifice in the bladder (*F*). *E*, treatment in the female by passing slender forceps through the urethra into the bladder to grasp the ureterocele and pull it out as far as possible; division with scissors, knife or, preferred, cautery, is shown. *G*, suprapubic excision of ureterocele. *H*, a running suture is taken about the base of the excised ureterocele; this is seldom required. Of these procedures, the simplest is *D*, yet the enormous size of the ureterocele in some patients makes suprapubic excision the safer and preferred procedure.

will not prolapse further than the triangular ligament (external sphincter).

Symptoms of ureterocele are the result of the low ureteral obstruction to which complicating infection is usually added, in short, the clinical
picture of ureterovesical junction stricture (q.v.). Prolapse into the deep
urethra may cause acute or chronic urinary retention. Should prolapse
occur in the female, the ureterocele presents itself as a smooth extruded
mucosa which is ballooned rather than everted as a urethra prolapses and
can usually be readily reduced into the bladder by pushing it back with
a blunt-tipped instrument such as a straight sound, rigid catheter or the
tip of a cystoscope.

Diagnosis.   Ureterocele is recognized cystoscopically as a ballooning
intravesical cyst which tends to stay constantly dilated. Some ureteroceles are so large as to fill the bladder completely. The ureterogram in
ureterocele may be that of the cobra-head or spring-onion effect in which
the intracystic mass is well outlined by excretory urography or it may
appear negatively in the cystographic shadow as a rounded filling defect
(Fig. 88).

Treatment of ureterocele is fundamentally that of relief of obstruction; in small ureteroceles this is by cystoscopic division with operating
scissors or a resectoscope but a large ureterocele filling the bladder or
which prolapses from the vesical outlet calls for suprapubic excision (Figs.
86, 88–89). In some instances the upper urinary tract damage is so
advanced as to demand ureteroheminephrectomy in reduplicated kidney
or even ureteronephrectomy.

Cystic dilatation of the lower end of the ureter has been described
but in many cases this is simply a sealed-off ureterocele, in which the
ureteral orifice is not found. The diagnosis may be made by cystoscopy
and excision is the treatment.

Blind-ending ureters may have a small or even normal-appearing

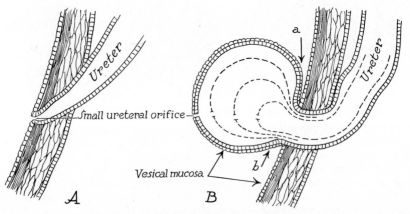

FIGURE 87.   Ureterocele. Genesis. In the author's experience the small ureteral orifices
are more often hidden on the posterior surface of the ureterocele (a, b).

orifice but the duct ends in a narrow fibrous cord a variable distance up. Unless cyst formation has occurred by partial sealing off of the duct, the condition is without clinical importance.

Congenital high insertion of the ureter is important as it may produce obstruction with hydronephrosis and its usual chain of symptoms (Fig. 234, also Chapter 5). The usual obstructive factor is mechanically a spur-valve formation which sometimes can be divided or other ureteropelvioplasty may save the kidney. When the renal damage is far advanced, nephrectomy is the treatment.

Postcaval or retrocaval ureter is limited to the right side and results from persistence of the early lateral fetal cardinal veins whose branches surround and lie largely anterior to the ureter. When it induces no obstruction it rarely causes symptoms. The uropathy and symptomatology are those of ureteral obstruction at the point where the ureter encircles the vena cava. *Symptoms* likewise are those of infection and ureteral obstruction, midabdominal pain being frequent. The *diagnosis* is made by

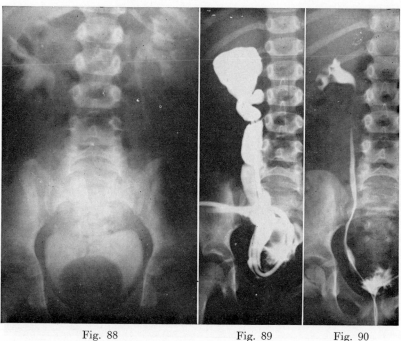

Fig. 88   Fig. 89   Fig. 90

FIGURE 88. Ureterocele in a twenty-two-month-old girl examined because of persistent urinary infection. Excretory urography showing a normal left upper urinary tract with a mildly dilated lower segment of a reduplicated right kidney. Negative shadow filling defect in the blatter outlines the ureterocele.

Figure 89. Urographic demonstration of the reduplicated upper half of the right kidney. This greatly dilated ureter opened into the ureterocele. Treatment: right ureteroheminephrectomy; transvesical ureterocelectomy.

FIGURE 90. Remaining lower right renal segment following ureteroheminephrectomy. Cure of infection.

ureterography which demonstrates the ureter swinging well to the midline and then reversing itself upward to the renal pelvis; when obstructed at the caval crossing, dilatation of the proximal ureteral segment and hydronephrosis result.

Treatment consists of disjoining the upper ureter at the pelvic outlet, mobilizing the duct from behind the vena cava and re-anastomosing it to the pelvis making sure that the suture line is oblique rather than transverse to leave a large ostium and avoid stricture.

Herniation of the ureter is rare. In several instances the ureter has been found in the inguinal canal and even down in a scrotal hernial sac to produce urinary obstruction and the usual chain of complications, notably infection, which chiefly cause the symptoms. The diagnosis is made by ureterography. Ureteral resection is the treatment when the

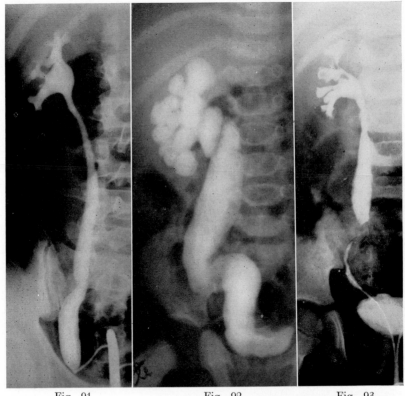

Fig. 91	Fig. 92	Fig. 93

FIGURE 91. Congenital ureteral stricture at the ureterovesical junction in a twenty-year-old man. Mild ureterectasis. Pyuria. Corrected by cystoscopic dilation.

FIGURE 92. Congenital ureterovesical junction stricture. Late.

FIGURE 93. Congenital tight ureteral stricture at the junction of the middle and lower thirds of the right ureter in a twelve-month-old boy with balanitic hypospadias. An initial excretory urographic study was carried out because in one in three cases of genital deformity, the upper urinary tract is also anomalous. The excretory study prompted retrograde urography. Cystoscopic ureteral dilation.

degree of renal damage warrants preservation of the organ; otherwise perform ureteronephrectomy.

III. ANOMALIES OF FORM, CALIBER AND STRUCTURE

Ureteral agenesis is associated with renal agenesis and occasionally occurs in hypoplasia of the kidney or of half of a reduplicated organ. There may be only a fine lumen or none, or the ureter may be simply a fibrous cord, and with or without an orifice or dimple in the bladder.

Congenital ureteral stricture occurs in about 0.6 per cent of all newborn, a ratio of 1:164 in 19,046 autopsies in infants and children. The condition, of unknown etiology, is simply an abnormal narrowing of the duct comparable to similar narrowing so often observed in the lower urinary, gastrointestinal, pulmonary, vascular, and biliary tracts. The ureterovesical junction is involved in over half the cases, the ureteropelvic in a little over a third, and about 10 per cent occur in the body of the ureter. In a fourth of the cases the stricture is bilateral and may be multiple but we have never encountered more than three congenital strictures in the same ureter. Strictures which we have clinically identified as congenital have been largely in patients under two years of age; they have been found many times postmortem in the fetus. The stricture may be sharply localized or extend over 1 to 2 cm. in length, may be broad caliber, or impassable, but in all events structurally shows only an abnormal narrowing of the normal ureteral caliber with absence of fibrosis except as secondary inflammation and infection have ensued.

These strictures all cause urinary obstruction and consequent ureterectasis and hydronephrosis above with a frightfully high incidence of secondary infection and its collateral pathologic and symptomatic manifestations.

Symptoms of congenital ureteral stricture are those common to upper tract obstruction together with reflex vesical irritation (see Chapter 5). In the absence of infection ureteral stricture may produce the clinical picture of chronic interstitial nephritis especially as the renal injury is evidenced by urinalysis and other laboratory studies. This illustrates the advantage and even necessity of carrying out at least a satisfactory excretory urographic study when the clinical picture of chronic nephritis is present.

Diagnosis. This is suggested by one or more of the presenting symptoms of upper urinary tract obstruction; the ureterogram showing the ureteral narrowing with proximal dilatation is definitive (Figs. 91–95). The chief differential consideration is ureterospasm but spasm seldom produces an identical urographic narrowing in all films of the same series or in films taken on different days unless there is a local causative pathologic process, the nature of which should be determined.

Treatment. In strictures of the lower ureter, periodic progressive cystoscopic dilation with bougies is frequently successful, carrying the dilation in young children to 8 to 9 F. caliber and in adults to 12 or 14 F.

at least.* This treatment is regularly unsatisfactory when the stricture is in the upper ureter or at the ureteropelvic junction.

When the condition fails to respond promptly to conservative cystoscopic dilation, it is patently a surgical problem. Ureteroplastic eradication of the obstruction may succeed but when renal damage is hopelessly advanced perform ureteronephrectomy, removing the dilated ureter to below the point of blockage. Sterilization of the urine completes the treatment.

Ureteral valves are transverse folds of redundant mucosa which have

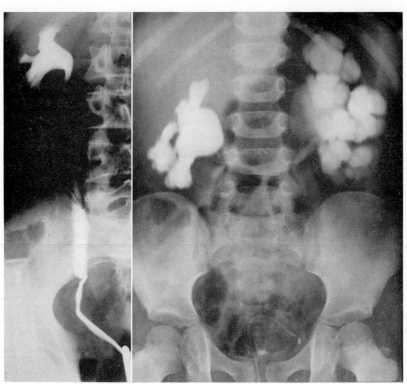

Fig. 94   Fig. 95

FIGURE 94.   Acquired ureteral stricture in a thirty-year-old man becoming symptomatically evident five years following appendical abscess which was separated from this area of the ureter only by the peritoneum. Treatment: cystoscopic ureteral dilation was successful.

FIGURE 95.   Congenital bilateral ureteropelvic junction stricture with advanced hydronephrosis, infection and diminution of renal function in a three-year-old boy examined because of persistent pyuria. Left nephrectomy was followed by right ureteropyeloplasty. Satisfactory result.

* A word of caution should be given against too frequent instrumental ureteral dilation such as once a week, week in and week out, as we have observed the practice of some alleged urologists to be. Rarely should cystoscopic ureteral dilation be performed oftener than once in three or four weeks and as progress is evident the intervals are increased to two, three, four, or six months, guided by the maintenance of an increasing caliber of the obstruction and improvement in the patient's general condition with disappearance of pain, hematuria, pyuria or other symptoms.

usually been made more prominent by their circular muscle fibers. They appear chiefly near the ureterovesical junction and are important only as they may produce obstruction, the uropathy and *symptoms* of which are those of ureteral stricture. The *diagnosis* is seldom made during life but the ureterogram demonstrating the lesions shows a transverse filling defect of the ureter at the point of blockage or a fusiform termination of a greatly dilated ureter above. In some instances the ureterogram has been not unlike that shown in Figure 94. In most of the recorded cases far-advanced renal injury has demanded ureteronephrectomy.

Congenital dilatation of the upper urinary tract is a manifestation of faulty neuromuscular development and nearly always the bladder is similarly involved. This is discussed in Chapter 9.

Congenital diverticulum of the ureter is extremely rare and is usually a manifestation of secondary ureteral budding or outpocketing (attempted bifid ureter), the principal uropathic consideration being secondary compression of the adjacent ureter with consequent urinary stasis and complicating infection with its own chain of symptoms. Abdominal pain, especially at the site of the ureteral diverticulum, is not uncommon. The diagnosis is made by ureterography and excision of the diverticulum is the treatment.

Congenital twist or torsion of the ureter occurs once in about 12,000 persons, the embryologic explanation being failure of the ureter to rotate with the kidney and when pronounced, the condition may cause obstruction and hydronephrosis. Stereoscopic urograms will demonstrate the site, nature and degree of the twist. Advanced obstruction calls for ureteronephrectomy.

Congenital ureteral kinks are indeed rare; by obstruction they produce symptoms commonly seen with other varieties of upper urinary tract blockage. With sharp sudden kinking, the renal colic of Dietl's crisis may occur. The diagnosis is made by urography, preferably stereoscopic, with the patient in upright and also Trendelenburg positions which will show the fixation of the kink. *Treatment* is ureterolysis with elevation of the kidney, together with cystoscopic ureteral dilation adequate to assure a channel which is free draining throughout. Complicating infection must be eradicated.

Vascular compression of the upper ureter by anomalous renal vessels has been discussed in preceding paragraphs in this chapter (page 142). Likewise the lower ureter may be blocked by anomalous vessels, chiefly the uterines where they cross the ureter just before entering the lower segment of the uterus.

EMBRYOLOGY OF THE BLADDER

The essentials have been given under Embryology of the Ureter (Fig. 96). The *urachus* passes from the uppermost portion of the bladder to the umbilicus, being formed as a condensation and fibrosis of the *allantois* or yolk stalk. Failure to close gives rise to urachus fistula or cyst formation (Fig. 97). *It is imperative to recognize that the bladder is primarily a hindgut derivative, receiving blood and nerve supply from the same segmental derivation, the latter being of great clinical importance in the diagnosis and therapy of neuromuscular vesical disease.* As a clinical corollary the rectal tone as determined by digital examination will usually reflect that of the vesical outlet.

Derived from the cloaca, the bladder is an entodermal structure surrounded by coats of mesenchymal muscular and areolar tissue. The trigone, on the other hand, is a wolffian duct derivative and largely of

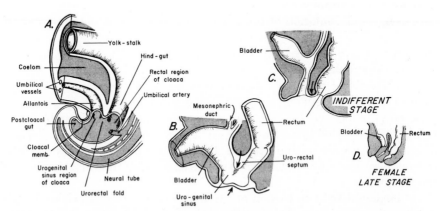

FIGURE 96.   Embryology of the bladder showing the primitive hindgut divided by the urorectal septum into the anterior vesico-urogenital segment and the posterior rectal segment. *A*, 8 mm. stage; age ca, 40 days (after Patten); *B*, 11 mm. stage; age ca, 6 weeks. Note the downward pasage of the urorectal septum. *C*, completion of hindgut division with establishment of separate rectal and urinary orifices. *D*, female: late stage.

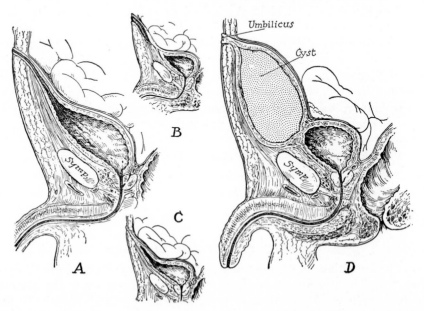

FIGURE 97.   Anomalies of urachus closure. *A*, patent urachus. *B*, blind external ending patent urachus. *C*, blind internal opening urachus. *D*, urachus cyst.

mesodermal origin. In infancy the bladder is an abdominal organ partly as a result of its tubular urachal derivation and partly because the distended viscus is too long for the comparatively small pelvis. Gradually it settles in the pelvis to reach its definitive adult position on the pelvic floor at about twenty years of age.

ANOMALIES OF THE BLADDER

These may be enumerated as follows:
1. Agenesis
2. Hypoplasia (dwarf bladder)
3. Reduplication
4. Diverticula
5. Exstrophy
6. Urachus cyst
7. Urachus fistula
8. Trigonal folds
9. Cloacal formation

Vesical Agenesis. Some fifty cases of this condition have been reported and usually as an associated lesion in monster formation. We found seven instances in 19,046 autopsies in children and, in each, other grave anomalies coexisted which would of themselves have been fatal. Vesical agenesis results from faulty development of the urogenital sinus with or without atrophy of the allantois.

Vesical hypoplasia or **dwarf bladder** is usually one of a number of serious malformations encountered chiefly in nonviable monsters and is of academic rather than clinical interest. Associated anomalies are nearly always incompatible with life.

Vesical reduplication may be complete or incomplete.

The *embryologic etiology* is unknown but obviously a splitting of the vesico-urethral anlage occurs. Grave anomalies almost always coexist not only elsewhere in the urinary tract but also in other systems. The urethra and penis may or may not be duplicated. The *diagnosis* is made by cystoscopy; cystography, particularly stereoscopic and including lateral and oblique views may beautifully show the vesical divisions. *Treatment* consists of excising the diseased segment of the reduplicated bladder or removal of the septum and complicating calculi, obstruction or infection.

Congenital vesical diverticulum should be diagnosed only in the absence of infravesical obstruction. The recognition of bladder neck obstruction is sometimes difficult in early infancy, yet diverticula have been found in the fetus as well as in the newborn; those occurring in the young constitute about 5 per cent of all diverticula (Fig. 98).

Most congenital vesical diverticula are found near the ureteral orifices, usually just above the orifice, medially or laterally; about 90 per cent in children are found just behind the trigone. Some believe all diverticula are congenital, but in any event they are most common when bladder neck or other infravesical obstruction exists, the diverticulum forming as a pouch blowout.

The *symptoms* of vesical diverticulum are largely those of initial urinary obstruction with difficulty, frequency and so forth, plus infection, hematuria, and often stone formation. Installment bladder emptying (pis en deux temps) is characteristic. Persistent pyuria is the commonest symptom directing urologic examination in which the orifice of the diverticular sac will be cystoscopically observed. The sac may be splendidly outlined by cystography including lateral exposures, and preferably stereoscopic (Fig. 98).

Treatment is excision of the sac, either intravesically or extravesically. If a ureter opens into the diverticulum, ureteroneocystostomy must be employed in addition to diverticulectomy if the kidney is salvagable. Obstruction at the bladder outlet or peripherally must be removed. Sterilization of the urine completes the treatment.

Bladder Exstrophy. This is characterized by absence of the anterior vesical and lower abdominal walls with eversion of the posterior bladder wall (Fig. 99). The anomaly is one of the worst afflictions of the human race, occurs once in thirty to forty thousand persons, but in our autopsy series in the young the incidence was one in 1002, the oldest child being three and a half years of age. In 32,834 autopsies in adults it occurred but once, in a thirty year old male, an observation which at once defines its vital (lethal) importance.

The ureteral orifices are easily seen in the widely open bladder and

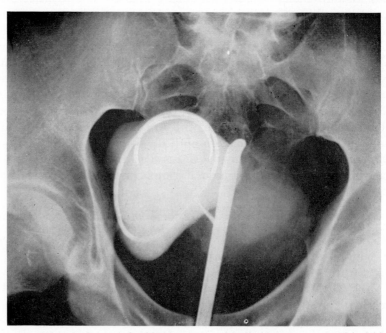

FIGURE 98. Diverticulum of the bladder urographically demonstrated. The shadow of media in the bladder itself can be faintly seen.

freely discharge urine externally, leaving the patient thoroughly soaked and foul smelling; friction of the water-soaked clothing against the tender, highly sensitive, easily bleeding exstrophic bladder urothelium and adjacent macerated skin causes great pain. Untreated, most of the patients are dead of pyelonephritis by the age of twenty-one, half die in early childhood, two thirds are dead by the tenth year.

In *incomplete exstrophy*, the defect is relatively meager and may be little more than a well-developed epispadias in which the pubis may be fully joined. In the usual exstrophy the pubes are widely separated (Figs. 100, 101). This causes the child to waddle or shuffle when he walks, owing chiefly to the outward rotation of the femurs. The umbilicus is usually somewhat lower than normal or may be obliterated entirely at the upper margin of the exstrophy. Malformations of the recti muscles and fasciae account for the large inguinal and/or femoral herniae so often present.

Genital anomalies are common, epispadias always being present. The penis is a rudimentary, broad, flat stump, slit or grooved above; the vesical

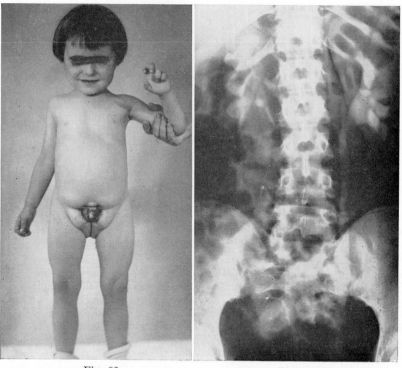

Fig. 99   Fig. 100

FIGURE 99.   Bladder exstrophy in a three-year-old girl. Ureterosigmoidostomy performed employing Higgins' technique.

FIGURE 100.   Excretory urogram made seventeen years later and after the patient shown in Figure 99 had given birth to a child. The upper urinary tract shows remarkably little dilatation. The pubis was absent. The blood Wassermann test was 4 plus at time of initial operation; antiluetic therapy apparently was successful.

and urethral sphincters are incomplete and lie widely open leaving the verumontanum easily visible on the floor of the male posterior urethra. The prostate is hypoplastic, the scrotum often cleft, and cryptorchism is frequent. In the female the clitoris is divided or cleft, and the labia minora separated anteriorly to leave the vaginal orifice widely exposed (Fig. 99). The urethra, when present, is laid wide open and is short. Coitus, pregnancy and delivery are possible (Fig. 100). Pronounced anomalies of the urinary and other system: exist in three fourths of the cases (Fig. 101).

The *embryologic explanation* of Patten and Barry is both the most recent and the most acceptable. Their theory is based on the development of the epispadias which regularly accompanies exstrophy.*

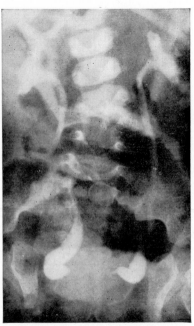

Figure 101.   Vesical exstrophy with associated congenital bilateral ureterovesical junction stricture and ureterectasis. Note absence of pubis.

* Patten and Barry believe that the starting point is the paired primordial genital tubercles, and the initial developmental disturbance involves the appearance of these paired primordia a little too far caudally with reference to the cloacal outlet (cloacal membrane). Such a relative displacement would cause the primordia to lie at the level where the urorectal fold divides the original cloacal orifice into the urogenital and anal outlet (Fig. 96). Under these circumstances the corpora cavernosa found just caudad to the urogenital outlet and the urethral groove would develop in their dorsal angle rather than in their ventral angle as is the normal. With this, failure of midline convergence of the displaced paired primordia accounts for the uncommon exaggeration of the associated anomalies in which the penis and clitoris are represented by separate halves, each molded about a single corpus cavernosum.

With this there is failure of the mesodermal ingrowth to form the anterior abdominal wall. Normally the mesodermal ingrowth occurs first just cephalad to the urogenital orifice when the paired primordia of the genital tubercle meet each other in the midline. If the paired primordia of the genital tubercle are caudally displaced, the crucial spot remains unduly long without mesodermal reinforcement. Under the circumstances, the urogenital

Symptoms of bladder exstrophy are those enumerated under Pathology. Rectal prolapse is often present and ascending renal infection through the exposed ureters will produce its own train of clinical manifestations. The *diagnosis* is made by inspection. The nature and extent of the accompanying herniae should be recognized.

Treatment is surgical and some variety of ureterosigmoidostomy is performed—transplantation of the ureters to the rectosigmoid—several techniques being available. The ureterosigmoidostomy should be performed by the end of the first year if possible, yet only if physical examination discloses a normal rectal sphincter. Prolapse or other rectal malformations susceptible to surgical treatment should be corrected prior to ureterosigmoidostomy. Unless a rectal sphincter capable of retaining urine in the bowel is present, ureteral transplantation will only aggravate the condition. Experience has shown that young infants withstand even radical urologic surgery well and in ureterosigmoidostomy, the ultimate surgical success will rest almost as much on preoperative and postoperative care and control of electrolyte balance and general fortification of the patient (whole blood transfusion and so forth) as upon the technique of the surgical procedure itself. The former formidable operative morbidity and the 20 to 25 per cent mortality has now been reduced in most clinics to not over 5 per cent, thanks to better surgical techniques, increased knowledge of biochemistry, and antimicrobial therapy.

Dilatation of the upper urinary tract is not uncommon following ureterosigmoidostomy and urinary back pressure above the site of ureteral transplantation may destroy the kidneys. Complicating infection, urosepsis and renal failure are the usual direct causes of death.

Urachal cysts are rare (1:5000) and result from failure of obliteration of the allantois; each end of the canal becomes closed (Fig. 97). With external rupture of the cyst, a persistent fistula opens at the umbilicus. With intravesical rupture an internal fistula into the bladder forms and if it is large may persist as a diverticulum in which even stone deposit may occur or neoplasm develop. In a few instances intraperitoneal rupture has occurred with disastrous results.

The *diagnosis* of urachal cyst may be suspected by palpation, first making sure the bladder is empty. Roentgenography with radiopaque medium injected into the cyst will demonstrate the size of the lesion. Excision is the treatment.

Patent urachus is found at autopsy in one in about 650 newborn children. It results from failure of the allantois to close and this is generally due to infravesical obstruction during fetal life. There is constant

---

membrane opening into the presumptive bladder region will be much longer than normal and tend to extend in the midline all the way to the umbilicus. This extension of faulty mesodermal covering is enhanced by the rapid absorption of the area between the urogenital orifice and the umbilical cord which occurs at this stage of development. Even slight retardation of mesodermal ingrowth at this critical time would cause delay in reinforcing this region sufficient to account for the characteristic extension of the exstrophic defect.

urinary drainage from the umbilicus which makes the diagnosis. Excision of the fistulous tract with removal of the bladder-neck or urethral obstruction is the treatment which is completed with sterilization of the urine.

Redundancy of the trigonal mucosa is extremely rare and is characterized by a mucosal transverse valvelike flap on the anterior trigone just inside the vesical outlet. This mucosal structure cusps over the vesical outlet when the patient tries to void and produces obstruction. The *diagnosis* is made by cystoscopy; lateral cystography may even show a filling defect of the bladder floor at the point of the mucosal flap. One must be sure that the flap is not simply a collapsed ureterocele redundancy obstructing the vesical outlet. *Treatment* is removal of the obstructing leaflet transurethrally when small or through the open bladder when large.

Persistent cloacal formation is discussed on page 187.

EMBRYOLOGY OF THE URETHRA AND THE REPRODUCTIVE TRACTS

In the male, the anlagen from which the urethra is derived are: (1) the long narrow portion of the vesico-urethral anlage above the wolffian duct; this forms the urethra down to and including the verumontanum and the utricle; (2) the urogenital sinus below this opening (Fig. 96). The *female urethra* is derived from (1) and lacks the verumontanum and associated structures.

The *urogenital sinus* begins at the openings of the wolffian and müllerian ducts and extends to the cloacal or urogenital membrane which separates the sinus from the cloacal fossa outside. About the fifth week the tissue bordering the external cloacal fossa on each side anteriorly grows forward into a rounded projection, the genital tubercle (Fig. 102). Patten in particular has stressed this bilateral origin of the genital tubercle and especially as it is concerned in the genesis of epispadias, hypospadias and vesical exstrophy.

The genital tubercle rapidly increases in size and differentiates into a distal knoblike end, the phallus, and a bulbous ventral expansion. As the genital tubercle grows, the urogenital sinus elongates with it; elongation is greater in the male than in the female. On its under surface the

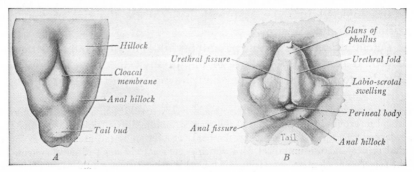

FIGURE 102. Embryology of the urethra. Region of the human cloacal membrane. *A*, at 3 mm. (Arey after Keibel; × 60). *B*, at 121 mm. (Arey after Otis.)

genital eminence is longitudinally grooved, the first indication of the *urethra* (Figs. 102, 103). By resorption, the urogenital membrane is perforated and the orifice of a ventral sinus, the *urogenital opening*, appears.

By *coalescence of the lips* of the newly formed urethral gutter, the urogenital membrane of the cloacal fossa closes from behind forward leaving a urethral tube which opens into the bladder at one end and externally at the meatus at the other (Fig. 103). The anterior part of the groove is the last to be closed over and, in hypospadias, explains the higher incidence of the glandular or balanitic variety (Fig. 116).

Development of urethral glands accompanies formation of the canal. The wolffian duct and the method by which it comes to open into the posterior urethra has been briefly discussed under Embryology of the Kidney, Ureter and Bladder (Figs. 60, 82, 104).

The *prostate* is derived as epithelial outpocketings arranged in five groups: the two lateral, the median, the anterior and the posterior (Lowsley, 1912). *Skene's ducts* are the prostatic homologue in the female (Johnson, 1922).

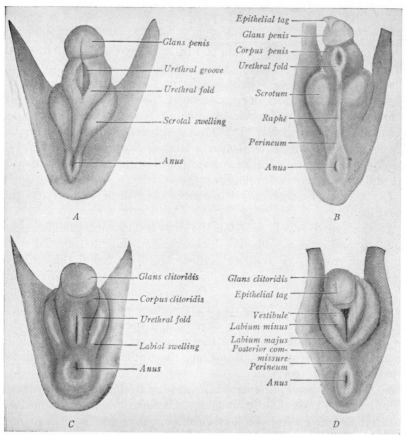

FIGURE 103.   Differentiation of the human external genitalia (×8). Arey after Spalding.
Stages at ten and twelve weeks; *A, B,* male; *C, D,* female.

The *bulbomembranous* glands of Cowper bud from the male deep bulbous urethra as epithelial nests, branch, and acquire a lumen lined with secretory epithelium. *Bartholin's glands* are the female homologue of Cowper's glands and open laterally into the vestibule (Fig. 104).

The many glands of Littré developed as tiny urethral offshoots appear in longitudinal rows throughout the length of the anterior urethra. The *lacunae of Morgagni* develop as small outpocketings of the fossa navicularis and are lined with nonsecretory epithelial cells. The anomalous development of the periurethral glands may result in cyst or fistula formation of clinical importance.

Coincident with the development of the urethra, the abdominal wall closes anteriorly as high as the umbilicus. The *genital eminence* or *phallus* forms at the junction of the urogenital membrane and the newly formed lowermost abdominal wall (ninth week). An undifferentiated sex organ at first, the phallus later becomes the male *penis* or female *clitoris* (Fig. 103). By the third month the penis has appeared as such at the tip of the phallus and the urogenital sinus has been drawn out with the formation of the penile urethra (Fig. 103). Simultaneously the penis is covered with skin. *Genital ridges*—the labioscrotal folds—appear laterally at the base of the phallus and extend posteriorly to unite in front of the rectum ultimately to form the scrotum in the male or the labia majora in the female. The *median raphe* marks the line of fusion. Thus the *pendulous* urethra is formed from the genital eminence and the *bulbous* urethra from fusion of the cloacal membrane which also forms the perineum. The *prostatic* urethra is a wolffian duct derivative as is the female urethra.

In the female, the urogenital opening remains as a cleft beneath and along the ventral surface of the cloacal tubercle. Unlike in the male, its walls do not fuse but remain open as the *orifice of the vestibule*. The groove on the female genital eminence closes without the formation of a canal and the *clitoris* is developed.

The sex can be determined in embryos of three months (56 mm.; Arey, 1946).

At the fourth week of fetal life the gonads are undifferentiated organs originating as mesothelial thickenings on the anteromesial surface of the mesonephrons or wolffian bodies. The mesothelial thickening increases in size to be the *germinal ridge* and contains the differentiated epithelial germinal cells embedded in its connective tissue, these cells arising by proliferation from the deep surface epithelium covering the ridge. From these germinal cells develop the spermatogenic cells of the testis and the graafian follicles of the ovary (six weeks). Should failure of urogenital union occur at this time, the testicle and epididymis will develop separately (q.v.).

At the fifth week, the wolffian and müllerian ducts traverse the germinal ridge longitudinally, it being unknown whether the müllerian duct originates as an independent development or as an offshoot of the wolffian duct. At any rate, the müllerian ducts open into the peritoneal cavity (celom) at their uppermost extremities and unite below to empty

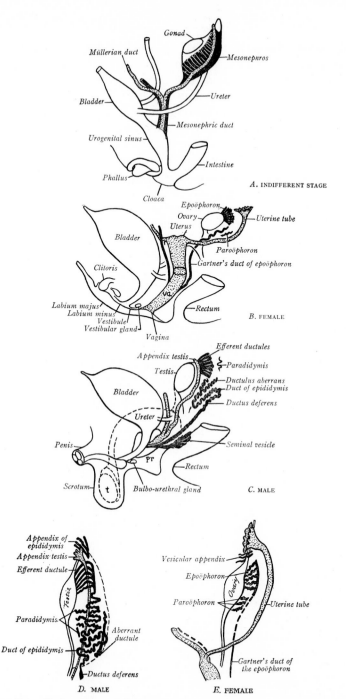

FIGURE 104.   Embryology of the genital tract.   Homologues in urogenital development. Diagrams depicting the transformation of the primitive genital system to the definitive male and female types. (Arey after Thompson.) The course of the mesonephric or
Gartner's duct is indicated in *B.* and *E.* While this structure usually disappears as such, in
about 5 per cent of females it persists as a fine patent tube. The persistence of Gartner's
duct in its embryologic association with the early kidney structure is advanced to explain
the appearance of ureteral ectopia in the vagina and more particularly in the cervix and
body of the uterus.

into the urogenital sinus (Fig. 104A), this lower opening persisting in the male as the *utricle* of the verumontanum. In the female, the müllerian ducts give rise to the fallopian tubes, uterus, and vagina, and in the male the prostatic utricle and testicular hydatids (Fig. 104).

Enlarging, the developing sex glands separate from the wolffian body to lie free in the peritoneal cavity attached only by a peritoneal pedicle which becomes the mesorchium in the male and the mesovarium in the female (Fig. 104). In the folds of the mesorchium is a band of muscular tissue, the genito-inguinal ligament or *gubernaculum*, which passes from the lower pole of the testicle to the uppermost scrotum and as the fetus grows and the trunk lengthens, the testicle progressively occupies lower levels and by the third month is near the internal inguinal ring.

A peritoneal pouch, the processus vaginalis, has by now grown downwards through the anterior abdominal walls towards the scrotum (Fig.

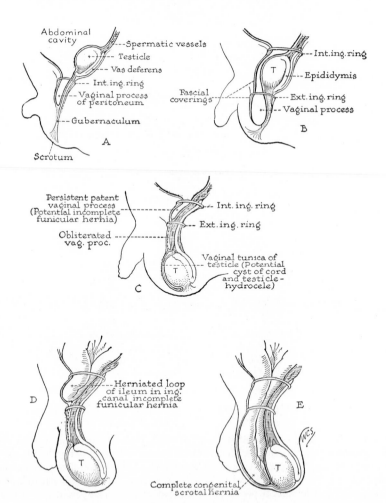

FIGURE 105. Descent of the testes showing how incomplete closure of the peritoneal pouch causes congenital hydrocele and hernia. (Jones-Shepard.)

105). At this time the inguinal canal is unformed so that descent of the testicle through it does not take place yet. In passing through the anterior abdominal wall, the processus vaginalis becomes covered with tissue layers and structures derived from the anterior abdominal wall—the cremaster and intervascular fibrous cord structures. Just before or during the first month of neonatal life, the testicle passes through the peritoneal evagination to reach the scrotum; later the processus vaginalis is obliterated above to leave the testis lying in its own cavity of peritoneal derivation. The serosal parietal layer lines the scrotal cavity as the tunica vaginalis, while the visceral layer covers the tunica albugina and surrounds the testicle and epididymis everywhere except at the head and tail of the epididymis. Failure of the processus vaginalis to close accounts for congenital hernia, and segmental closure gives rise to congenital hydrocele.

The cause of testicular descent is still unknown, the notion that the gubernaculum actively draws the testicle down being no longer accepted. Unquestionably endocrine factors play a part as often evidenced by the descent of a congenitally imperfectly descended testicle following the administration of anterior pituitary-like gonadotrophic hormone. Conversely, interference with or disruption of the descent mechanism can be produced experimentally by the administration of large doses of estrogen during late fetal development. Eleven anatomic factors which may predispose to cryptorchism are given on page 200.

TABLE 6. DERIVATIONS OF INDIFFERENT UROGENITAL ANLAGEN

MALE	INDIFFERENT TYPE	FEMALE
Testes	SEXUAL GLANDS	Ovary
Coni vasculosi and ductuli efferentes	WOLFFIAN TUBULES (SEXUAL GROUP)	Short tubules of the epoophoron
Paradidymis		Paroophoron
Duct of epididymis	WOLFFIAN DUCT	Main tube of epoophoron
Vas deferens		Gartner's duct
Seminal vesicle		
Epididymis appendix-upper end		Hydatid of Morgagni
Appendix of testes	MÜLLERIAN DUCT	Oviduct
Prostatic utricle		Uterus
		Vagina
Ureter	RENAL OUTGROWTH FROM WOLFFIAN DUCT	Ureter
Pelvis and collecting renal tubules		Pelvis and collecting renal tubules
Bladder	LOWER SEGMENT OF ALLANTOIS AND PART OF CLOACA	Bladder
Prostatic urethra	UROGENITAL SINUS	Urethra and vestibule
Prostate	(OUTGROWTHS FROM UROGENITAL SINUS WALL)	Para-urethral glands (Skene's)
Cowper's glands		Bartholin's glands
Penis	GENITAL TUBERCLE	Clitoris
Lips of urethral groove	GENITAL FOLDS	Labia minora
Scrotum	LABIO-SCROTAL FOLDS	Labia majora

In descending to the scrotum, the testis carries with it the epididymis, vas deferens, the testicular blood vessels, lymphatics, and nerves.

The seminal vesicles appear about the seventh week as outpocketings of the vas deferens (wolffian duct derivatives; Fig. 104C).

Derivatives of the indifferent urogenital anlage are shown in Table 6.

ANOMALIES OF THE GENITAL TRACT

Penis. Penile anomalies result from failure of normal development of the genital tubercles (phallus) and the segment of the urogenital sinus concerned with penis formation. Anomalies of the penis as a whole are rare. Grave penile anomalies are often associated with defects of the urinary or other systems which are incompatible with life.

Congenital absence of the penis occurs about once in about thirty million males and many urologists will never see one of these cases in their lifetimes. *Hidden penis* may suggest penile absence but the condition is usually one of relative micropenis buried in a great mass of pubic and subpubic fat. The chief concern in hidden penis is the occurrence of urinary obstruction consequent to penile and urethropenile angulation. Treatment consists of dietary loss of pubic fat and, if necessary, penoplasty to permit unobstructed urination.

Transposition of the penis and scrotum is exceedingly rare and is explained on the basis of retardation of genital tubercle development while the ventral labioscrotal swellings, now anterior to the tubercle, continue to grow normally. I have seen but one such case which was readily corrected by splitting the scrotum and moving it behind the penis.

Double penis is usually associated with vesical reduplication and is subject to great variation. Both urethrae may drain the bladder or, as in one reported case, the patient urinated through one urethra and ejaculated through the other. The usual treatment is amputation of the less useful segment.

Torsion of the penis is much more common than any of the previously mentioned abnormalities, the organ showing a clockwise or counterclockwise malrotation of the entire structure, usually with the urethral meatus pointing toward two or three, or nine or ten on the clock face. There is no treatment except to be sure the external urethral meatus is of normal caliber; in the several cases I have seen, congenital stenosis of the meatus coexisted and required meatotomy.

Megalopenis or *macropenis* is an hormonal manifestation in precocious puberty, is often found in congenital imbeciles, and in certain types of endocrine disturbances particularly in association with tumors of the hypothalamic region or especially of the adrenals.

Micropenis is an abnormally small organ, is seen in infantilism, hypogenitalism, or hermaphrodism, and is commonly associated with hypopituitary or hypopineal endocrinopathy as in Fröhlich's syndrome (dystrophia adiposa genitalis). The condition must be sharply distinguished from concealed penis in which the organ is buried in an excessively tight mons veneris and scrotum. There is no definitive treatment;

the administration of gonadotropic substances or testosterone will temporarily cause penile enlargement but this will regress to previous status with cessation of the therapy. The administration of testosterone will stimulate genital growth when there is testicular deficiency.

Precocious puberty not caused by tumors is discussed in Chapter 13, and as a result of adrenal lesions in Chapter 14.

Phimosis.   This is characterized by contraction of the prepuce sufficient to prevent its retraction over the glans (Fig. 106). The opening may be pinpoint, and in rare instances there is none (imperforate prepuce). In phimotic atresia the subpreputial surface is usually densely adherent to the glans penis (subpreputial adhesions) and, with segmatic retention, not only may secondary preputial calculi form, but stones passed from the upper urinary tract may be retained by the small preputial opening. In young boys the local irritation may induce masturbation. The small preputial opening may produce serious urinary obstruction with wide dilatation and injury of the proximal urinary tract. I know of five cases in which the pronounced phimotic obstruction was fatal; the entire upper urinary tract from the external meatus to the minor renal calyces was enormously dilated and the kidneys were reduced to thin shells. Preputial gangrene developed behind the stenosed prepuce with urinary decomposition and infection. Yet the small orifice may cause difficulty in voiding and the passage of a small stream.

Separation of the inner surface of the prepuce and the glans penis normally occurs by absorption of epithelium *in utero* or during the latter months of the first year but persistence of this union is pathologic. When the preputial orifice is minute, urination is accompanied by ballooning of the subpreputial cavity in which the retention and secretion

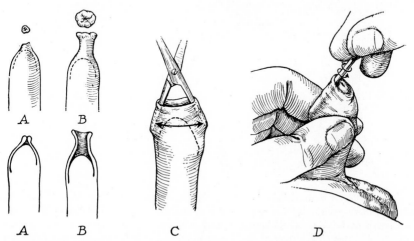

Figure 106.   Phimosis and adherent prepuce. *A,* redundant prepuce, schematically showing the elongated collarlike contraction the redundancy frequently presents. *A* (below), contraction of the preputial meatus when preputial adhesions exist. *B,* normal eversion after separation of preputial adhesions. Treatment: *C,* stretching of prepuce with hemostat. *D,* encircling preputial cavity with a probe to break down subpreputial adhesions.

of smegma and desquamation of epithelium commonly cause pronounced irritation even with ulcerative balanoposthitis. Congenital stenosis of the external urethral meatus commonly accompanies phimosis and here wide meatotomy should be done preferably at the time of neonatal circumcision. Sometimes subpreputial stones form in the postcoronal sulcus, these usually being calcific about a smegmatic nucleus (Fig. 237). The chief symptom of phimosis is dysuria with pain in the obstructed and inflamed prepuce.

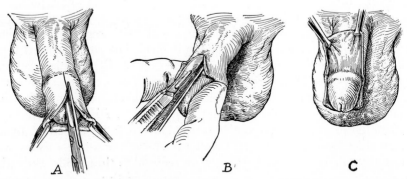

FIGURE 107.   Dorsal and lateral slits of the prepuce. *A*, dorsal slit employing two Allis clamps and scissors. *B*, employing a knife guided by a groove director. *C*, lateral slits made to obtain wide exposure of the glans and the postcoronal sulcus.

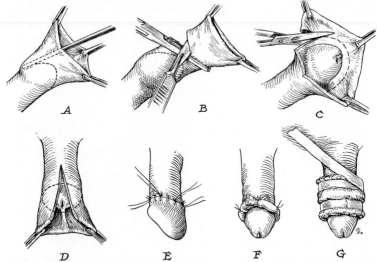

FIGURE 108.   Circumcision. *A*, freeing of subpreputial adhesions to well behind the corona. *B*, knife excision of the redundant prepuce. *C*, cosmetic resection of the prepuce with scissors. *D*, dorsal slit preparatory to excision of the redundant prepuce, this step being anticipatory of step *C*. *E*, suture of the skin to the post glandular mucosa; special attention should be directed to leave as long a collar of postcoronal mucous membrane as here indicated—at least 1 cm. *F*, four sutures placed equidistant about the circumference of the penis are left long to tie over a small petrolatum gauze dressing. *G*, the circumcision dressing should not be applied too tightly; the long tail of adhesive tape here shown is anchored to the abdominal wall and retains the dressing in place.

Treatment. Phimosis is largely preventable if early and periodic retraction of the prepuce is carried out by the mother or nurse. When the prepuce cannot be withdrawn behind the glans, dorsal or lateral slits (Fig. 107) should be made to enable free exposure. This can be carried out in the office and is less painful than stretching the preputial orifice with forceps. Moreover, dorsal slits should be immediate if severe infection exists, later to be followed by circumcision, or if the condition is not an emergency just a circumcision is needed.

Circumcision is the definitive treatment (Fig. 108). The chief indications for circumcision are: (1) a prepuce which cannot be freely retracted behind the glans, (2) fibrosis of the preputial orifice, (3) recurrent dermatitis of the prepuce, (4) persistent or recurrent balanoposthitis, (5) paraphimosis, (6) to promote local cleanliness and genital hygiene, and (7) prophylactic against cancer formation later. Most parents can be expected to appreciate the indications for circumcision on the basis of local cleanliness and genital hygiene and are naturally ready to adopt measures which may avert masturbation. Circumcision is usually advised on these grounds.

Circumcision can be performed in the newborn boy without anesthesia other than a sugar pacifier, and sutures are rarely required. Later anesthesia is necessary but local infiltration block anesthesia is adequate in most older patients. An adequate amount of prepuce must be removed so that the glans can be completely exposed behind the postcoronal sulcus.

In *atrophic phimosis* the prepuce is short, the orifice is tight and the treatment is dorsal slit.

A *short tight frenum* may (1) restrict retraction of the foreskin, (2) cause incurvation of the glans when erections occur or (3) be torn during strenuous intercourse. In two instances of the last type, the hemorrhage was brisk, voluminous and required vascular ligation for its control. The fold should be cut transversely and sufficient to insure free mobility of the prepuce.

ANOMALIES OF THE URETHRA

Complete absence or **atresia of the urethra** is, fortunately, most rare; urethral agenesis was found four times in 19,046 autopsies in children and urethral atresia in five. The condition often kills *in utero* by back-pressure damage of the kidneys or because the secreted urine distends the bladder to cause pressure on the umbilical arteries with pronounced embarrassment of the fetal circulation. Moreover, the distended bladder may cause dystocia. Most of these infants are stillborn, the greatest hope for survival in utero being secondary rupture of the bladder into the rectum or a persistent patent urachus to afford urinary drainage. In two neonatal males I saw, eight and twenty-four hours of age, with localized atresia of the urethra, there was a solid curtain blockage of the bulbous channel. By gentle instrumentation with small steel sounds, the obstruction was perforated and dilated sufficiently to permit an 8 F. catheter to be fastened in for twenty-four hours. This is done with full knowledge that urinary extravasation might occur and require prompt external urethrotomy, incision and drainage; intensive antibiotic therapy is given and a patent urethral canal is established at a later date.

Congenital cysts of the external urethral meatus are occasionally seen in young boys. There are no symptoms except as dysuria is produced by the small meatus. The diagnosis is made by inspection and excision or destruction of the cyst is the treatment.

Congenital Urethral Stricture. Stenosis of the external urethral meatus of the pinpoint variety is the commonest stricture, exists frequently yet unnoticed until urinary or urethral infection or dysuria develop, or instrumentation is attempted. It occurs in both sexes but is seldom detected in the female until instrumentation is undertaken. The tight orifice causes dysuria, frequency, urgency, and often urographically demonstrable back-pressure damage of the urinary tract above (Figs. 109, 110).

Ulceration of the stenosed external urethral meatus (ulcerative meatitis) is an extremely frequent condition in infant males, is rarely seen in females, results from congenital stenosis of the external urethral

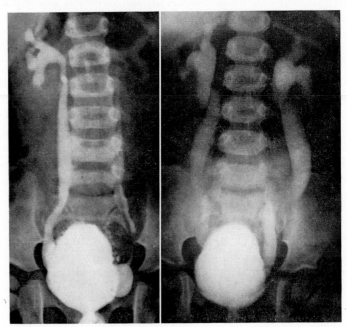

Fig. 109   Fig. 110

FIGURE 109. Advanced back-pressure damage consequent to congenital stenosis of the external urethra meatus in a five-year-old boy showing all of the characteristics back-pressure injuries to be expected with meatal obstruction: dilated urethra, trabeculated and sacculated bladder, left vesical diverticulum, dilated upper urinary tract on right outlined by vesicoureteral reflux and with slight reflux on the left.

FIGURE 110. Advanced back-pressure damage consequent to congenital stenosis of the external urethral meatus, in a seventeen-month-old girl examined because of persistent pyuria. Not only is the bladder irregularly dilated but also the infected upper urinary tract bilaterally.

meatus, causes urinary disturbances and bleeding, and is cured by meatotomy and the maintenance of a normal meatal caliber. The lesions are
usually superficial, extending about the meatus and slightly into it, seldom
over 3 to 4 mm. wide, and 1 to 2 mm. deep, with an acutely inflamed
periphery. In males, scab formation follows drying of the soft meatal
ulceration and with dislodgement of the scab or cracking of the ulceration,
hematuria or blood on the clothing alarms the parent. Because of local
moisture retention, ulceration occurs without scab formation in girls, and
in boys with a long prepuce which entirely covers the tip of the penis.
The condition is rare in infancy, occurs chiefly between the twelfth and
thirty-sixth month, but I have seen it much later. Back-pressure injury of
the proximal urinary tract is sometimes grave with wide dilatation,
diverticulum formation, advanced hydro-ureter and hydronephrosis (Figs.
110, 111). Chronic urinary infection often develops in these patients
with pronounced obstruction and urinary stasis. The *diagnosis* is readily
made by observation of the pinhole-size urethral meatus surrounded by a
small ulcerative area or the meatus may be entirely covered over by a
brownish-red scab which bleeds when it is broken. In some instances the
tightest portion of the constriction is 1 to 2 mm. inside the meatal opening.

Medicinal Treatment. Use of medicated diapers which have been
soaked in a 1:25,000 solution of Diaparene (1 tablet in 2 quarts of water),
and dried before using will control urinary decomposition—the ammoniacal diaper and ammoniacal dermatitis. The application of an ointment
of 5 per cent sulfathiazole in lanolin, or 5 per cent boric acid in lanolin
may be followed by temporary healing of the meatus but more scar tissue
is laid down and the pinhole meatus becomes smaller with subsequent

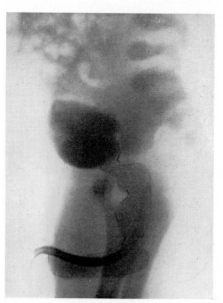

FIGURE 111.   Enormously dilated urethra behind congenital meatal stenosis in a two-
week-old-boy. Meatotomy.

recurrence of the ulcerative process and dysuria. This may be repeated several times with ever increasing obstructive uropathy.

Urologic treatment. Only wide *meatotomy* with the maintenance of a liberal size orifice (Fig. 112) is the certain permanent cure of ulcerative meatitis. Following incision of the opening, the mother or nurse should separate the incised margins every day and, at progressively lengthening intervals of seven, fourteen, and twenty-one days, the doctor should dilate the meatus with sounds or a hemostat, at least to a 20 F. caliber to prevent recontraction which may require another meatotomy. Undue bleeding after meatotomy is quickly stopped by gentle compression together of the incised margins between the thumb and forefinger for five minutes. No special dressing is required.

In the female, dilation with sounds usually suffices.

Congenital urethral stricture other than meatal stenosis may occur, chiefly in the membranous portion or at the penoscrotal junction. In the absence of a history of infection, instrumentation or trauma, the constriction is doubtless congenital and is simply an embryologic narrowing of the channel precisely as is found at the vesical outlet (contracture of the bladder neck), in the ureter, intestinal, biliary, pulmonary or cardiovascular systems, without sclerosis except as secondary infection has developed. The clinical aspects and treatment of urethral stricture in general are considered in Chapter 8. Periodic progressive dilation is the conservative and advocated treatment but when this fails or the canal is impassable, employ urethrotomy.

The *course of the urethra* may be anomalous, opening at the side of the penis, or rarely, in the groin, or as we have observed at autopsy may

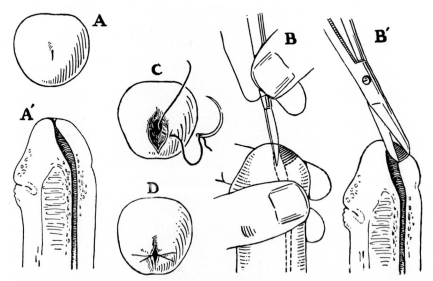

FIGURE 112.   Meatotomy employing both knife and scissors. If the tip of the penis is tightly grasped at the time the cut is made, the patient will feel no discomfort. Mucocutaneous suturing as shown in *C* is unnecessary in young boys.

follow a Z-course in the prostatic segment with wide dilatation of the urinary tract above.

Double Urethra (*Vera*) occurs only in true complete reduplication of the urethra and has even been found in the female. The urethrae may each drain its own bladder, a common bladder or, as has been reported, urination may occur through one urethra and seminal emission through the other. Double urethra must be distinguished from accessory local urethral canals which may be rudimentary or well developed and terminate in the bladder or prostatic urethra.

Accessory urethral canals are not unusual, may be situated dorsally or ventrally, and related or not to the true urethra. The condition is believed to result from the forward extension of, or splitting by the urorectal septum (Fig. 96). The accessory canal may extend back into the vesical outlet but most of them are located on the ventral surface of the urethra where they reflect abnormal closure of the urethral gutter and congenital urethral fistula formation. The ectopic opening may be at any point from the meatus to the triangular ligament but being distal to the membranous urethra, there is no incontinence. The dorsal variety (Fig. 113) is less frequent and does not produce incontinence.

Small *accessory periurethral ducts* are frequently observed opening in or about the urethra; these may join the urethra within the meatus or open externally to produce a fistula and reflect imperfect urethral gutter closure. They may become the site of cyst formation but more often are clinically important as they harbor infection. Frequently a thin mucosal wall separates the accessory urethral channels from the true urethra (Fig. 113). The *diagnosis* is suggested by the finding of two urethral meatuses, but usually requires instrumental and urethroscopic confirmation; by urethrography both the true and the accessory channel can be simultaneously demonstrated.

Treatment. When the accessory urethral canal harbors chronic infection or is associated with urinary leakage, it should be excised but

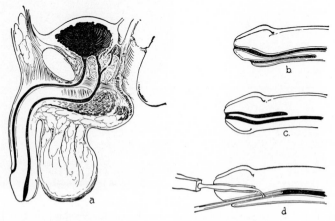

FIGURE 113. Accessory urethral canals. *a*, urethral reduplication. *b, c*, blind ending accessory channels. *d*, by incision both channels are made one. (Hinman.)

its obliteration may often be achieved by the injection of 5 per cent sodium morrhuate to the point of full (accessory) urethral expansion although other sclerosing agents may be used. Often it is possible by using the technique shown in Figure 113*d* to divide the membranous septum separating the true and the accessory canals, converting them into one channel with a common meatus. This office procedure is of special aid when the accessory canal opens at the usual position at the tip of the glans and the true urethral canal is balanitic.

Congenital urethral fistula results when the opening of the accessory canal is at any point from the meatus to the triangular ligament. The ducts of the periurethral glands vary in length from 2 to 10 mm., usually end blindly, but may join the urethra within the meatus and open externally to produce a fistula. They may harbor gonococci or other infection, or develop abscess.

Epispadias is the congenital absence of the upper wall of the urethra and in its advanced form it may be considered a first degree stage of vesical exstrophy (q.v.), and of which it is a regular accompaniment. The incidence of epispadias is about the same as that of exstrophy, one in 30,000 persons, but it was found four times in our autopsy series of 19,046 cases in children (1:4761). Yet I have seen twenty-three cases myself and have operated upon nineteen of them; five were males.

The *embryologic etiology* is that of vesical exstrophy (q.v.), the difference being solely one of degree. In the male the mildest form of epispadias is the *glandular* or *balanitic* variety in which the urethral opening is above and behind the glans (Fig. 114*B*). Exceptionally the meatal opening is stenosed. A dorsal groove usually indents the glans as far as its tip and causes this part to appear flattened out but the groove may stop at the corona or even proximally. In *penile* epispadias the

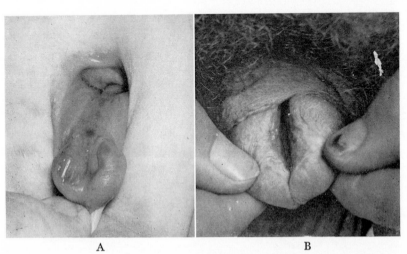

A   B

FIGURE 114.   *A*, epispadias in a ten-year-old boy; the urethral meatus is subpubic. No incontinence. Surgical correction. *B*, dorso-glandular epispadias in a thirty-five-year-old man.

urethral opening may be anywhere from the postcoronal sulcus to the suspensory ligament and is generally near the base of the penis (Fig. 114A). Here the entire penile dorsum is grooved to the tip or this may terminate proximally, the sulcus being covered by urethral mucosa and often dotted with the orifices of the ducts of the periurethral glands. As a rule, the organ is smaller than normal, spade-like in appearance, incurved upwards, and the prepuce hangs ventrally as a loose tag to leave the spatulous glans uncovered. Prostatic development is poor, often incomplete anteriorly, or may be entirely lacking. Although these patients may have intercourse satisfactorily, it is questionable that they are able to reproduce, usually because of inability properly to deposit the seminal charge in the vagina.

Complete epispadias occurs in both sexes. In the male the uncovered urethra opens to the bladder neck as a broad, deep funnel and variable degrees of vesical exstrophy are often present. When the vesical exstrophy is mild, or the lower abdominal wall is completely closed over the bladder, one may be able to insert the little finger into the bladder outlet for the pubic bones are usually not united and are often most rudimentary as in exstrophy. Incontinence is the rule.

In females, the epispadias is clitoric, subsymphyseal or complete according to degree (Fig. 115). The labia and pubic bones are widely separated as in complete exstrophy, and the bladder outlet stands widely patent. In complete epispadias in the female there is total incontinence causing excoriation of the skin by the continuous wetness. The patient of either sex, whether child or adult, and stinking with urine often suffers social ostracism. In the lesser degrees of epispadias in the female, the unrecognized lesion may cause her to be treated for enuresis.

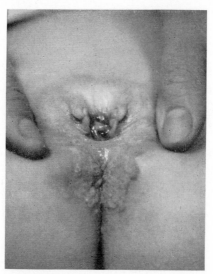

FIGURE 115. Epispadias in a three-year-old female with no urethra and total incontinence. Pronounced excoriation of the perineum. The clitoris is cleft and there is slight protrusion of the vesical membrane. Vaginal opening below.

The *symptoms* are those suggested by the anatomic findings, and the *diagnosis* is readily made by inspection (Fig. 115).

Treatment is by urethroplasty and fortunately in many of these cases a normally functioning bladder-neck control mechanism can be established. Experience has taught us to defer the operation until the child is over thirty months of age when conscious vesical control is normally established. Moreover, having had the urethroplastic repair, the patient is certain to have some difficulty learning to void and to control himself for it is a new and important experience he has previously been denied. In some of our cases it has taken as long as two years for perfect control to be established, yet the older and more cooperative the patient, the shorter will be the education in bladder control. Patient behavior and cooperation are the principal factors in achieving continence following a properly executed operation. Urinary control is stimulated postoperatively by practice of the start-stop-start urination exercise, wherein the patient as he voids starts the stream and then stops, starts again and then stops. Thus he learns not only the sensation of the desire to void and urination but also the associated mechanics of bladder emptying.

When the initial attempt at establishing control is unsatisfactory, the patient should be given the advantage of at least a second operative effort

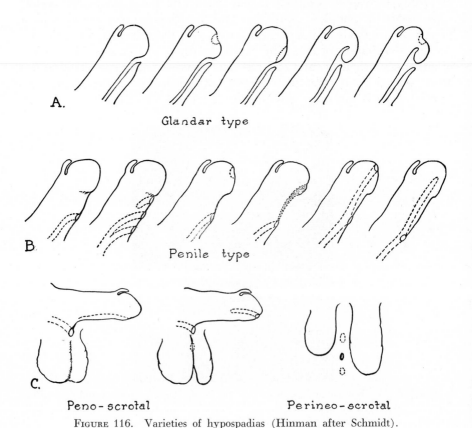

A.

Glandar type

B.

Penile type

C.

Peno-scrotal   Perineo-scrotal

FIGURE 116. Varieties of hypospadias (Hinman after Schmidt).

before considering ureterosigmoidostomy which, of itself, may be contra-indicated by lack of normal rectal control as often occurs in vesical exstrophy.

Hypospadias is a congenital defect of the anterior urethra in which the canal terminates ventral and posterior to its normal opening (Figs. 116–119). While the condition occurs in both sexes it is predominantly found in the male. Various reports of the incidence of hypospadias range from 1 in 160 to 1 in 1800; in our autopsy series of 10,712 boys there were seventeen cases, an incidence of 1 to 620. Yet our clinical experience suggests the condition is much commoner for many instances of balanitic hypospadias are totally overlooked. Except for stenosis of the external urethral meatus, hypospadias is the commonest urethral anomaly.

The *embryologic explanation* of hypospadias is an arrest in urethral groove closing from behind forwards to complete the closure to the tip of the glans. If the glandular or terminal segment of the urethra does not close, glandular hypospadias results.

In the male the hypospadiac meatus may be located at any point from near the frenum (balanitic) to the deep perineum; because the prostatic urethra is never involved as such in hypospadias, normal urinary control is maintained.

Hypospadias is an hermaphroditic manifestation in which the uro-genital derivatives in the male develop toward the female. Feminization of the male fetus in its early developmental period (one to eight weeks) logically explains the genesis of hypospadias as well as the congenital chordee (aplastic corpus spongiosum) which so regularly accompanies it and an occurrence not satisfactorily explained solely on the basis of failure of urethral gutter fusion. Experimental feminization of pregnant rats and other animals appears confirmatory of this while bifid scrotum and other pseudohermaphroditic stigmata so regularly present in hypo-spadias reflect the feminization and failure of proper midline fusion.

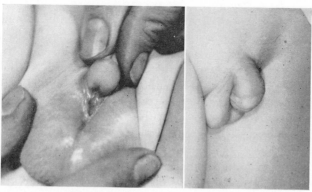

Fig. 117　　　　　　　　Fig. 118

FIGURE 117.　Deep scrotal hypospadias of mild pseudovaginal type with short incurvated penis in a seven-month-old boy.

FIGURE 118.　Midpenile hypospadias with pronounced chordee in an eleven-year-old boy. Correction of the chordee moved the urethral meatus backward to midscrotal.

There is no regularly operative hereditary influence in hypospadias although it has been traced through six generations and I have seen it in three generations. The likelihood of having hypospadiac or other mal-developments in subsequent children often deters parents of one such child from adding to their family; the genetic hereditary factors and percentage likelihood of repetition of this or other malformations in a subsequent child are given on page 123.

In more advanced hypospadias the utricle, a müllerian duct deriva-tive, is usually vaginaform, the depth of the pocket varying from 1 to 10 cm. Moreover, the orifice of the dilated utricle may obliterate or replace the verumontanum. Sometimes this müllerian outpocketing terminates in one or two fallopian tube-like structures (Figs. 140–142). The size of the vaginal pocket generally reflects the severity of the malformation of the external genitalia; the boy often looks more female than male, and to the anatomic condition the identification of *pseudohermaphrodism* (q.v.) is commonly applied.

The more proximal the hypospadiac urethral orifice opens, the greater will be the pseudohermaphroditic manifestations for in the scroto-perineal variety, the primitive scrotal folds are labialike, the urethra is correspondingly short, and vaginaform sacculation of the utricle is the rule. The more severe the hypospadias, the greater is the hypogonadism and prostatic underdevelopment. Penile hypoplasia is often present and the testes are smaller than normal, and commonly undescended.

The classification of the *degrees of hypospadias* in the male and the relative incidence are as follows:

Glandular or balanitic (40 to 50%), penile (25 to 30%), peno-scrotal, perineal or pseudovaginal (10 to 15%) according to location, yet as many as eleven varieties have been described. Multiple urethral open-ings occur in about 10 per cent of the cases, there is cryptorchism in about 15 per cent and in two thirds of these is bilateral.

Balanitic Hypospadias. The urethral orifice is at the site of the frenum, is usually abnormally small while the frenum is generally rudi-mentary or absent. With balanitic hypospadias, chordee is minimal or absent, urination is performed in the standing position and sexual inter-course and reproduction are normal. Meatal stenosis is the most im-portant condition in these cases and requires relief either by dorsal meatotomy (incision of the meatal roof) or by periodic progressive dila-tion with sounds. Attempts to radically "pretty up" the end of the penis in balanitic hypospadias is meddlesome surgery and is contraindicated; just be sure the meatus and entire urethra are normally patent.

The redundant preputial hood which incompletely covers the dorsum of the penis and is absent below may be removed by circumcision at a suitable time, but not until the patient is at least ten years of age when it will be definitely known whether or not this tissue may be required for a urethroplastic procedure, the need for which will occasionally be-come apparent later in the first decade. In the meantime for ritualistic circumcision, if desired, only a very small nick of foreskin is removed.

Penile hypospadias is characterized by ventral ectopic opening of the urethra at some point between the glans sulcus and the penoscrotal junction. The urethra may or may not be grooved from its opening forward to the tip of the glans. Occasionally penile hypospadias takes the form of a congenital fistula, the remainder of the canal proceeds forward to discharge some urine at the glans or, lacking a second meatus in the glans, the urethral canal may extend forward from the anomalous posterior orifice to end in a blind pouch (Fig. 116*B*). By lifting the penis the patient can usually direct the urinary stream from the standing position but he often sprays. Nevertheless, the broad, flattened, incurved glans and corpora together with the redundant hoodlike prepuce are cosmetically disturbing and may even prevent insemination. Congenital chordee is the rule in these cases, being increasingly pronounced the more proximal the hypospadiac opening is.

Scrotal Hypospadias. The penis is flattened, dwarfed, bent downward by congenital chordee and may even be attached to the scrotal raphe in webbed penis formation (cf. Fig. 121). Commonly the urethral meatus is stenosed to cause primary difficulty.

The *congenital chordee* in hypospadias results from hypoplasia and fibrosis of the corpus spongiosum which exists as a dense sclerotic band and usually extends in G-string effect from the frenum posteriorly as far back as the anterior portion of the ischiocavernosus muscles (Fig. 118). In the treatment of hypospadias, complete excision of this fibrous band is essential to afford the penis the chance to grow straight and to normal size for, unless this is achieved, subsequent plastic surgery is certain to fail of its objective (Fig. 121). The more advanced the hypospadias, the greater is the likelihood of malformation or hypoplasia of the corpora cavernosa and after puberty erections may be feeble or absent.

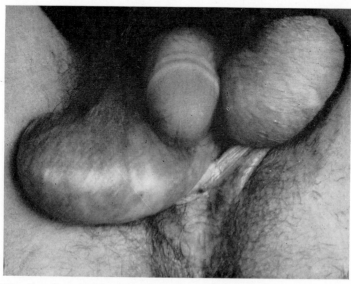

FIGURE 119. Pseudovaginal hypospadias with cleft scrotum in a twenty-year-old man.

In *penoscrotal* hypospadias the scrotum is cleft, bifid, or labiaform and especially in the pseudovaginal variety (Fig. 119). Rudimentary penis, cryptorchism, or other testicular anomalies as well as prostatic hypoplasia commonly coexist.

In *perineal* hypospadias, the genital development is thoroughly rudimentary with a clitoric type of penis which is often covered by a preputial hood or is engulfed in an overlying bifid scrotum, the whole picture strongly suggesting hypertrophy of the clitoris and labia. Congenital chordee is extreme and the testes are rarely normal, usually being hypoplastic or atrophic, or absent from the separated scrotal sacs. The urethral gutter may be absent or extend as a groove from the tip of the penis, is characteristically funnel-like, wide open, and aptly termed pseudovaginal. When the urethral meatus is well posterior in penoscrotal and perineal hypospadias, insemination will not occur because the sperm are ejaculated extravaginally. Sexual function is greatly diminished or absent and because of sterility or difficulty of coitus, reproduction seldom if ever occurs.

Because these patients cannot urinate in the upright position without spraying themselves and their clothing, the pseudohermaphroditic male will sit or squat to void and this increases his likeness to the female. While adrenal virilism in the female may cause changes simulating male pseudohermaphrodism, the vagina is present. Yet the hypertrophied clitoris or fused labia (q.v.) as well as a congenitally short urethra in the male may cause diagnostic error.

Determination of the true sex is extremely difficult in many cases of pseudohermaphrodism of the scrotoperineal or perineal hypospadiac variety. *It is most essential that the true sex be known as early as possible and always by the second year at least,* even if abdominal exploration and demonstration of definitive sex organs are necessary. By vaginoscopy in neonatal life a normal appearing cervix may be identified; the urethral opening will be proved to be hypospadiac. Visualization of a verumon-

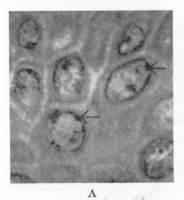 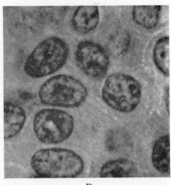

A   B

FIGURE 120. Genetic sex determination by examination of the malpighian layer of the skin. *A*, female with definitive chromatin mass in nucleus periphery. *B*, male; no definitive chromatin nuclear mass (see text; Barr).

tanum establishes the male dominance of the patient as will palpable testes. The findings of *testicular biopsy* are absolute.

Study of the chromosomal pattern of the nuclei of the cells of the malpighian layer of the skin gives strongly suggestive evidence of the true sex of the patient. According to sex, a difference is found in the nuclear structure, the skin nuclei from the female containing a mass of sex chromatin which is seldom seen in nuclei of skin specimens from the male (Fig. 120). Scrapings from the oral mucous membranes serve equally well for examination. The XX-chromosomes of the female produce in the periphery of more than two thirds of the epidermal nuclei a chromatin mass sufficiently large to be identified; the XY chromosomes of the male fail to produce a chromatin mass of sufficient size to be distinguished from the general chromatin. Thus the microscopic finding of these nuclear chromatin masses in over 60 to 70 per cent of the nuclei indicates the patient is a genetic female. While not an absolute test of true sex, this observation is at least indicative but, in the final analysis and particularly in pseudohermaphrodites, only *gonadal biopsy* is definitive.

Treatment of Hypospadias. This is surgical and is performed to enable the patient to reproduce, and to establish normal controllable urination in the standing position. We are less concerned with surgery as

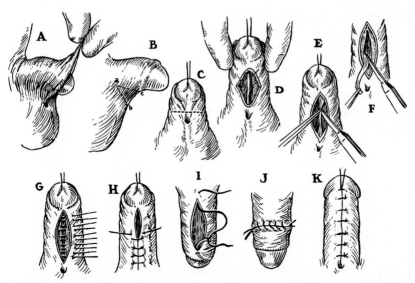

FIGURE 121. Hypospadias. Preliminary operation performed early to eliminate chordee and to permit the penis to grow. *A*, penoscrotal hypospadias showing the downward incurvation and the hooded prepuce. *B*, excision of restraining tissue in webbed penis. *C*, transverse incision of skin and subcutaneous fascia just anterior to the meatus. *D, E, F*, the sclerotic cord (aplastic corpus spongiosum) which causes the incurvation or chordee is excised. *G* and *H*, longitudinal closure of transversely incised wound to give penile elongation. The traction ligature through the glans is fastened to the lower abdominal wall to hold the organ in extreme retroflexion. *I, J, K*, longitudinal incision of the dorsal skin and penile fascia with transverse incision to foreshorten these structures, thus to help correct the ventral incurvation.

an antidote for psychologic problems. In *glandular balanitic* hypospadias the maintenance of free meatal drainage by meatotomy or urethral dilation is the treatment.

Penoscrotal hypospadias is best repaired in two stages, the initial procedure with correction of the congenital chordee being performed by the time the child is one year of age (Fig. 121). Later when he is four, five, or six years old or when there is sufficient tissue locally and the penis free of chordee is of sufficient size to carry out the urethroplasty satisfactorily, the corrective operation is performed. The importance of correcting the congenital chordee early cannot be overemphasized. Unless the organ can grow fairly straight and to a reasonably normal size, there is little object in attempting to make a new urethra to the glans penis for, though it may be a short curved water tube, it will be of no sexual (particularly reproductive) value.

In *perineal hypospadias* the chordee is corrected early. The urethral construction proper is begun when the child is four or five years old, building up the urethra to the penoscrotal junction from which point the canal is completed at a later date. With the Browne operation and following a preliminary satisfactory correction and straightening of the penis, it is possible in many of these cases to complete the entire surgical therapy in one stage. Similarly, *pseudovaginal hypospadias* may require a multiple stage surgical procedure which is begun when the child is four or five years old, having completed correction of the chordee at a much earlier age. In general, the surgical program is that just given for scrotal or scrotoperineal hypospadias.

Most unfortunate, many children suffer the disadvantage of having their malformation made the topic of dinner table, household and neighborhood conversation and deprecation and with which, at the time, the elders are much more concerned than is the patient. In my experience more psychic harm accrues to these children from what they hear at home in the discussion of their problem between the parents than from the derision given their malformation by unkind playmates. The attitude, instruction and training of the parents merits special consideration as it does in the clinical management of enuresis, masturbation, or other unfortunate behavior developments.

Operation is always advised on surgical rather than psychologic grounds and before operating for hypospadias the responsible party should be informed of the surgical difficulties and the high incidence of secondary infection and other complications which often make necessary two or more operations before a patent nonfistulous urethra is achieved. The surgical outlook today, however, is infinitely better than it was even ten years ago, this outlook resulting not only from improved technics, notably the Browne and Cecil procedures which I prefer, but also modern antimicrobial therapy.

Hypospadias in the female is discussed in Chapter 14.

Congenital urethral diverticulum is always almost a back-pressure blowout manifestation behind a peripheral obstruction, the most frequent being stenosis of the external urethral meatus. In their order of incidence, the site of congenital urethral diverticula are: (1) pendulous urethra, (2) penoscrotal junction, (3) region of the frenum, and (4) the bulbous urethra (Fig. 13). The cure is by excision as in the acquired variety (Chapter 8) and the maintenance of free urethral drainage.

Urethral Cysts.   Congenital cysts of the external urethral meatus have been described elsewhere (p. 174) but cysts may form at any point up to and including the vesical outlet. Several cases involving Cowper's glands, the prostate and/or the utricle have been described, some of these cysts enlarging sufficient to cause complete urinary obstruction. The *pathogenesis* of the occlusion is blockage of the ducts of the glands or cyst formation in epithelial cell nest inclusions along the urethra and consequent to incomplete urethral fold closure. The *symptoms* are those of obstruction, and the diagnosis may be suggested by palpation of the cyst but is confirmed by urethroscopy. Electrodestruction of the cyst is the treatment although some large cysts, particularly of the prostate and utricle, may require surgical excision.

Cysts may also occur externally along the medial genital raphe and especially in the region of the frenum.

Persistent Cloaca.   This is characterized by congenital intercommunication between the urethrovesical junction area or, more particularly, the prostatic urethra and the rectum in the male, and between the vesical and/or urethrovaginal and rectal segments in the female. It is one of the more rare yet severe of urogenital tract anomalies; complicating upper urinary tract back-pressure injury coupled with infection is often fatal. Moreover, grave urologic and nonurologic anomalies frequently coexist. The *pathogenesis* of the condition is shown in Figure 96 in which it will be noted that the urorectal septum fails to join the cloacal membrane. This leaves a connection between the bladder and rectum which is often misdiagnosed as congenital urethrorectal fistula and the *symptoms* of which are identical. Gas, feces and urine are passed both ways through the rectum, urethra and/or vagina according to sex. In the majority of these cases there is also imperforate anus and because of congenital urethral obstruction operating in utero, urinary drainage may take place through the urachus and umbilicus. Secondary renal infection and urosepsis is nearly always fatal. The *diagnosis* is made by endoscopic and urographic demonstration of the urorectal opening. *Treatment* is surgical with redirecting of the various malformed channels through properly located outlets, sometimes with the construction of new sphincters.

Congenital urethrorectal fistula is due to the same cause as persistent cloaca, namely, failure of the urogenital fold completely to separate the rectum from the posterior urethral segment of the bladder; the fistulous connection is nearly always in the anterior prostatic urethra or at the membranous junction (Fig. 122). The condition occurs about once in 5000 individuals and twice as often in males as in females with urethrovaginorectal fistula. The incidence of rectal atresia or imperforate anus in the newborn is one in 6500 and in the majority of these, urethrorectal fistula will also be present; serious urologic or nonurologic anomalies may co-exist elsewhere. Most of the twenty-nine cases of urethrorectal fistula that I have seen to date (1955) had previously been operated on for imperforate anus soon after birth, the surgeon thinking that when he struck urine on incising the anal occlusion, he had incised the posterior urethra or bladder. Yet in all cases the congenital urethral fistula pre-existed. By embryologic aberration, the fistula may even open in the anterior trigone or bladder floor (Fig. 123). The principal *symptoms* of urethrorectal fistula are the passage of urine by rectum and feces per urethram.

Diagnosis. A dye such as methylene blue or indigo carmine injected intravenously or into the bladder appears in the stool. The diagnosis is

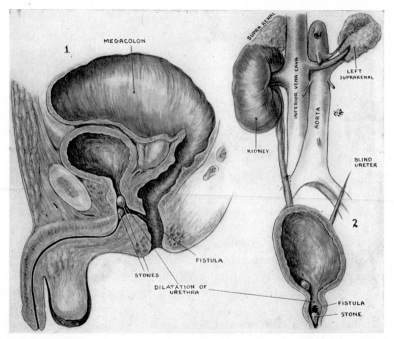

FIGURE 122.   Urethrorectal fistula in a four-year-old boy. A secondary stone formed in the prostatic urethra. There was also congenital absence of the left upper urinary tract.

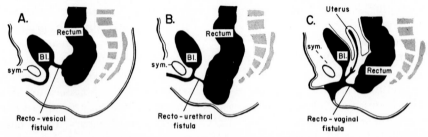

FIGURE 123.   Embryologic error giving rise to (*A*) rectovesical and (*B*) urethrorectal fistula. In each instance the anus is imperforate and in (*A*) the rectal pouch terminates high. *C*, in female with rectovagino-urethral fistula formation.

accurately made by urethroscopy when the fistulous opening on the posterior urethral floor will be identified. If operation is contemplated shortly,
a ureteral catheter can be passed through the urethral fistula into the
bowel and left indwelling as a surgical guide. Often the rectal orifice of
the fistula is just within or not over 2 cm. inside the anal ring. The anal
opening is tight and usually scarred.

Treatment is excision and closure of the fistulous tract; some modification of the Whitehead-Stone pull-through procedure works best.
Suprapubic cystostomy counterdrainage is first established following
which the rectum is mobilized to well above the fistula. The rectal cuff
is then pulled down so that the rectal orifice of the fistula is outside the
anal ring. The cuff is cut off and its proximal margins are sutured to
the cutaneous margin.

Congenital Valves of the Posterior Urethra.   These are deep mucosal
folds or redundancies located in the prostatic urethra, are usually attached
at one end to the verumontanum and pass anteriorly to the urethral
wall (Type 1) or back to the vesical outlet (Type 2). Occasionally the
valve formation is an iris diaphragm and rarely is imperforate (Type 3).
Various types of urethral valves are indicated in Figure 124; in two of our
patients the valves passed from the midverumontanum laterally to the
urethral walls as a modification of Type 1 valves. In these cases the ver-

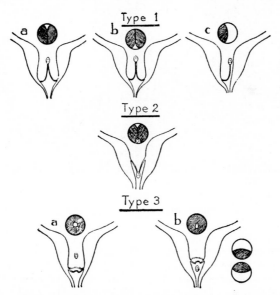

FIGURE 124.   Congenital valves of the posterior urethra. *Type 1: a,* two bifurcated
valves springing from the distal portion of the verumontanum; *b,* two fused valves in the
same position; *c,* unilateral valve in the same position. *Type 2:* bifurcated valve extending
from the proximal portion of the verumontanum to the lateral sides of the prostatic urethra
and roof. *Type 3: a,* iris valve below the verumontanum; *b,* iris valve above the verumontanum. The shaded circles represent the cystoscopic field seen in the region of the
valves. The vesical outlet and the prostatic urethra are shown to be dilated; the region of
the membranous urethra is indicated. (McKay after Young.)

umontanum is usually anomalous, being much larger and longer than normal. The condition is comparatively rare and is usually recognized late or not at all.

The condition is predominantly obstructive and because of its location produces vesical as well as bilateral upper urinary tract damage. Failure to relieve the obstruction and control complicating urinary infection leads to certain urosepsis and death. Some of the most extreme ureteral dilatations one will encounter are seen in these cases (Fig. 42).

Symptoms. The symptomatic picture in valvular obstruction is that of infravesical blockage in general and which has been discussed in Chapter 5.

The *diagnosis* is suggested by the history of urinary difficulty, chronic urinary infection, renal pain, pronounced and persistent gastrointestinal disturbances or, in advanced cases, urosepsis or uremia. In some instances of long-standing obstruction in the young the condition of *osteitis fibrosa*

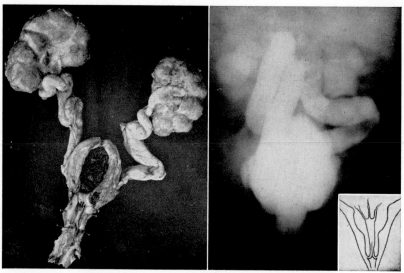

Fig. 125   Fig. 126

FIGURE 125.   Congenital valves of the posterior urethra in an eleven-month-old boy. The verumontanum is nearly four times normal size and length, and bifurcates anteriorly to form Type 1 valves. Three deep Type 2 valves are seen extending from the posterior verumontanum to the bladder outlet. There is marked hypertrophy of the bladder wall, four to five times normal thickness, and acute hemorrhagic decompression cystitis due to the sudden evacuation of the chronically overdistended viscus. The patient was admitted to the hospital because of constipation. An abdominal mass was thought to be filled constipated bowels but proved to be greatly distended ureters. The bladder was palpable to the umbilicus. Mechanically the overdistended bladder compressed the rectum to prohibit normal movements. By maneuvering the irrigating fluid, the obstructing valves were cystoscopically observed to balloon into cusp formation. The bladder urine was sterile. Uremic death occurred one week following cystostomy drainage. Extreme dilatation of the ureters and renal pelves with hydronephrotic renal destruction are notable.

FIGURE 126.   Cystogram of Figure 125 showing extensive dilatation of the entire upper urinary tract and the striking cystographic delineation of the posterior urethra behind the anterior (Type 1) valves. (Bellevue Hospital.)

cystica, commonly known as *renal rickets* or secondary renal hyperparathyroidism, develops (q.v.; Figs. 49–52).

The correct diagnosis is made by cysto-urethroscopy in which the valve leaflets are visualized and, by manipulation of the irrigating stream, can be made to wave back and forth in the fluid current (Fig. 125). The back-pressure effects on the bladder wall are evident—trabeculation, sacculation, cellule formation and, not infrequently, diverticulation and sometimes with secondary stone deposit. True valvular obstructions are not apt to be confused with the normal frenulae of the posterior urethra. By *cystography* the dilatation of the urethra and bladder neck behind the obstructing valves is often clearly delineated (Fig. 126).

The *prognosis* will depend upon the degree of renal damage and in advanced cases must always be guarded. Today the outlook is somewhat improved because of modern antimicrobial therapy but these agents will not restore destroyed renal parenchyma.

Treatment of urethral valves is their excision or division by transurethral resection which, in our experience, is preferable to the more radical suprapubic or retropubic attack. Following removal of the valves, cure cannot be claimed until the urine is sterilized and free drainage is established throughout the urinary system.

Congenital hypertrophy of the verumontanum is characterized by enlargement of the verumontanum two or more times, so that it occupies much or all of the prostatic urethra and may even extend back into the vesical outlet or forward into the membranous urethra (Fig. 127). The cause of the enlargement is not known. The symptoms, physical, laboratory and urologic findings are common to all infravesical obstructions. By urethroscopy the enlarged verumontanum is identified; the utricle is

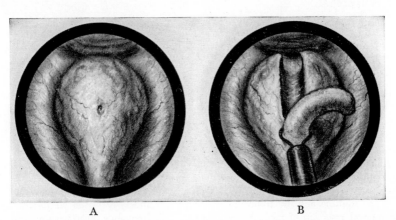

A   B

FIGURE 127. Hypertrophy of the verumontanum. *A,* cystoscopic appearance; often the organ fills the entire deep urethra despite liberal dilation with irrigating fluid. Unless the prostatic urethra is well distended at the time of deep urethroscopy, the verumontanum in all boys will appear abnormally large owing to the close proximity of the tissue to the objective lens of the instrument. *B,* author's method of treatment by transurethral electrocutting loop resection. It is unnecessary to remove the entire organ and as far as possible the ejaculatory ducts should be spared.

seldom made out in the hypertrophic mass. While the lesion may appear as a large ball and act in a ball-valve manner, usually it is greatly elongated and fills the prostatic urethra. But unless one is able to get a good panoramic urethroscopic view under fluid distention, even the normal verumontanum or one edematous from inflammation may seem unusually large. The hypertrophic verumontanum may cause a filling-defect shadow in the posterior urethrogram.

Treatment of hypertrophy of the verumontanum is transurethral resection in which most of the hypertrophic obstructing tissue is removed (Fig. 127B). As a rule, tissue remaining will shrink and contract. It is recognized that in this process, the ejaculatory ducts of the seminal vesicles may become occluded with resulting sterility but unless the obstruction is relieved, the patient may not live long enough for reproduction to become a problem. The hypertrophic verumontanum may also be removed by the suprapubic and perineal methods, but these are more traumatic, are of greater surgical risk, and have been largely replaced by the transurethral procedure.

Congenital Contracture of the Vesical Outlet. This is a variety of congenital urethral stricture comparable to congenital stenosis of the meatus at the outer end of the urethra (Figs. 128–130). It is sometimes manifest at birth but it may not become clinically troublesome until the patient is twenty or even thirty years of age. About 20 per cent of cases

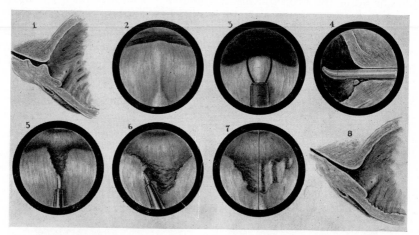

FIGURE 128. Congenital contracture of vesical outlet. *1*, sagittal view in contracted bladder neck with median bar obstruction in boys; there is pronounced elevation of the inferior lip of the vesical outlet. *2*, cystoscopic view of *1*, showing marked elevation of the bar in the midline and the frenulum which passes anteriorly to the verumontanum. *3*, transurethral resection of median bar with the high frequency electrocutting loop (Fig. 276). *4*, lateral view of *3*. *5*, employment of miniature electrocutting knife of the Collings' type for the eradication of median bar obstruction in young boys. *6*, the procedure in *5* is nearing completion. *7*, the left half shows the appearance of the newly made channel following the procedure shown in *5* and *6*; on the right are shown the furrows caused by the cutting loop as indicated in *3* and *4*. *8*, the appearance of the vesical neck following proper eradication of the obstruction; the posterior urethra is now isoplanic with the trigone which is the test of proper performance of the procedure.

of congenital contracture of the vesical outlet are found in females and a greater awareness and wider study of the vesical outlet in this sex will disclose many more cases than are now recognized. The lesion is simply a congenital narrowing of the bladder neck, the same as is commonly observed elsewhere in the urethra, ureters, biliary passages, cardiovascular system, and gastrointestinal tract. Histologic study of the vesical outlet in early noninfected cases often shows a submucous sclerosis. Commonly there is hypertrophy of the musculature of the vesical outlet but inflammatory fibrous tissue is not observed except as inflammation and infection have developed. It must be recognized that with mild congenital contracture of the vesical outlet, the patient consciously or subconsciously compensates against the blockage so that true clinical obstruction may not become manifest until the second to fourth decades. In some of these cases we have found the patient still wetting the bed in his twenties. Others, thirty-five or forty years of age, present all the cardinal symptoms of prostatic obstruction yet the gland feels normal or slightly less than normal size but the fibrotic vesical outlet is congenitally contracted.

As bladder neck congestion and inflammation appear in the growing patient, round-cell infiltration is not unusual and even calcific infiltration in the obstructing tissue has been observed. The entire circumference of

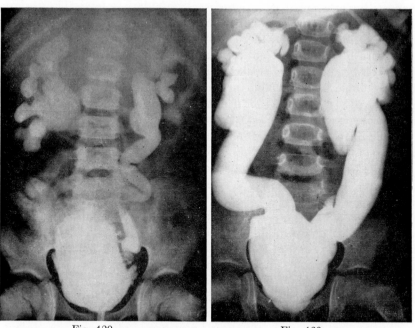

Fig. 129   Fig. 130

FIGURE 129. Congenital contracture of vesical outlet in a four-year-old boy with widely dilated infected upper urinary tract. Five ounces residuum. Suprapubic resection.

FIGURE 130. Congenital contracture of the vesical orifice in a five-year-old girl examined because of mild pyuria. No urinary difficulty. There is enormous dilatation of the upper urinary tract; the kidneys were reduced to thin shells. Suprapubic cystostomy drainage was instituted and six months later was followed by transurethral resection of the vesical outlet.

the vesical outlet is generally involved in a concentric collar-like manner. With the contraction there is usually elevation of the inferior segment of the bladder outlet from five to seven or four to eight on the clock face to produce a median bar behind which the trigone and bladder floor fall away (bas fond). Anteriorly, the prostatic urethra sharply rises from the proximal verumontanum to the crest of the median bar. Back-pressure changes of the bladder wall such as trabeculation, sacculation, saccule formation, and even diverticulum and secondary stone deposit are the expected developments (Figs. 129, 130).

Symptoms, therefore, are those common to all vesical obstructions; in children the urinary frequency or incontinence may erroneously lead to the diagnosis of enuresis. Chronic pyuria appears with the advent of infection and when this is acute the condition is usually and incorrectly diagnosed as "pyelitis." Suprapubic pain may result from vesical distention and renal pain from urinary back pressure or even from the effort to void.

The *diagnosis* of bladder neck contracture is made by urethroscopy in which, with a panendoscopic or direct-vision lens system, the concentric collar-like contraction of the bladder outlet is visualized, nearly always with considerable elevation of the inferior segment. The urethral floor immediately in front of the obstruction falls away rapidly while the trigone is hypertrophied and there is a variable bas fond. The residual urine in these cases is variable, from a half ounce to 30 ounces, and in complete chronic retention there is overflow or paradoxical incontinence. Contracture of the vesical outlet is differentiated by urethroscopy from valvular obstruction of the posterior urethra, congenital urethral stricture, congenital hypertrophy of the verumontanum and sphincterospastic neuromuscular disease of the vesical outlet. The last may require confirmatory neurologic examination and cystometric study (q.v.). The late atony of chronic infravesical obstruction and neurogenic atonic bladder is sometimes cystoscopically somewhat similar but in the last condition the trigone does not show hypertrophy as it regularly does in vesical neck contracture. The prognosis is identical with that of prostatic urethral valves just described.

Treatment. In some cases of mild contracture of the vesical outlet, periodic dilation or overdilation of the orifice will produce symptomatic relief and usually diminution of residuum. When these objectives are not achieved, the obstruction must be surgically removed. In our hands removal of the obstruction has been most successfully achieved by transurethral resection which causes the patient a minimal loss of blood and surgical trauma. We have also employed suprapubic removal of a V-wedge from the vesical outlet, either transvesically or as a retropubic procedure and lately have used Bradford Young's urethrovesicoplasty in several cases. But in most instances these methods have no superiority over the transurethral removal.

Congenital neuromuscular disease is the remaining important obstructive lesion at the vesical outlet and is discussed under neuromuscular diseases in Chapter 9.

Absence of the Prostate.   This most unusual condition is associated with other urogenital maldevelopments such as testicular agenesis, bilateral cryptorchism, exstrophy of the bladder, marked epispadias and pseudovaginal hypospadias. It occurs about once in 5000 newborn males. **Prostatic hypoplasia** is commonly observed in sexual infantilism and is correlated to underdevelopment of the remainder of the genital tract. **Isolateral congenital hypoplasia of the prostate** and the associated seminal tract is not infrequent in severe unilateral anomalies of the upper urinary tract, particularly renal agenesis.

Pseudohermaphrodism is a congenital condition of the external genitalia in which they resemble those of the gonadal sex opposite and has been classified as (1) complete, (2) internal and (3) external. In the *complete masculine* variety the sex glands are male and the sexual organs are female (Fig. 131). In the *complete female* type the sex glands are female and the external genitalia are male (Fig. 132) while the *internal masculine* type occurs in a male with fallopian tubes, uterus and vagina (Fig. 133) and the *internal feminine* variety is present in a female with both male and female sexual passages. In short, in external masculine pseudohermaphrodism the genitalia are male and the internal passages and glands are female; in the external feminine type, the female has female external genitalia but male gonads and internal genitalia. The problem of intersex is one of increasing interest particularly as new endocrinologic discoveries are made, new tests are devised for quantitative hormonal assay in the living human and, by synthetic chemistry, these hormones can be copiously produced for either replacement (e.g., testosterone) or stimulative (e.g., gonadotrophin) therapy.

Intersex.   The *male* type is the more common; here pseudovaginal hypospadias simulates a vulva in which the testes are usually absent and confirms the idea that hypospadias is an hermaphroditic condition (Figs. 131-134). A rudimentary cordlike structure represents the uterus and tubes. In the *external female* type the vulvar lips are often adherent or

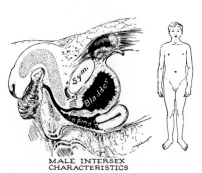

MALE INTERSEX
CHARACTERISTICS
Undescended testis.
Imperfect masculine development of urogenital sinus.
Imperfect feminine development of Muellerian ducts.

Fig. 131

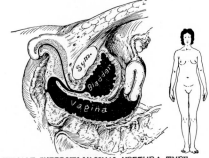

FEMALE INTERSEX VAGINAL URETHRA TYPE
CHARACTERISTICS
Normal ovaries and adrenals.
Muellerian ducts imperfect in descent and fusion.
Atypical masculinization of urogenital sinus.

Fig. 132

FIGURE 131.   Intersex in a male. (Figs. 131 to 134 courtesy of Dr. Frederick S. Howard.)
FIGURE 132.   Intersex in a female.

grown together to seal over the vagina or urethral orifice which may be common to both urethra and vagina, a mild variety of this condition being seen in congenital fusion of the labia minora (q.v.). Theories as to the cause of pseudohermaphrodism are largely concerned with overabundant secretion of maternal sex-opposite hormone affecting the male or female fetus.

In perineal and pseudovaginal hypospadias the local findings are often bisexual so that the true sex of the patient cannot be determined accurately without surgical exploration. Such cases present grave sociologic and legal questions in adulthood and particularly as to matrimony; the true sex of the individual should be known or determined early. The external examination may disclose no gonads and the genital morphology may be indeterminate. Here skin biopsy study of the chromosomal pattern of the malpighian layer may be highly suggestive of the genetic sex if not definitive (see page 184). Only laparotomy with gonadal biopsy is absolute, and advisedly should be made early, at least by the second year, not only for immediate identification of the sex of the patient but because in the future the surgeon's observations may be questioned. By this study in my own practice I have histologically confirmed three true hermaphrodites.

At the operating table the surgeon is often faced with a tremendous responsibility and a far reaching decision. He must take into consideration (1) whether the child has developed more like a boy than a girl and vice versa, (2) the comparative stage of development of the two sets of sex structures found, and (3) the past rearing of the child. When these factors are predominantly male, and usually there is other confirmatory evidence including hormonal assay studies, the female sex organs may advisedly be removed and vice versa. It has been my observation that in the cases thus "altered," the child adjusts better to a male existence than to the female life; and I have observed some lamentable examples of the last.

Sometimes intraperitoneal pneumograms with the pelvis well filled

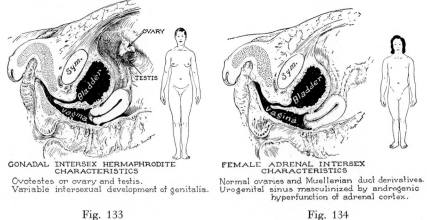

GONADAL INTERSEX HERMAPHRODITE
CHARACTERISTICS
Ovotestes or ovary and testis.
Variable intersexual development of genitalia.

FEMALE ADRENAL INTERSEX
CHARACTERISTICS
Normal ovaries and Muellerian duct derivatives.
Urogenital sinus masculinized by androgenic hyperfunction of adrenal cortex.

Fig. 133   Fig. 134

Figure 133.   Intersex. Gonadal hermaphroditic intersex.
Figure 134.   Female adrenal intersex.

with air may disclose abnormalities or even absence of the pelvic reproductive tract in the female and under certain circumstances these data may suffice to answer a current problem, but are not acceptable proof of the presence or absence, activity or morphology of a female gonad.

When the definitive decision has been made upon sound evidence and the child assigned to unisex, the opposite sex organs should be removed including the clitoris when indicated. Particularly in cases of adrenogenital syndrome, clitoric amputations have been performed when the organ was thought to be a penis.

In recapitulation, the sex of the patient must be determined early and accurately, preferably as soon after birth as possible, and certainly not later than the second year. Having determined the true sex and with matrimony a problem, the partner to be should be fully apprised of the facts.

Hermaphrodism defines the condition in which the individual is truly bisexual, possessing gonads and external genitalia of both sexes (Fig. 133). A classification of hermaphrodism follows:

1. Bilateral: There is a testis and ovary on each side.
2. Unilateral: A testis and ovary are on one side with either a testis or ovary on the other. Bilateral and unilateral hermaphrodism has been reported chiefly in the lower animals.
3. Lateral: An ovary on one side and a testis on the other. In these cases the female generative organs are sometimes ectopic with the uterus in the groin or scrotum and the testis ectopic.
4. Ovatestis: These gonadal structures are present on one or both sides.

Hermaphrodism is rare; I have had three clinical cases and have seen one in infancy at autopsy. Hermaphrodism is believed to result from maternal excess supply to the fetus of sex opposite hormones. Thus, in

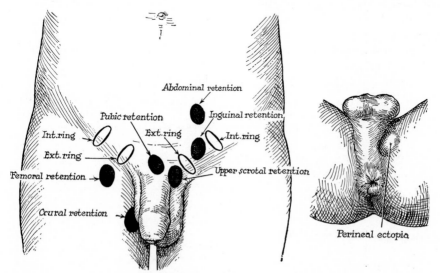

FIGURE 135.   Congenital testicular ectopia. The testicle may also be displaced into these unusual positions by trauma.

the masculine type which occurs most often, there is a small short penis, a hypospadiac meatus, the scrotum is cleft and bifid, the testes are generally in the inguinal canal or are abdominal, and a short small cordlike uterus and vagina with tubes and one or both ovaries are present. In the female type the clitoris is enlarged to penile size, the labial formation simulates a bifid scrotum, and may contain one or both testes or even herniated ovaries as well. Vaginal atresia is the rule. Acceptable diagnosis requires gonadal biopsy of both testis(es) and ovary(ies).

Treatment of the vagina in hermaphrodism or pseudohermaphrodism in the male will be largely guided by the collateral treatment. When the ovary, tube, and uterus are removed, most of the vagina down to the region of the utricle can be taken en masse, as I have done three times. The mere discovery of a vagina does not mean it must be removed and in most cases it can simply be forgotten and the hypospadiac defect properly corrected.

ANOMALIES OF THE TESTICLE

These are extremely common although some will pass wholly unrecognized except as discovered at operation as, for example, faulty urogenital union. Anomalies of the testis may be conveniently classified as indicated in Table 7.

Anorchism, congenital absence of the testis, is extremely rare, and is bilateral in a fifth of the cases. Anorchism may be classified according to (1) absence of the testicle only, (2) absence of the testicle, epididymis, and a portion of the vas deferens, and (3) absence of the entire spermatic tract. In unilateral anorchism the opposite testicle is often intra-abdominal.

In our series of 10,712 autopsies in boys, the testis was apparently unilaterally absent in eight cases (1:1339) and bilaterally absent in twenty-six yet it is possible that some small glands may have been overlooked. Certainly clinical experience does not lead one to suspect this high incidence. The *diagnosis* of anorchism properly cannot be made without full exploration of the entire area concerned in the initial gonadal

TABLE 7.   ANOMALIES OF THE TESTICLE

A. Anomalies in development	Anomalies in number...	1. In deficiency:	Absence or anorchism Fusion or synorchism
		2. In excess:	Polyorchism
	Anomalies in size.......	1. In deficiency:	Hypoplasia
		2. In excess:	Hypertrophy
B. Anomalies in position	Testicle undescended....	At some point in its normal course	Cryptorchism
		Outside its normal course	Ectopia
	Testicle descended......	Upside down	Inversion
		Hindside foremost	Retroversion

development up near the kidney and along the whole retroperitoneal course and inguinal canal through which the gonads normally descend. If the spermatic artery is found, trace it to its destination. There is no *treatment* except hormonal replacement therapy with testosterone, the dosage of which should be adequate but can be determined only by trial and evaluation.

Synorchism is fusion of both testes into one mass and may occur in the scrotum or abdominally. The diagnosis may be suggested by the absence of one testis from its scrotum and a double size lobulated testicular mass in the other scrotal pouch. There is no treatment.

In **polyorchism** or **supernumerary testes,** the presence of a third testicle is not to be confused with a small firm encysted hydrocele or spermatocele which may closely simulate a testis. The condition has been reported in about twenty cases, in some of which one of the testes had suffered from torsion of the spermatic cord. *Splenic rests* in the scrotum and along the cord have also simulated a third testicle, but ectopic adrenal rests are usually integral with the testis and epididymis or lie between them, and are not likely to simulate a third testicle.

Hypoplasia or **congenital atrophy** of the testicle is usually unilateral and compensatory hypertrophy of the mate generally coexists. The testis may be atrophic at birth from intra-uterine torsion of the spermatic cord or other trauma. Most undescended testes show some hypoplasia or atrophy which usually is proportional to the duration of the ectopia or imperfect descent. Hypoplastic testes are characteristically found bilaterally in congenital infantilism and associated with other endocrine disturbances, particularly of the pituitary. There is no treatment other than the adequate replacement administration of testosterone for, in most of these testes, the interstitial tissue is too meager or undeveloped to produce its own androgen in response to chorionic gonadotropin stimulation.

Imperfectly Descended Testicle.   This is also known as *cryptorchism* (hidden testicle) which describes the abdominal variety but now identifies all varieties of imperfectly descended testes. The testes fail to reach their normal destination in the base of the scrotum at birth in 1 to 3 per cent of all males and bilaterally so in about 10 per cent of all clinical cases. Right and left sided involvement are about equal. Although the testes are in the scrotum in only two thirds of premature newborn males, by the end of one year only 1 per cent remain imperfectly descended and half of these will descend at puberty with the greatly increased gonadotrophin hormonal stimulation occurring at that time. It may be accepted that if the testicle is to descend spontaneously, it will nearly always be completed by the first year and if not completed by puberty the likelihood of subsequent descent is scant.

According to the site of final resting place, undescended testes may be classified as (1) abdominal (lumbar or pelvic), (2) inguinal (in the canal), (3) subinguinal, prepubic, or upper scrotal. One hundred and ten of 23,529 (1:214) adult males examined post mortem showed cryptorchism, being bilateral in twenty-one, an observation of striking variance of bilaterality in the young. Notable in this study in adults is the high incidence of atrophy of the undescended testis which occurred in half of the cases, being pronounced in eighteen, in contrast to only three in a series of 217 infants and young cryptorchids similarly examined. In the adult group the location of the undescended testicle was intra-abdominal in only eight, at the internal inguinal ring in one, at the external ring in eight, in the inguinal canal in eighteen—the last being 28.1 per cent of the total number. In at least 90 per cent of permanently arrested testes, the glands are retained by adhesions or by anatomic factors as enumerated in second succeeding paragraph.

About 70 per cent of undescended testes are inguinal while about 25 per cent are abdominal and the remainder are perineal, pubic or are located in other unusual positions (Fig. 135). In 10,852 boys examined post mortem, there were 313 instances of cryptorchism or one in thirty-four, right and left sided incidence being about equal, and bilateral in 234. The testes were intra-abdominal in seventy-one, at the internal ring in twenty-two, in the canal in 170, at the pelvic brim in two, retroperitoneal in one, and at the external ring in twelve, and in an additional forty cases, the organs could not be found.

Etiology. The multiplicity of theories as to the cause of imperfect descent of the testis attests the answer is still unknown. It is recognized that the following anatomic factors, either singly or in combination, may predispose to cryptorchism:

1. An unusually long mesorchium (testicular mesentery) which allows the gland undue intra-abdominal freedom and renders engagement in the internal inguinal ring less likely.
2. Mesorchioperitoneal adhesions withholding the testis and preventing its descent.
3. An abnormal persistence of the plica vascularis which may anchor the testis high.
4. Short spermatic vessels or vas deferens.
5. The diameter of the testis and epididymis is greater than that of the inguinal canal.
6. Testicular fusion.
7. An absent, unusually long, or inactive gubernaculum.
8. Cremasteric hyperactivity interfering with descent. The paucity or even absence of the cremaster muscle in the cryptorchid is believed by some to be a factor, the effect of the cremaster being a downward milking action on the testis.
9. Maldevelopment of the inguinal canal with relative or absolute atresia.
10. Scrotal maldevelopment with absence of a testicular cavity.

Recent experimental observations suggest the gubernaculum plays no part of importance in testicular descent (Wells and State, 1947). Other experimental work suggests that (1) faulty genitocrural nerve function may be a factor by causing cremasteric muscle paralysis (Lewis, 1948), (2) that inguinal cryptorchism results from faulty muscular development of the groin coupled with failure of the gubernaculum to adjust itself to the muscular growth, this depending upon the development of the transversalis and internal oblique muscles and adjoining tendons which retain the testis high in the canal.

When the external oblique muscle is anomalous, low testicular retention occurs, an observation often made at operation in cryptorchism.

Today the *endocrine factors in testicular descent* have gained credence following the experimental work of Engle (1932) in rhesus monkeys. He found that the injection of prolan A—a chorionic gonadotrophin—caused the immature monkey testes to double in weight with increase of interstitial cell structure four to ten times, scrotal edema and tergescence, and premature descent of the testes from the external ring into the scrotum.

Following Engle's studies, Deming (1937) showed experimentally that following the injection of chorionic gonadotropin the testis of the immature rhesus monkey increases 50 per cent in size because of testicular interstitial cell enlargement and tubular enlargement in the epididymis, the vas deferens doubles in size and elongates, the vascularity of the cord is greatly increased, the cremaster muscle doubles in size, the dartos of the scrotum enlarges as does the inguinal canal, but the scrotal skin does not.

The fact that the testes sometimes descend spontaneously at puberty lends weight to the probable relation of an hormonal factor to migration of the gland but just how this occurs is still undemonstrated. Chorionic hormone (gonadotrophin) is present in greatest amounts in the fetus and for a week after birth, is almost entirely absent in boys from birth to about ten years of age, again becomes present in large amounts during adolescence and continues so until about the fortieth year when it quantitatively declines (Womack and Koch, 1932). A carry-over of high concentration of chorionic hormone has been advanced to explain descent during the neonatal period of most testes not properly descended at birth, as it may also occur with the sudden burst of hormonal elaboration as puberty approaches. To date, hormonal therapy in cryptorchism has not been successful in more than 5 to 8 per cent in large series of cases.

The *migrating testis* has unusual free mobility within the inguinal canal, the gonad being freely pushed up or down and even into the abdominal cavity. As the boy approaches puberty the organ usually becomes firmly anchored in the bottom of the scrotum and if it is not, the condition strongly predisposes to torsion of the spermatic cord (Chapter 8). Moreover, should pain develop in the migratory testis, orchiopexy should be promptly performed and bilaterally if both testes are freely movable.

Inversion and *retroversion* of the testis are rarely observed and are of little importance except as the condition may confuse palpation. Here the position of the epididymis will give the clue.

Ectopic or *aberrant* descent of the testis may be:
1. *Interstitial,* in which the ectopic gonad lies anterior to the aponeurosis of the external oblique muscle. This is the most common form of aberrant descent. After leaving the internal ring, the testis passes upwards and outwards to lie upon the aponeurosis; the gubernaculum can readily be identified. Completion of descent is blocked by absence

of a scrotal opening through anomalous development or is otherwise impervious.

2. In *femoral or crural* ectopy, the testis lies in Scarpa's triangle in a third of the cases.

3. *Penile* ectopy places the testis at the penile base or overlying the pubic bone; this is one of the rarest urologic anomalies.

4. *Perineal* ectopy. The gonad lies in the anterior portion of the perineum just lateral to the midline. The testis is usually attached by the gubernaculum to the spine of the ischium while the spermatic cord overlies Poupart's ligament. The condition is generally overlooked because of failure to examine the perineum and, because of this oversight, the testicle is usually designated erroneously as intra-abdominal. Therapeutically this is the easiest ectopia to correct because both the blood supply and the vas deferens are generously long. The testicle is simply mobilized from the perineum and placed in the scrotal depth.

5. *Transverse aberrant* testicular maldescent. Both organs descend through the same inguinal canal to the same scrotal sac or the testicle which has crossed over may be trapped in a hernial sac. In a pseudo-hermaphrodite, both testes and an infantile uterus were found in the same scrotal cavity (Hertzler).

Pathology of Cryptorchism.   In addition to the gonadal malposition, the most striking surgical finding is the associated congenital hernia which has been variously observed in 70 to 100 per cent of the cases; in my experience this is 80 per cent, the cause of the hernia being failure of the processus vaginalis to close. While most of these herniae can be detected by physical examination, in some it is demonstrated only at operation. The unfortunate consideration is that so many physicians fail to examine for, or even think of hernia in this connection, and are content fruitlessly and expensively to administer hormone therapy when the condition is obviously surgical from the start, the needless delay retarding or even stopping the further development and maturation of the testicle.

The most common congenital hernia accompanying cryptorchism is the indirect inguinal type although it may be sliding and even the cecum or sigmoid may join in the descent. About 15 per cent of these herniae are interstitial being (1) subcutaneous (between the superficial fascia and the external oblique muscles), (2) interparietal (between the external and internal oblique muscles), or (3) properitoneal (between the transversalis fascia and the peritoneum). In my experience about half of improperly descended testes lie in the superficial inguinal pouch anterior to the aponeurosis of the external oblique muscle. Sometimes the inguinal canal is completely blocked off which explains the undescent as does retention in an overly dilated canal. Maldescended in the inguinal canal, the testis is more subject to trauma by direct blow or by muscular contraction and is more likely to undergo torsion of the spermatic cord. At the opening into the scrotum (third inguinal ring of McGregor) the orifice may be narrow or completely shut off to explain failure of the testis to enter the scrotum, an interstitial or other ectopy developing.

The vessels of the spermatic cord are usually shorter than normal

although the vas deferens is nearly always of normal length. A long testicular mesentery or mesorchium attaching the epididymis to the testis is
commonly found, and, of itself, predisposed to torsion of the spermatic
cord, so often observed in cryptorchism. There is also frequently failure
of urogenital union in which the epididymis is not joined to the testis or
the vas deferens and epididymis are ununited (Fig. 139).

The *atrophy* so regularly observed in imperfectly descended testis
will be slight or pronounced, depending chiefly on the duration of the
anomaly but also on interference with its blood supply to produce
ischemia. Trauma or compression within the inguinal canal or blows to
the testicle when it overlies the pubis are additional potential injuries. The
cellular changes are chiefly atrophy of the seminiferous tubules involving
principally the spermatogenic cells which commonly disappear so that
about 90 per cent of testes undescended at puberty are sterile. The endocrine interstitial cells of Leydig may show little change except an increase
in fat or they may hypertrophy. Patients whose interstitial cells are preserved are rarely impotent in adulthood even though bilateral cryptorchism and sterility exist. Occasionally the Leydig cells are also destroyed,
the entire testis becoming a small fibrous mass. In bilateral cryptorchism
with injury or destruction of the interstitial cells, pronounced endocrine
disturbances generally occur, manifested by eunuchoidism or hypogenitalism. Somatic endocrinopathic changes seldom develop except in bilateral
cases. The normal mate of an imperfectly descended testis will show
variable hypertrophy.

It has been conclusively shown that the scrotum functions as a
testicular radiator in the cooler confines of which development and
maturation of the gonad normally take place (Moore, see Chapter 4).
The intrascrotal temperature is two to four degrees (Fahrenheit) cooler
than the intra-abdominal; normal testes placed intra-abdominal promptly
degenerate as a result of the increased heat. Even the continued wearing
of a scrotal suspensory with consequent increased testicular temperature
will induce infertility.

It has been amply demonstrated by comparative testicular biopsy
that both the normal testis and the cryptorchid develop essentially parallel until the age of four or five years. After this the cryptorchid gland
will not grow as rapidly in size or may even cease to grow, may degenerate with fibrosis, and will never match its normal mate in the size of
the tubules or in spermatogenesis (Figs. 136, 137). Sohvol observed three
types of testicular dysgenesis, the most frequent being (1) immaturity of
the seminiferous tubules in half the cases and occurring at or just following prepuberty. Less frequently (2) *congenital germinal aplasia* with
complete absence of spermatogonia has been found just before or during
the pubertal period. (3) Least frequent and most grave is the rudimentary
testis without Leydig or germinal Sertoli cells in the hypogonadal adult.
In short, the organ is congenitally dystropic from the beginning. Yet the
seminiferous tubular immaturity can usually be corrected by proper treatment of the cryptorchism with chorionic gonadotropin administration and
early surgical positioning of the gonad in the scrotum. But, in any event,

all three types of these organs are decidedly and congenitally abnormal. This may explain the higher than usual incidence of cancer in them as compared with the normally formed and normally descended organs, and explains the discouraging low rate of fertility in many of these patients when surgical treatment has been delayed until puberty or later.

The *symptoms* in cryptorchism are largely dependent upon the age of the patient and whether one or both gonads are involved. Local symptoms, except for the absence of the testis from the scrotum or complicating torsion of the spermatic cord, are usually lacking in infancy but in older boys there may be recurrent cramplike pains in the testis even with voiding; this usually reflects periodic moderate torsion of the spermatic cord. The inguinal testis may be painful when the legs are crossed or pain may arise from an accompanying hernia. The atrophic testis tends to become insensitive but may be the site of a dull or acute pain from nerve-end compression. Epididymitis of an undescended testis may suggest (1) torsion or (2) by pain reference, acute intraperitoneal surgical disease. *Endocrinologic symptoms* rarely appear except in bilateral cryptorchism and usually not until puberty approaches or postpuberty. Psychic disturbances are observed largely in older boys who sometimes develop a sense of sexual inferiority or general depression because of their anomaly to which only too frequently the attention has been directed by conversation within the family circle.

The *diagnosis* is made by palpation with which (1) the testicle can-

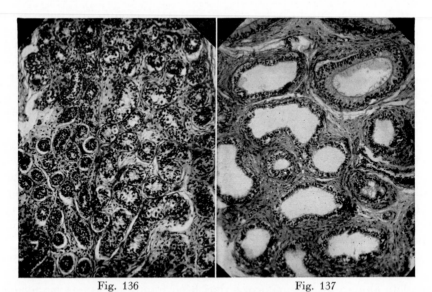

Fig. 136   Fig. 137

Figure 136. Imperfect descent of the testes. Histology. Normal testicle in a ten-year-old boy. Note the rich cellular structure with abundance of tubules and relatively scant interstitial tissues.

Figure 137. Inguinal testicle of a ten-year-old boy retained in the inguinal canal. The tubular degeneration and marked increase in interstitial tissue are remarkable and quite in contrast to the normal histology shown in Figure 136.

not be found in the scrotum, perineum, or, often, in the inguinal canal, (2) there is no history of orchiectomy or testicular trauma. Failing to palpate the testis, it may be assumed to be deep inguinal, intra-abdominal, or retroperitoneal. The scrotal development often gives the clue; in abdominal cryptorchism the isolateral scrotum is usually poorly developed and small and in congenital absence of the testis the isolateral scrotum is not developed at all.

In the study of the patient standing before the seated physician, to examine the right inguinal canal the examiner's left hand is placed on the outer buttock of the patient to give him support. The thumb of the right hand is firmly placed and held above the region of the right internal inguinal ring. The right index finger is then inserted into the inguinal canal, exploring the internal inguinal ring if possible. An extra-abdominal testicle may be palpable between the thumb and first finger and if it is not, an attempt is made by "stripping" to move the testis downwards in the canal, applying descending pressure by the thumb along the course of the canal. Thus a fixed testis will not noticeably move lower but with the stripping a migratory gland may be pushed into the scrotum between the thumb and index finger. Thus, it will be determined (1) whether a testis is in the inguinal canal, (2) the size, location and consistency of the gland, (3) if the gland is migratory (pseudocryptorchid) or true cryptorchid, and (4) if there is a hernia. In examining the left side the hands and positions are reversed. Often the *differential diagnosis* of complicating disease such as acute epididymitis, torsion of an undescended testicle or strangulated hernia accompanying cryptorchism will be made only at operation which, because of the presenting clinical picture, is urgent.

In ectopic testicle the *diagnosis* is made by noting the absence of the gonad from the scrotum and its location in the perineum, at the base of the penis, or its other location outside the usual course of descent. In any patient with cryptorchism *the perineum should be carefully examined.* These ectopic testicles are nearly always atrophic and may be insensitive.

Treatment. The objectives are (1) to encourage maximum fertility, (2) prevention of damage of the organ by trauma because of its abnormal position, (3) a satisfactory cosmetic result (which, of itself, will do much to improve the psychologic outlook), and (4) to forestall malignant changes. Unless early hormonal and surgical therapy succeeds in bringing the testicle permanently well down into its normal situation in the scrotum, aspermatogenesis becomes almost a certainty.

Treatment should begin early. For more than twenty-five years and as a result of personal histologic studies in the Pathology Laboratory of Bellevue Hospital, I have strongly advocated beginning treatment by the third year, especially in bilateral cryptorchism. Subsequent experimental and histologic studies have amply confirmed this recommendation (Engle, Robinson and others). In any event, the treatment must be undertaken by the fourth or fifth year at the latest if maximum benefits are to be obtained.

When there is demonstrable hernia the condition is surgical from the start. When there is no demonstrable hernia, a trial of hormonal therapy may be undertaken with the knowledge that it will promote normal permanent descent in about one in twenty of these cases.

When treatment is unduly delayed until puberty for example, as so many of the pediatric books in particular have recommended and unfortunately some still advocate, there is grave danger to the undescended organ by (1) torsion of the spermatic cord which the anomaly encourages, (2) trauma of the organ in the inguinal canal, (3) strangulation of an associated hernia, (4) the opportunity for fertility may be hopelessly lost and, finally, (5) neoplastic changes may occur. In those rare cases of spontaneous testicular descent following puberty, the weight of evidence and chance is that the organ is immature, congenitally defective and, in all likelihood, sterile. Ninety per cent of men with bilateral cryptorchism after puberty are infertile (MacCollum). This is a most discouraging prospect to encourage watchful waiting of these unfortunate boys during a period when much can usually be done to salvage to an appreciable degree the testicle and its fertility. The administration of chorionic gonadotropin renders it no longer necessary to wait until puberty to ascertain if the testicle will descend spontaneously because this phenomenon can be anticipated by a test series of injections of the hormone even at the age of two or three years.

In short, it would be well in all cases of cryptorchism to begin treatment immediately after the third birthday unless symptoms or conditions arising before this time demand earlier intervention.

When only one testis is normally descended, mechanical factors such as retaining fibrous bands or anomalous development of the gland or canal should be suspected. When the maldescent is bilateral, the failure suggests either bilateral mechanical (anatomic) hinderance or more likely *in utero* there was inadequate elaboration of chorionic hormone at the critical prenatal time (seven to nine months).

Conservative or Nonsurgical Treatment. The dangers and disadvantages of watchful waiting until after puberty have just been cited. When there is no hernia, the testicle, imperfectly descended or migratory, may be given a trial course with hormonal therapy as (1) definitive treatment, (2) as a diagnostic test and, when necessary, (3) as a step preparatory to surgery. The testes which descend with chorionic hormonal therapy are the ones which normally would descend during puberty. The interstitial Leydig cells of the testis are stimulated by chorionic gonadotropin to secrete increased amounts of androgen. Excess fruitless overtreatment is likely to produce the manifestations of pubertas praecox (q.v.) and will stimulate closure of epiphyseal bone centers to prevent normal body development and encourage a variable dwarfism.

For many years relatively small doses of gonadotropin substance (anterior pituitary-like hormone of pregnancy urine marketed under various trade names by various manufacturers: Antuitrin "S", Parke Davis Company; Follutein, Eli Lilly Company; A.P.L., Ayerst, McKenna & Harrison), have been used intramuscularly, 200 to 500 units two to three times a week, for a period of three or four weeks at least. Today the use of larger doses is advised and for shorter periods; I use 2000 units twice a week for five injections. In responsive cases congestive enlargement of the genitalia is noted by the end of the first week and if the testes are to be stimulated to descend by this method, they will be located in the scrotal depths by the third week. Should the testes appear normally descended before the last injections are given, the treatment is stopped. Failure to descend is both prima facie evidence of anatomic retention and that surgical treatment is necessary. Yet gonadotropin therapy is of no value in imperfectly decended testicle associated with pronounced testicular hypoplasia incapable of stimulation.

If the operation is performed promptly at the end of the therapeutic and diagnostic test, the temporarily engorged and enlarged structures encountered in the operation may be handled with much greater facility. This is of particular advantage in young boys in the intervascular dissection of restricting bands in the spermatic cord.

In unsuccessful hormone therapy, following withdrawal of the gonadotropin the enlarged congested genitalia return to their previous size. In another two to three months the course can be repeated but we accept the one trial period as definitive.

In some instances the administration of testosterone propionate has succeeded when chorionic gonadotropins were unsuccessful. The use of testosterone in this connection is advised against because it is replacement therapy and further lulls the androgenic elements of the testes into inactivity. Androgenic hormone is indicated only when the testes transplanted to the scrotum fail to develop. Moreover, when given in great excess, testicular atrophy may be caused as I have twice seen in young boys given excessive amounts of testosterone for the treatment of cryptorchism. Testosterone causes a reduction of spermatogenesis and excessive doses, aspermia and even agametogenesis.

Surgical Treatment.   When there is complicating hernia the cryptorchism is surgical from the start and in any event operation should be performed when one or two therapeutic tests with hormone therapy fail to achieve the desired result. Where there is complicating hernia, operation rather than a truss should be employed; parenthetically, *under no circumstances should a truss be permitted in undescended testicle.*

The most satisfactory operation for cryptorchid testis is some modification of the Torek procedure or other traction fixation to ensure firm anchorage of the testis in the depths of the scrotum (Fig. 138). This may involve suture of the testis to the upper inner thigh through a window in the lateral scrotal wall, or traction attachment to the thigh by the intermediary of silk thread and/or rubber band technic. The spermatic cord and testis must be completely mobilized and cord elongation achieved by careful intervascular dissection including retroperitoneal, if necessary, to bring the testis to the lowermost scrotum. Sometimes apparent achievement of the desired result is possible by bringing the testis and cord through the lower abdominal wall medial to the deep epigastric artery.

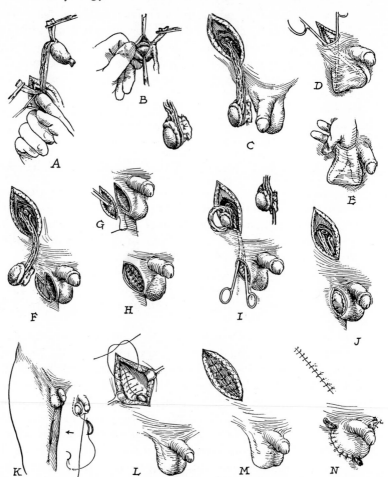

FIGURE 138.   Cryptorchism. Treatment by the Torek procedure. *A,* the hernial sac
is ready to be tied off. A finger introduced high into the inguinal ring will break down
adhesions and permit added lengthening of the cord to at least 1.0 or 1.5 cm. Should difficulty be encountered in obtaining sufficient cord length by the simple procedure just
described, open the internal inguinal ring upward 4 to 8 cm. to give free exposure of the
retroperitoneal space to mobilize the cord and especially the spermatic artery high. Sometime added cord length is gained by dividing widely the transversalis fascia as it forms the
floor of the inguinal canal, even cutting the deep epigastric vessels if necessary and bringing the adequately elongated cord and testis down through and out the lowermost angle
of this wound. *B,* opening of tunica vaginalis and its eversion behind the testicle to prevent
hydrocele. *C,* by intravascular dissection with the breaking down of restraining adhesions,
the spermatic cord has now been adequately lengthened. *D,* preparation of the scrotal
cavity to receive the testicle. It is extremely important that the dartos fascia be widely
divided in the scrotal depth. *E* to *J,* an opening is made in the lateral scrotum, the posterior
margin of which is sutured to a similar incision at the same level in the upper inner thigh.
The testicle is now brought down and through the scrotal opening and is fastened by two
or three fine silk sutures to the deep fascia of the thigh. The scrotal thigh wound is then
closed and the inguinal wound is closed as in herniotomy, with or, preferably, without
transplantation of the spermatic cord. In *K* is shown an alternate method for maintaining
traction of the newly mobilized testicle through the intermediary of a rubber band (after
Cabot). One suture anchored to the testicle in the lower pole of the scrotum is tied to one

When the testis cannot be brought down into the scrotum and yet appears worth saving, it may be brought down as far as possible at the first-stage procedure and months later re-operation performed to bring it the rest of the way to the scrotum. In my experience this is seldom successful. When the testis is congenitally atrophic, malformed, or is a small fibrous nubbin and obviously useless, it should be removed. In general, orchiectomy is preferable to leaving the testis in the groin or abdomen and certainly it should not be left lying over the pubic bone to be continually subjected to trauma. Because of the danger of neoplastic change, although comparatively remote, most of these organs which cannot be brought down into the scrotum should be removed.* Fortunately for the patient in whom orchiectomy under these conditions may incite psychogenic

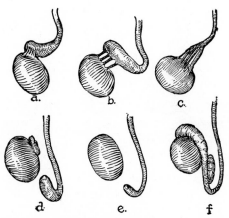

Figure 139.   Anomalies of urogenital union. Schematic presentation of some of the more common maldevelopments of urogenital union. *a*, epididymis detached from the testicle except at the globus major. *b*, epididymis attached to the testicle only by elongated ductuli efferentes. *c*, direct union of the vas deferens through ductuli efferentes to the testicle; the epididymis is absent. *d*, the body of the epididymis is absent; failure of union of the vas and testicle. *e*, globus major and body of the epididymis are absent. *f*, accessory epididymis forming on the globus minor of its mate (Hinman after Hinkey and Lubash).

---

* The incidence of cancer in imperfectly descended testis has been statistically cited as twenty-two times greater than in normal testes (Dean, 1940). Comparatively, new growths of the testicle are so rare as to merit scant special consideration. On a statistical basis, the danger of malignant change in a testicle should not alone be adduced as an indication for operation in cryptorchism. Orchiopexy per se does not prevent testicular cancer, for there have been reported several cases of neoplasm developing in testes surgically placed in the scrotum. This illustrates the proposition that these testes are congenitally abnormal in their internal morphology and structure.

end of the rubber band while to the other end of the band is tied a second suture which, in turn, is fastened lower down to the skin of the thigh. This permits free movement of the leg yet maintains traction. This traction pressure must not be great or either the suture in the testicle or in the thigh will pull out; usually the former gives way. *N*, closed wounds; a small petrolatum gauze wick is temporarily placed in the posterior space between the scrotum and thigh. In young boys it is well to restrain the legs for three or four days following this operation so that the anchorage of the testicle and/or the scrotal anastomosis with the thigh is not disrupted.

changes, plastic or metal testicular prostheses are available for implantation in the scrotum.

Treatment of *abnormally mobile testes* is orchiopexy, securely anchoring the gland to the lowermost scrotum. This alone will prevent torsion of the spermatic cord.

Treatment of *ectopic testicle* is surgical with mobilization of the gland from its ectopic site and implacement in its normal position in the scrotum and by the third year. As a rule this is simple to do; endocrine therapy is valueless in these cases.

Failure of urogenital union is extremely common in imperfectly descended testes in many of which a congenital discontinuity of the

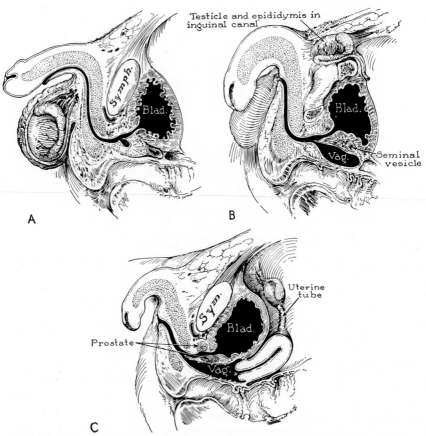

FIGURE 140.   Anomalies of the utricle; these are most commonly observed in advanced hypospadias. *A*, in penile hypospadias with slight enlargement of the utricle reflecting a minimal degree of feminization. *B*, greatly dilated utricle in penoscrotal hypospadias accompanied by incompletely descended testes, and hypoplasia of the penis, prostate, and seminal vesicles which reflects greater feminization than in *A*. *C*, extreme feminization in which the penis resembles a large clitoris and the urethral meatus is perineal. An atrophic testis and a rudimentary epididymis lay in contact with the uterine tube in the pelvis, the uterus being well developed and the vagina present. Prostatic underdevelopment with absence of seminal vesicles and vasa. (Howard.)

spermatic transportation tract accounts for isolateral sterility even though the gonad is normally spermatogenic (Fig. 139). The principal types of malunion are those in which (1) the epididymis and vas deferens are descended into the region of the scrotum but the testis is absent (anorchism); (2) the testicle is present but undescended; the epididymis is partially descended into the scrotum; (3) only the vas deferens is present in the scrotum, and (4) the testicle and epididymis are descended but are widely separated by a long mesorchium; here the epididymis usually precedes the testicle in the descent process and this is the usual condition often observed in high inguinal or abdominal testicle. All of these malunions are potential factors in the development of torsion of the spermatic cord (Fig. 191).

Adrenal rests are occasionally encountered along the course of the spermatic cord and, in two instances we have seen, rested between the epididymis and testicle.

Aplasia or **agenesis** of the isolateral spermatic tract is occasionally observed in renal agenesis or pronounced hypoplasia. *Aberrant wolffian duct remnants* are present in the epididymis as the hydatid of Morgagni and the paradidymis or organ of Giraldes, the first being attached by a blind duct to the head of the epididymis and the latter similarly attached to the tail of the epididymis. Occasionally these testicular appendages

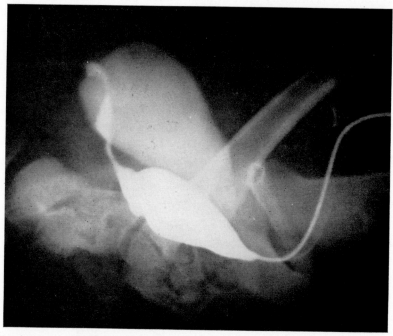

FIGURE 141. Congenital diverticulum of the utricle in an eighteen-month-old boy with penoscrotal hypospadias examined because of persistent pyuria of one-year duration. Lateral view of combined utriculogram and cystogram, a medium of lighter density being injected into the bladder. A curious fallopian-tube-like termination of the utricle is notable, this being the male homologue of the uterus.

undergo torsion to cause great pain and simulate torsion of the spermatic cord.

Anomalies of the vas deferens are concerned largely with its absence or aplasia in similar isolateral status in the upper urinary tract—especially renal agenesis or aplasia. These vasal anomalies are also observed as a part of faulty urogenital union described in the third previous paragraph, and may account for isolateral sterility.

Anomalies of the seminal vesicles occur chiefly when the isolateral upper urinary tract is maldeveloped. Vesicular malformations are rarely of clinical importance except as factors in isolateral sterility. In rare instances the seminal vesicles may become cystic and by extravesical or extra-urethral compression cause bladder neck obstruction. The *diagnosis* is made by urethrography or seminal vesiculography and by rectal palpation.

The **utricle,** the *uterus masculinus,* is a midline fusion development of the müllerian ducts and may be extremely deep with spacious dilatation or diverticulum formation or may form a cyst extending up between the seminal vesicles beneath the bladder base (Figs. 140–142). By distention and compression, the utricular cyst may cause bladder-neck blockage. The usual form, however, is that of a pocketing or small diverticulum of the utricle which opens into the urethra through the verumontanum and is not only commonly seen in hypospadias but the more advanced the hypospadias, the greater the anomaly of the utricle. This further reflects the feministic influence in hypospadias. Infected, the utricle sac becomes a urethral diverticulum and continues to pour infection into the urinary tract. The *diagnosis* is made by urethroscopy with catheterization and radiographic demonstration of the injected sac (Fig. 141). As a corollary, urethroscopy and examination of the verumontanum and its utricle should be performed in all cases of more pronounced hypospadias. The treatment is perineal excision of the sac.

Anomalies of the female external genitalia are discussed in Chapter 14.

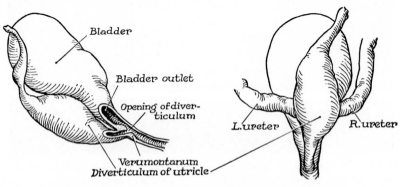

FIGURE 142.   Schema of local pathology for Figure 141.

CHAPTER 7 *Infections of the Urinary Tract*

URINARY infection is by far the most common urologic disease. It results from bacterial invasion, its chief predisposing factor is urinary obstruction, and singly but most often together these two conditions comprise over 90 per cent of major urologic problems. In urinary infection the kidney must always be considered to be involved until proved otherwise; more often than not the initial bacterial invasion is via the kidney(s). Bacteria are regularly present in the urine and, except in rare "pure" bacteriuria, pus cells are always found. Variable hematuria ranging from scant microscopic to gross hemorrhagic is generally demonstrable and in pyelonephritis the demonstration of pus casts makes the diagnosis. Urinary infection may be wholly asymptomatic or may make the patient desperately ill or even kill him. Uremia is the cause of death in about a third of the cases, hypertensive vascular disease secondary to the inflammatory renal damage is a cause of death in a sixth of the patients, and in the remainder complicating interstitial nephritis or even unrelated disease terminates the picture.

Unfortunately even today the wholly inadequate and pathologically incorrect diagnosis of "pyelitis"—either acute or chronic—is generally made when a laboratory reports the presence of pus in the urine, no matter how carelessly or casually the specimen was taken. Repetitiously confirmed studies have shown that in renal infection the usual lesion is an interstitial suppurative nephritis in conjunction with which infection and inflammation of the pelvis is clinically, if not pathologically, unimportant. Until an accurate anatomic diagnosis can be made it seems best to designate the urinary infection simply as pyuria, acute or chronic, for sometimes an infection is confined solely to the lower urinary tract. Urinary infections are here classified as (1) nontuberculous which is the usual variety, (2) tuberculous, and (3) unusual (parasitic, mycotic, syphilitic, etc.).

213

The commonest invading organisms are Escherichia coli and micro-cocci (Staphylococcus aureus and Streptococcus). The bacilli commonly arrive urogenously and show predilection for the drainage elements of the kidney, notably the pelvis and collecting tubules, while staphylococcic and streptococcic infections are mostly hematogenous with predilection for the cortical glomerular or secretory elements of the kidney.

NONTUBERCULOUS URINARY INFECTION

The *incidence* of urinary infection is highest before the age of two and after forty years. Occasionally it appears in the newborn and neonatal period in which age group the mortality has been as high as 40 per cent, but thanks to improved antimicrobial therapy fewer patients of all ages today die from urinary infection than did even twenty years ago. Exten-sive studies of the urologic problems of infants and children have shown that this group is subject to nearly every urologic disease known to adults. In the young, in incidence, urinary infection is by far the most common urologic disease and unrecognized, improperly or inadequately diagnosed, neglected or insufficiently treated with failure to sterilize the urine, com-monly leaves the young patient with a low-grade, smoldering, chronic pyelonephritis. With recurrent acute attacks and advanced interstitial tissue injury, cicatricial contraction of the kidney occurs with widespread damage or even total destruction of the parenchyma. With advancing disease, chronic pyelonephritis develops most commonly unilaterally in males and bilaterally in females without predisposition for one side or the other. Progressive destructive injury of the kidney(s) by infection and its variable reparative scar not only vastly reduces their function but ac-counts for the clinical manifestations so commonly recognized later as Bright's disease or chronic interstitial nephritis. In this disease, arteriolar sclerosis plays a nefarious role, especially in the genesis of hypertensive vascular disease. This is not intended to convey that all cases of Bright's disease have their genesis in chronic pyelonephritis of childhood but there is increasing evidence that this is so in a most substantial number so afflicted.

Predisposing Factors. The predisposing factors and accessory causes which (1) prepare the soil for the bacterial invasion and enable it to gain a foothold, and (2) help to perpetuate an established infection, are sche-matically shown in Figure 1 and Table 8. The *age factor* has been indi-cated in the preceding paragraph. The *sex incidence* is variable, urinary infection being recognized more often in infant girls than boys (3:1), and attributed largely to ascending diaper infection. In hematogenous renal infection at all ages, the sex incidence is about equal as is the severity of the disease. *Heredity or familial influence* has not been observed in urinary infection.

Mechanical Factors. Obstruction merits the greatest consideration as an associated etiologic agent, not only in the initial occurrence of urinary infection but in its perpetuation. Uncomplicated obstructive uropathy is discussed in Chapter 5. Urinary tract blockage of whatever cause, includ-

TABLE 8. ETIOLOGIC FACTORS IN URINARY INFECTIONS*

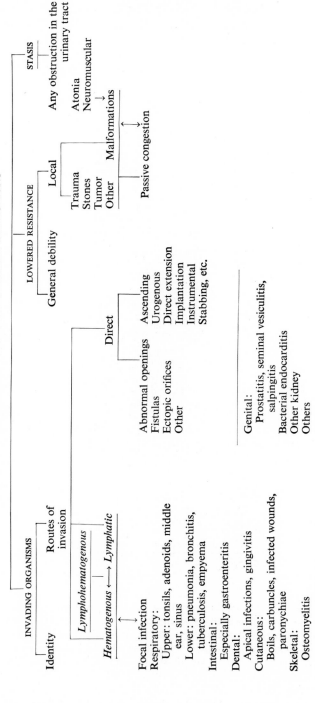
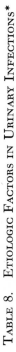

INVADING ORGANISMS

Identity

Routes of invasion

Lymphohematogenous

Hematogenous ⟷ Lymphatic

Focal infection
Respiratory:
Upper: tonsils, adenoids, middle
  ear, sinus
Lower: pneumonia, bronchitis,
  tuberculosis, empyema
Intestinal:
Especially gastroenteritis
Dental:
Apical infections, gingivitis
Cutaneous:
Boils, carbuncles, infected wounds,
  paronychiae
Skeletal:
Osteomyelitis

Direct

Abnormal openings
Fistulas
Ectopic orifices
Other

Ascending
Urogenous
Direct extension
Implantation
Instrumental
Stabbing, etc.

Genital:
Prostatitis, seminal vesiculitis,
  salpingitis
Bacterial endocarditis
Other kidney
Others

LOWERED RESISTANCE

General debility

Local

Trauma
Stones
Tumor
Other

Malformations

Passive congestion

STASIS

Any obstruction in the
urinary tract

Atonia
Neuromuscular

* Modified after Vose.

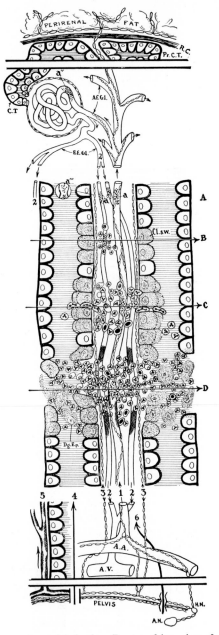

FIGURE 143.   Schema of renal infection. Routes of invasion of the renal parenchyma.
1,2,3, hematogenous. *A.A.*, arcuate artery giving off interlobar branches (1) which ultimately pass to the glomeruli as the afferent glomerular arteries (*Af.Gl.*). Leaving the
glomeruli, the efferent glomerular vessels (*Ef.Gl.*) pass downward as nutrient vessels of
the parenchyma, ultimately to become large veins (2) and finally empty into the arcuate
vein (*A.V.*). Retrograde extension of bacteria by pyelovenous or pyelotubular backflow
from the pelvis may occur.
     3. Lymphogenous. Through the lymphatics of the pelvis, or those which surround the
arteries and collecting tubules (Kumita), or those which penetrate the renal capsule
(*R.C.*) from the perirenal fat. *H.N.*, hilar lymph node; *A.N.*, aortic lymph node.

ing neurogenic, induces congestion in the proximal tract, and especially the kidney. The resistance or defensive mechanism of the congested tissues is variably reduced, especially in the rich endothelial cell structures of the capillary network. Debilitated, these injured cells fail to phagocytose and destroy blood-borne or urogenous invading bacteria, so that these organisms are enabled to pass through the walls of the capillaries and small blood vessels to establish themselves in the interstitial tissue of the kidney (Fig. 143). Most of these obstructions in children are associated with anomalous development as in the congenital forms of ureteral stricture, contracture of the bladder outlet, stenosis of the external urethral meatus, for example. As a corollary, while urinary infection does not appear early in more than half of all children with congenital urinary tract obstruction, we found the incidence of congenital obstruction to be twenty times as high in children with chronic urinary infection as in those without obstruction. In adults the more usual obstructive lesions are acquired such as stricture, stone, or prostatism, or as neuromuscular vesical disease, for example, as following cord injury, cord tumors, or in tabes dorsalis. These have been shown in Figure 41.

In the absence of obstruction most urinary infections are self-limited and clinically disappear in a week to ten days irrespective of treatment, but if the urine shows infection after three to four weeks of intensive medical treatment, a complete urologic examination is called for (see Indications for Urologic Examination, Chapter 2). Moreover, in persistent pyuria, and even though the urine is sterilized by modern antimicrobials,

---

4. Intratubular. Spread by retrograde extension (reflux) through the tubules from the pelvis.

5. Extension from the pelvis by vascular thrombosis.

6. By rupture through the pelvis with direct intertubular (interstitial) extension or extravasation. This is probably rare. Bacterial invasion of the kidney by eruption from neighboring foci or by surgical attack is not shown.

Pathologic sequence of infection:

A. Bacterial embolism in interlobular arteriole *a*, interlobular efferent vessel *a′*, glomerular arteriole *a″* or lymphatic vessel *a‴*. An extensive process of this nature is shown in Figure 154.

B. Early cellular reaction to the bacterial invasion. Note that the lesion is at first limited to the interstitial spaces of the kidney and the interstitial reaction is a perivascular leukocytic infiltration. Cloudy swelling (*Cl.sw.*) of the epithelial cells of the adjacent tubules occurs (Fig. 144). Symptoms are probably uncommon at this stage.

C. An advanced stage of *B.* Leukocytic infiltration and cloudy swelling increases; polymorphonuclears, lymphocytes, plasma cells, and large mononuclears are the cells regularly found. Histosections of this stage frequently show polymorphonuclears extruding between the swollen epithelial cells into lumen of the tubules (Figs. 144, 146, 147).

D. Late stage of *C* with massive focal suppuration. Vascular thrombosis, extensive leukocytic infiltration, destruction of the adjacent tubules (*Dg.Ep.,* degenerated epithelium) with discharge of purulent debris into collecting tubules and into the pelvis (Figs. 146, 147).

The above schema indicates why, in so-called pyelitis, the interstitial lesion is so much more important than mere inflammation of the pelvis. It also demonstrates how most of the pus found in the urine originates in the interstitial lesions rather than in areas of mucosal inflammation.

C.T., convoluted tubule. *Pr.C.T.,* proximal convoluted tubule.

at least a satisfactory excretory urographic study should be made before the patient is discharged as cured to be certain that no stasis producing lesion or condition persists in the urinary tract, the previous persistence of the infection *a priori* suggesting such a condition is probably present. By this examination one will be less apt to overlook obstruction, calculus, diverticulum, prostatism, hydronephrosis or tumor. Generally, by the time it is recognized in chronic pyuria, the obstructing lesion will have caused residual urine in the bladder or kidney pelvis.

Toxemia and Trauma. Toxic injury of the renal tissues reduces their resistance to infection just as congestion does, and makes the organ more vulnerable to invading bacteria. Examples of toxic injury are the infectious diseases (scarlet fever, measles, tuberculosis, typhoid fever, diphtheria, endocarditis, pneumonia, gastroenteritis), and chemical irritation. One of the commonest types of renal injury by inflammation is that seen in long-standing, smoldering, asymptomatic kidney infection in which, with local debilitation by obstruction for example, an acute flare-up or grave exacerbation of the infection occurs to augment the damage. Recurrences of this character often cause them to be improperly designated as episodes of "acute pyelitis"; the "pyelitis of pregnancy" is a classical example of this and, in some instances, the "pyelitis of deflorescence" or "bride's pyelitis" may be. Even though the initial invasion was unilateral, the longer the toxic agent persists, the greater the certainty of eventual bilateral involvement.

Similarly, *trauma* by external violence, renal stone, or by instruments induces variable congestion and comparable local debility in the renal parenchyma; in severe traumatic injury the tissue damage may be pronounced and extensive. In either event, a fertile field is furnished for bacterial enlodgement and propagation.

BACTERIOLOGY

The bacterial invaders in the usual nontuberculous urinary infections are most simply classified according to their gram-stain characteristics (Table 9).

The gram-negative bacilli Escherichia (E. coli communis and coliform group) are reported in 50 to 75 per cent of the cases of urinary infection, but it is probable that in many of these the laboratories have failed to distinguish between a rather wide variety of gram-negative bacilli including Aerobacter aerogenes or Bacillus lactis aerogenes, Pseudomonas aeruginosa, Proteus, E. typhosa, Shigella, Salmonella, and paratyphoid group organisms, designating all of them as E. coli. These gram-negative bacilli are most commonly found in the urine in the early stages of ascending or urogenous infections, and affect fundamentally the drainage elements of the urinary tract, particularly the renal pelves and medullary tubules. These organisms may reach the kidney hematogenously. Colon bacilli may be hemolytic—thought to be more virulent—and nonhemolytic, believed to be more tenacious. Urine badly infected with these organisms has a fetid, dead-mouse odor which, of itself, suggests the diagnosis although a urine comparably infected with Proteus may have a similar or dead fish stench.

The gram-positive cocci are predominantly hematogenous invaders, and characteristically first attack the secretory elements of the cortex, notably the glomeruli and adjacent convoluted tubules. In the gram-positive group of organisms, micrococcus forms predominate, chiefly *Staphylococcus pyogenes* (aureus, albus, hemolytic or nonhemolytic) which are of highest incidence—30 to 50 per cent. Some strains of staphylococci are urea splitters to produce stinking ammoniacal urine. Staphylococcus albus is not to be considered lightly as a contaminant; it may be as gravely important as Staphylococcus aureus. *Streptococci* may be hemolytic or nonhemolytic; Streptococcus viridans is occasionally encountered. Streptococcus faecalis (enterococcus), an encapsulated streptococcus whose normal habitation is the bowel, is found in about 10 per cent of urinary tract infections in children. Its precise identification is imperative; these organisms are generally difficult to eradicate being unresponsive to most drugs; Terramycin and mandelic acid are the drugs of choice. In a study of 100 strains of streptococci from the urine of children, Porch found 70 were Streptococcus faecalis. *Alcaligenes faecalis,* also of intestinal origin, is occasionally present but usually as a secondary invader. Other gram-positive cocci include the pneumococcus, Micrococcus tetragenus, Streptococcus lactis (nonpathogenic) and, rarely, Streptothrix.

It is fundamental that the invading organism(s) be accurately identified in order to prescribe the medication most likely to be effective against the various bacterial groups having specific drug sensitivities (see Table 9).

A *changing bacteriology* is commonly observed during the course of a urinary infection, first staphylococcic, for example, then colon bacillary or mixed, later Proteus, Pseudomonas, Aerobacter, or streptococcic and so forth. This is confusing to the unwary, the reason for the changes seldom being evident; the convenient theory of bacterial mutations is both inadequate and unproved. The necessity for repeated urine cultures is obvious if the physician's efforts are going to keep up with the infection and the antimicrobials given according to existing bacteriologic indications and drug sensitivity.

PATHOGENESIS

As indicated in Figure 143 and Table 8, routes of invasion of the kidney are: (1) hematogenous, (2) urogenous, (3) lymphogenous (lymphohematogenous), and (4) direct extension.

Hematogenous. This is the usual route of invasion, the bacteria being carried by the blood to the renal cortex, especially the glomeruli, and the interstitial vessels between the convoluted tubules. Later the microorganisms are transported by the glomerular efferent nutrient vessels to the other portions of the kidney, particularly the interstitial tissues between the tubules of the medulla (Figs. 143–147).

Hematogenous infections are initially bilateral; unilateral clinical disease suggests either an overwhelming bacterial invasion or diminished

TABLE 9.   ANTIMICROBIAL THERAPY

INFECTION OR DISEASE	1 a,g SULFAS TRIPLE OR SULFISOXAZOLE (GANTRISIN)	2 a,g NITRO- FURANTOIN (FURADANTIN)	3 a,f MANDELIC ACID	4 c,d,e PENICILLIN G
Gram-Negative Bacilli: Escherichia coli	B	A	C	
Aerobacter aerogenes	B	C		
Proteus vulgaris	B	B		
Pseudomonas aeruginosa	B	C		
Salmonella- E. typhosa				
B. dysenteriae	B			
B. Friedländer	C			B (4 & 6)
B. Brucella	B			
Gram-Positive Cocci Streptococcus: Beta hemolytic	C		C	A (4 & 6)
Alpha hemolytic			C	B (4 & 6)
Faecalis	C		A	A (4 & 6)
Viridans				B (4 & 5; 4 & 6)
Staphylococcus: Aureus; Albus	B	C	C	B (4 & 5; 4 & 6)
Pneumococcus				A
Gram-Negative Cocci Gonococcus	B			A
Tuberculosis				
Syphilis				A i
Chancroid				
Lymphogranuloma venereum				B
Granuloma inguinale				
Dose: Grams in 24 hours Infants and Children	0.5–4.0	0.06–0.3	1.0–10.0	0.1–1.0
Adults	2.0–8.0	0.4–0.8	10.0–15.0	1.0–5.0

In severe illness initial doses may be doubled, then reduced to "regular."
Key: A, B, C: indicates order of choice.
Blank spaces mean of little or no value.
Combined therapy if infection severe or resistant shown in parentheses, e.g., (6 & 8— Streptomycin and Achromycin).

    a. Oral only.
    b. Intramuscular only.
    c. Both routes.

IN UROGENITAL TRACT INFECTIONS

5	6	7	8	9	10	11
a,j ERYTHRO-MYCIN	b STREPTO-MYCIN OR DIHYDRO-STREPTO-MYCIN	c,d,e,g CHLOR-TETRA-CYCLINE (AUREO-MYCIN)	c,d,e,g TETRA-CYCLINE (ACHRO-MYCIN)	c,d,e,g OXYTETRA-CYCLINE (TERRA-MYCIN)	c,g CHLORAM-PHENICOL (CHLORO-MYCETIN)	b NEOMYCIN (POLY-MYXIN B)
	C, b (6 & 8)	B	B	B	B	
	B (6 & 8)	B	A	B	B	
	B				C	B
	B			A(B,6 & 9)	B	A
	B (6 & 1)				B(10 & 1; 9 & 10)	
	B	B	B	B	B	B
		B	B (8 & 10)	B	B	
	B (6 & 8, 9)	B	C	B		
A	B (5 & 6)	B	C	C	C	
A	B	B	C	C	C	
A	B	A	B			
B						
A (5 & 6)	B	B	C	C		
A	C	B	B	B		
A		B	B	B	B	
	A h					
						B
	B	A		B	A	
		A		B	A	
	B	A		B	A	
0.25–1.5	0.05–0.5	0.25–1.5	0.25–1.5	0.25–1.5	0.25–1.5	0.25–1.0
1.0–4.0	0.5–1.5	1.0–5.0	1.0–5.0	1.0–5.0	1.0–5.0	1.0–3.0

d. Oral dose four times and intravenous half the intramuscular dose.

e. May be given intravenously also.

f. As calcium mandelate tablets or syrup equivalent.

g. As capsule, tablet, drops, or suspension equivalent.

h. Combined with PAS (para-aminosalicylic acid) and isoniazid.

i. Use other antibiotics and arsenicals when patient is hypersensitive to penicillin and cannot be desensitized.

j. Novobiocin (Albamycin, Cathomycin) similarly used.

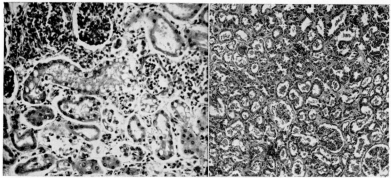

Fig. 144   Fig. 145

FIGURE 144.   Moderately advanced stage of acute renal infection showing hydropic degeneration and disintegration of the tubules with extensive interstitial perivascular leukocytic infiltration. There is also moderate leukocytic infiltration of the glomeruli. This stage is comparable to level *B* in Figure 143.

FIGURE 145.   Late stage of acute renal infection showing generalized interstitial inflammatory involvement with tubules filled with leukocytes.

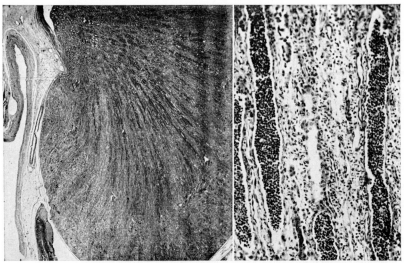

Fig. 146   Fig. 147

FIGURE 146.   Acute pyelonephritis. Cross section of kidney showing the medullary rays formed by tubules packed with leukocytes en route to the bladder. A section of one papilla as well as a segment of the upper ureter is seen; these structures show relatively mild inflammatory reaction. Seven-month-old girl.

FIGURE 147.   Collecting tubules of medulla packed with leukocytes en route to the bladder. Moderate degeneration of the renal parenchyma. This indicates how, in most renal infections, pus reaches the urine; doubtless over 90 per cent of the pus in the urine originates in the interstitial parenchymal lesions.

resistance of the invaded kidney by the congestion of toxemia, urinary stasis or pre-existing disease such as urinary calculi or hydronephrosis.

The extent and degree of renal injury in hematogenous infection will depend upon the magnitude and localization of the bacterial embolism. In the usual event, there is myriad of microscopic lesions, generally bilateral, and spread throughout the kidney but predominantly in the cortex. If large vessels are occluded, a large wedge-shape *infarction* develops which may become clinical *abscess* or *carbuncle*. The studies of Longcope and others strongly suggest that renal infections are generally hematogenous and the gastrointestinal tract is the most frequent primary focus.

Ascending Renal Infection. *Urogenous.* Here bacteria reach the kidney via the ureter against the normal urine flow (reflux); this mechanism is favored by obstruction at the bladder outlet or peripherally. There may also be vesico-ureteral spread by regurgitation in which opening of the ureterovesical valve for urinary ejaculation and contraction of the bladder are simultaneous; infected bladder contents are forced into the presumably uninfected upper urinary tract. While the theory of renal infection by urogenous retrograde extension from the bladder is the oldest, there are today no substantial data concerning the relative incidence of this mechanism as compared to the hematogenous, nor general agreement as to its relative clinical importance. On the other hand, the generally unsuspected high incidence of colon bacillemia for example, is impressive.

Lymphogenous Route. There is little precise knowledge concerning this; it seems probable that most renal infections thought to be lymph borne are in fact lymphohematogenous, the bacteria absorbed from external genital or lower urinary tract foci, for example, are passed to the regional lymphatics which eventually empty into the thoracic duct to reach the blood stream to be carried throughout the body and particularly to the kidneys. There is reason to believe that this is the usual mechanism operating in the production of *urethral chill* following instrumentation, and in the so-called deflorescence pyelitis in which bacteria are absorbed by the lymphatics from the lacerated hymen. Thus *trauma* may occasionally be a factor whether by instrumentation, traumatic perforation, surgical attack, or calculus in the renal pelvis.

Direct extension rarely occurs from an adjacent suppuration as in appendiceal abscess or a primary perinephric abscess. Bacteria may reach the kidney by *direct implantation* despite most careful technique of cystoscopy and ureteral catheterization. Yet the organisms thus introduced are of little moment unless free urinary drainage is impaired.

Spread of infection within the kidney is by direct interstitial extension, progressive vascular thrombosis, through the tubules and vascular tree (hematogenous) and/or by pyelovenous backflow (Figs. 20, 31).

PATHOLOGY

The clinical symptomatology and the renal changes in urinary infection are not necessarily reciprocal. A wide range of complicating and associated lesions due to infection may cause the identical clinical picture. Pathologically, these different conditions are identified as pyelonephritis, infected hydronephrosis, pyonephrosis, renal thrombosis, embolism or infarction, carbuncle (solitary abscess), perinephritis, perinephric abscess. Bacteremia may be mild; pyelitis as a sole anatomic lesion has never been acceptably demonstrated in the human; our knowledge of this stage of renal infection has been gained by animal experimentation. The definitive differential diagnosis rests upon complete urologic examination.

The usual renal lesion in pyelonephritis—clinically and loosely designated as pyelitis—is an interstitial suppurative nephritis; the routes of invasion and progressive stages of the infection are schematically shown in Figure 143, the legend of which tells the story. It will be noted that most of the pus which appears in the urine comes from the lesions in the interstitial spaces of the parenchyma, the leukocytes having extruded themselves between the swollen tubular epithelial cells and into the lumen and on down to the bladder.

Section of the hematogenously infected kidney discloses a swollen, congested organ with innumerable minute scarlet or chocolate color wedge shape hemorrhagic areas on the surface just beneath the capsule, in the cortex and, to a lesser extent, in the medulla. Some of these foci may be yellowish with suppuration. Numerous wedge-shaped, gray or yellowish gray streaks, the so-called *septic infarcts,* are seen radiating from the medulla to the cortex. The cut surface is wet and the capsule usually strips easily unless scar of previous infection is present. The pelvic changes range from catarrhal redness and moderate edema to widespread hemorrhage and ulceration. Advanced pelvic changes generally reflect urinary obstruction or pelvic stone.

Mild or moderate urinary infections commonly pass unrecognized and no permanent renal damage may result. More severe infections not only cause symptoms but heal with variable renal scarring, the tubules

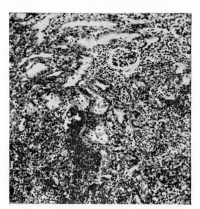

FIGURE 148.   Late stage of acute renal infection in which (in lower half of section) there is gross suppuration while above there is extensive parenchymal degeneration with loss of normal renal architecture. Above, a degenerated glomerulus is seen.

often becoming blocked by fibrosis (stricture) or they may become totally blocked off or disconnected, and bacteria thus withheld become therapeutically impregnable (Figs. 148, 149). This alone explains the persistence of infection in many cases despite intensive and rational treatment, the tubular stasis favoring perpetuation of the infection. The glomeruli of these tubules generally later become hyalinized. The outer layer of Bowman's capsule which surrounds a normal glomerular tuft and capsular space is replaced by sclerosis (periglomerular fibrosis). The late hyalinization of the capillaries has been attributed to compression of the afferent and efferent arterioles by (1) the capsular fibrosis, (2) adhesions between the glomerular capillaries and the sclerotic capsule, or (3) endarteritis obliterans. All of these conditions are factors in the progressive renal injury and in the genesis of vascular hypertensive disease (Fig. 149).

Even though the tubules are blocked, some glomerular function may continue and produce cystic dilatation of the tubules which together with continuing infection and sclerosis, progressively and irreparably injure the organs. The variably occluded tubules strictured in the corticomedullary zone and filled with hyalinized secretion may simulate the picture of colloid goiter. In the early stage of these changes there may be no symptoms but as the disease progresses, corticomedullary zone sclerosis may produce a clinical picture simulating Bright's disease or chronic interstitial nephritis. Glomerular destruction, widespread sclerosis, and chronic inflammatory infiltration continue with obliterating endarteritis, vascular fibrosis; increasing functional and architectural loss of renal units is the usual progress (Fig. 148). The glomeruli are not always greatly altered histologically, for some patients may die in renal failure (uremia) with normal appearing glomeruli. Nevertheless, the proximal tubules in these patients regularly show atrophy and dilatation.

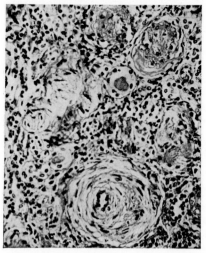

FIGURE 149. Chronic pyelonephritis. Arteriolar thickening, glomerular hyalinization, interstitial round-cell infiltration and fibrosis, tubular atrophy, hyaline casts.

In pyelonephritis the tubules suffer greater injury than the glomeruli. The renal architecture is altered to present a granular somewhat wrinkled surface, diminished in size, and the pelvis becomes contracted and irregular (Figs. 150, 151). Ultimately fibrolipomatous changes ensue in the peripelvic fat and also in the perinephric fat; the last constricts the kidney and pelvis, often with ureteropelvic outlet stricture or blockage, to form infected hydronephrosis.

Thus in chronic pyelonephritis tubules are blocked off by sclerotic repair, are dilated and the vascular supply is interfered with. Terminally chronic pyelonephritis proceeds to hydronephrosis when obstruction exists or to renal atrophy in the absence of obstruction.

Histology in Ascending Renal Infection. The invading bacteria— predominantly strains of the gram-negative colon group—cause variable inflammation of the renal pelvis, with lymphatic and vascular extension to the peripelvic and perirenal fat and other adjacent structures as well as to the medulla, usually to incite wide parenchymal involvement when urinary stasis exists. In ascending infection the glomeruli are involved much less often and seriously than in hematogenous infection but early in the pathogenesis the interstitial tissue is also invaded and later his-

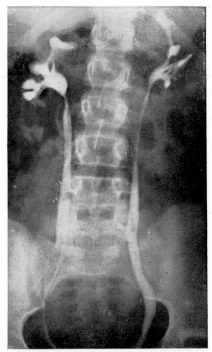

FIGURE 150. Chronic pyelonephritis. Terminal urographic changes in twenty-three-year-old girl periodically observed for ten years. The initial lesion was bilateral uretero-vesical junction stricture which responded well to conservative dilation. Progressive decrease of renal function throughout the clinical course. Uremic death. There is contraction of the kidney with narrowing of the calyceal necks and irregular calyceal dilatation with ureterectasis.

tologically simulates the lesion in blood-borne infection. Thus the urogenous lesion early becomes an interstitial suppurative nephritis rather than a simple pyelitis. From this point the histologic changes are the same as occur in hematogenous infection.

SYMPTOMS

Acute Renal Infection. The *symptoms* in the different varieties of acute renal infection (e.g., pyelonephritis, abscess, carbuncle, infected hydronephrosis, pyonephrosis) are fundamentally the same in patients of all ages; urotoxic gastrointestinal manifestations are most prominent in infants and young children but may also be disturbing in older patients of all ages.

Children under Two Years of Age. In this, the diaper age, the symptoms are predominantly systemic rather than local with fever, apathy, gastrointestinal disturbances (vomiting, diarrhea, distention, constipation), and even delirium or prostration. Early dysuria or frequency are seldom noted. *A shaking chill in an infant or a young child signifies either acute urinary infection or malaria.*

The *diagnosis* is made by examination of a properly collected specimen of urine; anemia and leukocytosis usually coexist. The specific *treatment* is fundamentally that employed in adults for the particular type of invading bacteria and associated pathologic factors. But the general condition of the young patient generally merits stricter attention than does the choice of antimicrobic therapy.

Older Children and Adults. In these age groups the systemic symptoms and clinical considerations are essentially the same as in the younger group. Usually the onset is abrupt with chilliness or real chills and fever.

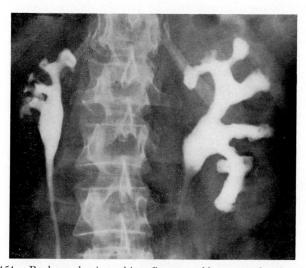

FIGURE 151. Pyelography in a thirty-five-year-old woman showing irregular renal sclerotic contraction especially on the right (hypoplastic kidney), with pelvic distortion on the left, the curious patchy irregularity suggesting pyelitis cystica.

In half the cases there are no urinary symptoms (frequency, dysuria, burning, tenesmus, urgency, and the like) or localizing signs such as renal pain or loin tenderness, and in these patients the initial diagnosis is too often grippe although pneumonia may be suspected. Gastrointestinal disturbances with nausea, vomiting, constipation, diarrhea may develop as may neurologic symptoms with irritability, headache, malaise, photophobia, and even toxic meningismus. Meningismus too often causes examination of the spinal fluid to precede urinalysis. When the urinary infection is secondary to another disease such as tonsillitis, pharyngitis, pneumonia, or enteritis, the general symptoms may overshadow any urinary tract manifestation.

Chronic Urinary Infection.   There is commonly a recognized antecedent urinary infection but in many patients the discovery of the chronic condition is made by urinalysis at the time of a school or insurance medical examination for example, or when urinary symptoms such as frequency, hematuria, dysuria exist, or there is pain in the renal region or along the ureter. A low-grade fever may be present or the patient may experience great lassitude or suffer malaise, poor appetite, indigestion, biliousness, chronic gastritis, constipation, failure to gain or even loss of weight and anemia. These symptoms often completely misdirect attention to the gastrointestinal and other tracts. In children with these secondary toxic urinary manifestations, anemia is the rule and often developmental retardation as well. Headache, irritability, apathy, nervousness or insomnia are common urotoxic manifestations particularly in older patients and there may even be urotoxic "rheumatism."

Course of the Disease.   *Acute urinary infection* developing in the absence of urinary obstruction or stasis is apt to be self-limited. With stasis, the infection lingers though asymptomatic. The rapidity of the extension and tissue damage will be largely determined by the nature and severity of the associated etiologic factors which are generally stasis producing but there may be an active bacterial feeder focus elsewhere. Unrecognized or inadequately treated, the acute urinary infection becomes largely asymptomatic, gradually progressing to chronic infection.

Chronic Urinary Infection.   By accepted definition, a condition which persists longer than four weeks, is chronic. When the renal destruction is not halted, ultimate death in uremia or urinary sepsis must be anticipated. Alertness of the patient's doctor should forestall such an ending which must be looked upon as the fruit of medical neglect. During this period of progressive injury of the urinary tract by infection and especially in the kidney, recurrences of acute urinary infection are common and must be considered simply as exacerbations of an asymptomatic smoldering infection which too often exists unrecognized. A long interval between disappearance of infection (negative culture) and a subsequent attack always suggests a new infection has occurred.

The lives of innumerable patients of all ages are dotted with recurrent attacks of "acute pyelitis" which are simply exacerbations of previously incurred infection and invited by debility of the patient or an attack of sinusitis, pharyngitis, dental apical infection, enteritis, or the advent of acute urinary obstruction. The pyelitis of pregnancy is believed to be of this type—the exacerbation of a low-grade smoldering urinary infection ("pyelitis") carried since childhood.

DIAGNOSIS

The diagnosis of either acute or chronic urinary infection is suggested by consideration of the symptoms as previously enumerated. *Abdominal palpation* may reveal one or both kidneys enlarged or tender, especially in the costovertebral angle. Overlying protective abdominal spasm may preclude satisfactory abdominal examination. The diagnosis is made positive by the demonstration of bacteria and, almost always, pus in the urine; *pus casts mean pyelonephritis*. Red blood cells may be present. In short, urinalysis of a properly collected specimen is the keystone of the diagnosis and, by subsequent urinalysis, the progress and success of treatment is determined. The examination of a gram-stained centrifuged urine sediment will give a quick indication as to the nature of the infection, whether gram-positive coccic or gram-negative bacillary, a point of prime concern in the initial selection of medication. The results of urine culture and sensitivity tests will not be known for at least twenty-four hours and generally longer.

A *complete urologic examination* is demanded in persistent acute urinary infection lasting seventy-two hours despite intensive antibacterial therapy as it is in chronic pyuria not cured by intense present-day treatment in three weeks. The test of cure is negative culture (preferably two) of properly collected specimens.

It is axiomatic that persistent urinary infection is perpetuated by urinary stasis until proved otherwise; a major objective in the urologic examination is to demonstrate the cause and nature of the associated obstructing lesion(s).

In the urologic examination in chronic pyuria has been found practically every condition known to exist in the urinary tract, most often obstruction, stone, tumor, or neuromuscular disease. The fundamentals of complete urologic examination are given in Chapter 3. Cytoscopic examination, divided renal function tests, collection of ureteral specimens for comparative examination, and the urographic findings will be of invaluable diagnostic aid and will indicate whether the renal interstitial damage is mild or is far advanced with scarring and renal distortion— particularly of the pelvis—secondary obstruction or complicating stone, for example (Figs. 140, 150). The examination will show whether conservative medical or surgical treatment is called for.

PROGNOSIS

Uncomplicated urinary infection rarely causes death in older patients but is sometimes fatal in infants, particularly in the neonatal period. Formerly the infant mortality from urinary infection was 20 to 40 per cent, but it is now not more than 2 or 3 per cent, and in the fatal cases the major surgical uropathy usually present has been renal thrombosis, advanced infected hydronephrosis, pyonephrosis, renal carbuncle, or perinephric abscess.

TREATMENT

The objective is to kill all the invading bacteria in the urinary tract without injuring the host, the last consideration being very real in the extremely delicate patients of the neonatal and early diaper age. The advent of sulfonamide and antibiotic therapy during the past few years has completely revolutionized the medical treatment of all varieties of urinary infections in patients of all ages.

The perfect urinary antiseptic has not yet been discovered. The "wonder drugs" have wide areas of failure among various strains of the same generic organisms, the development of drug resistance is high, the incidence of side reactions such as nausea, vomiting, diarrhea, and dermatitis is relatively high, while several cases of complicating fatal ulcerative staphylococcus enteritis have been reported. The last condition results from grave alterations in the intestinal bacterial flora. The drug susceptible gram-negative bacilli which normally inhabit the intestinal tract, especially Bacillus lactis aerogenes, are inhibited or killed off and the Staphylococcus gets the upper hand while the advent of Monilia with diarrhea and itching of the rectum and anus is frequent. Any medication causing such reactions should be stopped at once. The administration of Mycostatin will usually control such monilial disturbances.

In some infections the co-administration of sulfonamides and antibiotics or of two different antibiotics may be more effective than the use of a single medication. This has been employed chiefly in combating Proteus by the use of large doses of penicillin (a million units or more at a time) and 1 to 3 gm. of streptomycin or dihydrostreptomycin a day. Gantrisin (sulfisoxazole) and Chloromycetin (chloramphenicol) have also been effective in combination against Proteus in drug ratios of two to one and for periods of ten to twenty days. Streptomycin or dihydrostreptomycin and Terramycin in combined therapy have been found effective against Brucella organisms (q.v.). The Enterococcus is best attacked by Terramycin and mandelic acid; often it is most tenacious and difficult to eradicate. Other drug combinations for antibacterial attack are given in Table 9.

Treatment of Acute Urinary Infection. Put the patient to bed and keep him there until the temperature has been normal thirty-six to forty-eight hours. If fever recurs when he gets up, put him to bed again. Patients who have been extremely sick or who have suffered severe toxic prostration may wisely be kept in bed an even longer time than just indicated. A hot pad over a tender renal area may afford relief from pain. In unilateral infection, a small pillow placed under the isolateral loin may straighten the ureter and improve urinary drainage.

1. *There is no special diet.* Let the patient take what food he will, but his intake will be largely liquids. As he improves, his normal appetite

will return unless medications are permitted to make him sick. If this occurs, change to another drug.

2. *Give fluids generously*. If the patient is not nauseated nor vomiting and can take fluids by mouth, have a five-year-old child take at least 1200 cc. in twenty-four hours, and an adult 2200 to 2500 cc. according to size. If the patient is vomiting, give the fluids intravenously or by hypodermoclysis. The choice and variety of fluids available and the amounts to be given in various age and weight groups are shown in Table 10.

3. *Combat acidosis or alkalosis* when the carbon dioxide combining power estimation indicates their presence. This is discussed and outlined in Chapter 4.

4. *Clean out the intestinal tract* by laxative and, if necessary, by colonic irrigation; be sure the patient has at least one satisfactory bowel movement daily.

5. *Treat and remove, if possible, any primary foci of infection* (see the listing of these under Treatment of Chronic Urinary Infection).

TABLE 10. FLUIDS FOR PARENTERAL ADMINISTRATION (PEDIATRIC QUANTITATION AFTER NELSON, 1950)

FLUID	INDICATION	ROUTE Sc. = subcutaneously Iv. = intravenously Bm. = Bone marrow			QUANTITY Infants and Children	Adults cc. (Iv.)
Physiologic saline	Dehydration; mild alkalosis or acidosis when renal function is adequate	Sc.	Iv.	Bm.	Iv. fluid at one time in vol. not greatly exceeding 10 cc. per lb. of body weight nor faster than 10 cc. per min. Same vol. may be given into bone marrow at ½ the speed.	1000–1500
5% glucose in water or saline	Ketosis; dehydration; inadequate oral intake		Iv.	Bm.		1000–1500
Ringer type of solution	Dehydration, mild acidosis	Sc.	Iv.	Bm.	Vol. and rate subcutaneously limited by rate of absorption. If fluids are given cont., the daily vol. = approx. 2½ to 3 oz. per lb. of body weight for small infants.	1000–1500
Concentrated glucose or sucrose (20 to 50%)	As a diuretic temporarily to reduce high intracranial pressure; hypoglycemic shock; toxemia		Iv.	Bm.	10–50 cc. at a time.	50–100 at a time
⅙ sodium-r-lactate	Acidosis (CO₂ above 20–25 vol. per cent)	Sc.	Iv.	Bm.	Cc. molar lactate = wt. in kg. $\times$ 0.3 $\times$ CO₂ deficit. Dilute with 5 parts sterile water.	same
Sodium bicarbonate	Acidosis (CO₂ below 20–25 vol. per cent)		Iv.	Bm.	Cc. 5% solution = 20 (wt. in Kg. $\times$ 0.026 x CO₂ deficit).	same
Plasma	Shock; burns; hypoproteinemia; edema; to avoid hypoproteinemia when entire fluid intake is by parenteral routes		Iv.	Bm.	May be used in normal strength or if dried plasma is used it may be concentrated 3 to 4 times blood normal.	250–500 at a time
Whole blood	Anemia; to supply antibody and complement; to supply carbonic anhydrase in premature infants		Iv.	Bm.	Always type and cross match. 15 cc. per kg. of body weight raises blood count by approx. one million.	500–1000 as needed

6. *Antimicrobial Therapy: Chemotherapy.* This is largely by the administration of one of the *sulfonamides*, either as a single drug such as sulfisoxazole (Gantrisin) or as a triple sulfonamide.

When sulfonamides are used the urine should be alkalinized with 10 to 15 grains of sodium bicarbonate daily (nitrazine paper indicator). Because of their cumulative action, these compounds must not be used when the renal function is low or the patient is uremic. Urinary output must be maintained as evidenced by accurate measurement. Sulfadiazine, sulfathiazole, and sulfamerazine combined in equal parts to make 0.5 gm. tablets (the triple sulfa) may be employed on the basis that the dangers of toxic injury or of acetylated crystalline precipitation in the tubules is less than that of a comparable dose of any one of these drugs alone. With the increased dosage made possible thereby, a higher blood level is obtained.

The sulfa drugs cause a relatively high incidence of reactions (nausea, vomiting, diarrhea, dermatitis, anemia) and must often be discontinued because of unfavorable reaction or bacteriocidal ineffectiveness. These drugs are available in suspension or emulsion forms for children or other patients who cannot swallow pills. As a rule, a five-year-old child can take 0.5 gm. of Gantrisin four times a day, and an adult 1.0 to 2.0 gm. four times a day for a week, at the end of which time a recheck urine culture is made. If the urine is not sterile then, the therapeutic course should be repeated, often with a different antimicrobial (Table 9).

Furadantin (nitrofurazone) has been particularly effective against two thirds of strains of Escherichia coli, is less effective against Micrococcus pyogenes, and is variably inhibitory of Proteus. It is excreted in high concentration in the urine. It has the advantage of wide spectrum activity, freedom from causing blood dyscrasia, crystalluria, moniliasis with gastritis, pruritus ani, and Staphylococcus enteritis. These patients seldom have complicating headache, dizziness, paresthesia, or dermatitis with itching as so often occurs with other potent antiseptics. Many patients become nauseated or vomit when taking Furadantin but this is generally worst the first thirty-six hours and if the medication can be continued beyond that period, the nausea usually passes off. The medication should always be taken after meals, with a glass of milk or, in any case, only with something in the stomach and *never on an empty stomach.* The drug has no cumulative effect and may be taken for long periods. The initial dose is one and a half or two times the average dose for twenty-four hours, continuing with the smaller calculated dose.

Mandelic acid therapy, the successor of the now abandoned ketogenic diet (acid) therapy, is employed far less than previously, having been largely replaced by sulfonamide and antibiotic therapy. When given according to strict bacteriologic indications, however, and with proper acidification of the urine, mandelic acid will sterilize the urine in two thirds to three fourths of the patients in whom it is employed provided there is no urinary stasis.

Mandelic acid requires limitation of fluids to achieve a twenty-four hour urine output of 1000 to 1200 cc. daily, a pH of 5.5 or less, and a high drug concentration in the urine preferably 1 per cent and, in any event, over 0.5 per cent. The urine titer is easily determined by methyl red indicator or, even simpler, the use of nitrazine test paper (Squibb). Children especially dislike the taste of mandelic acid preparations and may refuse to take the drug. In adults the calcium mandelate tablet, given to a limit of 10 to 15 gm. per day, is probably the most effective medication against Streptococcus faecalis. Urinary acidification may be enhanced by the coadministration of enteric-coated tablets of ammonium chloride or ammonium nitrate (8 gm. a day), and/or a high acid-ash diet.

Methenamine (urotropin) is practically never used today as an antiseptic.

Arsenical antiluetic compounds, neoarsphenamine and Mapharsen, have cured many chronic indolent Staphylococcus infections resistant to other treatment. The *modus operandi* is unknown. A course of treatment consists of five or six doses of 0.15 to 0.2 gm. of neoarsphenamine given intravenously every other day. Discontinue the treatment if one course is unsuccessful in sterilizing the urine.

Antibiotics. These may be administered intensively in acute urinary infection and have the advantage that in nauseated or vomiting patients most can be given intramuscularly or even intravenously (Table 9). When the stomach quiets down, the antibiotic can be given by mouth. The bacterial sensitivity tests will suggest the proper antibiotic to be given to the patient although at the outset and before the test is made, most of the broad spectrum products may be given until additional laboratory data and sensitivity test results are known. An immediate Gram stain of urine sediment will indicate whether bacillary or coccic organisms or both are the invaders. For example, penicillin is generally useless in primary Esch. coli infection, while Aureomycin is less effective against gram-positive coccic invasions than against most gram-negative bacillary forms (Table 9).

The antibiotics are frequently ineffective in sterilizing the urine but this is usually the result of (1) haphazard administration, these antibiotics being given without previous knowledge as to the invading bacteria or their probable therapeutic value as determined by sensitivity tests; (2) inadequate doses, or (3) administration for too short a period. When properly given, antibiotics are generally effective in their immediate attack upon acute urinary infection as they are in chronic urinary infection, especially in conjunction with urosurgery. Today surgeons can confidently perform many radical yet necessary operations which only fifteen years ago they would not have dared to undertake because of the unfavorable outlook through complicating infection.

Penicillin. At this time, drug sensitivity tests show that at least 90 per cent of the strains of organisms formerly sensitive to penicillin are now penicillin resistant. The field of usefulness of this antibiotic is reduced by this much and informed physicians employ it less and less. Carroll found only 6 per cent of urinary staphylococci in his patients were sensitive to penicillin, and my experience is similar. When penicillin is used it should be given in large doses up to a million units a day intramuscularly; oral penicillin is of questionable value and in the intestinal tract is believed by many observers to increase sensitization of the patient to the drug. I seldom employ it.

Erythromycin has considerably displaced penicillin as the antibiotic of choice in coccic infections. It is already evident that Erythromycin—as has penicillin—will lose much of its effectiveness through bacterial mutations and the acquisition of drug fastness by the bacteria. At the present writing, Erythromycin is effective in three fourths of micrococcic infections. The only prophylaxis against the development of drug fastness appears to lie in combined therapy, Erythromycin and streptomycin being used together more and more.

Novobiotin, marketed under the trade names Cathomycin and Albamycin, has proved effective in eradicating therapy-resistant staphylococci and streptococci. The dose is that of Erythromycin.

Aureomycin is a broad spectrum antibiotic effective against many of the gram-negative bacillary invaders of the urinary tract but may be ineffective not only against some strains of Esch. coli but more especially against many strains of Pseudomonas aeruginosa (pyocyaneus) and Aerobacter aerogenes, while Proteus is practically totally immune. For the last, use Novobiotin and streptomycin.

Terramycin (oxytetracycline) is effective in much the same bacterial range as is Aureomycin but may also cause disturbing nausea and diarrhea. It is effective in about a third of the cases of staphylococcic infections but is losing ground in this respect. Enteric disturbances especially diarrhea are of high incidence with Terramycin despite antimonilial (mycostatin) co-therapy. Several cases of ulcerative Staphylococcus enteritis have been reported following the continued administration of Terramycin.

Chloromycetin (chloramphenicol) has essentially the same antibacterial status as Aureomycin but in general I prefer Chloromycetin despite reported instances of aplastic anemia following its use.

Achromycin (tetracycline), also a broad spectrum antibiotic, is the choice against Aerobacter aerogenes organisms. These simulate Esch. coli, are highly therapy resistant and, unfortunately, are showing a rapid incidence increase as evidenced in hospitals over the country maintaining reliable bacteriologic laboratories. Nowhere is the need for precise bacterial identification in urinary infection exhibited more effectively than in the recognition of the various strains of gram-negative bacillary organisms. For example, the few drugs to which Aerobacter responds are largely ineffective against Proteus or Pseudomonas, and vice versa.

Streptomycin has been used chiefly against the tubercle bacillus but it is also effective against many gram-negative bacilli. Unless it is effective within seventy-two hours, however, the bacteria generally develop strong drug resistance to streptomycin. It tends to cause vestibular nerve damage which dihydrostreptomycin is less likely to do, but the latter commonly induces rapid drug resistance and sometimes auditory nerve damage as well. These compounds must be given intramuscularly, 0.5 gm. b.i.d., in acute infection, or twice this quantity two times a week intramuscularly in chronic urinary tuberculosis. The two drugs may be given together with a corresponding reduction of dosage of each and comparably reducing the likelihood of eighth nerve injury.

Neomycin (Polymyxin B) is the only compound enjoying high effectiveness against Pseudomonas aeruginosa (pyocyaneus) but, because it is both nephrotoxic and neurotoxic (especially eighth nerve), its use is limited to grave infections in hospitalized patients. It is given intramuscularly and the injection is painful.

The bacterial spectra of the drugs and antibiotics most frequently employed in the treatment of urinary infection and their dosage are shown in Table 9.

Causes of Therapeutic Failure. These are repeated here. The most common reasons for antimicrobial failure are (1) lack of precise knowledge of the bacterial invader(s) and their drug sensitivity; (2) inadequate drug dosage, (3) administration for too short a time, and (4) coexisting urinary obstruction with urinary stasis either from early prostatic hyperplasia or strictures of renal tubules in chronic pyelonephritis, for example. Often the function of the gravely diseased chronic pyelonephritic kidney is so low that it cannot excrete or even circulate adequately the antibacterial medication in bacteriostatic quantities. Finally, an unrecognized focus of infection (teeth, tonsils, sinus, osteomyelitis, prostate, pelvic disease, cervix, skin, etc.) may be continually feeding the urinary infection hematogenously or by other routes.

Establishment of Urinary Drainage. In vesical distention associated with acute renal infection, indwelling catheterization for a few days may temporarily turn the tide as may ureteral catheter drainage of an obstructed infected kidney. The need for the establishment of drainage as well as far more radical surgery—immediate or later—will be determined by the findings on complete urologic examination. This will also show whether (1) one or both kidneys are involved and if one must be operated upon or, possibly, removed, and (2) the other kidney can be expected to support life.

Surgical treatment in acute urinary infection is distinctly an urgent consideration and, as far as possible, should be conservative. A hopeless or life-threatening pyonephrosis, for instance, must be removed if there is a reliable kidney on the other side. In advanced infected hydronephrosis due to ureteropelvic blockage, it is usually better to establish temporary urinary drainage by conservative nephrostomy or pyelostomy for example, and later correct the obstructive condition when the status of both the patient and the kidney is more favorable.

Treatment of Chronic Urinary Infection. Intelligent treatment demands an accurate urologic diagnosis and less than this means haphazard and, often, fruitless therapy. Multiple etiologic factors are commonly present in these cases—stone, obstruction, diverticulum, to name a few—and unless all are corrected, the chances of sterilizing the urine are vastly reduced even with large doses of medication and for long periods. Note again that no patient is cured until the entire urinary tract drains properly and the urine is sterile as shown by two negative cultures of aseptically collected urine (Chapter 3).

The treatment of chronic urinary infection may be outlined as follows:

1. A large fluid intake
2. Elimination of constipation
3. Diet for nutrition including added vitamin therapy
4. Eradication of focal infections
   a. Furuncles, boils, carbuncles, paronychia, infected wounds, etc.: open drainage
   b. Infected tonsils and adenoids: tonsillectomy and adenoidectomy
   c. Infection of sinuses and ears: open drainage
   d. Osteomyelitis: surgical treatment
   e. Abscessed or pulpous teeth: extraction
   f. Respiratory or kindred infections: medical treatment
   g. Genital infections (rare): chiefly cleanliness (see Chapt. 8).
   Most of the infections just enumerated will readily respond to bacteriologically indicated antibiotic therapy and correspondingly reduce the indications for surgical drainage or treatment.
5. Medication (mandelic acid, sulfonamides, antibiotics)
6. Elimination of urinary stasis
   a. *In the upper urinary tract:* Ureteral stricture: progressive dilation, incision, ureteral meatotomy, ureteropelvioplasty or resection; ureteral anomalies: ureteroplasty, ureteroheminephrectomy, etc.; ureteral stone: intra-ureteral manipulation, ureterolithotomy;
   b. *In the lower urinary tract:* Phimosis: dorsal slit or circumcision; urethral stricture: meatotomy, dilation, urethrotomy; urethral stones: crushing or removal; urethral diverticulum: diverticulotomy (conversion of sac into part of the urethral lumen), diverticulectomy; congenital valves of the posterior urethra, congenital hypertrophy of verumontanum, contracted vesical outlet, median bar obstruction, prostatic enlargement or cyst: transurethral resection, or suprapubic excision; vesical stone: litholapaxy, cystolithotomy; bladder diverticulum: diverticulectomy; intravesical obstruction such as mucosal folds at bladder outlet, ureterocele, trigonal hypertrophy sufficient to cause blockage or trigonal curtain: transurethral resection or suprapubic excision.
   c. *Neuromuscular disease:* Establishment of free drainage by indwelling catheter, cystotomy; antiluetic therapy when due to syphilis; transurethral or suprapubic resection of vesical neck when chronic sphincterospasm, muscular hypertrophy, or secondary sclerosis of the bladder outlet exists.
7. Drainage of the kidney by ureteral catheter, or of the bladder by temporary indwelling catheter.
8. Surgical treatment. This may require nephrostomy drainage, incision and drainage of suppuration in or about the urinary tract; decapsulation for renal abscess, including cortical concurrent with perinephritis; nephrotomy for stone, recurrent abscess of kidney, hemorrhagic type of pyelonephritis (in the last two nephrectomy is usually neces-

sary); nephrectomy for diffuse suppurative pyelonephritis with destruction of kidney, renal carbuncle (occasionally), atrophic pyelonephritis, pyonephrosis, infected hydronephrosis when ureteropelvioplasty is contraindicated, technically impracticable or has failed, persistent uncontrollable hematuria, or tumor.

Surgical treatment is required in a fourth to a third of cases of persistent urinary infection in patients of all ages. The indications for urosurgery are given in the preceding paragraph. In adults with persisting urinary infection of renal origin, 15 to 20 per cent will require nephrectomy.

RENAL LESIONS CHARACTERIZED BY ACUTE OR CHRONIC URINARY INFECTION

Infected hydronephrosis is one of the most common of major urologic conditions. The pathogenesis of hydronephrosis has been discussed in Chapter 3 and in all of these cases secondary infection (1) may be intensified, (2) accelerates the hydronephrotic destructive process, and (3) commonly destroys the organ. The symptoms of infected hydronephrosis are those due to obstruction itself (see Chapter 3) together with the systemic urotoxic manifestations of the infection and renal injury. There may be only a low-grade malaise with anemia, mild gastrointestinal disturbances or, more severe, colicky renal pain in the loin, urinary frequency or dysuria reflexly produced or resulting from secondary infection of the bladder, particularly at the vesical outlet. The symptoms of infected hydronephrosis demand a complete urologic examination in which pyelographic study will establish the anatomic diagnosis and comparative renal

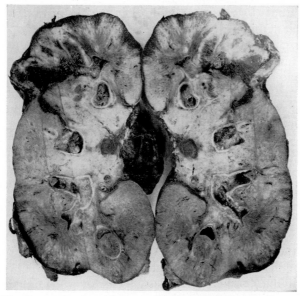

FIGURE 152. Pyonephrosis with generalized renal destruction by suppuration.

function tests will indicate the capacity of the "better" kidney to carry on should removal of its mate be necessary.

Treatment of infected hydronephrosis may at first be medical with the objective of sterilizing the urine by antibacterial therapy and thus preparing the patient for the necessary definitive surgical correction of the obstruction and associated conditions. Often in such patients temporary nephrostomy must be employed until the condition of the patient permits the corrective surgery to be carried out. In infected hydronephrosis of half of a double kidney, ureteroheminephrectomy is often curative and will preserve a sound functioning segment of renal tissue.

Pyonephrosis is the total or almost complete loss of renal function by suppurative destruction of the parenchyma. Pyonephrosis is generally the end stage of chronic pyelonephritis or infected hydronephrosis, the organ usually becoming enlarged and lobulated with universally suppurating parenchyma and pus-filled and often ulcerating pelvis (Fig. 152). Secondary perirenal fibrolipomatosis is usually found and by contraction may compress the kidney sufficient to obstruct its vascular supply and compromise the adjacent upper ureter with stricture or extra-ureteral compression blockage. Microscopically the tissue shows complete suppurative disorganization (Fig. 148).

Unfortunately the terms infected hydronephrosis and pyonephrosis are often interchangeably applied but pathologically they are two entirely different lesions; in pyonephrosis the organ is converted into a mass of focal abscesses.

Symptoms of pyonephrosis are similar to but are usually more severe than those just enumerated under infected hydronephrosis; in the young the inadequate diagnosis of "hyperacute pyelitis" is frequently made. There is a chronic form of pyonephrosis in which the symptoms are predominantly systemic consequent to urotoxemia.

Diagnosis. Urography in pyonephrosis nearly always demonstrates widespread ulceration of the kidney pelvis, sometimes simulating that seen in advanced caseous renal tuberculosis (cf. Fig. 163).

Treatment in pyonephrosis is nephrectomy as soon as the condition of the patient will permit, and assuming that an adequately functioning opposite kidney will remain.

ACUTE HEMATOGENOUS RENAL SUPPURATION

Acute Diffuse Suppurative Nephritis. This is also known as the *pyemic kidney*, the lesions being part of a systemic pyemia. The bacterial localization generally takes place in the terminal arterial circulation to form septic infarcts (Figs. 153, 154). The primary focus is often a bacterial endocarditis or pulmonary embolism. The overwhelming systemic toxemia of the disease commonly causes the renal lesions (which are always bilateral) to be overlooked and the diagnosis correspondingly delayed until the outlook is hopeless. The overwhelming bacteremia is usually gram-positive coccic, either streptococcus or staphylococcus, and, if recognized in time, it is conceivable that intensive antibiotic therapy might offer therapeutic hope but most of these cases are recognized only at autopsy.

Acute Focal Suppurative Nephritis.   This condition is an overwhelming hematogenous infection similar to acute diffuse suppurative nephritis except that it is more often unilateral. The kidneys show wedge-shaped suppurative infarcts most commonly due to streptococcic or staphylococcic hematogenous invasion, and secondary perinephric abscess is frequent. Several focal abscesses in the kidney commonly coalesce to form larger abscesses which, in turn, may rupture into the pelvis or extend to the perirenal tissues; secondary pelvic ulceration may occur. The patient is extremely ill from urotoxic absorption and generally has a pain in or about the renal area.

The *diagnosis* is made by complete urologic examination when intensive antibiotic therapy fails to improve the condition. Divided renal function tests will usually disclose a kidney of little or no function on the involved side. When the renal mate is proved sound, removal of the suppurative kidney is the *treatment*. Naturally, this is done with some trepidation because of the danger that the remaining kidney may become

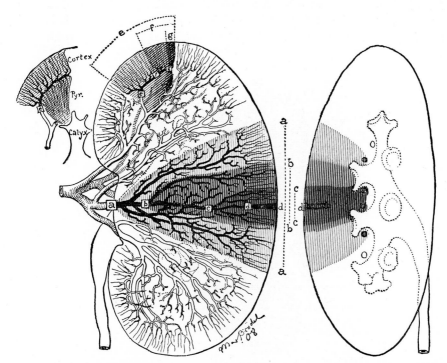

Figure 153.   Vascular distribution of the kidney and the formation of arterial infarcts (*a–g*). The infarcts are conical with the apex at the point of bacterial mass attack and enlodgement. The base is at the renal surface. The closer the vascular infarction approaches the renal pedicle, the larger will be the involved parenchymal lesion. (From Kelly-Burnham, courtesy D. Appleton & Company.)

similarly involved or, if the patient survives, may develop advanced chronic interstitial nephritis.

RENAL INFARCTION AND THROMBOSIS

These lesions result from severe hematogenous infarction or embolism with subsequent vascular plugging, sometimes in the vessels as they approach the kidney. Infarction is usually metastatic from acute or chronic endocarditis but occasionally complicates phlebitis. In **renal infarction** pyelonephritis develops first with thrombosis of the vessels within the parenchyma, beginning with those of the glomeruli. Thrombosis thus beginning in the kidney is designated as primary to distinguish it from the secondary variety following phlebitis of the vena cava, ovarian, spermatic, suprarenal, or accessory renal vessels, or results from prolonged pronounced inflammation of the renal pedicle as it lies within an acute perirenal phlegmon.

Renal thrombosis is predominantly a condition of infancy and here the nature of the lesion is usually unrecognized and the patient succumbs early. Initially the physician is generally satisfied with the diagnosis "pyelitis." Enterocolitis is the most frequent primary focus but other focal lesions such as measles, diphtheria, omphalitis, and cutaneous infections have been identified. The renal involvement in thrombosis is bilateral in about half the cases and sex distribution is equal. A portion or all

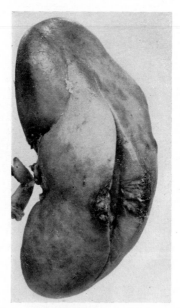

FIGURE 154. Septic left renal infarction in a nine-year-old girl who had been treated a month for "persistent acute pyelitis" before urologic examination was sought. The temperature curve had been of the septic typhoidal type. The removed kidney reveals multiple septic infarcts with the formation of one moderate size carbuncle and several smaller focal abscesses. It is likely that earlier surgical intervention with decapsulation and the establishment of drainage would have saved the kidney.

of the kidney may be involved, often with secondary thrombotic extension
to the other kidney, spermatic or ovarian vessels. I successfully performed
nephrectomy for renal thrombosis in two boys thirty-three days and
twelve days of age respectively, making the urographic diagnosis preoperatively in the second case.

Symptoms. The sudden appearance of sharp pain in the loin with
hematuria, tenderness, and sudden enlargement in a child with iliocolitis,
pneumonia, or phlebitis at once suggests the diagnosis of renal thrombosis.
The pain may radiate to the thigh or genitalia and reflex anuria may
ensue. There is vomiting, constipation or diarrhea, and collapse, usually
with fever. The course of the disease is rapid. The urine shows blood,
albumin, pus, casts and the function of the involved kidney is vastly
reduced or nil.

The *diagnosis* is suggested by the pyelogram in which the renal pelvis
is distorted, compressed or obliterated. Spread of the urographic medium
to the pulpacious thrombosed parenchymal areas may occur. Immediate
nephrectomy is the *treatment.*

Renal Carbuncle. This is a massive localized parenchymal suppuration consequent to bacterial metastasis in which localized vascular thrombosis or infarction is the initial renal lesion. Abscesses of variable size
follow (Fig. 156). As in the development of perinephric abscess, an antecedent history of cutaneous infection, paronychia, or osteomyelitis, for
example, is obtained, a staphylococcal infection being the usual type.

When the initial thrombosis or infarction occurs in one of the
arcuate vessels of the corticomedullary zone, the lesion shows wide in-

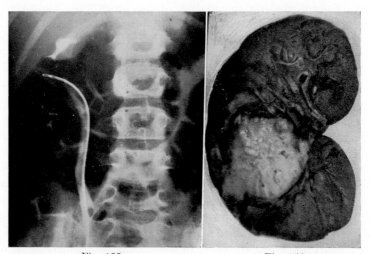

Fig. 155   Fig. 156

FIGURE 155. Massive carbuncle of the right kidney in a four-year-old girl with
"persistent acute pyelitis." In this pyelogram the pelvis, except part of the superior calyx,
is completely blotted out by the compressing suppurative mass.

FIGURE 156. Renal carbuncle. Massive suppurative area within the kidney substance; urographically, such a lesion commonly suggests renal neoplasm (cf. Fig. 155).

volvement of both cortex and medulla. In nearly every case the cortical involvement is the more advanced and by eruption often incites perinephric abscess the symptoms of which may be the first to direct attention to the involved kidney (Figs. 155, 156). The symptoms are those of acute renal infection to which are usually added the signs and symptoms of acute perinephritis or perinephric abscess (q.v.).

The diagnosis is made by urologic examination in which the plain urogram or "scout" film generally shows lateral curvature of the spine away from the lesion. The renal pelvis shows variable compression and in some cases complete obliteration (Fig. 155).

Perinephritis. This is inflammation of the fatty tissues about the kidney and is always secondary to infection elsewhere; it may be an extension from cortical infection but is sometimes direct primary metastatic. Staphylococcus aureus is the bacterium most often found; perinephritis often proceeds to suppuration—clinical perinephric abscess—but may resolve without much sclerosis or, with dense scarring, contracting fibrolipomatosis appears.

In mild perinephritis there is only a slight ache or pain in the loin and even this may be overlooked, the systemic symptoms commonly causing the diagnosis of grippe to be made. In *severe* perinephritis there is regularly pain in the loin and the *diagnosis* will largely be made on this finding alone in the presence of a normal urine which may be bacteria-free.

Treatment. The pain and toxic malaise of perinephritis usually respond well to salicylates or acetophenetidin, but codeine or morphine may be necessary. Heat to the loin often gives relief. Intensive antibiotic therapy is predicated on the basis of a Staphylococcus aureus infection for which penicillin or Erythromycin is most likely to be effective.

Perinephric abscess is often a late development of acute hematogenous perinephritis. It also occurs by direct extension of cortical abscess, by lymphatic extension from renal infection, from appendiceal or other pelvic abscesses, ascending along the periureteral structures or from pulmonary suppuration as in empyema. Its genesis is sometimes associated with trauma, stone, or tumor which may cause obstruction or rupture of the kidney. Common sites of perirenal abscess formation are schematically shown in Figure 157.

Symptoms. Fever, pain, gastrointestinal upsets, and occasionally urinary disturbances, especially frequency, are the outstanding symptoms in perinephric abscess. Without localizing signs the *diagnosis* is usually influenza or grippe; following a prodromal period of malaise there appear chills, high fever, sweats, anorexia, nausea or vomiting, headaches, sleeplessness, delirium, or convulsions. In the young, pronounced toxemia may suggest encephalitis or meningitis. Perinephric abscess may produce, both by local activity and by symptomatic reference, the symptoms of lower urinary tract, orthopedic, intra-abdominal, neurologic, or respiratory disease.

Perinephric abscess generally appears in the patient previously in robust health. The pain may be absent or extreme, dull, aching, shooting or stabbing, and localized over the affected loin or isolateral abdomen and costovertebral angle. It may radiate to the epigastrium, groin, genitalia, thigh or, with subphrenic involvement, to the shoulder. By reflex psoas spasm, the erroneous diagnosis of hip joint, knee, spinal or other orthopedic disease is made. Movement of the spine causes great pain, and the isolateral thigh is kept flexed as a protective mechanism against psoas spasm. In about 10 per cent of the cases the erroneous diagnosis of intraperitoneal disease is made, most often appendicitis, and perinephric abscess is particularly apt to simulate retrocecal appendicitis. In mild cases the condition may exist for weeks. As a rule, however, the course is progressive with increasing fullness in the side. With spread of the abscess it may point in the loin or, by retroperitoneal passage downward, appear in the groin or scrotum.

Diagnosis. There are few diseases in which the diagnosis may be more difficult, particularly in the absence of a palpable mass in the loin and with no urinary symptoms, the generalized toxemia overshadowing any urologic manifestations. The primary focus, especially when cutaneous, may have existed three or four months previously. A rigid abdomen is found in about two thirds of all cases and may suggest peritonitis, but there is no rebound tenderness. Flexion of the thigh exists in about half the cases, the patient walks lame, with the spine rigid and the body bent forward or toward the side of the lesion, sometimes with a supporting hand on the hip.

The *laboratory examination* may show variable urinary changes but, most important, a positive culture of Staphylococcus aureus is generally obtained. Leukocytosis may be high but usually runs around 10,000 to

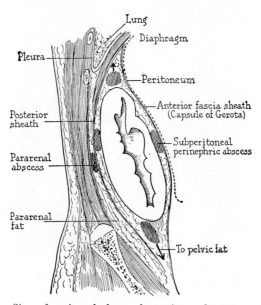

FIGURE 157. Sites of perirenal abscess formation and avenues of extension.

15,000 cells per cmm., chiefly polymorphonuclear. Blood culture may disclose a bacteremia, nearly always staphylococcic.

Urography. Obliteration of the isolateral psoas muscle outline is noted on the plain urogram with isolateral concavity of the lumbar spine due to erector spinae muscle spasm (Fig. 158). The urogram often shows displacement of the kidney, usually laterally, and frequently with alteration or compression of the renal calyces and pelves. A urologic examination will often disclose antecedent disease such as hydroureter, hydronephrosis, pyonephrosis, stone, or neoplasm.

The *differential diagnosis* must include influenza—the commonest erroneous diagnosis—malaria, typhoid, gastroenteritis, meningitis, encephalitis, tuberculosis, pneumonia, empyema, intercostal neuralgia, endocarditis, appendicitis, cholecystitis, splenic or hepatic tumor, fecal accumulations in the colon, hypernephroma, Echinococcus cyst, lumbago, or disease of the spine, sacroiliac joint, hip joint, or even of the knee.

The *treatment* of perinephric abscess is early and liberal incision with free drainage of all pockets. The kidney must be explored for carbuncle or cortical suppuration and, if the renal disease is extensive enough, nephrectomy is usually necessary. Surviving without nephrectomy, the patient may subsequently suffer (1) atrophic nephritis due to perirenal sclerotic contraction, (2) ureteral stricture and infected hydronephrosis,

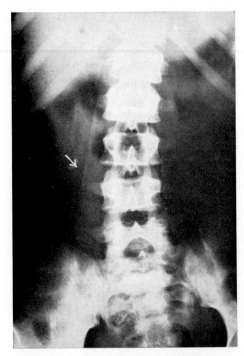

FIGURE 158. Perinephric abscess. Suggestive diagnostic findings in the plain urogram: (a) lateral scoliosis away from the side of the lesion (left), and (b) the disappearance of the shadow of the isolateral psoas muscle. Arrow points to the margin of the right psoas muscle which is distinct.

or (3) pyonephrosis may result from periureteral sclerosis. In short, perinephric abscess is a serious disease and its combat by antimicrobials alone may only serve to mask the true picture while suppuration and tissue destruction progress.

INFECTION OF THE URETER AND BLADDER

Ureter. The degree of ureteral inflammation will vary with the nature and severity of the bacterial invasion, whether primary hematogenous, renal descending, or urogenous ascending from the bladder. In mild infection the inflammation is limited to the mucosa and submucosa but in more severe involvement, extends through to the muscularis and even with ulceration, the healing of which produces stricture. In *chronic ureteritis* the submucosa and muscularis are involved chiefly with irregular dilatations and narrowings and, when the inflammatory process is pronounced, variable atonia results. Inflammation interferes with the neuromuscular mechanism so that peristalsis is diminished and maybe even cease, producing ureteral atonic dilatation. Severe chronic inflammation of the ureter and its sheath may convert the channel into a greatly thickened, somewhat right atonic tube, a centimeter or more in diameter. Secondary peripelvic or peri-ureteral scarring with liposclerosis and fibrolipomatosis variably constrict the ureter to cause secondary obstruction and hydronephrosis.

Diagnosis. The diagnosis is made by urologic examination including ureterography in which the degree of ureterectasis and ureteral peristalsis will be determined. *Treatment* is that of the primary condition and in advanced renal disease ureteronephrectomy may be necessary. Simple stricture in the lower segment of the ureter usually responds satisfactorily to periodic progressive cystoscopic dilation. In any event, antimicrobic therapy is intensively administered to eradicate all infection and sterilize the urine.

Pyoureter. This signifies a pus-filled, sausage-shaped, diverticulum-like ureteral sac which continues to pour infection into the urinary tract. Most often it is an infected dilated ureteral stump remaining after nephrectomy. Usually the ureterovesical orifice is small but may even be occluded. Pyoureter is caused chiefly by ureteral atony due to obstruction, the absence of peristalsis resulting from inflammatory injury of the intramural nerve supply of the duct. Chronic pyuria and often variable urinary toxemia are the *symptoms*, although localizing pain may be present. The *diagnosis* is made by urologic examination in which the dilated pus-filled sac or infected ureteral stump can be urographically delineated. Excision is the *treatment* which is completed by sterilization of the urine.

NONTUBERCULOUS INFECTION OF THE BLADDER (CYSTITIS)

This may be classified as nonbacterial or bacterial, the last being the usual type.

Nonbacterial Cystitis. The *chemical* variety is most commonly observed following irrigation of the bladder with irritant antiseptics but was frequently seen in the past from the administration of methenamine (formaldehyde cystitis). *Mechanical* or *traumatic* cystitis is produced by instrumentation, calculi, or foreign bodies. *Parasitic* cystitis is not unusual in the tropics, especially in schistosomiasis. *Allergic* cystitis is extremely rare. In a case of angioneurotic edema suddenly appearing in an eight year old boy and causing pronounced urinary frequency and distress, the cystographic outline induced by the enormous blebs looked exactly like that seen in moderately well developed myxosarcoma of the bladder in the young. It spontaneously and completely disappeared within one week.

Treatment of chemical and other nonbacterial forms of cystitis requires only removal of the irritant agent or other cause rather than antimicrobial therapy.

Acute Bacterial Cystitis.   This is not a primary or isolated lesion and must always be considered as a symptom and not as a disease. Except in the rare cases of hemorrhagic infarction or suppurative thrombophlebitis of the bladder wall, cystitis is never a solitary urinary tract lesion and must always be recognized as a complication of infection or inflammation elsewhere, generally in the kidney or adjacent urethra including the prostate. Any condition which produces vesical congestion predisposes to cystitis, urinary stasis being the commonest cause; stasis may result from mechanical obstruction at any point from the vesical outlet peripherally or from neuromuscular vesical imbalance. Foreign bodies are occasionally introduced into the bladder and may induce inflammation which always invites infection; stones and tumors may do the same. Constipation predisposes to cystitis by causing congestive engorgement of the lower vesical veins. Whether or not prior inflammation has been engendered, the bacterial infection arrives descending from the kidneys, ascending from the urethra, or by direct extension from adjacent suppuration as in pericystitis or appendiceal abscess, through vesical fistulae, by instrumentation, or the introduction of foreign bodies. Gram-positive staphylococci and streptococci and gram-negative E. coli and associated members of the gram-negative bacillary group are the most common invaders. Proteus ammoniae bacilli and other urea decomposing organisms are occasionally found but rarely in a person who has not had previous instrumentation. Tuberculous vesical inflammation is almost always secondary to renal tuberculosis (q.v.).

Pathology of Acute Cystitis.   This shows variable changes in the bladder wall structure depending on the type and intensity of the infection, and its associated predisposing factors, such as urinary stasis or the presence of calculus, foreign body, or tumor. Progressive pathologic changes observed are congestion, edema, ecchymosis, desquamation, muco-purulent exudation, ulceration, hemorrhage, pseudomembrane or villus formation, incrustation or, rarely with deep ulceration, perforation. This full progression seldom occurs and generally can be stopped by prompt and proper therapy. Healing of intense cystitis usually involves deposit of fibrous tissue in the bladder wall which eventually may lead to its contraction with diminution of the bladder capacity.

A localized variety of cystitis termed *urethrotrigonitis* is extremely frequent in patients of all ages and especially in young girls. Sometimes the condition is purely a congestive one but in most cases there is complicating infection. Too frequently this localized lesion with the urinary disturbance it often engenders causes a diagnosis of pyelitis or cystitis to be made.

Symptoms and Diagnosis. The symptoms of frequency, painful urination, and pyuria suggest the diagnosis cystitis which can be confirmed by cystoscopy. In severe cystitis frequency is accompanied by urgency and often the patient wets his clothing. In acute inflammation of the bladder outlet there is burning, scalding, or tenesmus on urination, often with suprapubic pain or tenderness. Sometimes the pain is most severe at the end of the penis, tip of the urethra in the female, or in the perineum or rectum. Hematuria, usually terminal, is common in acute cystitis and there may be terminal hematuria and spasm on voiding. In severe cystitis systemic symptoms will depend upon the amount of urotoxic absorption but are usually mild and may be thought to be only those of grippe.

The *cystoscopic diagnosis* in acute cystitis is made by observation of the disappearance of the normal outlines of the mucosal vascular network. Variable edema, vesicular or bullous, may appear and submucosal hemorrhages or ecchymoses may develop. Granulomatous changes indicate chronicity. One rarely performs cystoscopy in acute cystitis except when necessary for the diagnostic study of acute renal infection, prostatitis, or stone to which the vesical condition is secondary, and only when the infection remains persistently acute or abscess is suspected.

Treatment of acute cystitis is attack upon the causative factor, whether it be bacterial, chemical, obstruction, foreign body, and so forth. Rest in bed and the application of heat locally will give some relief. The following prescription is an excellent one to make the bladder more comfortable; for children the dose is appropriately reduced.

R

Codeine Sulfate	gr. vi
Tinc. Hyoscyamus	oz. 1½
Liquor Potassii Hydroxide	dr. 2
Syrup of Acacia	q.s. ad. oz. iv

M. and Sig.: One teaspoonful every four
to six hours as necessary
for relief of discomfort.

The following medication will give relief from acute vesical distress and frequency but is slightly less effective in severe vesical disturbance than the previous medication containing codeine.

R

Papaverine Hydrochloride	gr. ½
Extract Hyoscyamus	gr. ½
Pulvis Takadiastase	gr. v
Phenobarbital	gr. ⅓
Alcaroid	gr. xxx

M. et ft. d.t.d. #50
Sig.: i p.c. t.i.d.

Commonly used, but still less effective than either of the two medications just given are the "alkaline mixtures" which most pharmacies carry in stock and varying in composition from locality to locality. Most of them contain potassium citrate and tincture of hyoscyamus.

Heat locally such as hot sitz baths, hot rectal irrigations, or hot water bag suprapubically may afford some relief. Local measures other than the removal of foreign bodies, calculi, or obstruction are not necessary. A large fluid intake may temporarily increase the patient's frequency. Acute cystitis due to infection should be promptly combated by appropriate antimicrobial therapy as described under acute urinary infection.

Hemorrhagic infarction of the bladder wall by massive bacterial embolism, usually streptococcic, occurs chiefly in infants and is generally rapidly fatal. But small lesions may heal with eruption of the necrotic wall abscess into the bladder.

Suppurative thrombophlebitis of the bladder wall is almost always a secondary vascular extension from an adjacent infection or thrombophlebitis. The onset is rapid, the systemic manifestations are overwhelming, and the diagnosis is generally overlooked. Intensive antibiotic therapy with the maintenance of free vesical drainage offers the only hope of cure.

Chronic cystitis signifies a bladder inflammation which has persisted longer than four weeks. It is one of the most frequent and loosely made of all urologic diagnoses. The condition may follow inadequately treated acute cystitis but most commonly results from unrecognized persistent pyelonephritis, prostatic lower urinary tract obstruction, or is perpetuated by chronic extravesical urinary infection of one type or another, including tuberculosis. The mucosal changes in chronic cystitis vary with the degree and duration of the infection and the accessory etiologic factors, and range from roughly granular congested mucosa to a subacutely inflamed, variably edematous surface showing multiple flakes of mucopus or even superficial ulceration. Occasionally phosphatic incrustations occur and later petechiae, submucosal hemorrhages, venous dilatation, and inflammatory granulomas are cystoscopically observed. In infravesical obstruction, trabeculation, sacculation, and/or diverticulum formation reflect back-pressure changes and damage. With stones or foreign bodies present, areas of mucosal gangrene or phosphatic incrustation may be seen. The ureteral orifices reflect inflammatory changes in the lower ureters as well as in the adjacent bladder wall, may stand widely open or may be closed by sclerosis, or even retracted upward. Degenerative mucosal changes such as cystitis cystica, cystitis glandularis, leukoplakia, malacoplakia, occasionally result from long-standing chronic vesical inflammation (q.v.), as may variable fibrosis in the bladder musculature. The last may lead to sclerotic atrophy or inflammatory atonia.

Symptoms of chronic cystitis are those of acute cystitis only milder (q.v.). There may be only persistent frequency of urination.

Diagnosis. This is made by cystoscopic study of the bladder wall changes, the nature of which has been enumerated in the second preceding paragraph. At the time of the cystoscopic study the upper urinary tract should also be investigated. The detection of neuromuscular vesical disease as an etiologic factor in cystitis must not be overlooked (Chapter 9).

Treatment of chronic cystitis rests upon correction of the cause; usually this implies eradication of renal infection together with the establishment of free urinary drainage and/or correction of other coexisting uropathy. In fulfilling this treatment, follow the outline for treatment of chronic urinary infections as given earlier in this chapter. It is amazing how many cases of "chronic cystitis" are symptomatically cured solely by adequate dilation of a tight or strictured urethra.

Interstitial cystitis is a chronic, patchy submucous cystitis, also known as elusive ulcer, Hunner ulcer, or interstitial panmural cystitis, and affects chiefly women. For this reason, discussion of the condition is given in Chapter 14.

In **cystitis emphysematosa** there are numerous small gas-filled vesicles and cysts in the bladder wall and its mucosa; the cause is unknown; it is seen most often in diabetic patients with a complicating ammoniogenic urinary infection. There is no treatment other than correction of any demonstrable etiology.

Chronic urethrotrigonitis is most common in women, the high incidence being explained by the brevity of the female urethra. It may follow an acute urethrotrigonitis or may be the principal manifestation of infection elsewhere in the urinary tract, chiefly renal, may develop insidiously, or even as a congestive process in the absence of infection. Stricture of the urethra, congenital or acquired, is the common underlying cause, particularly in infants and children. The lesion is the most frequently observed one in persistent enuresis in the young, and it is often seen in young boys with chronic prostatitis. There is congestion and sometimes edema of the trigone and vesical outlet and with extension into the posterior urethra for at least a centimeter. Generally the mucosa appears dull red and granular; occasionally in long-standing cases both granulomatous changes and small polypoid excrescences may be seen, especially about the bladder neck. In more acute cases there is bullous edema with or without ulceration and incrustation.

It is believed by many that this inflammatory lesion in the posterior urethra and bladder neck, particularly in young girls, is associated with infection of urethral gland follicles of the area and serves to perpetuate urinary infection, particularly of the ascending urogenous type.

Symptoms are those noted under acute cystitis which in many cases is acute urethrotrigonitis. In chronic urethrotrigonitis the symptomatology is similar but milder, urinary frequency and/or urgency, and sometimes "enuresis" being the complaints.

The persistence of the symptoms of irritation of the vesical outlet calls for thorough urologic examination in patients of all ages and urethrocystoscopy will establish the diagnosis.

Treatment. Dilation of the urethra and bladder outlet to a size a little above normal for the age and general urethral development of the patient is the best treatment. This is followed by endoscopic application of silver nitrate 2 to 4 per cent directly to the anterior trigone and vesical outlet. Occasionally in obstinate cases electrocoagulation of the granulomatous excrescences is helpful. When this simple treatment does not achieve the desired result, a complete urologic examination should be made to be certain that pyelonephritis, hydronephrosis, ureteral stone or other obstruction has not been overlooked, the treatment of which is essential to the over-all cure.

Pericystitis. This is inflammation and infection of the fatty areolar envelopes surrounding the bladder, is a frequent occurrence, may be acute or chronic, localized or diffused. The bacteria may arrive by the lymphogenous or hematogenous routes, by direct extension from bladder wall suppuration, from the reproductive tract, or from trauma or extravasation. Suprapubic tenderness or rigidity may be felt, the underlying infection giving a woody texture to the tissues, and rectal examination may disclose a similar involvement of the vesical floor. The clinical picture is that of the associated urologic infection, usually with systemic manifestations. Gastrointestinal upsets, chills and fever, and urinary disturbances are frequent and reflect the acuteness of the condition.

In *chronic pericystitis,* secondary contracture of the bladder wall within the fatty fibrotic capsule may occur to cause a diminished bladder capacity with urinary frequency. Incision and drainage of suppurative areas together with intensive antibiotic therapy is the treatment. The mortality is high and the prognosis is bad.

Omphalitis is inflammation of the umbilicus and may be important as a primary focus of renal infection, especially in the newborn and infants. Abscess of the urachus may develop secondarily.

Unusual mucosal changes in the urinary tract are rarely of clinical importance except as they reflect chronicity of infection. The more important of these are multiple mucosal cystic lesions recognized as pyelitis, ureteritis, cystitis, urethritis cystica or glandularis respectively, leukoplakia and malacoplakia. Of themselves they cause few or no symptoms and may involve any portion of the urinary tract from the renal calyces to urethral meatus.

The *cystic changes* (epithelial-lined submucosal cysts) are believed to develop as epithelial cell nest inclusions as a result of chronic toxic irritation from inflammation. They are to be distinguished from edematous blebs and glandular polyps which they most closely resemble. They are recognized in the bladder cystoscopically, and in the ureteropyelogram they cause a rather characteristic filling irregularity of the ureteral and pelvic outlines (cf. Fig. 151). There is no satisfactory way of destroying all of the cysts but every attempt should be made to sterilize the urine.

Cystitis, ureteritis, and/or pyelitis glandularis is a metaplastic change of transitional mucosal epithelium into cylindrical epithelium with the formation of glandular acini which may harbor infection and engender urinary re-infection. Occluded, these acini may form cysts or infected crypts and involve any portion of the urinary tract.

Leukoplakia is a metaplasia of the transitional epithelium to the squamous type forming a patch of cornified, greatly thickened, elevated, whitish or celery white epithelium, and is definitely a symptomatic precancerous condition. There is no treatment except sterilization of the urine to remove possible bacterial irritation. Should the lesion appear to grow or ulcerate, excise it at once as it is probably cancer.

Malacoplakia is an extremely rare formation of yellowish or grayish convex, elevated, soft patch of bodies originating in the submucosa and containing large peculiar cells, each with a large vesicular nucleus containing refractile bodies of unknown composition (Michaelis-Gutmann bodies). It is of no clinical importance and there is no treatment.

URINARY TUBERCULOSIS

In most parts of the United States the incidence of urinary tuberculosis is gradually diminishing, doubtless as a result of the remarkably improved therapy of pulmonary tuberculosis. In 1900 the death rate from tuberculosis was 194.4 per 100,000 population but in 1945, only 40.1 per 100,000 population, a four fifths reduction. Surgical renal tuberculosis is predominantly a disease of early adulthood, two thirds of all cases occurring between the ages of twenty and forty. Unfortunately the occurrence of tuberculosis in children's hospitals has not materially declined. In New York I found that one in every sixty cases of so-called chronic pyelitis in children was in fact caseous renal tuberculosis. The condition occurs twice as often in males as in females and somewhat more often on the right side than on the left. Natural immunity to tuberculosis is negligible, but the development of the chronic renal ulcerative variety rather than acute miliary tuberculosis suggests an unusual degree of acquired resistance. In short, urogenital tuberculosis is still a potentially fatal condition which must ever be kept in mind in all patients with urinary infections of any kind.

Acute miliary tuberculosis is but part of a rapidly fatal generalized hematogenous form of the disease, is found particularly in the young, causes bilateral renal involvement and has carried a high death rate although active streptomycin therapy now produces cures in many patients who formerly would have died.

Chronic Renal Tuberculosis. This is usually of the erosive type (ulcerative, caseocavernous, ulcerocavernous, pyonephrotic) but in patients with unusual resistance the infection may appear as a diffuse nodular or sclerotic form. Although the clinical picture in each pathologic grouping is not necessarily the same, identical treatment is required.

Pathogenesis. In all varieties of urogenital tract tuberculosis the kidney must be considered to be involved, and is nearly always the initial site for dispersion of tuberculosis to the remainder of the genitourinary apparatus. Unquestionably the pulmonary and/or intestinal tract is the usual portal of entry of the infection; when urogenital and skeletal tuberculosis coexist, it is probable that they are both secondary to the same initial focus. Osseous tuberculosis is demonstrable in a third of the cases of urogenital tuberculosis and pulmonary tuberculosis—active or arrested —in about 40 per cent.

The routes of invasion of the kidneys by tubercle bacilli are the same as in nontuberculous infection but the hematogenous route predominates. Doubtless lymphatic transmission commonly occurs or there is combined lymphohematogenous invasion. Ascending primary urogenous tuberculous infection may be disregarded.

As shown by Medlar et al. (1948) nearly all renal tuberculous lesions are bilateral and other urogenital tract organs are always involved. Tubercle bacilli having reached the kidney, the development of clinical tuberculosis will depend upon the virulence of the bacteria on the one hand and the local resistance of the patient on the other. Unsuspected renal invasion is found in practically every patient dead of pulmonary tuberculosis although clinical renal disease may not have been evident or recognized. Minute miliary lesions may heal but it has never been proved that an established major ulcerative tuberculous renal lesion will heal spontaneously.

As the tuberculous infection in one kidney becomes established, extension to other portions of the kidney occurs as well as downwards with involvement of the ureter, bladder, and eventually the genital tract in the male and commonly the remaining upper urinary tract in both sexes (Figs. 159–165). Tubercle bacilli like other bacteria will not pass through the uninjured kidney and when tubercle bacilli are found in the urine, an established infection must be accepted.

Microscopically the renal lesion is fundamentally similar to tuberculous lesions elsewhere with lymphatic infiltration, epithelioid and giant cell deposit. While these lesions may be healed by sclerosis, the tendency

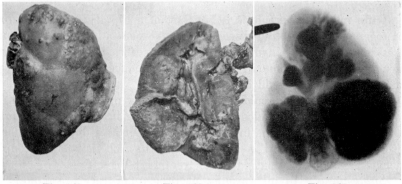

Fig. 159   Fig. 160   Fig. 161

FIGURE 159. Renal tuberculosis in a six-year-old girl examined because of "chronic pyelitis." Diffuse spread of cortical tubercles particularly over the superior renal pole; adherent perinephric tissue laterally.

FIGURE 160. Section of kidney (Fig. 159) disclosing large caseocavernous abscess. Throughout the kidney are diffusely scattered macroscopic abscesses.

FIGURE 161. Postoperative pyelogram of Figure 159 showing not only a large tuberculous abscess but the urographic changes consequent to pelvic and parenchymal ulceration (Fig. 160).

is toward the development of central necrotization about which a marked polymorphonuclear infiltration develops and, as the process extends, there is tubular invasion with the passage of bacilli, pus, and usually red blood cells into the urine just as occurs in nontuberculous infection. The infection spreads through the kidney predominantly by intrarenal lymphatics rather than by intratubular or hematogenous extension, although these at times obviously play a part. Extension to the subcapsular tissues and perirenal fat occurs through intrarenal lymphatic connections to engender tuberculous perinephritis with pronounced fibrolipomatosis.

As the ulcerative process in the parenchyma extends, a break through into the pelvis occurs, frequently at the papilla. With this ulceration into the pelvis, secondary tuberculous pyelitis develops often with superficial pelvic ulceration. From this stage infection spreads widely throughout the kidney as well as to the lower urinary tract with tuberculous involvement of the upper ureter first and then the lower segment of the ureter, and finally the middle ureteral segment and the bladder (Figs. 162–165). As attempts at sclerotic renal repair are made, some freely draining caseous cavities may fill in by granulation or even be relined by epithelium. In some ancient tuberculous kidneys with considerable reparative activity, there is pronounced tuberculous pyelitis, ureteritis, and surrounding peripelvic and perirenal liposclerosis.

With tuberculous stricturization of the pelvic outlet or upper ureter, tuberculous hydronephrosis develops and this may progress to tuberculous pyonephrosis—the usual late surgical kidney. In these advanced cases, section of the organ discloses little or no remaining cortex, and the entire kidney is often transformed into a collection of large caseous abscesses

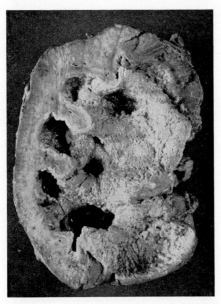

FIGURE 162.   Late caseous (inspissated; noncavernous) renal tuberculosis with total renal destruction.

separated from one another by the remnants of the interlobar vascular divisions (Fig. 162). With inspissation of caseous pus of the abscess, it becomes putty-like and sometimes infiltrated with lime which will cast an x-ray shadow (cement kidney). Complicating mixed infection may superimpose an acute inflammatory process on the more indolent tuberculous one. Rarely such a kidney becomes spontaneously sealed off to cease discharging tubercle bacilli and tuberculous debris into the ureter. This is known as *autonephrectomy,* and explains some apparent spontaneous cures of surgical renal tuberculosis. The organisms are merely walled off, are living, and ever ready for activation with eruption or with trauma of the kidney and particularly for hematogenous systemic spread to cause generalized miliary tuberculosis.

Unfortunately the "better" kidney, considered not infected with tuberculosis as far as is clinically possible to tell, suffers a variable toxic nephritis from its involved mate and this, long continued, leads to a sclerotic nephritis with diminishing renal function and ultimately death from renal failure. Occasionally such involvement of the better kidney has misdirected attention from the more seriously involved organ. Urinanalytic findings from the better kidney injured by toxemia may suggest nephritis: albumin, tubular epithelial cells, hyaline and granular casts, and occasionally red blood cells. With removal of the tuberculous mate, this toxic nephritis disappears and rehabilitation of the better kidney occurs to support life except as previously unrecognized latent tuberculous infection may become activated and destroy the second organ as not infrequently happens.

With downward extension of the tuberculous infection, *tuberculous*

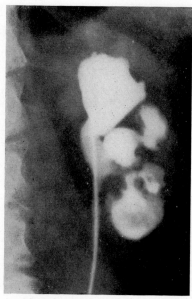

FIGURE 163. Far advanced tuberculous pyonephrosis in a seventy-year-old female. Note evidence of widespread pelvic ulceration.

ureteritis develops with thickening, irregular dilatation, and narrowing of the channel, fibrolipomatous periureteritis, and finally the duct may be converted to a semi-pipestem structure (Fig. 164).

In the *bladder* the initial changes are most pronounced around the ureteral orifice of the involved kidney with congestion, edema, and later the formation of miliary tubercles. This process then spreads to become universal over the bladder wall and especially around the second ureteral orifice from which this kidney may secondarily become invaded by the ascending route. Serpiginous tuberculous ulceration may appear later with scarring, occasionally granulation tissue proliferation, trigonal ulceration, generalized cystitis, sclerotic attempts at healing, and the production of a widely patulous somewhat retracted ureter—the golf-hole ureter. In late *tuberculous cystitis*, the organ is irregularly contracted, highly sensitive, often deeply ulcerated, and bleeds freely (Fig. 165).

Urethral tuberculosis is found in about 2 per cent of all cases of far-advanced renal tuberculosis and generally as a terminal development. Histologically and clinically the condition is similar to that observed in the proximal urinary tract.

Symptoms of Renal Tuberculosis. Too often the symptoms of renal tuberculosis cause the physician to be satisfied with a diagnosis of chronic urinary infection or, worse yet, chronic pyelitis. Because of the vesical

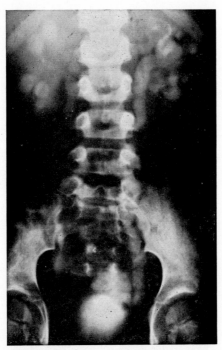

FIGURE 164. Advanced bilateral renal tuberculosis in a six-year-old boy dead in uremia one year later. The widespread pelvic and parenchymal ulceration as well as ureteral dilatation and vesical irregularity are characteristic of the disease. Sanatorium treatment.

symptoms, notably pronounced urinary frequency, in more than half of the cases the initial diagnosis of cystitis, acute or chronic, is made. This vesical irritability and frequency is simulated only by nontuberculous interstitial panmural cystitis—Hunner's ulcer (q.v.). Bladder irritability, renal pain, urinary frequency and hematuria will occur in at least 90 per cent of the patients and secondary urotoxic manifestations may be observed in the gastrointestinal tract and central nervous system with variable fever, usually low grade.

As vesical ulceration and contraction occur, the frequency of urination is greatly increased, sometimes to as much as every fifteen to twenty minutes day and night. With the exhaustion contributed to by the disease and especially by the loss of sleep, the patient rapidly declines and dies. In most instances death is due to renal failure from advanced bilateral renal involvement or from advanced involvement on one side with fatal urotoxic damage of the opposite kidney. Only rarely do patients with active renal tuberculosis maintain the picture of good health. In some instances "silent" renal tuberculosis occurs, the parenchymal lesion being walled off from the pelvis. There is a good chance that soon or late the infection will erupt with tuberculous spread to the entire urogenital tract.

Diagnosis. The history, especially with repeated painless hematuria, and pyuria, may suggest the diagnosis of renal tuberculosis particularly if active pulmonary tuberculosis is or recently has been present. The pulmonary involvement is suggested by a history of chronic cough, hemoptysis, wet pleurisy, lymphadenitis, persistent low-grade tempera-

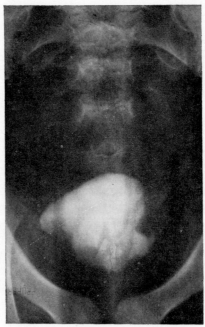

FIGURE 165. Vesical tuberculosis, cystographically demonstrated. Pronounced vesical irregularity; right renal tuberculosis.

ture, rapid pulse, or a subnormal physical development. Demonstration of tubercle bacilli in the urine clinches the diagnosis.

Tuberculous foci may be found in the chest, cervical glands, chronic fistulas, osseous swellings, or joint involvements. The tuberculin skin tests, von Pirquet and Mantoux, may be positive but are not reliable guides and may even be negative although active renal tuberculosis exists and vice versa. Occasionally the enlarged tender kidney can be palpated or costovertebral angle tenderness is found. Palpation of a tuberculous epididymis should at once suggest renal tuberculosis. While excretory urographic study may suggest the diagnosis, a cystoscopic examination is far more reliable, particularly with ureteral catheterization, divided renal functional and bacteriologic studies and retrograde pyelography. Cystoscopy will give the definitive clue when tuberculous lesions are observed in the bladder, or the characteristic ulcerosclerotic pelvic urographic changes are found, often with evidence of parenchymal cavitation (Figs. 161, 163, 164). The cystoscopic and urographic pictures in tuberculous and nontuberculous urinary infection may be strikingly similar and only the finding of extra-urinary tuberculosis or tubercle bacilli in the urine suggests the clue.

Examination of the Urine for Tubercle Bacilli. By simple acid-fast stain of a properly collected and centrifuged urine from patients with urinary tuberculosis, the organisms can be demonstrated in nearly 90 per cent of the cases. The urine is centrifuged at 2500 revolutions per minute for fifteen minutes and the supernatant fluid is poured off. The sediment is then taken up with a pipette and smeared on the glass slide, is stained by the steaming acid-fast method and examined. The *guinea-pig test* is performed by injection of 1 to 2 cc. of the suspected urine into the animal. When positive, the test shows tuberculous involvement at least of the regional glands but this takes six weeks. *Bacteriologic culture* for tubercle bacilli has largely replaced the guinea-pig test; the results are known in three weeks. In most cases the presumptive diagnosis can be made by clinical and urographic observations alone.

In the urologic examination it is extremely important to determine that the apparently uninvolved kidney is in fact free of tuberculous infection and that its function is adequate to support life when its mate is removed. Clinical tuberculosis will be manifested in the "good" kidney in a third of the cases showing pus in the urine at the time of the initial examination and even though no tubercle bacilli are obtained from this side.

Urography. The ureteropelvicalyceal changes demonstrated by excretory urography and suggestive of renal tuberculosis include (1) an irregular pelvic and juxta-ureteral dilatation, (2) failure to demonstrate all the calyces on one side with an irregular outline caused by parenchymal erosion or necrosis, (3) reduced or no renal excretion on the diseased side. *Demonstration of a sound opposite kidney is the most important achievement of excretory urography.*

The pelvic changes consequent to ulceration are the striking findings of retrograde pyelography and here the earliest alteration is the urographic fringing of the calyces (Fig. 163). Irregular urographic shadows peripheral to the calyceal outlines suggest parenchymal abscess and may occur in only one portion of the kidney while the remainder of the pelvic outline is normal. With advancing caseocavernous ulceration the pyelogram is characterized by an irregular moth-eaten, fuzzy pelvic outline indicative of the parenchymal necrosis (Figs. 163, 164). Deformity of the pelvis and ureter by sclerosis may be observed as well as tuberculous stricture, secondary hydronephrosis or, in the late stage, pyonephrosis. Frequently, however, the pyelogram is indistinguishable from that of advanced chronic nontuberculous pyelonephritis. The pelvic changes in renal brucellosis (q.v.) may closely simulate those of renal tuberculosis.

Secondary calcium deposit in the caseous area at once suggests tuberculosis.

In the *ureterogram* the tuberculous ureter appears as an irregularly strictured and dilated channel, the initial and greatest involvement being near the kidney, later near the bladder, and ultimately with alteration of the entire structure (Fig. 164). Retrograde pyelography is urged in every case except when rendered impossible by sclerotic obstruction of the ureteral orifice or inability to find it even with chromomeatoscopy. Here the excretory urographic study must be relied upon even though it is less satisfactory. *Great caution should be exercised in performing nephrectomy solely because of the excretory urographic findings.*

Treatment. Renal tuberculosis is neither an isolated nor a self-limited disease, and demands prompt treatment. Surgical treatment of renal tuberculosis by nephrectomy is practically never an urgent procedure. The therapeutic results are vastly improved if the patient has the benefit of medical treatment for three to six months before nephrectomy is performed. In the medical regimen the patient receives sanatorium rest and care or its equivalent. The administration of streptomycin has completely revolutionized the treatment of tuberculosis in all fields and nowhere is this more promising and satisfactory than in urogenital phthisis.

MEDICAL TREATMENT OF UROGENITAL TUBERCULOSIS. This is employed both in (1) the preoperative preparation for nephrectomy when surgical treatment is indicated and feasible, and for (2) the treatment of bilateral renal tuberculosis when surgery is contraindicated or the prognosis is otherwise grave. As a corollary, *the surgical prognosis is best in those patients who have had ample preoperative medical treatment.* The medical treatment has proved especially efficacious in the treatment of genital disease with surprisingly prompt closure and healing of tuberculous scrotal fistulas as well as striking improvement in tuberculous foci in bone and lung. Today dihydrostreptomycin, para-aminosalicylic acid (PAS), and isoniazid are used chiefly, the average dosage and duration of treatment being given in Table 9. Unfortunately, for medical or economic reasons the preoperative course of sanatorium treatment cannot always be given and the patient is operated upon shortly after the diagnosis is made.

SURGICAL TREATMENT OF RENAL TUBERCULOSIS. *Nephrectomy should always be performed in unilateral tuberculosis when the condition of the patient and of the opposite kidney permits.* In general the excretion of a deep indigo carmine of at least 10 per cent phenolsulfonphthalein in fifteen minutes from a tuberculosis-free kidney justifies removal of its mate. *Nephrectomy is not an emergency procedure in renal tuberculosis!* The operations usually carried out are nephrectomy or nephro-ureterectomy or, for relief of intolerable vesical tuberculosis in patients in whom nephrectomy is contraindicated, cutaneous ureterostomy. The last puts the bladder at rest, permits the vesical lesions to subside, and affords quick symptomatic relief.

Nephrectomy for renal tuberculosis is *contraindicated* in (1) advanced interstitial nephritis, (2) hypoplasia or absence of opposite kidney, (3) active tuberculosis elsewhere, and almost always in (4) bilateral renal tuberculosis. A pyonephrotic or hydronephrotic tuberculous kidney causing fever or uncontrollable bleeding must be removed promptly despite an early tuberculosis in the opposite kidney. Secondary perirenal suppuration on one side may demand surgical intervention. With these exceptions, bilateral renal tuberculosis is a nonsurgical condition to receive intense medical treatment.

In some instances an apparently localized tuberculous process in a kidney has been subjected to partial renal resection, but this procedure is still *sub judice* and certainly not one for general employment.

Tuberculous infection of the lower urinary tract and especially of the genital tract may require a special attention. This is concerned chiefly with tuberculous epididymitis which demands epididymectomy and, if the testicle is involved, orchiectomy as well. The vas deferens is simultaneously removed to the external inguinal ring. Excision of tuberculous prostate and seminal vesicles is not an acceptable procedure today. With these and other tuberculous complications, give the patient full benefit of intensive antimicrobial therapy and rest. Fortunately today, at least half of all clean wounds of nephrectomy for tuberculosis will heal by primary union. Some of these wounds, apparently healed, will break down in two to four weeks and, with rehealing, leave one or more discharging fistulas, the origin of which is generally the ureteral stump or remaining infected perirenal fat. This calls for antimicrobial treatment.

With successful surgery a prompt gain of weight generally occurs and is likely to be permanent. Vesical symptoms begin to abate shortly but will persist more or less permanently in a fifth of the cases. This applies chiefly to urinary frequency and dysuria. Pyuria remains for some time although no tubercle bacilli are demonstrable. Toxic nephritis, tuberculous or nontuberculous infection of the remaining kidney must be ruled out and when this can be satisfactorily done, the persistent pyuria comes from infection of the bladder, ureteral stump, posterior urethra, prostate, or genital adnexa.

Symptoms persisting longer than two years postoperatively may be considered permanent. Nearly always this means tuberculosis in the remaining kidney. Persistence of tubercle bacilli in the urine indicates active ulceration, electrocoagulation of which in the bladder will sometimes afford relief. With persistence of intolerable vesical irritability, as often as every fifteen to twenty minutes and with a bladder capacity of only 15 to 20 cc., cutaneous ureterostomy is indicated rather than local treatment of the tuberculous bladder. Hydraulic overdistention of the scarred weakened bladder may crack or rupture the viscus with profuse hemorrhage, urinary extravasation and/or disseminate acute generalized miliary tuberculosis. With activation of tuberculosis of the only kidney or of lesions elsewhere, a downward course to fatal termination sets in.

Prognosis. In renal tuberculosis the prognosis is favorable only with early nephrectomy in unilateral surgical disease; a surgical mortality of not over 3 per cent should be expected. In general, the older the patient the better the prognosis because of the greater tendency to resistance to the disease by localized fibrosis. Two thirds of all children with tuberculosis under two years of age die early and this trend is observed in renal tuberculosis in older children. In 1380 statistically studied cases of all ages, Nesbit (1948) found that only half of the patients were alive five years after nephrectomy. Emmett and Kibler (1938) found that when the "good" kidney was free from pus, the chance of a five-year cure was 43.5 per cent but when the urine from this kidney was free from pus cells and tubercle bacilli, the five-year outlook was 50 per cent. In short, in renal tuberculosis which is fundamentally a bilateral disease, the best we can hope for is a 50 per cent chance of cure. Without operation, two thirds are dead within five years and not over 5 per cent will live more than ten. *With operation,* nearly two thirds will be alive at the end of ten years. In those not surviving ten years, tuberculosis of the other kidney or of the lung is the usual cause of death, yet miliary tuberculosis or intercurrent nontuberculous infections will kill many. Streptomycin and other medical therapy, chiefly para-aminosalicylic acid and isoniazid, augur well to improve this prognostic outlook.

UNUSUAL INFECTIONS OF THE URINARY TRACT

Brucellosis (undulant fever) may cause important urologic lesions resembling tuberculous disease especially in the kidney, bladder, prostate, and testes and, because of its unusualness, it fails to be correctly recognized. It is primarily an infectious disease of animals (goats, sheep, cattle, swine) and is transmissible to man in whom the three types of infection have all been identified. The usual type is Brucella melitensis, the goat being the dominant reservoir of infection in spreading its disease through its unpasteurized milk. The second type, Brucella abortus, causes contagious abortion in cattle (Bang's disease) and has been known to do the same in the human. About 4 per cent of cattle are known to be thus infected. The third type, Brucella suis, causes infectious abortion in swine, the general incidence of the infection being 5 to 15 per cent of all hogs. The geographic occurrence largely follows the commercial use of these animals: goats, chiefly Central and South America, North Africa and the Mediterranean borders, the Near and Far East; dairy cattle, throughout the world; swine, Central America, South America, and in the United States chiefly in the midwestern states, particularly Iowa and southern Minnesota. The infection in man respects no age but most of the observed patients have been adults.

Pathology. The infection spreads chiefly by the lymphatics and produces tuberculosis-like or sarcoid-like granulomatous disease in infected organs with collections of round and plasma cells surrounding and interspersed between myriad epithelioid cells, often with associated Langerhans' type of giant cells. Necrosis is usually absent or but slight.

The special urologic interest of brucellosis centers about renal infection by these organisms, the changes in the kidney, the symptomatology of the disease and the urologic findings including the pyelographic, closely simulating or even being indistinguishable from these findings in urinary tuberculosis. The difference is that tubercle bacilli are absent and Brucella organisms are present. Brucellosis should be especially considered in the differential diagnosis of chronic inflammatory urogenital tract disease when the patient is a farmer, dairyman, stock breeder, packing-house worker, butcher, or veterinarian.

In short, the bacteriologic examination of aseptically collected urine makes the correct diagnosis. These organisms are gram-negative, non-sporulating, nonmotile bacilli or coccobacilli. In addition to culture, identification of the Brucella organism by the agglutination test is highly reliable especially when positive in high titers. The cutaneous sensitivity test and complement fixation test also become positive when the infection is well established. The sedimentation test is normal or only slightly elevated and the leukocyte count is normal or shows mild lymphocytosis. Secondary anemia may exist.

Any portion of the urogenital tract may be invaded in brucellosis, the manifestations being those observed in either tuberculous or nontuberculous infection of the particular inflamed structure. Abscess may occur in any organ; skeletal involvement is frequent, especially in the lumbosacral area.

Treatment. Fortunately brucellosis usually responds favorably to intensive antimicrobial combined therapy. Combinations of triple sulfonamides (or of sulfadiazine) and streptomycin or dihydrostreptomycin have worked well as has dihydrostreptomycin and chlortetracycline (Aureomycin) or oxytetracycline (Terramycin), but apparently the triple combination of dihydrostreptomycin (0.5 gm. intramuscularly every six hours), Aureomycin (0.5 gm. orally every six hours) and triple sulfonamide (4 to 6 gm. in twenty-four hours) has given the lowest relapse rate (3 to 5 per cent). In children the dose is appropriately reduced. The physician must be alert to the possibility of eighth (auditory) nerve injury by the dihydrostreptomycin or of gastrointestinal disturbances by any or all of these drugs. In the event of such complications, the dose must be reduced or stopped for a few days and, if possible, then resumed. During medical therapy the patient is best kept in bed with a high fluid, nutritional, and vitamin intake, and the drug dosage maintained for eighteen to twenty-one days which is usually long enough. Suppurative lesions whether in the testicle or kidney, for example, require excision of the hopelessly involved organ(s) at which time the previous diagnosis of tuberculosis may be changed to brucellosis.

Syphilis. Urogenital tract syphilis in infants and children is usually congenital while in adults it is nearly always acquired. Syphilis of the reproductive organs is briefly discussed in Chapter 8. *Syphilitic nephritis* is rare, and renal gumma is even more rare. Renal gumma in the young is nearly always an autopsy finding while in adults it may urographically simulate renal tumor by compression or distortion of the pelvic outline. Structurally renal gumma resembles gumma elsewhere, usually being nodular with a grayish vascular, more or less fibrous network, which surrounds and encapsulates it and its necrotic or caseous center. With ulceration into the pelvis, gumma may simulate tuberculosis both symptomatically and urographically. Antisyphilitic treatment is the indication and today is done largely by massive doses of penicillin.

Syphilis of the bladder is evidenced by patchy inflammation, ulceration or granulomatosis of the mucosa. The dominant symptoms are frequency, dysuria, pain, hematuria, and pyuria. The diagnosis is made by cystoscopic observation of punched-out ulceration, papillary villi, granulomatosis, and is confirmed by a positive Wassermann test. Luetic cystitis merits little consideration in the differential diagnosis of urinary infection. The disease is usually cured by antiluetic therapy; the last may also cure bacillary and coccic nontuberculous infection.

Thrush (Candida albicans) infection is not uncommon in adults, particularly adult women, but a few cases have been reported in children; I have recognized four instances in the young. It is amazing that it is not more often diagnosed in view of the high incidence of monilial vaginitis in which the infection extends through the urethra to the bladder to produce the symptoms of cystitis. Cystoscopically the vesical lesion appears as soft, pearly white, slightly elevated patches resembling coagulated milk, yet densely adherent to the mucosa. Removal of these patches causes bleeding. The filament and yeast-like cells of the mold will be identified in tissue removed from the patch and even in the catheterized urine specimen itself; on Nickerson's medium the monilia grow as small brownish or black colonies. In addition to establishing free urinary drainage by dilation of the tight urethra, administer antibiotics and arsphenamines which have shown some value. Urinary alkalinization together with sulfonamide treatment has worked as has streptomycin and even the instillation of 1 per cent gentian violet in the bladder. Vaginal suppositories of Mycostatin (500 mg.), used once daily, will usually control the infection and diminish urinary frequency. Be sure that cross reinfection between man and wife is not occurring.

Echinococcus Disease. This results from infection with the cysticercus stage of the dog tapeworm, Taenia echinococcus, and for this reason is extremely common in countries where the inhabitants live in intimate contact with animals, particularly sheep and dogs.* A sixth of the Iceland population is thus infected and it is only slightly less common in Argentina, Australia, France and Greece. It is comparatively rare in the United States, some 500 cases having been reported, but it has often been found in Puerto Rico. Most of the cases found in the United States have been immigrants infected in other lands, and infected adults commonly give the history of passing hydatids since early childhood.

While the renal infection is usually hematogenous, it may be by direct spread from hepatic Echinococcus disease and in 3 per cent of the cases is bilateral. As the cyst enlarges both pelvic and parenchymal compression occurs with alteration of the vascular supply and pelvic outlines, and secondary infection usually produces pyonephrosis. The symptoms are tumor, pain, dysuria and, occasionally, hematuria. The pain which usually appears late, is a dull ache but may be sharp and colicky with renal ptosis or ureteral obstruction by the passage of hydatid debris. Following cyst rupture, spontaneous healing may occur.

Diagnosis is made by the discovery of the ova, hooklets, or scolices in the urine. A palpable mass in the loin or persistent vesical disturbances demand complete urologic examination in which renal neoplasm is the usual preoperative diagnosis. Urographically tuberculosis, solitary cystic renal disease, polycystic disease, and/or neoplasm may be suggested by the pelvic deformity. A high eosinophilia up to 10 per cent or more is commonly found and suggests the parasitic nature of the disease. The complement fixation test for Echinococcus is positive in 85 per cent of the cases and becomes negative upon cure of the patient.

Treatment. Nephrectomy is the treatment, medical therapy being wholly ineffective. In some instances of massive cystic involvement of

---

* Zoologically the adult Taenia echinococcus is interesting with its four suckers situated behind a double row of hooklets encircling the head, with which it attaches itself to the intestinal wall. The worm is 3.5 to 5.5 mm. long, has but a few segments in the terminal spine of which are numerous ripe ova encased in a gelatinous membrane capsule. Periodically these ova are discharged into the intestinal tract and are passed by rectum.

The life cycle of the parasite requires two hosts. The adult worm lives in the duodenum of the dog, wolf or other carnivorous animal, the ova being discharged in the stool to contaminate grasses, drinking water, green vegetables or animal foods, and is thus taken into the intestinal tract of herbivorous animals or man. In the intestine of the secondary host, the gelatinous shell of the ova is dissolved by the digestive juices to liberate the ova, the larvae of which then penetrate the intestinal wall where they are carried by the portal circulation to the liver and eventually to the heart. Thence by the blood stream they are carried to the lungs, brain, kidneys or elsewhere, renal invasion occurring in about 5 per cent of the cases. In the kidney the embryo grows to form a cyst which, until large, causes no symptoms. Rupture of the cyst into the renal pelvis discharges blood and scolices which appear in the urine. In the germinal lining of the cyst wall are small buds or capillary sprouts representing the brood capsules for the formation of new cysts containing scolices. As the daughter cysts are developed and following rupture of the mother cyst, new cysts are formed. Occasionally cyst rupture is accompanied by pronounced allergic reaction with urticaria, prostration, and occasionally death. In about a third of infected patients the cysts die off spontaneously.

and around the kidney, marsupialization of the infected mass with suture of the cystic margins to the skin and chemical destruction of the cyst wall with phenol has been successful. Let a cyst rupture during nephrectomy, however, and all hope of cure is lost. A preoperative injection of 1 or 2 per cent formaldehyde into cyst cavities for five minutes destroys the parasites. Lower bowel involvement occurs in about 4 per cent of the cases. In some instances, Echinococcus involvement of the retrovesical tissues, especially the seminal vesicles and peritoneal cul-de-sac, has been identified and has caused urinary obstruction by pressure on the vesical outlet or lower ends of the ureter. Here, surgical excision, extirpation or marsupialization of the bladder base, with subsequent chemical destruction of the cystic infection, is the treatment. In this last group of cases, an example of which we saw at Bellevue Hospital, the findings on rectal examination may suggest the diagnosis.

Schistosomiasis (bilharziasis) is caused by the trematode *Schistosoma haematobium* (discovered by Bilharz, 1851) which in some countries commonly invades the urinary tract. In Egypt two thirds of the laboring population is infected and in a tenth of these the disease or its complications are fatal. In one district 79 per cent of the school boys were infected. It is rarely seen in the United States except in immigrants bringing their disease with them. The male and female parasite exists in symbiosis, the ventral surface of the male (15 to 18 mm. long and 1 mm. wide) enveloping the body of the female (18 to 22 mm. and 1 mm. wide). They attach themselves by two suckers, one at the extreme anterior end and the other a short distance behind. Transmission and development of the parasites require an intermediate host without which the life cycle ends. The oval yellowish-brown ova possessing a terminal spine are voided in the urine, fall into stagnant fresh water, swell and liberate motile em-

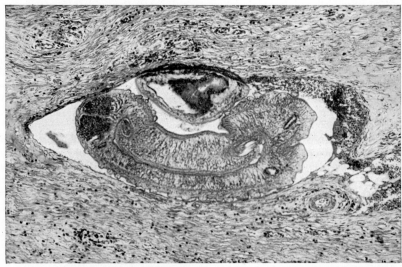

FIGURE 166.   Adult worm of S. haematobium within a vein of the bladder wall. (Courtesy Armed Forces Institute of Pathology, Washington, D. C.)

bryos (*miracidia*) which develop further and in thirty to forty hours are taken up by the fresh water snail, Bulinus. Sporozoites are formed in the snail following which, by sexual reproduction, bifid-tail cercariae are discharged into the water. These, in turn, penetrate the skin to reach the liver through the portal circulation where they nest and mature. Leaving the liver in pairs and with a peculiar ability to travel against the blood flow, they reach the vesical veins which are the sites of predilection. The female then gives off ova which gain entrance into the bladder by eruption. The ova are passed per urethram and the cycle begins again.

The bladder wall is greatly thickened and congested, ulcerated, or papillomatous; ova are generally found in the ulcerative lesions. The cystoscopic picture may suggest chronic cystitis although parasitic ulcerative papillomatosis may be mistaken for malignancy.

The *symptoms* of vesical schistosomiasis are those of acute cystitis with pain in the bladder or urethra, frequency, dysuria and, characteristically, terminal hematuria. Cystoscopic observation of ova ulcerating into the bladder has been reported by many and a high eosinophile count suggests the diagnosis which is clinched by demonstration of ova in the urine. A complement fixation test prepared from infected snail's liver has proved more than 80 per cent accurate.

Treatment. The accepted specific treatment of bilharziasis has been antimony given intravenously as Fuadin.* Recently Aureomycin has been employed in many cases and even more successfully than Fuadin which it seems likely to replace. The test of cure is the complete disappearance of ova from the urine with healing of the bladder.

Actinomycosis. This is caused by the *ray fungus* which most commonly causes lumpy jaw in cattle. Renal involvement which is quite rare is a hematogenous spread, the organisms gaining initial entry to the gastrointestinal or respiratory tract from which they hematogenously reach the urinary tract and especially the kidney. In the kidney a chronic granulomatous lesion develops which clinically resembles caseous tuberculosis. Small pathognomonic yellowish bodies aptly called sulfur granules are found in the purulent center of the lesions. The diagnosis rests upon the identification of myceliobacillary or coccoid forms in the urine; the pyelogram suggests tuberculosis. The course is usually rapidly fatal, no regularly satisfactory medication being known. The administration of disodium formaldehyde sulfoxylate diamino-diphenylsulfone (Diasone, Abbott) has cured actinomycosis of the jaw. On the other hand, nephrectomy to be successful must be accomplished without spilling of infection. In most cases the diagnosis is made at autopsy.

Other rare parasitic urinary tract infections have been identified: These are (1) the mycoses: coccidioidal granuloma which affects the kidney as part of a systemic infection; Aspergillus fumigatus causes a blackish urethral discharge; Penicillium glaucum; (2) the parasites: Dioctophyma renale is a long nematode invading the kidney; (3) protozoa: amebae invade the bladder and kidney during the course of enteric amebiasis. All of these are characteristically tropical infections.

* Fuadin or stibophen (sodium antimony-III-bis-catechol-2,4-sodium disulfonate).

CHAPTER 8

*The Male Reproductive Tract**

THE GENITALIA mean "sex" to all people from early childhood and, if we are to believe our psychiatrist colleagues, it is the greatest driving force of human beings, especially males. Consciously or unconsciously, in both sexes, the genitalia—their morphology, development, idiosyncrasies and diseases—receive an amazing amount of energetic attention. The young child is first intrigued with the discovery of his genitals, especially the penis; the adolescent is usually shy, reticent, and somewhat confused concerning his; the teenager or early adult, spurred on by his androgens, usually learns the amusement features of the apparatus; the young groom displays his reproductivity, while the oldster must too often be content with his memories.

During this life cycle, sexual psychosomatic problems are extremely common and are apt to be more disabling than organic genital tract disease. With this background of human development and behavior, it is not surprising that a large portion of a physician's patients will be concerned with these problems in which sexual neurosis may well do more physical, social and economic damage, disorganize families and disrupt more lives than will relatively severe organic disease properly treated.

In the present chapter we are concerned with the more usual inflammations and infections of the male reproductive tract.

THE PENIS

Skin. The commonest diseases of the penile skin are redundancy, phimosis, adhesions, paraphimosis, balanitis, balanoposthitis, herpes, erythema, intertrigo or chafing, scabies, and syphilis. Localized or phlegmonous infection with or without ulceration or gangrene is occasion-

---

* The applied anatomy of the male genital organs has been given in Chapter 4, Embryology and Anomalies in Chapter 6, Injuries are discussed in Chapter 10, Tumors in Chapter 12, and Urology in the Female is presented separately in Chapter 14.

266

ally observed in adults but is extremely rare in the young. Infections and inflammations of the penile skin usually result from phimosis, lacerations, abrasions, urethritis, periurethritis, or appear as postoperative complications. Even mild inflammations or infections commonly cause marked edema of the lax penile skin, and subcutaneous infections tend to spread rapidly. Today, when circumcision is so universally practiced in the United States as an obstetric encore, the incidence of penile cutaneous lesions in boys is diminishing and by the same token reduction of penile cancer in adults may be anticipated.

Redundancy of the prepuce is normal in infancy and early childhood but the foreskin should be freely retractable behind the glans, both for hygienic cleansing and to lessen the incidence of paraphimosis (Fig. 106). Preputial redundancy is important when (1) the prepuce cannot be retracted, (2) there is subpreputial retention of smegma or other irritating debris causing chronic local inflammation and/or predisposing to cancer, (3) interference with the discharge of urine results in its retention and decomposition, (4) it retains gonorrheal or other urethral discharge, or (5) hides underlying chancroid, chancre or neoplasm. The *symptoms* are chiefly those of local irritation with sometimes dysuria. Circumcision is the recommended treatment particularly when the prepuce is not freely retractable (Fig. 108).

The *nonoperative treatment* is that of *preputial adhesions* in which the visceral surface of the penis is bound to the glans penis by epithelization which is physiologic in infancy, absorption taking place during the latter months of the first year of life normally, when these adhesions may be easily broken up. These delicate adhesions may fail to separate or, made fibrous by retention of irritant secretions, will firmly bind the prepuce and glans together, generally most tenaciously in the corona glandis. In dense preputial adhesions the tip of the prepuce is infolded rather than normally everted (Fig. 106). In infants and young boys preputial adhesions may usually be readily broken up by slow and gentle retraction of the prepuce over the glans, or by stretching the prepuce with a hemostat or encircling its inner surface with a probe (Fig. 106). When the adhesions are dense, bleeding may occur, especially in older patients. Following retraction of the tight prepuce, well anointed on both sides with Vaseline, the structure is slid back and forth a few times to make sure it goes easily over the glans when it is then restored to normal position. Failure to restore the prepuce invites paraphimosis (q.v.).

Phimosis. Because this is usually congenital and predominantly a childhood problem, it has been considered in Chapter 6.

Short frenum has been discussed in Chapter 6.

Cysts of the prepuce originating as epithelial inclusion formations sometimes follow improperly performed circumcision, especially in the region of the frenum.

Paraphimosis (Spanish collar) is the compression or strangulation of the glans penis by the prepuce and can occur only when the tight foreskin is left retracted behind the glans (Fig. 167), or it may follow traumatic swelling of the glans as in masturbation. It is frequent in the uncircumcised. In the development of paraphimosis primary and secondary constricting rings develop which compress the dorsal veins and lymphatics to increase local swelling which, in turn, increases the constrictions. In the examination, the penile skin should be drawn backward to show the entire continuity, a constricting band commonly being found about 2 cm. behind the glans with both proximal and distal edema.

The vascular involvement may lead to thrombosis or gangrene of the cutaneous elements (Fig. 167*A*); the glans does not suffer because its blood supply is through the corpus spongiosum. In less violent swelling, *chronic paraphimosis* may ensue, or the acute swelling and infection with ulceration of the prepuce may result in cellulitis, erysipelas, gangrene of the penis, inguinal adenitis, or even phlebitis extending into the deep pelvic vessels. Pain and swelling are the chief *symptoms*. When preputial necrosis and gangrene occur, sloughing and extensive hemorrhage may result.

The *diagnosis* is made by inspection (Fig. 167). *Treatment* will depend upon the degree of penile strangulation.

Conservative treatment is applicable in moderate acute paraphimosis seen early. The penis behind the obstruction is elevated with the first two fingers of each hand and by exertion of continuous pressure with the

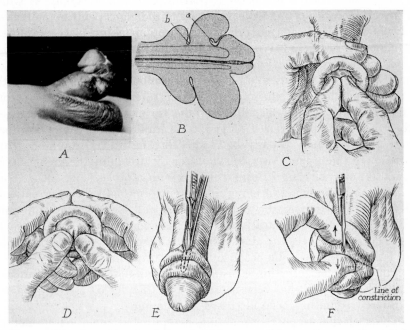

Figure 167. Paraphimosis. *A*, in a forty-four-year-old man; the secondary constriction as well as early preputial gangrene are well shown. *B*, schema showing primary (a) and secondary (b) contraction rings. *C*, *D*, two methods of manual reduction of prepuce; squeezing edema from glans; *E*, dorsal slit, grooved director inserted beneath the contraction rings from behind; the rings are then incised against the instrument. *F*, dorsal slit through contraction rings without a guide with special care not to incise the glans.

two thumbs on the glans, it can be slowly squeezed or pushed through the constricting preputial ring (Fig. 167C, D). Gentle squeezing of the swollen prepuce will often compress some interstitial edema behind the constricting ring to facilitate the digital reduction. A hairpin or grooved director may be placed under the constricting skin as a shoehorn to encourage reduction of the prepuce. In the acute process requiring more radical treatment, a dorsal slit should be performed at once incising completely through all the constricting rings. Unless the constricting bands are widely severed, the treatment fails.

If the prepuce is bluish black and cold, debridement of the necrotic tissue should await demarcation. Later when the condition of the tissues warrants and the infection has subsided, circumcision is performed.

The local injection of hyaluronidase has been successful in some cases in bringing about helpful quick diminution of the local edematous swelling.

Posthitis, Balanitis, Balanoposthitis. Posthitis is inflammation of the prepuce; *balanitis* is inflammation of the glans penis and almost always accompanies posthitis, the combined lesion being known as *balanoposthitis* which may be due to any local irritation or inflammation. It is common in infants with ammoniacal diaper, in fat boys with phimosis, and in older patients with faulty local hygiene. It is a frequent finding in older boys addicted to excessive masturbation, although the habit may be engendered by the irritation of an unrecognized balanoposthitis.

The local signs and *symptoms* of balanoposthitis are variable according to the severity of the local inflammation. The prepuce is red and swollen, there is local itching and burning, often with secondary herpes. As the inflammation and swelling intensify, a thin sticky yellowish or whitish yellow discharge appears, often to be incorrectly diagnosed gonorrhea. This yellowish discharge stains the clothing and by drying may seal the meatus and prepuce.

Soft *verrucae*, often called venereal warts, sometimes form on the mucosal lining of the irritated moist subpreputial cavity (see p. 271).

Phlegmonous balanoposthitis is usually caused by a hemolytic streptococcus and the onset is sudden with rapid local penile swelling and pain. Penicillin or erythromycin when given in time may check it promptly.

In balanitis, dorsal slits should always be performed when necessary to give free drainage.

Diphtheritic balanitis is caused by the diphtheria bacillus and characteristically causes local superficial ulceration on both the glans and the prepuce. The local symptoms of pain, swelling and dysuria are acute and the bacterial toxemia is profound. Diphtheria antitoxin is the treatment.

In *chronic balanoposthitis,* the thickened prepuce more or less firmly bound to the glans by adhesions calls for circumcision.

Ulceration of the meatus, also known as *ulcerative meatitis* and consequent to congenital meatal stenosis is discussed in Chapter 6.

Herpes of the penis usually follows the dorsal penile nerve distribution but may be found on the mucosa behind the corona glandis or on the prepuce. Sometimes the arrangement is crescentic or circular, the lesions being similar to herpes elsewhere and appearing as small superficial red spots which become vesiculated, rounded, translucent, and rupture leaving a superficial ulceration, or uneventfully heal. Inguinal adenitis appears only with secondary infection of the herpes. A slight itching or burning sensation is the chief symptom.

The cause of herpes is unsettled. Phimosis and masturbation predispose to it. It is believed by some to be caused by a filtrable virus (0.25μ diameter) but many urologists believe prostatitis plays a part, the therapeutic test of prostatic massage often lending weight to this assumption. In short, most penile herpes promptly disappear following prostatic massage, this being the only effective active treatment known. Penicillin, a sulfonamide, local cleansing or a dusting powder of zinc stearate may help. Circumcision is indicated when phimosis or a long prepuce accompanies recurrent herpes.

Parasitic infection of the cutaneous genital covering is not uncommon, particularly in adults. *Scabies* (parasite Acarus scabiei) shows a predilection for the penis as well as the wrist and between the fingers. The spot of invasion is marked by a vesicle or a papule in the center of which are small black dots—the excreta of the female nits.

Treatment is first a thorough bath followed by anointing the entire body with an ointment of 15 per cent precipitated sulfur or similarly using a 1 per cent ointment of the gamma isomer of hexachlorcyclohexane in a vanishing cream base (trade name Kwell, Commercial Solvents Corp.). Previously infected clothing or linen must be sterilized or discarded.

Pediculosis pubis is recognized by the ova or nits which attach themselves to the pubic hair and make the diagnosis. Treatment demands a thorough washing of the parts and complete drying, followed by a liberal application of 10 per cent ammoniated mercury; infected clothing or linen must be sterilized or discarded.

Tinea cruris or *inguinal ringworm* is due to the parasite *Epidermophyton inguinale* (floccosum) and is always complicated by eczema intertrigo described in the following paragraph. It is unusual in young patients, and in older males it is commonly recognized as gym itch or jock itch. It appears chiefly over the inner side of the thighs where the scrotum is in contact, may spread to the groin and involve the apposing surfaces of the penis and scrotum, and even the axilla as I observed in two children. The lesions begin with one or more small red raw elevated patches which spread peripherally with sharply defined margins, elevated slightly with inflamed borders and central healing as the lesion extends. The involved surface becomes covered with brown and scaly patches but papules, vesicles, ulcerations, or incrustations are common and there is maceration of the apposing moist surfaces. Itching is the chief *symptom*. The *diagnosis* is made by inspection and the demonstration of the etiologic parasite in scales scraped from the margin of the lesions. *Treatment* is by painting the involved areas with tincture of iodine which is usually curative although 1 per cent aqueous gentian violet is equally effective and far less irritating. All previously infected clothing must be sterilized or discarded.

Erythema intertrigo may exist only as a hyperemia of the genital and perigenital skin but is often accompanied by superficial maceration when the moist cutaneous surfaces are continuously in apposition. It is extremely common in infants in whom urinary decomposition results from failure to change soiled diapers. The direct *etiology*, however, is unknown and the condition is observed in patients of all ages and in both sexes. The involved areas are hyperemic, the skin becomes macerated, serous exudate appears and pyogenic infection may be superimposed. A feeling of heat and soreness are the chief symptoms. *Diagnosis* is made by inspection and should not suggest syphilis. *Treatment* of intertrigo is absolute cleanliness with thorough baths using soap and water followed, when the skin surfaces are thoroughly dry, by a dusting powder such as two parts zinc stearate and one part boric acid. When pyogenic skin infection coexists, painting with a 1 per cent aqueous solution of gentian violet is usually curative.

Tuberculosis of the penis is extremely rare and occurs chiefly in late urinary tuberculosis as a spread from and about the urethral meatus. Many tuberculous infections along the line of circumcision have occurred when a tuberculous rabbi sucked the wound for hemostasis. The *treatment* of cutaneous genital tuberculosis is medicinal as described under nonoperative treatment of renal tuberculosis (q.v.).

Chancroid or *soft chancre* is caused by the bacillus of Ducrey, is almost always acquired by sexual contact, is characterized by one or more circumscribed ulcers about the corona or elsewhere on the penis. The initial lesion is a small nonindurated vesicle, papule, or pustule which ulcerates with marked collateral secondary inflammation and pronounced inguinal adenitis. Chancroid in contrast to chancre is usually painful, yet the two may co-exist. The *differential diagnosis* rests upon darkfield examination and a Wassermann test or its equivalent and when syphilis is ruled out, intensive administration of streptomycin or Aureomycin is the treatment of chancroid.

Condylomata acuminata (verrucae or venereal warts). These benign papillomata which behave like a dermatitis are not due to venereal disease but rather to persistent inflammation or irritation in the presence of moisture. A long or tight prepuce is the chief predisposing factor and, under analogous conditions, the condition is sometimes seen in women. The warty lesions are usually multiple and occur chiefly behind the glans or on the prepuce and perifrenal area. Local irritation is the chief symptom.

Treatment is removal of the growth. A mixture of salicylic acid, 1 dram, in glacial acetic acid, 1 ounce, is specific; a drop is put upon each wart and more than one treatment may be required. The application of 25 per cent podophyllin (resin of podophyllin peltatum) ointment cures condyloma acuminatum. This is extremely tissue destructive and none should be spilled on adjacent normal tissues which are best protected by an application of Lassar's paste. Extensive lesions should be treated piece-meal and soaks of equal parts of hydrogen peroxide and distilled water should be applied to the treated area four or five times daily, beginning twelve hours after the application of podophyllin. The next application should not be made in less than forty-eight hours and not until local reaction from the previous application has subsided. In most instances it is best to wait five to seven days between treatments.

I have removed localized pedunculated verrucae by ligating the bases with silk thread after which the wart dries and falls off.

Syphilis.   *Chancre*, the primary lesion, is usually acquired by sexual contact, normal or erotic; many instances have been reported of its acquisition from the rabbi's mouth at the time of ritualistic circumcision, by criminal or illicit exposure to an adult in the family or elsewhere, but *syphilis in children is congenital in 90 per cent of cases.* Syphilis may be acquired at the same time as chancroid or gonorrhea or the patient may even be a triple loser. The commonest sites of primary chancre are the genitalia, mouth, face, neck, and anus. The initial lesion is an indurated, heaped-up ulceration which is painless except when secondarily infected, and regional adenitis regularly coexists. The demonstration of Treponema pallidum by darkfield study and a positive Wassermann reaction confirms the diagnosis.

Secondary cutaneous genital syphilides and *mucous patches* are often accompanied by *condyloma latum.* Penile or genital *gumma* or other tertiary manifestations are rare. These are discussed in books on syphilis and dermatology. Today, the accepted treatment is enormous doses of penicillin, a million or more units a day being given for five to ten days.

Lymphangitis is manifested as an inflammatory thickening of the dorsal lymph cord and is common with severe infections of the glans and penis, especially with chancroid or chancre. The lymphatic induration

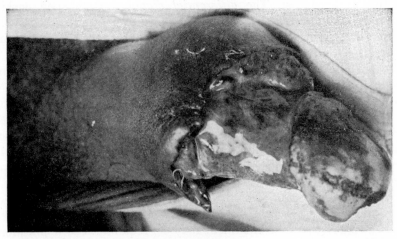

FIGURE 168.   Spontaneous fulminating streptococcic gangrene of the penis with consid-erable loss of tissue.

may simulate thrombosis of the dorsal vein, aptly described as feeling like a pipe cleaner. Inguinal adenitis is usually present. The treatment is that of the primary condition following which the lymphangitis disappears.

Cellulitis of the penis is generally secondary to virulent infection of the prepuce or to severe periurethritis, being evident as a brawny edema and subsides with adequate treatment of the cause. It is far less serious than penile gangrene about to be described and so often accompanying similar scrotal phlegmon.

Phlegmon of the penis is a comparatively rare condition resulting from bacterial invasion, usually streptococcic, although various anaerobes have been found (Fig. 168). Local trauma or inflammation, dermatitis or a severe systemic infection may predispose.

A peculiar acute fulminating phlegmon, *streptococcus penile and scrotal gangrene*, is believed to result from bacteria introduced by friction of the clothing (Figs. 168, 169). With infection, there is prompt rapid and extensive swelling involving the entire cutaneous covering. Extensive thrombosis occurs with consequent gangrene in two to four days; there is grave systemic toxemia, particularly with similar involvement of the scrotum which so commonly coexists. Inguinal adenitis is comparatively rare. The general *symptoms* are those of sepsis, a sharp chill often heralding the onset to be followed by high temperature, general malaise, acute gastrointestinal disturbances, prostration, and sometimes toxic neurologic manifestations. The *diagnosis* is made by inspection in which the penile and/or scrotal skin in the early stages of the infection is reddish purple but in twenty-four to forty-eight hours shows scattered patches of gangrene which by coalescence can convert the entire genital covering to

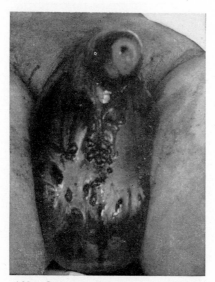

FIGURE 169.   Streptococcic gangrene of the scrotum.

gangrenous skin with demarcation. Absence of antecedent urethral disease usually rules out urinary extravasation.

Treatment.   Following assurance of free urinary drainage by a well-anchored balloon catheter, removal of the gangrenous penile skin to the boundaries of normal skin is required. This may leave the organ stripped bare to the penile fascia; when involved the scrotum is similarly treated to leave the testicles hanging freely (Fig. 170). The intensive administration of penicillin or Terramycin in the early stages may check the gangrenous process and require only stab incisions for surgical drainage but the patient is rarely so fortunate. In any event, the massive administration of bacteriologically indicated antibiotics should be carried out together with sufficiently bold cutaneous debridement. During convalescence wet dressings of potassium permanganate 1:5000, 1 per cent sulfathiazole solution, or zephiran chloride 1:5000, until the involved areas are covered with granulations, will stimulate early healing. Spontaneous rapid epithelization of the skin occurs so that skin grafting is unnecessary.

The *mortality* in severe cases used to be about 40 per cent, but has now been sharply reduced to about 20 per cent by the advent of modern antimicrobial therapy. The responsibility of the physician is indeed grave for the early recognition, prompt and proper treatment of this extremely serious fulminating condition.

Cavernositis.   This is an infection of the corpora cavernosa or corpus spongiosum, and in the acute form is most commonly caused by virulent gonorrhea. It may occur with trauma complicated by infection, periurethral phlegmon, urinary extravasation, hematogenous infection, and certain blood dyscrasias, especially leukemia, or after circumcision under

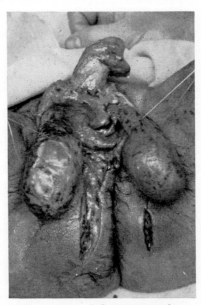

FIGURE 170.   Streptococcic gangrene of the scrotum after removing necrotic tissue.

local anesthesia when the drug has been injected too deeply, too vigorously or in too great concentration.

The lesions appear as localized tender indurated masses in the cavernous bodies which may produce urethral compression with painful or difficult urination, or induce persistent priapism. Like periurethral abscess, a cavernosus abscess may rupture into the urethra. *Treatment* is incision and drainage together with antimicrobial therapy.

In *diffuse* or *pancavernositis* there is widespread involvement of the cavernous bodies, the initial infection being hematogenous and usually associated with fatal pyemia, which in turn produces the clinical picture of sepsis.

Chronic cavernositis, manifested by generalized induration and scarring, is rare and usually follows acute cavernositis. The lesion may result from traumatic (1) penile laceration, (2) masturbation, (3) intercourse, or (4) "breaking" an erection; also from (5) extensive periurethritis with or without abscess, or (6) a healed gumma.

Plastic induration of the penis involving chiefly the corpora and also known as Peyronie's disease, is a patchy or localized manifestation of chronic cavernositis as described in the preceding paragraph. The condition is neither rare nor serious, is seen chiefly in men over fifty-five years of age, may be due to the causes of chronic cavernositis just given or may appear for no accountable reason. The sclerosis with the formation of hard, almost cartilage-like, plaques (0.5 to 1.5 cm. or more in diameter and 2.0 to 5.0 mm. thick), irregular in outline and often sharp edged, may begin in or near the cavernous septum, but is usually most pronounced beneath Buck's fascia (Figs. 33, 34). The condition though harmless causes penile distortion, usually painless, with curvation upwards, downwards or laterally. The chief complaint may be difficulty in coitus. The diagnosis should be easy to make since the conditions the plaques might simulate—chondroma, malignant tumor, fibroma—are exceedingly rare in this location while Peyronie's disease is not.

Treatment is unsatisfactory, excised scar being replaced by even more scar. Radiation therapy helps little. The administration of alpha tocopherol (vitamin E, 300 to 400 mg. a day) offers some hope for improvement as it does in the treatment of Dupuytren's palmar contracture, to the likeness of which Peyronie's disease has been noted. On alpha tocopherol, it usually takes three to four months of continuous medication before notable improvement in the lesion occurs, and often there is no change. The important thing is to be able to assure the patient he does not have cancer! The local injection of hyaluronidase and metacortin into and about the fibrous plaques is alleged to encourage their softening and even disappearance.

Gangrene of the penis results from vascular obstruction or thrombosis which may follow accidental injury but more commonly is caused by a string, thread, or hair tied about the organ or when the penis is introduced through a ring or neck of a bottle, for example (Fig. 217). Massive gangrene of the penis seldom results from extravasation, or gangrene of the glans from paraphimosis. With vascular blockage from whatever cause, massive thrombosis ensues with subsequent necrotic ulceration. The organ becomes painful, swollen, reddish brown, and, with gangrene, bluish black, and anesthesia follows. It is painless, and cold to the touch. The *diagnosis* is made by inspection and *treatment* is removal of the cause when constrictive or traumatic. The incised gangrenous portion does not bleed. The application of hot wet dressings will indicate the viability of the involved tissues; in many cases amputation is required, the resection being carried well into healthy tissue. Meanwhile, antimicrobials are given to combat local infection.

Noma is a rare variety of penile gangrene which results from massive thrombosis of hematogenous origin and is observed almost entirely in early infancy. The *treatment* is a combination of that employed in penile gangrene and penile cellulitis and the outlook is always grave.

DISEASES OF THE MALE URETHRA

Urethritis. Inflammation of the urethra may be nongonorrheal or gonorrheal. The usual nongonorrheal variety is commonly designated as nonspecific; tuberculous urethritis as a phase of genital tract disease is briefly discussed under tuberculosis later in this chapter.

Nongonorrheal or *simple urethritis* may result from sexual exposure although it is often secondary to the local irritation and uncleanliness of phimosis or may even be hematogenous from a distant focus. Masturbation and balanoposthitis are common predisposing causes. The usual etiologic organisms are staphylococci but many varieties of cocci as well as colon and diphtheroid bacilli have been found. Nongonorrheal gramnegative coccic forms, usually extracellular and believed to be degenerative staphylococci, are frequently observed in nongonorrheal urethritis in adults. The infection may involve only the distal inch or two of the urethra or may extend back to the prostatic urethra, the involvement usually being slight. Yet clinically evident posterior urethritis, prostatitis, or epididymitis may develop.

The onset of the disease is variable, three to twelve days or even longer following sexual exposure. A urethral tickling with painful urination is noted, and a thin purulent urethral discharge is seen which in a day or two becomes thicker. With a long foreskin or phimosis, edematous swelling and balanoposthitis appear, may be the initial symptoms and cause the underlying urethritis to be overlooked. The disease usually runs a mild course and disappears spontaneously in one to two weeks with local cleanliness and treatment, but with complicating prostatitis, stricture or periurethral abscess, it may persist much longer. The *diagnosis* of acute gonorrhea may be suggested but microscopic examination of the discharge or of the centrifuged urine sediment will disclose the etiologic agent, gram-negative or gram-positive cocci together with diphtheroids being most often found. This will be confirmed by culture. If the infection has extended to the deep urethra and prostate, both the first and second glasses of voided urine will contain shreds. The condition must be distinguished from Reiter's syndrome (q.v.) and gonorrheal urethritis.

The *treatment* of simple urethritis is identical with that of gonococcic urethritis (q.v.), and usually runs a shorter course, and more readily responds to treatment. But it may be more tenacious than gonorrhea.

Gonococcus urethritis, also known as specific urethritis, is caused only by the gram-negative diplococcus of Neisser and except in the very young is almost always acquired by sexual contact. The incidence of gonorrheal infection in the United States has declined remarkably since the introduction of sulfonamide and antibiotic therapy. By achieving rapid cure the mass disseminators of infection have been controlled in large measure; this applies more to the willing amateurs and victory girls than to the professionals of the street or brothel, the incidence of both gonorrhea and/or syphilis in the last group being as great as ever, i.e., nearly 100 per cent.

The *incidence* of gonorrhea in young boys is still considerable in the country at large, and in girl infants and young children is twenty to thirty times greater than in boys.

Although gonorrhea is essentially a disease of young and middle aged adults, it is no respecter of old age and many instances have been observed in early infancy, as young as four days, and I have seen gonorrheal epididymitis at three weeks. The sexual impulse progressively develops throughout childhood, becoming more active as puberty approaches, and in many children intercourse is stimulated by the desire to emulate acts observed in elders. Several epidemics of urethral gonorrhea in boys' schools have been spread by sodomy, the focal offenders often showing paralyzed anal sphincters with papillomatous growths. Accidental infection of the male urethra is indeed rare but spread of the disease to females by linens, towels, bed pans, douche apparatus, and by undetected methods is not uncommon.

The gonococcus is soon killed by complete drying but will live a long time outside the body when kept moist at room temperature; this explains most linen and toilet infections.

Pathology of Gonococcus Urethritis. With inoculation of the meatus with gonococci, backward extension by surface progression of the infection occurs, the organisms thriving on the columnar epithelium of the anterior urethra. They do less well on the transitional epithelium of the posterior urethra and almost never grow on the squamous transitional epithelium of the bladder. Penetration of the epithelial cell lining of the urethra is variable, but may extend deep to the corpus spongiosum. Deep invasion of the urethral glands of Littre also occurs. Myriad desquamated epithelial cells are found in the discharge.

In the *healing process* there is regeneration of epithelial cells, chiefly the squamous variety. The deeper periurethral invasion heals by sclerosis and when there has been a pronounced localized lesion, the scarring may lead to clinical stricture. With extension to the deep urethra, not only is the mucosa acutely inflamed but prostatic invasion is manifested by prostatitis. Similarly the glands of Cowper between the layers of the triangular ligament are sometimes involved, but extension of gonococci to the seminal vesicles is of much lower incidence than formerly believed. Infection from the posterior urethra may extend down the canal of the vas deferens to incite epididymitis. Fortunately with present-day antibiotic therapy, gonorrhea usually can be cured so promptly that posterior urethritis and its associated potential complications are rarely seen. So striking is this that most urologists do not see more than one or two cases of gonorrheal infection a year, most patients thus infected being treated by their family physician or prescribed for by the corner druggist.

Symptoms. The *incubation period* in gonorrheal urethritis is usually four to eight days during which a slight smarting on urination is noted. In a day or two a thin mucopurulent discharge appears and rapidly becomes thickly purulent and greenish-yellow to leave a similar colored stain on the linens. The meatal lips become intensely red, swollen and everted and, reflexly by local irritation, recurrent and extremely painful priapism often develops. A long prepuce of phimosis usually shows balanoposthitis with pronounced edema. Inguinal adenitis does not occur in gonorrheal urethritis unless there is balanoposthitis and especially with mixed infection. There are seldom systemic symptoms in the absence of complications.

Gonorrhea tends to run a self-limited course but this may be over many months, dependent upon the adequacy of treatment and the development of complications, chiefly urethral stricture and prostatitis.

Diagnosis. The demonstration of the gram-negative intracellular diplococcus of Neisser in the urethral discharge establishes the diagnosis. A history of recent sexual exposure is usually obtained. Gonococci can also be demonstrated by culture which is a most precise bacteriologic procedure. Other gram-negative organisms which may morphologically simulate gonococci are Micrococcus catarrhalis and degenerated forms of staphylococcus. With the development of gonorrheal prostatitis or other complications, the gonococcus *complement fixation test* becomes positive, but with present-day therapy this diagnostic measure has been largely discarded.

When the infection is limited to the anterior urethra, the first glass of voided urine will be flaky with shreds and pus but the second glass will be clear. When the infection has reached the prostatic urethra the first glass will show shreds as will the second glass also and, with complicating prostatic infection, there will be many pus clumps.

Complications. Generally these reflect inadequate or improper treatment. The more commonly observed are balanoposthitis, periurethritis, stricture, prostatitis, prostatic abscess, epididymitis, ophthalmia and arthritis; these may occur in patients of all ages. I have operated for gonorrheal prostatic abscess in a twenty-eight months old boy. With proper prophylactic care at the time of delivery, *gonococcus ophthalmia* has largely been eradicated. With present-day therapy, gonorrheal *arthritis* is a rarity; I have not seen a case in nearly twenty years although before this time at Bellevue Hospital in New York there was always a ward full of these patients, and another full ward devoted solely to gonorrheal epididymitis. These rooms are now empty of these cases.

Proctitis is spread by infected clothing, careless toilet maneuvers, infected rectal thermometers, or by sodomy. Gonococcus *septicemia,* endocarditis, pericarditis, and meningitis are now rare complications.

Treatment of Acute Gonorrheal Urethritis. PROPHYLAXIS. Today the intramuscular injection of 300,000 units of penicillin immediately before or immediately after sexual exposure is generally accepted as competent prophylaxis against gonorrhea and syphilis. Hygienic therapy includes cleanliness, rest, and a nonirritating diet. *Alcohol and sexual excitement are prohibited until the patient is cured.* The epidemiologic aspects of gonorrhea are extremely important not only in children's hospitals and especially among little girls, but also for those who live under poor housing conditions with atrocious crowding and the carelessness of infected elders in the household.

Local genital cleansing with soap and water with wide retraction of the prepuce and washing away of all underlying debris is imperative. While a discharge is evident, the patient should wash his hands after every urination and should avoid putting his fingers to his eyes. Let him sleep alone and be sure that his personal toilet articles, especially towels and wash cloths, are used by no one else, and the bowels move every day.

Specific Treatment. Chemotherapy by the administration of sulfonamides and antibiotic compounds has successfully replaced all previous forms of treatment. This at once relieves the tender infected urethra from the repetitious trauma of urethral injections as well as variable injury from the chemical itself. Nor is infection mechanically pushed back into the deep urethra as so commonly happened with careless injection. Today the urethra receives no instrument until it is apparent the patient is cured. Only with unusual delay in achieving cure or the development of some localizing complication, should instrumental examination or investigation be performed.

Sulfonamide Therapy. Sulfisoxazole (trade name Gantrisin) or one of the triple sulfonamides may be employed, giving the patient an initial dose of 6 grams the first day in divided doses, followed by 4 grams daily in four divided doses thereafter until the disease is cured. Within forty-eight hours the discharge should be greatly reduced and cure is usually achieved in six days. Gram stain should be made of any urethral shreds and, if after four or five days there is no evidence of gonococci, a small sound may be passed into the urethra to activate any dormant, hidden or walled-off foci in the urethral glands. If there is still no evidence of infection, the patient is probably cured (see test of cure).

Antibiotic Therapy. Soon after its introduction in 1941, penicillin became the recognized treatment of gonorrhea, particularly in the Armed Services, a daily dose of 100,000 to 300,000 units intramuscularly being given for five to eight days. In most cases all evidence of the disease has disappeared by the fourth day and many one-day cures are achieved.

With its wide use penicillin has encountered a notable increase in bacterial insensitivity to it among the population at large. For this reason other antibiotics, chiefly Aureomycin and Terramycin at present enjoy a greater vogue. For most rapid results these are given intramuscularly 100 mg. a day to a young boy and 200 mg. twice a day to an adult, together with an auxiliary oral intake of 1.0 to 1.5 gm. a day for one week.

As a rule, on antibiotic therapy, discharge disappears within twenty-four hours with sometimes apparent cure of the infection. The antibiotic therapy should be continued for at least a week and if, at the end of this time, Gram stain examination of the urine shreds or centrifuged sediment shows no gonococci, a week without treatment is observed during which time a liberal alcoholic intake is prescribed to activate any hidden infection.

If the patient appears cured after the initial course of therapy, a sound is passed to the triangular ligament to stir up any latent infection and if none appears and all tests of cure (q.v.) are observed, the patient is discharged. Gonococcus culture is confirmatory.

Chronic gonorrhea reflects improper treatment of the acute disease. It is manifested by a mild purulent or mucoid discharge or only shreds in the urine, especially in the morning, and which represent the overnight collection in the urethra. If the infection is gonorrhea, the gonococci should be demonstrable in the gram-stained urethral specimen but relatively few will be intracellular. Sulfonamide or antibiotic therapy is employed precisely as in acute gonorrhea and the same tests of cure are observed. If a mild mucoid discharge persists and no gonococci can be found, it is most unlikely that the infection is gonococcic and will usually disappear spontaneously or following one or two instillations of a mild astringent solution such as silver nitrate 1:5000 or zinc sulfate 1:400. Dilation of the urethra with sounds to at least 26 F. caliber in an adult will stir up any lingering nongonococcic infection in the urethra and periurethral glands.

Test of Cure. If the first and second glasses of the voided urine are clear, sparkling, and without shreds, it is probable that the patient is cured. Failure of activation of latent infection by the passage of urethral sounds, or the injection of silver nitrate solution (1:2000) vastly enhances the probability of cure. The complement fixation test is of little value as it seldom becomes positive in uncomplicated anterior gonorrheal urethritis. It means nothing unless it becomes negative after having previously been positive and, having been so, usually remains positive for four to six weeks following clinical disappearance of the gonorrhea.

Reiter's Syndrome. This triad of abacterial urethritis, conjunctivitis, and arthritis, although usually unrecognized for what it is, has been reported in about 300 cases. It was initially described by Reiter (1916) after his observation of it following an attack of bloody diarrhea in a soldier. It has even been reported in a boy of four years. Many more cases will be recognized in the future as clinicians become aware of its manifestations.

The *cause* is unknown; viruses, dysentery bacilli, pleuropneumonia organisms, and even spirochetes have been thought to be etiologic. In recent years with greater study of the condition, a high incidence of inflammatory and obstructive lesions in the upper urinary tract have been observed.

Symptoms. The disease generally begins with a clear viscid urethral discharge, rarely mucoid or mucopurulent, together with a purulent conjunctivitis, later to be followed by arthritis. The conjunctivitis may be the first of the symptom triad to appear. The discharge usually follows coitus by four to thirty days and shows few or no organisms in the smear. There is frequency of urination, dysuria, pyuria and urethral discharge; sometimes a diagnosis of "pyelitis" is made. Conjunctivitis is often followed by photophobia or iritis, keratitis and iridocyclitis. With this, arthritis appears, usually in the knee, ankle, or wrist, commonly migrating. The joint becomes swollen, hot and tender, often with hydrarthrosis but seldom bone destruction. Sites of involvement are multiple in a fourth of the cases. Apparently the urethral infection does not extend to the scrotal contents for orchitis and epididymitis have not been observed. Malaise, low-grade fever, occasional nausea with gastric distress, leukocytosis, and an increased sedimentation rate are present. The disease may have a remittent course but spontaneous cure usually takes place within three to six months although it may persist longer. Apparently the disease directly causes no deaths.

Treatment. There is no specific therapy. When gram-positive cocci are demonstrated in the smear, give erythromycin and penicillin, and when gram-negative coliform organisms are found, give Aureomycin, Chloromycetin and/or Gantrisin. Treat complicating prostatitis, stricture or periurethritis in the usual manner. Before the patient is discharged, a satisfactory excretory urographic study should be made to be certain no upper urinary tract disease exists, which so often passes unrecognized, and may be serious, especially when obstructive. The arthritis and conjunctivitis are treated according to standard practice.

When the urethritis is viral or abacterial, employ Aureomycin 200 to 300 mg. intravenously once daily or orally 2 to 3 gm. per day.

Periurethritis and Periurethral Abscess. Most often these conditions are complications of bacterial urethritis, chiefly gonococcic but may result from trauma or be associated with urethral calculi or foreign bodies. A diffuse or localized inflammatory infiltration of the corpus spongiosum occurs, its severity depending upon the intensity of the disease. While the condition when mild heals by absorption of the inflammatory debris, in more pronounced infection healing is by sclerosis which produces clinical stricture.

Symptomatically, *periurethritis* is evident as a mild local inflammation with variable chordee and pain on urination. By irritative reflex from the inflamed urethra, distressing priapism may occur. A small nodular lesion is often best palpated against a sound in the urethra and may feel like a small pea; sometimes two or more of these infiltrated nodules will be palpable.

Treatment. While heat locally and anodynes may give symptomatic relief, intensive antibiotic therapy according to the infection as determined by bacteriologic study of the urine should be started at once and in large doses as in the treatment of gonorrhea (q.v.). Stricture formed by sclerotic healing of the lesion requires periodic dilation of the urethra with sounds, at least to 26 F. and preferably eventually to 30 F. caliber.

Periurethral abscess develops as a progressive stage of simple periurethritis. It may visibly extend externally or rupture intra-urethrally but seldom externally. There is local pain and swelling with dysuria and frequency as well as systemic manifestations caused by absorbed toxins from the lesion.

The *diagnosis* is suggested by history and symptoms, is confirmed by palpation, and fluctuation may be noted. Should the lesion break loose, it may become grave periurethral phlegmon within twenty-four hours.

Treatment. A small periurethral abscess often responds promptly to intensive antibiotic therapy while large abscesses require external incision, especially when pointing to the skin. Incision of palpable abscess, the intensive administration of antibiotic compounds according to bacteriologic indication and the maintenance of urethral drainage by the gentle passage of a sound if necessary, may be expected to be curative. A month later sounds should be passed to be sure there is no stricture and, if there is, periodic progressive dilation should be carried out at least to 30 F. caliber in an adult.

Stricture of the Urethra. By definition this is a pathologic diminution of the lumen or of the distensibility of the channel and may be (1) congenital, (2) caused by the insults of infection, particularly when improperly treated, or (3) by trauma. Not only the length but the caliber of the urethra alters with penile growth; the normal urethra of a one-year old male should comfortably accommodate a 10 F. instrument, at five years a 15 F. sound, at ten years an 18 F. sound, and at twenty years a 26 F. or 28 F. sound can normally be passed to the bladder without difficulty unless the meatus is unusually small.

In *congenital stricture* the local etiology does not include periurethritis, the lesion simply being a narrowing but, with infection, periurethritis may be added to the picture. Congenital stricture has also been referred to in Chapter 6.

Most *acquired strictures* result from gonorrhea improperly treated. *Traumatic* stricture is identical with inflammatory stricture except (1) as to etiology, and (2) operation is more often required (see Chapter 10).

Pathogenesis of Stricture. The usual urethral inflammatory process alone seldom causes stricture but rather an intense localized lesion, or improper treatment is responsible. In nongonorrheal inflammatory stricture, the character of the urethral epithelium is of less importance than in the gonorrheal variety but the changes produced are fundamentally the same as in gonorrhea.

Because of the absence of glandular structures in the mucosa of the membranous urethra and the transitional cell epithelium, inflammatory stricture of the membranous and posterior urethra is practically unknown. By contrast, the innumerable glands and crypts interspersed between the columnar cells lining the anterior urethra offer a favorable habitat for infectious foci, particularly gonorrheal, and in the bulbous portion. Excepting congenital stenosis of the external urethral meatus which is the commonest form of urethral stricture, about a third of all strictures will be found in the pendulous urethra and a third in the bulbous portion, and a third in the bulbomembranous segment (Fig. 32). In 1244 cases of gonorrheal stricture in adults I reported, the lesions were located in the pendulous urethra in 242, in the bulbous segment in 206, in the bulbo-membranous portion in 247, in the membranous urethra in 99, and none in the prostatic urethra; in the remainder the locations were multiple.

In the development of inflammatory stricture there is first a soft periurethral infiltration which will eventually be transformed to scar or stricture if not promptly treated by bacteriocidal agents such as sulfona-mides or antibiotics together with adequate urethral dilation with sounds to promote resorption of the infiltrate. The amount of sclerosis will depend upon the extent and intensity of the urethral infiltration and the quality of treatment, gentle periodic progressive urethral dilation with sounds being the important favorable factor. Like all scar tissue, urethral stric-ture manifests an inherent tendency to contract and, if neglected, pro-duces urinary obstruction of increasing gravity. Most traumatic strictures are single and are located chiefly in the bulbomembranous urethra (strad-dle injuries), and show an even greater tendency to sclerotic contraction and therapy resistance so that most of them must be cut rather than dilated. The changes in the uninfected urinary tract above the obstructing stricture are described in Chapter 5 and complicating infection is dis-cussed in Chapter 7.

Symptoms. Urinary frequency with dysuria and straining to void is the usual initial manifestation of urethral stricture including congenital stenosis of the meatus. The stream is often intermittent and urination is a painful act, commonly accompanied in children by crying. As the urinary difficulty progresses there is terminal dribbling which results from (1) the tightening stricture with retention of urine behind it and (2) the faulty action of the accelerator urinae muscle in turn produced by periurethral sclerosis in the posterior corpus spongiosum. A few drops of urine retained in the canal subsequently leak out to wet the clothing. A mild mucoid or mucopurulent discharge is often present, the so-called *gleet.* As the stricture progresses, pain or burning on urination is added and even hematuria may occur. Gastrointestinal or associated disturbances result from urotoxemia. With the increasing difficulty of urination and straining, the development of hernia is frequent and I have seen scrotal hernia of this cause. Soon or late infection develops with chronic pye-lonephritis, although it is commonly passed off as a simple "pyelitis."

Diagnosis. Stricture of the external meatus is recognized by inspec-tion. The palpation of sclerotic nodules along the canal suggests deeper stricture, the presence of which is confirmed by (1) the passage of sounds which are grasped, or (2) by urethroscopy. When a tight meatus is present, first perform liberal meatotomy so that instrumentation is not impeded at that point.

The passage of a small olivary bulb may elicit a "hang" at the point of stricture on its withdrawal. A urethrogram will demonstrate stricture (Fig. 171).

In tight stricture one may be unable to pass even a filiform. But in most instances the strictured area is tortuous rather than tight and large instruments will often pass where small ones fail (Fig. 172). By urethroscopy one visualizes the blanched-out scarred area at the stricture site; this may be only a short localized sclerotic ring or it may extend over an area one, two or more centimeters long. Strictures designated as broad caliber will relatively impede the urinary outflow and induce prostatic congestion—if nothing worse. In the male with clinical urethral stricture, prostatitis is practically always present as is urethrotrigonitis in the female similarly afflicted.

Coexisting periurethral abscess will be recognized by palpation, and urography will show stones in the urethra or elsewhere in the urinary tract (Fig. 235). In all except mild cases, the urine showes variable albumin, pus, blood, and generally bacteria. The phenolsulfonphthalein test and blood chemistry studies will reflect the amount of renal damage; the blood pressure may be elevated.

Treatment of Stricture. The *prophylaxis* against stricture is proper treatment of acute urethritis, or avoidance of urethral trauma in carrying out instrumental urologic investigation.

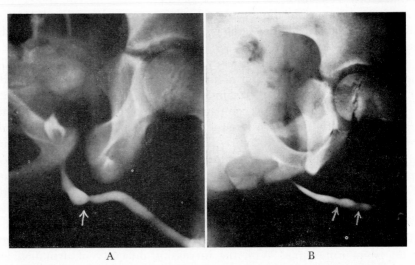

A   B

Figure 171. *A*, gonorrheal stricture of the urethra in an eight-year-old boy urologically examined because of enuresis. Gonorrheal infection at two years of age. In the above urethrogram the narrowing at the site of stricture in the bulbous urethra is clearly shown; in the dilated posterior prostatic urethra, the negative shadow (filling defect) of the verumontanum is evident. *B*, two irregular congenital strictures of the anterior urethra in a two-year-old boy demonstrated by urethrography. The external urethral meatus was also tight.

The *nonoperative treatment* of all types of stricture is gradual, progressive and persistent dilation of the urethral scar (Fig. 16). This will control all strictures and cure some. The instrumenteur must guard against traumatic dilation either by prematurely attempting the passage of instruments too large for the stricture lesion or passing them too often. Seldom should dilation be done oftener than once a week and better once in ten days to two weeks, gradually lengthening the intervals to three, four, six, or eight weeks or longer as progress is made. *The stricture will be cured only when it remains dilated.*

Surgical Treatment. Failure of conservative instrumental treatment demands the stricture be cut. Stricture of the pendulous urethra not accompanied by periurethral abscess should be cut on the roof by *internal urethrotomy.* In internal urethrotomy of the young, the small size of the urethra may require the use of the Campbell instrument rather than the Otis type of urethrotome.

Strictures of the deep bulbous and bulbomembranous area, especially when complicated by periurethral abscess, should be cut by perineal section (external urethrotomy). Most traumatic strictures require cutting and, in some, resection of the scarred segment of the urethra is beneficial. Even following incision of the stricture, periodic dilation with sounds must continue beginning on the fifth to seventh postoperative day in order that the ends of the divided stricture band may heal widely separated. Unless this is done, subsequent stricture will be worse than that preceding operation. To repeat, the stricture is cured only when it remains fully dilated.

Prognosis. This parallels the persistence and intelligence of treatment. Unfortunately the establishment of comfortable urination causes many patients to neglect further treatment with which neglect the stricture contracts, blockage recurs, urinary infection appears or exacerbates and the continued combined obstructive uropathy destroys the kidneys.

Complications. Fistula may develop unless the urethra is kept ade-

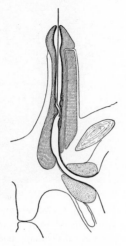

FIGURE 172. Stricture of the urethra. Passage of filiform as guide for tunnelled sounds.

quately dilated following external urethrotomy. *Chronic prostatitis* will disappear following the establishment of free urethral drainage and sterilization of the urine. *Renal failure* through infection and back-pressure injury (urosepsis, uremia) kills most of these gravely ill patients unless pneumonia intervenes.

Periurethral Phlegmon (urinary extravasation). This is an extensive fulminating phlegmon originating in or about the urethra, is usually accompanied by massive genital and perigenital gangrene and, until the introduction of sulfonamide and antibiotic therapy, entailed a 40 per cent mortality (Fig. 173); it is now half this. The lesion is peculiar to males, is almost always associated with periurethral abscess, and especially with stricture, but may follow periurethral abscess or trauma otherwise uncomplicated.

Pathogenesis. With periurethral suppuration or with inflammatory or traumatic rupture of the urethra, the initial process is a cellulitis which extends, guided by the perineal genital or pelvic fascia into the areas indicated in Figures 34, 174 and 175. The triangular ligament is the dividing line. Phlegmon or extravasation originating on the pelvic side of the triangular ligament engenders retroprostatic, perirectal and ischiorectal infiltration and sometimes perivesical and prevesical involvement, and even perforation of the peritoneum. When the phlegmon originates anterior to the triangular ligament it is guided by Colles' fascia into the perineum, over the scrotum and penis, and suprapubically beneath Scarpa's fascia (Fig. 174). Extravasation originating within the triangular ligament may extend either way.

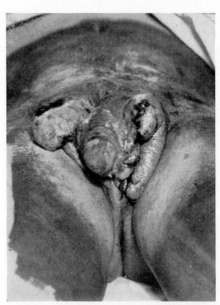

FIGURE 173. Periurethral phlegmon (urinary extravasation) (cf. Fig. 169). Postoperative appearance in a forty-two-year-old man in whom extensive excision, scrotal bisection, and perineal urethrostomy vesical drainage had been carried out.

In adults stricture is the original site of urethral necrosis in 85 per cent of the cases of extravasation while in children the initial lesion is generally a traumatic rupture of the urethra or is idiopathic, as in two infants I saw three and six weeks of age. As cellulitis develops there is extensive vascular thrombosis and gangrene quickly ensues (Fig. 173). Streptococci, staphylococci, colon bacilli, and Clostridium perfringens have been most often found in the tissues but anaerobic bacteria are blamed by many for the occurrence of gangrene. Phlegmon may occur with or without extravasation of urine.

Symptoms. The toxemia of the phlegmonous cellulitis overshadows all other symptoms except urinary retention when it exists. The onset is sudden, often with acute dysuria which is immediately followed by extensive swelling of the scrotum or penis or both, and the evidence of virulent cellulitis. The commonest urethral symptoms are frequency, dysuria, a diminished stream, hematuria, and burning on urination; the patient may develop acute urinary retention. Chills and fever reflect the toxemia which when mild may produce mental confusion with even delirium and coma. The gastrointestinal disturbances are often hyperacute and alarming—vomiting, especially protracted vomiting, and abdominal distention.

Diagnosis. This is made by inspection when one sees a bulging perineum and greatly swollen purplish brown scrotum which looks as though it were about to burst (cf. Fig. 169). There may be greenish-black areas of gangrene and the characteristic stench of decomposing flesh. In extensive phlegmon not only are the scrotum and penis involved but also

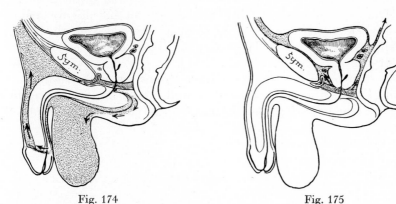

Fig. 174   Fig. 175

FIGURE 174. Schema of spread of infection in urinary extravasation in periurethral phlegmon. When the primary focal lesion is anterior to the triangular ligament a course bounded by Colles' and Scarpa's fasciae is pursued.

FIGURE 175. Schema of spread of infection in urinary extravasation in periurethral phlegmon when the extravasation originates on the pelvic side of the triangular ligament. Retroprostatic, perirectal, and ischiorectal infiltrations are most commonly observed although perivesical and especially prevesical involvement may occur. Rupture into the peritoneal cavity was observed in three cases. When the extravasation originates within the triangular ligament, the phlegmonous spread occurs in either direction, most often externally.

the groins and suprapubic area. Development of a black patch of gangrene over the glans penis forebodes death. The edematous cellulitis of the denser phlegmonous tissues may feel somewhat boardy and the investigation generally discloses obstruction.

In the *differential diagnosis* periurethral phlegmon is distinguished from diabetic gangrene by the urinalysis; other conditions to be considered are the massive edema of nephrosis, nephritis, and cardiac failure although this should offer little difficulty. A fulminating streptococcic scrotal gangrene most closely simulates urinary extravasation but in the first there is no history of antecedent genital disease or stricture and perineal involvement is unusual and secondary to the genital inflammation.

Treatment. The establishment of free urinary drainage by external urethrotomy (perineal cystostomy) is first followed by wide debridement of the gangrenous tissues (Fig. 173). Meanwhile the patient's general condition is fortified by the copious administration of fluids and whole blood, and the intensive and generous administration of wide spectrum antibiotics such as Aureomycin, Chloromycetin, or Terramycin, of a known effectiveness against streptococci and gram-negative bacilli.

The demonstration of gas bacillus infection in the tissues calls for gas-bacillus antitoxin and immediate administration of penicillin. The advent of antibiotic therapy has reduced the mortality a half. In 135 cases, including two infants I reported in 1929, a fourth were dead twenty-four hours postoperatively, with an over-all mortality of 42.9 per cent. With sulfonamide and antibiotic therapy added to surgical treatment, in a subsequent series of 103 cases treated without antibiotic therapy at Bellevue Hospital, the mortality was 38 per cent and this was reduced to 20 per cent in an additional 75 cases by the added employment of sulfonamides and penicillin. The longer the disease has existed, the poorer is the prognosis.

Diverticulum of the Urethra. These lesions are epithelial-lined outpocketings or sacs springing from the urethra and are often congenital (Fig. 176). The following classification (Watts) adequately indicates the etiology.

    1. Congenital diverticula
    2. Acquired diverticula
        a. from dilatation of the urethra due to
            (1) urethral calculus
            (2) urethral stricture
        b. with perforation of the urethra resulting from
            (1) injuries to the urethra
            (2) rupture of abscesses into the urethra
            (3) rupture of cysts into the urethra

Congenital urethral diverticulum has been observed in the newborn; I have seen it in the balanitic region in a seven-day-old male. Sacculation or enormous dilatation of the utricle is not strictly a diverticulum. Urethral outpocketings to form diverticula seldom if ever occur in the absence of distal urethral obstruction; the resulting urinary back pressure causes the blowout. This obstruction is often a urethral stricture, predominantly congenital, and includes stenosis of the external urethral meatus.

Symptoms. In urethral diverticulum the chief symptomatic complaint is dysuria or complete urinary stoppage. As the patient voids the sac becomes distended with urine and after the last is passed, the contents of the sac variably dribble away to wet the clothing. With infection the sac content is often thick and foul. There may be pain in the urethra or perineum, a stone may form in the diverticulum and persistent pyuria is common. Sexual disturbances do not occur unless the utricle of the verumontanum is involved or seminal ejaculation is interfered with as it may be in diverticulum of the deep urethra.

The *diagnosis* is suggested when the distended urethral sac can be palpated, and is confirmed by cysto-urethroscopy. Urethrography will disclose the location, size and outline of the sac; lateral and oblique views, preferably stereoscopic, should be made.

Treatment. The urinary stream is diverted by suprapubic or perineal cystostomy following which the urethral sac is excised. When a deep urethral sac cannot be excised, the roof of the diverticulum is widely removed to convert it and the posterior urethra into a large common cavity. Treatment is incomplete, however, unless all urethral obstruction such as stenosis of the meatus, stricture or stone is removed. Postoperative dilation of the urethra must be regularly performed to ensure against stricture.

Urethral Fistulae. Some of these are consequent to congenital distal

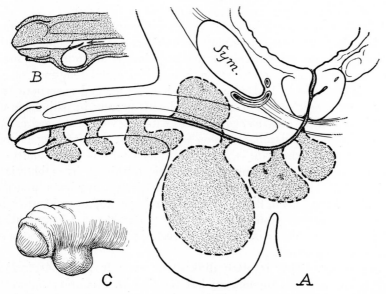

FIGURE 176. Diverticulum of the urethra. The several potential sites of sacculation are indicated. *B*, flap-valve covering diverticulum. *C*, diverticulum of frenal area.

obstructions, but more often follow transverse rupture of the urethra or occur with stones, stricture, or foreign bodies, or a periurethral abscess which ruptures externally. The chief symptom is ectopic urinary drainage. The diagnosis is made by inspection. Treatment demands elimination of the urethral obstruction, drainage of the suppuration, removal of foreign bodies or stone, after which the urethra usually closes promptly. If the fistula is long standing and well scarred, it should be excised. Temporary cystostomy counterdrainage is essential. Following operation, periodic dilation of the urethra at lengthening intervals will prevent urethral blockage by stricture. The urine must be sterilized.

Priapism. This is prolonged penile erection which is usually painful and does not disappear following sexual gratification. Etiologically priapism may be classified as follows (Hinman):

1. Due to nervous causes:
   a. from ascending peripheral stimuli
   b. from direct stimuli
      (1) to the spinal cord center
      (2) to the nervi erigentes
      (3) to the pudic nerves
   c. from descending cerebral stimuli
      (1) direct
      (2) indirect
2. Due to local mechanical causes:
   a. thrombosis (inflammatory or associated with blood dyscrasia, especially leukemia)
   b. hemorrhage or hematoma
   c. new growth of the penis
   d. inflammatory swelling and edema of the penis

Priapism may occur at any age; in the young it is most commonly secondary to prostatitis consequent to habitual masturbation. Transitory priapism is often a reflex manifestation of phimosis, stenosis of the meatus, urethritis, urethral or vesical stone, prostatitis, rectal tenesmus or parasites. It is common in leukemia in which the engorged cavernous spaces are filled with myelocytes or other blood cells present in pathologic numbers. *Thrombosis of the cavernous spaces* causes severe prolonged priapism and here trauma and inflammation are frequent predisposing elements. Pain is the chief symptom, is principally perineal and occasionally there is difficult urination which may require vesical drainage by catheterization or cystostomy. The *diagnosis* is made by the history, inspection and palpation. Palpate the spleen, do blood and neurologic studies to identify blood dyscrasia or nervous system disease, and perform rectal examination to identify any thrombosis of the pelvioprostatic venous plexus. Sometimes no cause can be found.

Treatment. This is often difficult or even fruitless. *Aspiration* of the clots has been satisfactory in but few hands. *Radiation therapy* has caused subsidence of the priapism in some instances as has the administration of spinal or general anesthesia, or of curare (intracostin) as a vascular antispasmodic to improve the local circulation. Incision of the corpora and evacuation of the clots is distinctly a last resort measure.

INFLAMMATORY DISEASES OF THE SCROTUM

Most lesions of the scrotum in adults result from infection of the testicle or epididymis or are secondary to urethral, rectal or perirectal disease while in young boys these conditions are largely caused by inflammation of external origin. Superficial cutaneous lesions of the scrotum are the same as of the penis and the description need not be repeated here; *intertrigo* is the most common. Sebaceous cysts (wens) developing as post-inflammatory or as inclusion nodules, are extremely common, often multiple and, while not serious, are a great cause of worry to their possessor. They are easily excised.

Scrotal edema is usually associated with cardiac or renal disease but it may be a part of the clinical picture in severe anemia, leukemia or other blood dyscrasias, abdominal tumor or filariasis. In short, advanced scrotal edema is usually due to constitutional disease, but it may be secondary to inflammation of adjoining or underlying structures. Noninflammatory edema occurs frequently in premature infants and usually lasts the first eight to ten weeks of their lives.

Because of the laxity of the scrotal skin, edema rapidly progresses to startling dimensions causing the skin to become extremely tense, shiny, and in severe cases almost translucent. The penis is usually similarly involved, but in massive scrotal edema the penis may be partially invaginated as it sometimes is in extensive hydrocele, and by distortion and displacement cause severe interference with urination. The urine runs over the scrotum and macerates the tissues in which infection and ulceration commonly follow. These debilitated tissues are particularly prone to infection and, with cellulitis, pain is increased and the systemic symptoms of toxemia appear. Massive scrotal edema may also cause inconvenience in walking, or pain by the mass weight or tension of the skin. In the young the delineation of the lesion in an otherwise healthy child differentiates noninflammatory genital edema from sclerema but when acute infection exists, erysipelas, streptococcic genital gangrene, or urinary extravasation (phlegmon) must be considered in the differential diagnosis; their distinguishing characteristics are described elsewhere in this chapter.

The *treatment* of scrotal edema is treatment of the cause. High support of the scrotum by an adhesive scrotal suspensory is employed in bed patients and, when the edema has subsided, an ordinary scrotal suspensory or an athletic supporter may be substituted. Should tense edema sufficiently devitalize the skin to cause ischemic necrosis or secondary infection to produce cellulitis, the tissues must be widely incised, debridement of necrotic scrotum performed, and antibiotic therapy intensively administered, employing a broad spectrum compound such as Terramycin or Aureomycin. Surgical intervention need not be employed in massive penile or scrotal edema caused by nephrosis because these patients are highly susceptible to bacteriemia and peritonitis. Sulfonamide compounds and antibiotic therapy judiciously employed prophylactically will largely prevent grave cellulitis complications or control them.

Scrotal cellulitis and suppuration may result from superficial infection or from periurethral phlegmon or suppurative lesions within the scrotum. With cellulitis the scrotum becomes greatly swollen, dark red, or reddish purple or purplish yellow, the process extending to the base of the scrotum and, if severe, to the adjacent tissues. The scrotum should be kept well supported and dry to prevent local maceration of the tissues by moisture; antibiotic therapy may cause prompt recovery from the cellulitis or, should incision and drainage be necessary, help to control the infection.

Erysipelas of the scrotum may also extend to the penis. The scrotum becomes enlarged two or three times the normal size and, by toxic absorption, the patient is sick. Intensive Aureomycin or erythromycin therapy is the treatment.

Diphtherial cellulitis of the scrotum has been observed in a few boys as has diphtheria of the penis. The Klebs-Löffler bacillus is found in the inflammatory exudate and diphtheria antitoxin is the specific treatment.

Scrotal gangrene is caused by interference with the cutaneous blood supply and may result from cellulitis, extensive noninfectious edema, or intrascrotal suppuration. The etiologic factors may be (1) chemothermal or mechanical injury; (2) certain systemic diseases such as diabetes; (3) cardiorenal conditions accompanied by extensive scrotal edema; (4) infected, traumatic or surgical wounds of the scrotum. The lesion is common with urinary extravasation. Atrophic disturbances of the scrotal skin are frequent with spinal cord lesions, particularly traumatic injury, and predispose to scrotal infection and gangrene.

Scrotal gangrene usually appears in a patient previously in good health. The onset is abrupt with chills, fever, acute intestinal upset with nausea and vomiting and pronounced swelling of the genital skin which proceeds to gangrene within forty-eight hours. The process usually becomes demarcated at the scrotoperineal junction but commonly involves a portion or all the penis. The etiologic bacteria may be isolated but the mode of inoculation is unknown, it being assumed that the organisms are rubbed in by friction of the clothing. Urethral disease plays no part. As gangrene progresses, the skin falls away leaving the testicles hanging freely. The *diagnosis* is made by inspection, the gangrenous skin showing patches of deep purple, blue, black, or dark green. The *treatment* is debridement (complete removal) of the gangrenous tissues together with intensive antibiotic therapy, especially Aureomycin and erythromycin in combination. In scrotal gangrene simple incision is inadequate.

Streptococcic penile and scrotal gangrene has been described on page 273.

Elephantiasis. *Nonparasitic* elephantiasis of the scrotum sometimes follows excision or postoperative sclerosis of the inguinal lymph nodes into which the scrotal lymphatics drain. This is well demonstrated in granuloma inguinale. There is enormous swelling of the scrotum, the edematous tissues having a brawny hardness as distinguished from the softer edema in cardiorenal disease, for example. This brawniness is attributable to fibrous infiltration and cutaneous hyperplasia, the skin becoming leathery and coarse. The cutaneous blood supply is generally maintained so that gangrene seldom occurs. Progressively the scrotum enlarges, becoming spheroform with great bulging below and often invaginating or completely engulfing the penis above. This causes urinary difficulty and maceration of the tissues as the urine runs down over them. Scrotal enlargement is the chief symptom but there is sometimes discomfort or pain. The diagnosis is made by inspection and excision of most of the scrotal skin is the treatment.

Parasitic elephantiasis is extremely common in certain Asiatic countries, especially India, although many cases are seen in Puerto Rico, for example. The condition results from infection with the nematode *Filaria bancrofti*, an organism which requires two hosts—man and certain mosquitoes, chiefly Culex—to complete its life cycle. The filaria is blood-borne but gets into the lymphatics to plug the regional lymph nodes. The resulting obstruction to lymph flow causes elephantiasis of the genitals and may similarly involve the lower extremities. The appearance of the scrotum in filarial and the nonparasitic elephantiasis described in the preceding paragraph is identical. The differential diagnosis is made by the demonstration of filaria in the blood stream, a high eosinophilia at once suggesting the parasitic etiology. At present the only drug successful in the treatment of filariasis has been Hetrazan (1-diethylcarbamyl-4-methyl-piperazine dihydrogen citrate), the dose for adults varying from 0.5 to 2.0 grams per kg. body weight three times daily for periods of five to twenty-two days with repeated nocturnal microfilarial blood counts. When these blood studies strongly suggest that the filariae have been killed, treatment is stopped. Cosmetic and symptomatic relief of the genital elephantiasis may be obtained by extensive resection of the scrotum, excising well into the adjacent uninvaded skin and removing the entire covering down to the tunica vaginalis. Sometimes skin grafts are necessary but restoration of the scrotal skin usually takes place unaided.

HYDROCELE

Hydrocele of the tunica vaginalis is an abnormal collection of fluid within the cavity of the tunica vaginalis and is the commonest tumor of the male reproductive tract (Figs. 177, 178). The condition may be congenital or acquired, acute or chronic. *Acquired* hydrocele usually results from infection (especially of the epididymis) or trauma, either direct or from wearing a truss. Normally a few drops of fluid are found within the cavity of the tunica vaginalis for the protection of the testicle. When the funicular peritoneal process fails to be obliterated from the internal inguinal ring to just above the epididymis, a variety of abnormalities result, particularly congenital hydrocele and hernia. In the female a similar condition occasionally exists when the process surrounds the broad ligament in the canal of Nuck.

Hydroceles may be classified according to location; the various types are schematically shown in Figure 177.

Hydrocele of the Testis. A. *Hydrocele within the tunica vaginalis.* 1. *Congenital hydrocele* results from incomplete or unnatural closure of the processus funicularis (Fig. 177), and is the commonest variety observed in the young but it may persist into later life. A hernia generally coexists. Studies (Allen and Rinker; Bruskewitz and Ewell) of the lymphatics of the tunica vaginalis have shown they develop late and if communication between the tunica vaginalis and the peritoneal cavity closes before the lymphatics are completely developed, the child will have a congenital hydrocele. This is believed to explain the frequent disappearance of congenital hydrocele in infants because these lymphatics continue to develop after birth.

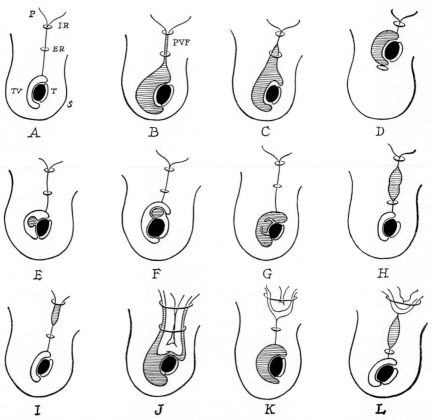

FIGURE 177.   Hydrocele. The various types are schematically shown. *A*, normal relationships. *P*, peritoneum; *IR*, internal inguinal ring; *ER*, fibrous cord (obliterated funicular process) and external inguinal ring; *TV*, tunica vaginalis; *T*, testis and epididymis; *S*, scrotum. *B*, congenital hydrocele. *PVF*, patent processus funicularis. *C*, infantile hydrocele. *D*, hydrocele of imperfectly descending testis. *E*, localized hydrocele of testis (tunica albuginea and tunica vaginalis). *F*, hydrocele of epididymis. *G*, bilocular hydrocele. *H*, hydrocele of cord. *I*, hydrocele of hernial sac. *J*, with hernia (congenital type). *K*, hydrocele of tunica vaginalis and hernia. *L*, of cord and hernia.

The reducibility of congenital hydrocele distinguishes it from the acquired variety. The aperture through which the hydrocele connects with the peritoneal cavity is sometimes so small that reduction of the fluid mass appears impossible, yet overnight the sac is perceptibly smaller. Upon resumption of an upright position, the hydrocele again becomes enlarged and tense. The cord is thicker on the side of the peritoneal communication and when the peritoneal opening is large, hernia epiplocele is generally found. Congenital hydrocele always suggests some anomaly of the testicle. Imperfect descent of the testis is a common accompaniment of congenital hydrocele; the organ may be in the upper scrotum, in the inguinal canal, or may periodically disappear into the abdomen.

In *infantile* hydrocele the processus vaginalis is closed off from the peritoneum in the region of the internal ring and renders the congenital hydrocele irreducible, the differential diagnostic point (Fig. 177). Sometimes infantile hydrocele is confined to the inguinal canal, the swelling becoming progressively less as the process extends upwards.

In *inguinal* hydrocele, the sac may be (1) congenital and filled with fluid derived from the abdominal peritoneum, or (2) infantile with fluid of local origin. It is distinguished by an improperly descended testicle, and torsion of the spermatic cord and hernia are frequent complications. The inguinal hydrocele presents a smooth rounded tumefaction in the groin which, with evidence of an imperfectly descended testicle, makes the diagnosis. The appendix has been found in the neck of the hernia sac in some of these cases and in the female the end of the fallopian tube may block the neck of the sac in the canal of Nuck.

2. *Acquired Hydrocele. Acute* hydrocele results from scrotal trauma or epididymitis and may occur at any age, the onset being abrupt with swelling and pain.

Chronic or *idiopathic* hydrocele is frequently observed in older boys and is common in adults (Fig. 178). While the direct etiology is usually unknown, observations at the operating table indicate that epididymitis is the most frequent cause of acute or chronic hydrocele. The epididymitis is usually low grade and mild, nontuberculous-nongonorrheal and, unnoted, often follows urethral instrumentation in the presence of infection. The changes in the epididymis in chronic hydrocele may result from pressure alone. Trauma is doubtless a factor in some instances, the tunica vaginalis being injured by falls, kicks, or being struck, or hydrocele may occur with local surgical injury of the tunica vaginalis as in herniotomy, varicocelectomy or orchiopexy. To forestall hydrocele consequent to surgical injury, in operating for hernia or varicocele, stay well away from the upper boundary of the tunica vaginalis and in orchiopexy and other operations on the testicle except removal, evert the tunica vaginalis behind the cord before closing the wound.

B. *Encysted* hydrocele of the testis and epididymis is a retention cyst which is or has been in communication with the seminiferous system. It is, therefore, almost unknown in boys since its formation is largely dependent upon spermatogenesis, and in adults it is recognized as *spermato-*

cele. Usually the cyst fluid is teeming with spermatozoa. The clinical manifestations are those of hydrocele and excision is the treatment.

Hydrocele of the Cord.   The condition is almost always *congenital,* appears early and is composed of one or more sausage-shaped cysts closed off from the tunica vaginalis below, from the peritoneum above, and is usually confined to the inguinal canal. The *acquired* variety is generally of traumatic origin. The cyst mass may be moved up and down within the inguinal canal but cannot be pushed into the abdomen. Sometimes the hydrocele is situated alongside the testicle and suggests spermatocele. I have found as many as four separate cyst compartments and have seen a pedunculated encysted intra-abdominal hydrocele of the cord at two and a half years. These cysts rarely disappear spontaneously and should be resected.

Pathology of Hydrocele.   Uninfected hydrocele fluid resembles blood serum with a specific gravity of 1.020 to 1.026, contains fibrin, albumin (4 to 6%), paraglobulin, and occasionally cholesterin; with infection, bacteria, or with trauma, red blood cells may also be present.

Except in congenital hydrocele the epididymis is seldom normal (atrophic, hypertrophic, sclerotic, or indurated) and in the congenital variety is usually widely separated from the testicle by a long mesorchium (testicular mesentery). Persisting hydrocele may cause secondary pressure atrophy of the testicle, either directly or more often by compression of the vascular supply.

In long-standing disease the tunica vaginalis generally loses its normal pallor, adhesions form from epithelial thickenings of the hydrocele sac and densely bind it to the tunica albuginea. Such a thick hydrocele

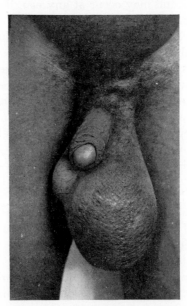

Figure 178.   Hydrocele of tunica vaginalis causing pronounced scrotal enlargement. Transilluminated.

sac may prohibit transillumination. Occasionally inflammatory hydrocele masks tuberculous epididymitis or testicular tumor.

Symptoms. Pain and swelling are the outstanding symptoms of *acute* hydrocele, the degree of pain depending chiefly upon the intra-vaginal tension produced by the rapid formation of the encysted fluid but may also be caused by an unrecognized epididymitis or orchitis (e.g., mumps). Often the pain is referred to the groin or lower loin. A rapidly swelling tense scrotum may produce a dragging sensation by mass weight.

In *chronic* uninfected hydrocele the development of the cyst pro-gresses much slower and is usually asymptomatic except for the mass or an underlying epididymitis.

Diagnosis. A pear-shaped scrotal tumor tapering upward toward the inguinal ring suggests hydrocele of the tunica vaginalis (Fig. 178). The mass is usually smooth and firm, but lobulation may be present. The congenital variety is reducible and the cough impulse of the complicating hernia is commonly present. The spermatic cord feels normal above the limits of the swelling but in long-standing chronic hydrocele is likely to be greatly thickened. When it can be felt, the testicle is usually behind and below the center of the hydrocele mass. A thickened epididymis is noted and in soft hydrocele fluctuation may be elicited. Clear hydrocele fluid transmits light, but the transillumination may be poor or absent when the tunical sac is greatly thickened or the fluid contains consider-able blood.

Differential diagnosis may be extremely difficult. Hydrocele must be differentiated from hernia; they frequently coexist. In infants and young boys the hernia contents in the scrotum will also transilluminate except

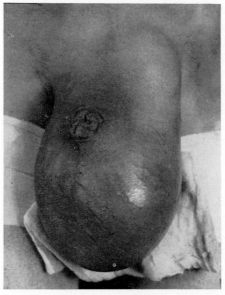

FIGURE 179. Hematocele filling tunica vaginalis following a kick in the scrotum. Note tense shiny overlying skin. Treatment was evacuation of clots and bloody fluid.

when strangulated. Only congenital hydroceles disappear early. Hernia
is a tympanitic reducible mass or the cough impulse can be obtained. In
palpation of the mass, if the fingers can get above it, it is not a hernia.
In hydrocele or cyst of the cord at the external inguinal ring, grasp the
testis between the thumb and first finger, gently draw it downward. If
the swelling is a hydrocele of the cord, it will move downward with the
cord.

For practical purposes **spermatocele** may be considered a variety of
hydrocele; the aspirated fluid looks like barley water and contains
spermatozoa. In **hematocele** there is a history of recent injury, superficial
ecchymosis may be present and there is failure of transillumination (Fig.
179). **Chylocele** is usually associated with tropical filariasis.

Neoplasms of the testis often grow rapidly under the guise of hydrocele and so important is the correct diagnosis in these cases that
aspiration of the hydrocele in order to palpate the testis satisfactorily is
permissible. When tumor alone exists, the mass is solid, hard, feels much
heavier than does a normal testicle and does not transilluminate. Involvement of the lower cord by tumor spread may be noted.

Treatment. Most congenital hydroceles disappear spontaneously
after birth as do some acquired hydroceles in early infancy. Surgical
treatment is indicated when the hydrocele remains tense, increases in size
or causes pain. Open operation is the treatment of choice and is demanded
in persistent congenital hydrocele as well as hydroceles in adults. Aspiration and injection has been advised by a few enthusiasts but it is not
recommended for general use because of its potential dangers in the hands
of the untrained. The spermatic vessels may be punctured to incite massive hematocele; bowel in an unsuspected hernia may be punctured and
the sclerosing solution running up into the abdomen may cause irritation,
necrosis or perforation of the bowel when the congenital funicular connection is not recognized.

Pyocele is the filling of the cavity of the tunica vaginalis with pus,
may follow abscess of the testicle or epididymis and even extend upwards
to cause peritonitis. Rarely, especially in the young, pyocele may follow
extension of peritonitis down the patent funicular process to the scrotum.
Treatment is incision and drainage of the tunica vaginalis with orchiectomy if indicated. Antimicrobial therapy will control the infection and
promote healing.

THE TESTICLE

Orchitis or inflammation of the testicle often develops as (1) a complication of mumps, (2) the result of trauma, (3) secondary to epididymitis, (4) metastatic or hematogeneous orchitis associated with systemic
febrile disease such as smallpox, influenza, malaria, pneumonia, tuberculosis or septicemia. These last varieties (4) are indeed rare. When due
to infection, staphylococci, colon bacilli, B. mucosus capsulatus (Klebsiella
pneumoniae), or typhoid bacilli are usually the cause. *Traumatic* orchitis
is discussed in Chapter 10. Pathologically orchitis is predominantly an

the first day and 100 mg. per day the following three or four days with gradual withdrawal as progress indicates.

Syphilitic orchitis is generally recognized as a congenital infection in which the testicles become smoothly enlarged, hard, rounded ("pigeon egg" or "billiard ball"), freely movable and, pathognomonic, insensitive. It may suggest a tumor. The epididymides feel hard. The condition is bilateral and histologically shows interstitial fibrosis with destruction of the spermatogenic cells and tubules. Interstitial keratitis with a positive Wassermann test may direct attention to the congenital infection which otherwise usually passes unnoted. Antisyphilitic therapy is indicated.

Torsion of the Spermatic Cord. Commonly known as torsion of the testicle, the condition is an axial rotation or twisting of the cord upon itself, with cutting off of the blood supply to the testicle, epididymis and other strangulated structures (Fig. 181). Unless relieved, testicular gangrene results, although in mild cases there may be only atrophy. In severe cases, the local pain is pronounced and systemic symptoms may be alarming. The condition is predominantly one of young boys, more than a fifth of the reported cases occurring during the first decade. The average age of the more than 500 recorded cases is approximately fourteen years, the youngest occurring in a child four hours old. I have twice seen it in the newborn and in each instance the onset occurred during the first day of life and required orchiectomy. The left testicle is involved more often

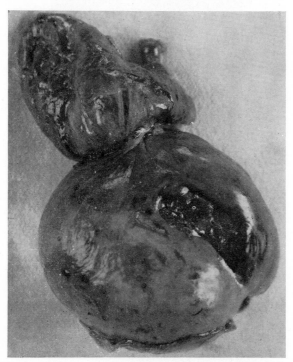

FIGURE 181. Torsion of the spermatic cord in a fifteen-year-old boy, the twist including the cord and adjacent head of the epididymis. Onset while playing basketball.

than the right, and several cases occurring bilaterally have been observed; I have seen three cases of the last.

Unfortunately, the possibility of occurrence of this important condition is insufficiently appreciated by physicians in general, the initial diagnosis usually being epididymitis or simple orchitis; conservative treatment by rest in bed permits loss of the organ by gangrene when it could probably be saved by prompt correct recognition and surgical treatment.

The *causes* of torsion of the spermatic cord are unknown. Nearly every case presents some local congenital malformation, the most common being abnormal mobility of the testicle and an unusually spacious scrotum. Additional factors are (1) elongation of the globus minor of the epididymis, and (2) an abnormal attachment of the mesentery and vessels to the lower pole of the testicle and globus minor which causes the gland to be anchored only by a narrow pedicle rather than a broad band. It is doubtful if a normally placed testicle with a normal mesorchium can be twisted. Sudden muscular exertion or a violent straining appears to be the usual direct etiologic factor inducing an irregular contraction of the cremaster muscle. Several instances of torsion have occurred during sleep; I have observed the results of this occurrence in three patients.

The rotation may be only a quarter turn although as many as five complete turns have been recorded. As a rule, on the right side the twists

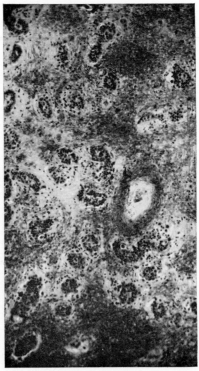

FIGURE 182. Testicle necrosis following torsion of the spermatic cord. Histology. All landmarks are lost.

are counterclockwise, and on the left, clockwise. Except in early infancy, the twist occurs within the tunica vaginalis and in the spermatic cord at or just above its junction at the testicle. In two cases I observed in the newborn the twist occurred outside the upper pole of the tunica vaginalis so that this structure as well as its glandular contents were involved in the hemorrhagic gangrenous process.

Pathology. The changes in the testicle resulting from torsion depend upon the acuteness and completeness of the vascular obstruction, the process usually progressing from hemorrhagic infiltration to gangrene of the organ within forty-eight to seventy-two hours. On section the testis appears as mahogany or bluish-black, resembles an organized blood clot and when cut does not bleed. *Microscopically* hemorrhagic infarction is seen throughout and, with infection, suppurative inflammation (Figs. 182, 183). Atrophy is almost certain when no infection is present and may progress to total disappearance of the organ (Fig. 183). Gangrene or secondary atrophy has been reported in 86 per cent of the cases not relieved immediately. The changes in the involved segments of the epididymis are like those in the testicle. Above the twist the spermatic cord may be slightly edematous or normal while below it is bluish-black or gangrenous.

Symptoms. In *acute torsion* the onset is abrupt with exquisite testicular pain and local swelling. The reflex contracture of the cremaster and the cord shortening by twisting elevates the testicle. Abdominal pain, nausea and vomiting occur and, with necrosis, chills and fever. Unrelieved, the local process becomes more severe and painful but in two or three days, as gangrene occurs, the organ is less sensitive and ultimately relatively anesthetic. Symptomatically, torsion of the spermatic cord may

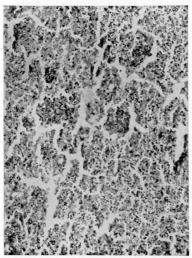

FIGURE 183. Late testicular atrophy with fibrosis following torsion of spermatic cord. Widespread testicular destruction with disintegration of the tubules.

closely resemble strangulated hernia, which offers the chief difficulty in differential diagnosis.

In rare instances, the testicle unwinds itself with subsequent recurrence of torsion; this is called *relapsing* or *chronic torsion*, and the attacks are comparatively mild. Yet, grave testicular injury with subsequent atrophy occurs. Some older patients have learned to untwist the testis.

Diagnosis. While the history and physical findings should suggest the diagnosis of torsion of the spermatic cord, it is usually recognized only at operation. If one will keep torsion in mind, it will more often be correctly diagnosed when there is an "epididymitis" without urethral infection, or "orchitis" in which there is neither an antecedent history of injury nor present evidence of mumps. The diagnosis of torsion is especially likely when (1) an epididymo-orchitis on one side is accompanied by a freely movable testicle or evidence of a long gubernaculum on the other side, (2) when there is an antecedent history of unusual testicular mobility on the side acutely involved, or (3) when there has been periodic disappearance of the testicle into the region of the external ring or even into the inguinal canal. In acute torsion of the spermatic cord there is redness, edema and swelling of the scrotum usually extending beyond the midline, the mass being three to four times normal size and exquisitely tender until the onset of gangrene. Unless superimposed acute hydrocele prohibits satisfactory palpation, the testicle and the epididymis can seldom be differentiated in the inflammatory mass. *Elevation of the testicle increases the pain in torsion (Prehn's sign), but gives relief in epididymitis.* In inguinal torsion of the spermatic cord, the condition may simulate strangulated hernia but the absence of fecal vomiting and absolute constipation rule out strangulation. The inguinal testicle may also suggest epididymitis of an undescended testicle, or testicular neoplasm. In a five-months-old boy whose acute clinical picture was that of torsion of the right inguinal testis, strangulation of a small loop of bowel resulted from tight compression by the undescended testis jammed with the gut in the internal inguinal ring.

Treatment. Immediate operation offers the only hope of preservation of the gland when it may be found possible to untwist the testicle and fix it to the lower scrotum. Variable atrophy will follow. In 90 per cent of the cases orchiectomy for testicular gangrene will be necessary.

Prophylactically, suture of the abnormally mobile testicle to the bottom of the scrotum (orchiopexy) will prevent torsion. Eversion of the tunica vaginalis should simultaneously be done to prevent hydrocele formation.

Torsion of the testicular and other spermatic tract appendages may precisely simulate torsion of the spermatic cord except they are less frequent and clinically less severe. This unusual condition is predominantly a disease of prepubertal boys, about sixty cases of torsion of the testicular appendage having been reported to date. The appendages varying from 2 to 15 mm. in length are composed of blind-ending fragmentary canals. The testicular appendage more commonly known as the *hydatid of Mor-*

gagni, or the sessile hydatid, is a vestigial remnant of the müllerian duct and is analogous to the fimbriated end of the fallopian tube. This pea-size reddish lobule, an almost constant organ, is attached to the upper pole of the testicle or to the upper anterior epididymo-testicular groove.

The cause of torsion of these appendages is unknown; following the twist the necrotic process is similar to that of the testicle in torsion of the spermatic cord.

Chronic or *relapsing* torsion of the hydatid has been observed in which periodic twisting and subsequent untwisting occurred. Symptoms and physical findings are precisely those described under torsion of the spermatic cord, but in general are less severe.

Diagnosis. Torsion of the spermatic cord, epididymitis, acute or- chitis or strangulated hernia are the usual erroneous diagnoses. Unless hydrocele prevents satisfactory palpation of the underlying structures, a bilobate mass can sometimes be felt in the upper testicular area, while the spermatic tract, testicle and lower epididymis are normal.

Differential Diagnosis. While by symptomatology and palpation it is generally quite impossible to differentiate preoperatively between tor- sion of an appendage and torsion of the spermatic cord, this is not too important since both demand immediate operation. Yet a patient with torsion of the testicular appendage will come to the physician's office for help while, if he has torsion of the spermatic cord, he will call the doctor to him. *Orchitis* is ruled out by the absence of mumps or general systemic disease such as influenza or typhoid, and *acute epididymitis* should not be considered in the absence of urethral discharge, prostatitis, or other evi- dence of genital infection. *Tuberculous epididymitis* implies demonstrable tuberculosis elsewhere. The acuteness of the condition generally rules out *tumor*. The gastrointestinal symptoms of strangulated hernia with tymp- anitic percussion note over the involved site is absent in torsion of the testicular appendix.

Treatment is surgical and immediate with ligation and excision of the twisted appendage. The tunica vaginalis should be everted behind the cord to prevent postoperative hydrocele. The *prognosis* is excellent.

Torsion of the appendix of the epididymis (organ of Giraldes) and of the vas aberrans are pathologically, clinically, and therapeutically simi- lar to torsion of the testicular appendix, but even more rare, and merit no further description here.

Epididymitis. This is the most common disease of the testicle and is relatively frequent in males of all ages, particularly young adults; it may occur in earliest infancy. I have seen it at ten days, two weeks, and three weeks.

Three general varieties are recognized: (1) gonorrheal, (2) nongon- orrheal-nontuberculous, and (3) tuberculous. The last is discussed under tuberculosis of the male reproductive tract later in this chapter.

Gonococcic Epididymitis. This used to be extremely common as a complication in about one in four cases of acute gonorrheal urethritis and a fourth of which progressed to abscess. But with the reduced incidence of gonorrhea consequent to present-day antimicrobial treatment engendering no therapeutic trauma by urethral infections, gonococcic epididymitis is now seldom seen by urologists. In short, it is nearly always the result of improper treatment of gonorrheal urethritis, with extension of the urethral infection to the prostatic segment and down the lumen of the vas deferens to the epididymis. It is probable that extension through perivasal lymphatics also occurs. The epididymitis makes its appearance early, usually between the second and fourth week of the urethral disease, and is predisposed to by forceful urethral injections, the passage of instruments, sexual excitement, alcoholism or direct trauma to the testicle.

Pathogenesis. Gonococcic epididymitis is an acute fulminating process accompanied by marked swelling and edema of the epididymis, collateral congestion of the testicle and variable acute hydrocele. The tunica vaginalis may be filled with yellow fibrin. The disease begins in the globus minor or tail of the epididymis, gradually extending to involve the entire organ with the development of first an acute catarrhal inflammation, progressing to localized necrosis of tubules with the formation of minute focal abscesses (Figs. 184, 185). There is dense acute inflammatory infiltration with suppuration proportional to the virulence of the bacterial attack. With resolution, inflammatory debris is absorbed and later replaced by scar tissue which occludes a variable number of epididymal tubules to cause sterility through prohibiting passage of spermatozoa to the vas deferens (Fig. 185).

Symptoms. These are chiefly pain, scrotal swelling and fever. There is usually a prodromal ache in the groin or discomfort along the spermatic cord and, as the disease develops, pain is increased and often extends over the hip or to the back, rectum, or lower abdomen. Pain in the spermatic cord is caused mostly by the drag of the testicle but may also result from edematous swelling of the cord within its sheath and in the inguinal canal. Elevation of the testicle relieves most of the pain and the patient, in walking, likes to support the scrotum manually. Systemic symptoms of

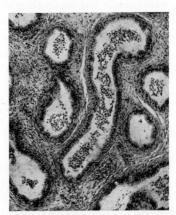

FIGURE 184.   Acute epididymitis. Histology. Early stage of acute epididymitis with generalized suppuration; both the lumina of the tubules and the interstitial spaces are infiltrated with leukocytes.

toxemia (chills, fever, headache, nausea or vomiting, etc.) variably appear but will subside as the disease improves.

Diagnosis. This is made by demonstration of gonococci in the urethral discharge in the presence of an acutely swollen and tender epididymis. The epididymis can usually be distinguished from the uninvolved testicle even though the scrotum is enlarged, inflamed, edematous and tender. Similarly the spermatic cord is swollen and thickened and the vas deferens may be inflamed and sensitive. Examination of the prostate and seminal vesicles often gives a clue, especially when the isolateral vesicle is enlarged, indurated, and tender, but the vesiculitis may be bilateral or even contralateral. The complement fixation test is nearly always positive in gonococcus epididymitis.

Although the morbidity is considerable, there should be no mortality. About 40 per cent of those with bilateral disease and a fourth of those with unilateral gonorrheal epididymitis will become sterile.

Treatment. Prompt and intensive administration of antimicrobials with the onset of gonococcic urethritis may be expected to prevent epididymitis (see Treatment of Gonorrheal Urethritis). Should epididymitis appear, elevation and immobilization of the testicles gives greatest relief and this is best accomplished with a scrotal suspensory such as that developed on the Urologic Service of Bellevue Hospital, New York (Fig. 186). With rigid splinting and elevation of the scrotal contents and an ice cap locally, pain will usually be relieved at once. The patient with acute epididymitis should be kept in bed for two days after the temperature has become normal; recurrence of pain or fever upon arising demands continued bed rest and antibiotic therapy. If pain and temperature do not disappear within three days after institution of treatment, epididymotomy is demanded even though there are no local signs of abscess.

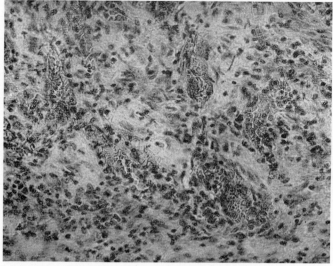

FIGURE 185. Late scarring following acute epididymitis. There is invasion of new capillaries and the deposit of scar.

Pain is a much better surgical indication for epididymotomy than temperature, and operation to be effective must be performed without great delay. The surgical risk is negligible and immediate relief of pain occurs. With massive epididymal suppuration, epididymectomy should be performed and if the abscess has extended into the testicle, orchiectomy.

Nongonorrheal-nontuberculous Epididymitis. This is the commonest type of epididymitis encountered today, and is the usual unrecognized cause of hydrocele. The most frequent invading bacteria are staphylococci, Aerobacter aerogenes, streptococci, and colon bacilli of frequency in the order named. Micrococcus catarrhalis and Friedländer's bacillus, B. mucosus capsulatus, have also been found. The infection may be blood-borne in pneumonia, influenza, and acute tonsillitis, or from peritonitis, hepatic phlebitis, or severe intra-abdominal infections but these are rare. Instrumentation in the presence of urinary infection is probably the commonest single exciting cause of epididymitis, the activated organisms reaching the epididymis via the vas deferens or by the hematogenous or lymphatic route.

The *pathogenesis* of nonspecific (nontuberculous-nongonorrheal) epididymitis is precisely that described under gonococcic epididymitis except there is a fourfold greater tendency to suppuration.

Symptoms. Nongonorrheal-nontuberculous epididymitis simulates acute gonorrheal epididymitis and may be just as severe but is usually milder with less pain, swelling and systemic manifestations. Yet, it is apt to be more tenacious than gonorrheal infection, and in this manner may simulate tuberculous epididymitis.

Diagnosis. The diagnosis of nongonorrheal-nontuberculous epididy-

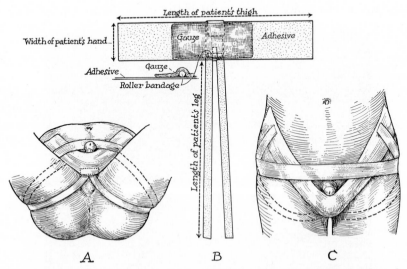

Figure 186. Scrotal suspensory made of adhesive tape. This bandage has been found the most satisfactory for its purpose. In applying this support, the small roller bandage is placed high in the scrotoperineal angle and effectively prevents the scrotum and its contents from slipping downward.

mitis is suggested by the history and is made by palpation as in gonorrheal epididymitis, but there is no urethral discharge or only a mucoid or muco-purulent discharge that contains no gonococci, but rather staphylococci or other invading nonvenereal organisms. An overlying hydrocele may prohibit satisfactory palpation of, and distinction between, the testicle and the epididymis. With resolution of the disease to the chronic stage, the scrotum becomes normal unless spontaneous rupture of an abscess engenders a scrotal sinus. The sinus and a thickened or even beaded vas deferens may suggest tuberculosis, but, when tuberculous, there are other demonstrable tuberculous foci in the body especially in the kidney.

Differential Diagnosis. Tuberculous epididymitis is discussed later in this chapter. *Torsion of the spermatic* cord is generally diagnosed as acute epididymitis or epididymo-orchitis. Torsion demands prompt recognition and immediate operation while epididymitis may usually be satisfactorily treated conservatively over a much longer period of time. *Tumors* of the testicle and of the epididymis may simulate orchitis or epididymitis and not be correctly recognized until operation. When the differential diagnosis is in doubt, operate. Explore the scrotum to be sure that a malignant lesion is not being overlooked or a salvable testicle is not permitted to progress to gangrene.

Treatment. This is the same as outlined under gonococcic epididymitis except that suppuration occurs four times more often in nongonorrheal epididymitis and correspondingly more often requires epididymectomy. Fortunately intensive sulfonamide and, more particularly, antibiotic therapy may be expected to check the infection and forestall abscess in these cases and bring about a high average of satisfactory cure. When intensive antibiotic therapy produces no improvement within forty-eight hours, surgical exploration is demanded. With suppurative invasion of the testicle, it must be removed together with the epididymis.

THE SPERMATIC CORD

Funiculitis (inflammation of the spermatic cord) most often results from extension of infection from the posterior urethra, and is usual in epididymitis and suppurative orchitis. It may arise as an outward extension of a pelvic phlegmon or abscess, or as the traumatic variety especially following herniotomy. In the Orient an epidemic form of *hematogenous funiculitis* caused by a particular streptococcus has been observed.

Acute funiculitis causes edematous swelling of the cord, the vas deferens is enlarged, indurated, and may be tender; local swelling causes pain and toxic absorption to produce mild malaise. Palpation of a swollen tender spermatic cord makes the *diagnosis*, particularly when urethritis, prostatitis and seminal vesiculitis coexist. In *chronic funiculitis*, the cord is boggy with an increase of connective tissue and may simulate hernia. Scrotal suspension is the treatment in both acute and chronic forms; the administration of antimicrobials is beneficial. Should local symptoms persist or frank suppuration appear despite scrotal suspension, an ice cap and medication, incise and drain.

Vas deferentitis is associated with epididymitis and funiculitis, the infection traveling through the lymphatics of its sheath or through the lumen and in either direction. The enlarged indurated vas is often beaded or nodular.

Hydrocele and *cysts* of the cord are described under hydrocele; *torsion* of the spermatic cord has been discussed under torsion of the testicle.

Varicocele is characterized by elongation, dilatation and tortuosity of the veins of the pampiniform plexus and may be (1) *primary,* spontaneous or idiopathic, or (2) *secondary,* symptomatic or obstructive (Fig. 187).

Primary varicocele is the usual variety and appears chiefly in young adults (Fig. 187). It is generally induced by faulty sexual hygiene and especially habitual masturbation, repressed sexual desire, or habitual unwholesome sex thinking which maintains a more or less constant pelvic congestion inducing congestive prostatitis as well. The condition is seldom seen in prepubertal boys but nearly all older patients with varicocele are unmarried; marriage cures the vast majority and particularly the psychologic morbidity. Anatomic factors held as etiologic are the great length of the valveless left spermatic vein and its emptying into the left renal vein at a right angle. The right spermatic vein has valves and opens into the lower vena cava.

Secondary or symptomatic varicocele results from obstruction of the spermatic vein by intra-abdominal tumors, particularly of the kidney, but trauma, cyst, large retroperitoneal or other compressing lesions may be

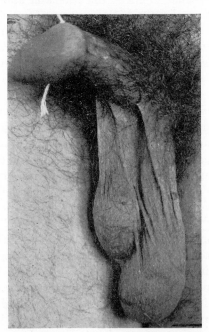

FIGURE 187.   Varicocele with elongation and varicosities of left spermatic cord, causing this testis to hang down considerably below its mate.

etiologic. In two unusual instances in older boys, varicocele resulted from blockage of the renal vein by an aberrant lower polar renal artery; in one of these cases the spermatic vein entered the renal vein against the outward flow of blood from the kidney. Varicocele on the right side always suggests intra-abdominal pressure or *situs inversus*.

Pathology. Venous dilatation and tortuosity with variable phlebitis and fatty atrophy characterize the changes in the spermatic vein and the vessels of the cord. Secondary trophic shrinkage of the testicle commonly results from the vascular interference.

Symptoms. The onset is usually insidious and small varicoceles generally cause more distress than large, the chief complaints being those identified with sexual neurasthenia. A constant dragging ache or pain in the testicle or groin, and local venous swelling are the principal specific symptoms. The *diagnosis* is readily made by inspection of the relaxed scrotum with a low hanging testicle, often with the outline of tortuous veins visible against the scrotal wall (Fig. 187); palpation of the typical "bag of worms" confirms the diagnosis.

Treatment. Usually a snugly fitting suspensory to elevate the low hanging tender testicle and correction of the sexual outlook and habits will cure. When this treatment is inadequate or the dragging testicular pain is unduly disturbing, operation should be resorted to but only when other measures fail. The best operation is that which suspends the testicle high and completely relieves all drag on the vas deferens; for this the procedure of Vincent is, to my notion, the best.

THE PROSTATE

Inflammations of the prostate gland in their acute or chronic manifestations comprise a large portion of the problems encountered by the urologic specialist, and occur with an amazingly high incidence in general practice. Acute prostatitis is observed only one tenth as often as so-called chronic prostatitis, and in general may be considered a specific disease. Chronic prostatitis, on the other hand, may reflect a wide range of uropathy, often grave, and in which the prostatic manifestations are purely secondary and comparatively insignificant, but receive continued treatments month after month and chiefly by prostatic massage ad nauseam, both unwarranted and ineffective. Yet these patients really need a complete urologic investigation and establishment of the fundamental diagnosis!

Acute Prostatitis. This is inflammation of the prostatic parenchyma and may exist as a nonbacterial congestive process produced by sexual overindulgence or by chronic excessive masturbation, and in males of all ages including young boys. In former days of high incidence of gonococcic urethritis, about half of the cases of acute prostatitis were gonorrheal. In most instances today prostatitis results from *bacterial* invasion; a non-gonorrheal urethritis caused by streptococci, staphylococci, diphtheroids, pneumococci, colon bacillus, B. mucosus capsulatus is commonly demonstrable. Bacteria invade the prostate (1) through the urethra from below,

(2) from the urinary tract above as in pyelonephritis, (3) hematogenous from focal infections especially of the dental structures or respiratory tract, or (4) during a systemic infection such as influenza. Bacteria may be introduced into the posterior urethra with foreign bodies, or even the passage of instruments. In hematogenous infection gram-positive cocci are most often found.

Prostatitis is a catarrhal inflammation of the acini and interstitial tissue of the gland; usually both elements are involved and the changes will vary with the virulence of the infection or inflammation. Congestion, inflammatory swelling and edema are noted and when the inflammation is severe enough there is edematous periprostatitis. In the acute stage the leukocytic infiltration is predominantly polymorphonuclear, while in resolution and in chronic prostatitis the cells are chiefly lymphocytes, and an increase in connective tissue occurs.

Symptoms. These generally lead to the diagnosis of acute cystitis or acute pyelitis. In the absence of pronounced urinary disturbances the initial diagnosis is usually grippe because of the chills, fever, general aches and malaise. The common local symptoms are frequency, urgency, burning, dysuria, and pain in the perineum, along the urethra, in the groin, loin, back, suprapubic area, or rectum. Tenesmus at the end of urination is frequently noted and there may be terminal hematuria. As a rule the acute disease lasts but a few days, subsiding as it responds to treatment. *Prolonged acute prostatitis* is prostatic abscess which is frequently heralded by acute retention, or only a partial retention may develop. In some boys, the irritation of prostatitis reflects itself as enuresis.

Diagnosis. This is suggested by the history and confirmed by rectal examination in which the tender variably swollen gland is palpated, often with edematous periprostatitis and obliteration of the sharp margins. The first and second glasses of voided urine are cloudy with pus and shreds. In *prostatic abscess* the gland is large and tense. Be sure the bladder is emptied before making the rectal examination. There is localized or general fluctuation only when the abscess is extensive or near the surface. Occasionally an abscess will rupture into the urethra upon rectal prostatic examination. In young boys most prostatic sarcomas have been operated upon under the erroneous diagnosis of prostatic abscess.

Treatment of Acute Prostatitis. Rest in bed, a liquid diet, adequate bowel elimination, heat to the pelvic regions as hot sitz baths or rectal irrigations and abstinence from alcohol and sexual excitement are most effective. To this is added intensive antibiotic therapy appropriately chosen for its specific bacterial effectiveness. With extreme urinary distress, the alkaline mixture of codeine and Hyoscyamus given on page 247 or an opium suppository (extract of opium and belladonna $\overline{aa}$ gr. ½) may be resorted to. When this conservative therapy is ineffective, prostatic abscess is almost always present, as it is when complicating acute retention requires catheterization. Prostatic abscess is best treated surgically by perineal prostatotomy.

With relief of symptoms and continued antimicrobial therapy, the prostate should be left alone for a month. Gentle massage may then be cautiously employed as described under treatment of chronic prostatitis.

Chronic Prostatitis. This may follow acute prostatitis or its onset may be insidious and cause unknown. In many instances the early stages are purely congestive, nonbacterial and frequently result from chronic habitual excessive masturbation especially in young males.

The dominant *histologic findings* in prostatitis are periacinitis with inflammatory infiltration and scarring. Ultimately this causes prostatic fibrosis which frequently becomes manifest as contracture of the bladder neck or median bar obstruction, and by producing residual urine and continued congestion at the vesical outlet maintains the progressive vicious cycle of urinary blockage.

Symptoms. Chronic prostatitis may cause no symptoms. Urinary frequency is the commonest complaint and results from hyperirritability of the inflamed mucosa of the vesical outlet and posterior urethra. Mild dysuria and even terminal hematuria may occur. Often there is referred pain to the perineum, lumbosacral area, down the thighs, or to the frenal area of the penis. A low-grade intermittent gleety mucous urethral discharge is of great concern to many patients with chronic prostatitis. Sexual capacity may be diminished.

Diagnosis. By rectal examination the gland is usually found variably enlarged and/or indurated and the seminal vesicles may be palpable. Usually the induration is of somewhat irregular distribution. Prostatic excretion obtained by digital expression shows pus in varying quantities, either as scattered leukocytes or large clumps, the amount found usually reflecting the intensity of the inflammation. The etiologic bacteria will be found in these smears and may be precisely identified by culture. Urethroscopic study shows the posterior urethra to be inflamed, edematous and granular; sometimes there are adherent flakes of mucopus. The verumontanum is frequently swollen, irregular, or considerably enlarged. Comparable inflammation of the anterior trigone is often noted. Cysto-urethroscopy is performed only when symptoms of deep urethral irritation exist, or the condition fails to be cured by four to six weeks of the usual recognized therapy.

Chronic prostatitis which stubbornly persists despite the usual treatment merits a complete urologic examination in which it will probably be found that there exists previously unrecognized contracture of the vesical outlet, sometimes congenital; chronic pyelonephritis or even chronic nephritis; urinary tract stone, infected hydronephrosis; ureteral or urethral stricture for example, and the prostatic changes are not only secondary but are relatively insignificant. In fine, and until proved otherwise, *chronic prostatitis should be looked upon not as a specific disease but rather as a concomitant manifestation of other more serious uropathy elsewhere!*

Treatment. At the outset of treatment, the nature of the infecting organisms should be determined and suitable antimicrobial therapy given to help achieve urinary sterilization as promptly as possible. When masturbation is the etiologic factor in chronic prostatitis, cessation of the habit must be encouraged but this will largely depend upon the patient himself.

The active treatment of chronic prostatitis is prostatic massage, gently performed and not oftener than once a week and usually for not more than four to six weeks (Fig. 6). In the absence of other uropathy, prostatic inflammation may be expected to respond satisfactorily with adequate co-treatment of the etiologic factor whether it be faulty sexual hygiene, extra-urinary focal infection, gonorrhea or urinary infection. To repeat, failure to achieve cure of chronic prostatitis in four to six weeks demands a complete urologic examination, the findings of which will direct rational future treatment.

Enlargements and tumors of the prostate are discussed in Chapter 12.

Seminal Vesiculitis. Inflammation of the seminal vesicles is usually secondary to posterior urethritis and is a frequent accompaniment of prostatitis. In the past the vesicles have too often been innocently accused of inciting clinical manifestations of which they were blameless. They have been called the male pus tubes, and an important focus of dispersion in both gonorrheal arthritis and in nongonorrheal rheumatic manifestations. Subsequent studies have largely absolved the seminal vesicles of much of this responsibility and their importance in clinical urology today is correspondingly reduced. But this does not overlook the fact that the seminal vesicles may become (1) the seat of infection, (2) greatly enlarged and indurated, (3) highly congested, (4) overdistended with seminal fluid which they elaborate as nutrition for spermatozoa and for their transport in emission, and (5) may even become the site of cystic or malignant disease.

Symptoms of seminal vesiculitis when present are indistinguishable from those of prostatitis; low backache, perineal distress and vesical neck irritability are common manifestations.

Treatment is the same as of prostatitis. Gentle massage or stripping down of the vesicles is performed in conjunction with similar gentle prostatic treatment. Antimicrobial therapy is co-administered for bacteriocidal purposes to cure latent infection in the vesicles.

VERUMONTANUM (Colliculus Seminalis)

Verumontanitis always accompanies posterior urethritis in the male, prostatitis or seminal vesiculitis; the organ has been referred to as the mirror of the seminal vesicles. Habitual excessive masturbation is the commonest cause of symptomatic verumontanitis in young males but the organ is most frequently inflamed as a result of genital or urinary tract infection. The *symptoms* it produces are indistinguishable from those of prostatitis or posterior urethritis except painful seminal ejaculation which is largely attributed to verumontanitis. Moreover, by referred pain as evidenced by the therapeutic test, distressing low backache, particularly lumbosacral, has been frequently observed to disappear following proper treatment of the inflamed verumontanum.

The *diagnosis* of verumontanitis is made by urethroscopy which reveals the congested, irregularly swollen verumontanum to which flakes of mucopus are often attached (Fig. 188). The granular surface bleeds easily, may show erosions and, in long-standing cases, granulomatous changes or warty papillomas may be observed. Inflammation of the prostatic utricle (*utriculitis*) is a common accompaniment and in some instances a small granulomatous polyp may be seen protruding from the orifice. *Treatment* of verumontanitis is that of the prostatitis, striking symptomatic improvement often follows the passage of sounds and the instillation of two to three drops of silver nitrate (1.0 to 4.0%). The topical application of silver nitrate (5 to 10%) to the verumontanum alone may be required. In more stubborn cases, urethroscopic electro-coagulation of the diseased verumontanum is sometimes necessary but only after failure of more conservative treatment and assurance that other

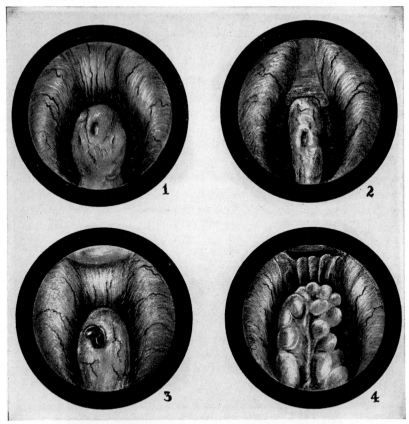

FIGURE 188. Verumontanitis; endoscopic appearance. *1*, normal; *2*, verumontanum extending back into the bladder outlet in a six-year-old boy with enuresis; *3*, granuloma of the utricle in a five-year-old boy with enuresis; *4*, cystic enlargement of the verumontanum in an habitual masturbator aged seven years and examined because of enuresis.

and possibly more important uropathy has not been overlooked (Fig. 188).

INGUINAL LYMPHATICS

Inguinal adenitis may be secondary to any infection of the superficial tissues below the hips which includes such diversified lesions as balanitis, scabies, furunculosis, eczema, intertrigo, or other infected lesions of the genitals or lower extremities. Thus, in inguinal adenitis without genital cutaneous infection, look between the toes for bacterial or parasitic infection. An overlooked paronychia of a toe may exist. The superficial inguinal glands are three groups: below, above, and external to the saphenous opening, while the deep glands lie beneath the superficial group, and are situated about the femoral veins near the saphenous opening. The lymphatics of the urethra drain into the deep inguinal nodes while the lymphatics of the penile skin drain into the inguinal nodes. In urethritis, inguinal adenitis will be found only when balanitis exists.

In acute inguinal adenitis the nodes become large and painful, and even may become matted together in a chain, the condition progressing to suppuration with fluctuation. In subacute adenitis, the nodes are distinctly enlarged and tender, and in the chronic or usual form the glands are more discrete and not painful.

Treatment of acute inguinal adenitis is rest in bed, an ice bag to the groin, and adequate antimicrobial therapy. Frank abscess must be incised and drained. Suitable local treatment of the primary inflammatory process in the genitalia or lower extremity is essential. Chronic adenitis requires no treatment except when tuberculous and then the treatment employed in urogenital tuberculosis is indicated (Chapt. 7).

Chancroidal bubo or suppurative adenitis represents a lymphatic extension from a genital chancroid which is usually in the postcoronal sulcus of the penis. The inflamed inguinal glands rapidly suppurate and the abscess must be drained. Fortunately, intensive treatment with antibiotics especially Aureomycin may be expected to cure promptly the bubo and its complicating adenitis.

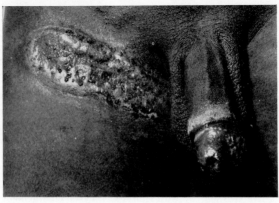

Figure 189.   Granuloma inguinale. Cured with tartar emetic injections.

Lymphogranuloma venereum (lymphopathia venereum, lymphogranuloma inguinale) is a comparatively rare variety of venereal lymphadenitis caused by a filtrable virus which produces initial herpetiform papules or erosive oval shaped lesions with a nonindurated base, usually quickly healing and involving the genitalia primarily with secondary inguinal adenitis and systemic spread. The infection is usually acquired by sexual contact, the portal of entry being through abrasions in the vulva, coronal sulcus or elsewhere on the penis or urethra, males being infected more often than females. The incubation time is two to twenty-one days. Rectal infections are acquired by sodomy, lymphatic spread or, in the female, by perineal spread from the vulva. Blockage of the inguinal lymphatics may cause elephantiasis of the penis and scrotum. Urethritis, prostatitis and vesical inflammation may produce urinary disturbances while conjunctivitis, ophthalmia, hepatic abscesses, dermatitis, and migrating polyarthritides have been observed as well as perirectal abscess and rectal stricture. The *diagnosis* is suggested by the presence of inguinal, axillary or cervical adenitis, vague urogenital or rectal disturbances with unexplained erythema nodosum or joint pains. Fistulas develop in and about the involved areas. The diagnosis is confirmed by the intradermal Frei test and the complement fixation test. In some cases carcinoma of the rectum cannot be ruled out without biopsy examination. Intensive therapy with Aureomycin has been most successful, the average dose in adults in the early stages of the disease being 2 to 3 gm. daily for 1 to 4 weeks and in older lesions a total of 75 to 100 gm. has been necessary for cure.

Granuloma inguinale is a superficial ulcerative lesion of the genital skin with complicating inguinal adenitis and commonly involvement of the inguinal skin as well (Fig. 189). The disease is caused by intracellular monocystic Donovan bodies, the transmission apparently being by sexual contact in most instances. Enormous edema and enlargement of the genitals may occur; in one of my cases the scrotum reached nearly to the knees. The diagnosis is made by observation of the patient and demonstration of the Donovan bodies in the smear stained with Wright's blood stain. Streptomycin has proved to be satisfactory therapy in adults, a total of 20 to 30 grams being given in five to ten days. Good results have also been obtained with Aureomycin in doses of 3 to 5 grams a day for two weeks. About 10 per cent show relapses and have to be treated by larger doses for a longer time than the first course.

TUBERCULOSIS OF THE MALE REPRODUCTIVE TRACT

This is always secondary to tuberculosis elsewhere and practically every case of genital tuberculosis is secondary to renal tuberculosis. A prevalent notion among urologists is that the genital lesion is almost always primary in the epididymis and is hematogenous, the relative infrequency of palpable tuberculous prostatitis and seminal vesiculitis being adduced to reinforce this theory. When tuberculosis of the prostate and seminal vesicles precede the epididymitis, the lesion in the genital tract is almost always secondary to renal tuberculosis.

Tuberculous Orchitis. This may be hematogenous as in miliary tuberculosis of the testicle as part of the generalized disease but otherwise must be considered secondary to tuberculous epididymitis. The testicular invasion progresses to variable ulceration and caseation with symptoms of orchitis accompanying those of the coexisting epididymitis. The testicular enlargement may be palpated but great caution should be exercised lest tubercle bacilli be squeezed into the general circulation. The treatment is orchiectomy with removal of the epididymis and scrotal vas deferens at the same time.

Tuberculosis of the Epididymis. This may occur in males of any age; I have seen it in advanced degree in a twenty-four-month-old boy with early renal tuberculosis and to which the epididymal lesion was secondary. The incidence of tuberculous epididymitis is highest in the period of greatest sexual activity (20 to 45 years). It is usually secondary to tuberculosis of the prostate and/or seminal vesicles and follows extension of the infection through the vas deferens or lymphatics of the spermatic cord, this variety almost always being secondary to renal tuberculosis. With tuberculosis elsewhere in the body, trauma to the epididymis or testicle may predispose to a local metastatic infection but the injury usually serves to draw attention to a pre-existing asymptomatic infection.

In a study of 5424 autopsies at Bellevue Hospital in patients over sixteen years of age, Medlar et al. (1949) found urogenital tuberculosis in 3.1 per cent of all of the cases; in 4.5 per cent of those dead with unhealed pulmonary tuberculosis but who had died of other causes, and in 26 per cent of those dead of tuberculosis. Forty-five per cent of the group with urogenital tuberculosis died of generalized miliary tuberculosis. Renal lesions were twice as frequent as prostatic, and three times that of seminal vesicular or epididymal tuberculosis. The clinical diagnosis had been made in only eighteen of these cases of urogenital tuberculosis which indicates that advanced tuberculous disease may be present without significant urologic symptoms.

In epididymal tuberculosis, the lesion characteristically begins in the globus minor or tail of the organ and spreads to the rest of the organ and in 20 per cent of the cases invades the testicle. The lesion may be caseous or tuberculosclerotic, depending largely on the resistance factors of the patient. *Secondary scrotal* fistulas commonly develop and even bilaterally. Irregular induration or beading of the vas deferens is generally observed especially in the segment of the duct near the epididymis. The entire spermatic cord may be thickened and the tunica vaginalis shows scattered tubercles or old tuberculous adhesions. Often overlaying hydrocele prohibits satisfactory palpation of the testicle and epididymis.

In *acute tuberculous* epididymitis the symptomatology is identical with that described under acute gonorrheal epididymitis; it is often impossible to distinguish between the epididymis and testis in the acute inflammatory mass. Suppuration, scrotal fistulization, and discharge of most of the inflammatory debris may occur and variable tuberculo-sclerotic healing follow.

Chronic tuberculous epididymitis may follow an acute process or as more commonly happens, develops insidiously with only mild nodular, painless or only slightly painful, changes in the organ. The tendency is always toward caseation and scarring with ultimately secondary invasion of the testicle.

Symptoms in both acute and chronic epididymitis are identical with those in the nontuberculous processes which have been described. Aspiration of hydrocele fluid for diagnostic aid is justifiable. The history and presence of tuberculosis elsewhere in the body and particularly in the urinary tract should at once suggest the tuberculous nature of the genital infection. If epididymitis is of less than one month duration bilateral involvement favors tuberculosis.

In the *differential diagnosis* of tuberculous from nontuberculous epididymitis, the following conclusions of Stevens (1923) are a substantial guide: "If the epididymitis is of less than one month's duration (1) bilateral involvement favors tuberculosis; (2) a previous orchiectomy or epididymectomy almost invariably means tuberculosis; (3) a scrotal sinus of over a month's duration is probably tuberculous; (4) clinical tuberculosis elsewhere in the body means genital tuberculosis in over 90 per cent of such cases. When the swelling is of more than one month's duration, the rectal examination is of most aid for the older the lesion, the more definitely involvement of the prostate and seminal vesicles point to tuberculosis."

The *prognosis* in surgical genital tract tuberculosis when treated by removal and medical therapy (see treatment of renal tuberculosis) is usually good in the absence of active tuberculosis elsewhere, especially pulmonary or renal. Complicating extrapulmonary tuberculosis always classifies the disease as far advanced.

Treatment. When hopelessly advanced tuberculosis elsewhere in the body is not a contraindication, epididymectomy and, if necessary, orchiectomy also, is the treatment. Sanatorium care or its equivalent as discussed under surgical treatment of renal tuberculosis is most desirable, both preoperatively and postoperatively. Preoperative treatment with chemotherapy (isoniazid, PAS) and streptomycin should be pursued for three months, and if it fails to achieve striking improvement, epididymectomy is indicated. When unilateral epididymitis is accompanied by palpable prostatic and seminal vesicle tuberculosis, vasectomy on the opposite side will usually prevent extension to that epididymis.

Tuberculosis of the vas deferens is a regular accompaniment of tuberculous epididymitis whether the infection begins in the latter organ or in the prostate and seminal vesicles. Beading or irregular nodulation of the vas is not pathognomonic of tuberculosis and frequently occurs in chronic nontuberculous infection. In tuberculosis of the vas, as in the ureter, the central portion of the duct is the last to show pronounced changes. Excision of the tuberculous vas deferens at the time of epididymectomy is the *treatment*, removing the vas at least as high as the external inguinal ring.

Tuberculosis of the prostate and seminal vesicles usually follows urinary tuberculosis and is rarely secondary to hematogenous tuberculosis of the epididymis or to retrograde extension. There is nodular induration and thickening of these organs with more or less sclerotic periprostatitis and periseminal vesiculitis; occasionally with caseation it may produce a palpable abscess. The *symptoms* of tuberculous prostatitis and seminal vesiculitis are indistinguishable from each other and are generally overshadowed by the symptoms of urinary tract involvement, particularly about the vesical outlet (see tuberculosis of the kidney and bladder). Rupture of prostatic or seminal vesicular abscesses causes perineal fistulization and tuberculous urethral stricture may develop, notably in the deep segment. Lattimer has called attention to the beefy redness and occasional ulceration of the deep urethral mucosa in early cases of prostatic tuberculosis, while in chronic cases dilatation and trabeculation of the prostatic urethra, "golf hole" dilatation of the prostatic ducts sometimes to the extent of forming small diverticula, are suggestive of the disease.

Diagnosis is made by rectal examination and the demonstration of urogenital tuberculosis elsewhere. Extreme gentleness should be exercised in the palpation of the lesions to prevent traumatic dissemination of tubercle bacilli into the blood stream.

Treatment. Prophylactic vasectomy will usually prevent epididymitis if it does not already exist, and removal of an involved epididymis is frequently followed by striking improvement in the prostatovesicular disease. Excision of the prostate, seminal vesicles, vasa and epididymides is no longer recommended as treatment but rather the intensive chemotherapy and antibiotic therapy as described under medical treatment of renal tuberculosis (q.v.). In patients of all ages with tuberculous prostatovesicular infection, the prognosis is poor and should be guarded.

HORMONAL DISTURBANCES CAUSED BY GONADAL DISORDERS

Because these disturbances practically always begin in the prepubertal period, they must be considered predominantly as childhood problems. It is recognized that hormonal disturbances may result from disease beginning after puberty, but such changes are predominantly the result of adrenal tumors and other lesions which are discussed in a separate chapter. Here we are concerned with gonadal disorders not etiologically related to adrenal disease.

In recent years enormous progress has been made in the recognition and treatment of many hormonal syndromes, biologic assay has been developed, and to some extent the synthetic chemistry of hormones. *Androgen*, the male sex hormone is secreted by the testis in the male and by the adrenal cortex in both sexes. *Testosterone* is elaborated by the interstitial cells of Leydig of the testicle which are stimulated to androgen production by the luteinizing hormone of the anterior pituitary, while the *follicle stimulating hormone* (F.S.H.) of the anterior pituitary stimulates the tubules of the testis to induce spermatozoa production at puberty. The interdependence of the testicle and pituitary gland is evidenced by testicular atrophy following destruction of the anterior pituitary while, with castration, hypertrophy of the anterior pituitary cells occurs. Moreover, hyperactivity of the anterior pituitary is manifested by sexual precocity through the intermediary of ACTH (q.v.) while deficiency dysfunction causes adiposogenital dystrophy. The thymus atrophies at puberty. In myxedema and cretinism of hypothyroidism, variable testicular atrophy occurs, while in imperfectly descended testicle the administration of thyroid will often stimulate descent.

In the female the ovaries are stimulated by the gonadotropins of the anterior pituitary hormone, the follicle stimulating element of the hormone acting on the ovary as puberty approaches to cause the production of estrogen which influences female sex development and at puberty stimulates the graafian follicles to periodic ovulation.

The transition to full hormonal activity at puberty begins two or three years previously at a premenstrual level. But at puberty and thereafter during the reproductive life of the female, the luteinizing hormone and luteotrophic hormone of the anterior pituitary influence the corpus luteum to produce progesterone and the recurrent endometrial changes associated with menstruation. At least six hormones of anterior pituitary origin have been identified; the follicle stimulating hormone (F.S.H.), the luteinizing hormone (L.H.), the luteotrophic hormone (L.T.H.), a growth hormone, a thyrotrophic hormone, and the adrenocorticotrophic hormone (ACTH). Both boys and girls excrete about the same amounts of estrogen until the seventh year; testicular androgens are not excreted in perceptible amounts until the eighth or ninth years. Prior to this time the adrenals supply at least two thirds of the androgens in the male and normally all of it in the female. The quantitative urinary excretion of these steroids in children and adults is shown in Table 11.

Sexual Precocity. This is observed chiefly in females who have premature menstruation and often precocious development of the genitals and breasts. Normally girls develop sexually about two years earlier than boys, and children in the United States mature about two years ahead of those in other countries including Europe. In sexually precocious boys, seminal emissions may occur as early as the second or third year but this condition is usually associated with suprarenal, pituitary or gonadal endo-

TABLE 11. NORMAL AVERAGE URINARY HORMONE EXCRETIONS PER TWENTY-FOUR HOURS (AFTER SECKEL ET AL., 1949)

Age, years	2 to 5	6 to 10	11 to 16	11 to 18	Adult	Adult
Sex	Both sexes	Both sexes	Female	Male	Female	Male
17-Ketosteroids mg.	0.15 to 2	1.5 to 2.6	2.6 to 6.3	2.6 to 8.1	5 to 15 (9)	8 to 20 (14)
Androsterone mg.		0.1 to 0.3	0.3 to 0.7	0.5 to 3.0	0.5 to 1	1 to 11 (5.5)
Estrogens I.U.	ca. 10	10 to 25	90 to 400	25 to 65	Up to 600	Up to 100
Pregnandiol mg.	0 to trace	0 to trace	0 to plus	0	3 to 50	0

crinopathy. This is discussed at greater length under tumors of the adrenal cortex, of which it is a frequent manifestation. When precocious puberty results from endocrinopathy, the changes are usually hetero-sexual as in adrenal disturbances. Some of these children are more intelli-gent than their chronologic age, some are normal, while many are subnormal.

Apparently most of the cerebral, pineal and other adjacent hypo-thalamic tumors operate through stimulation of the nearby anterior pituitary yet, in patients with pituitary or pineal tumors for example, not more than a third of them show genital changes.

In the Female. In most instances of apparent sexual precocity in this sex, the condition is simply a precocious physiologic development of sexual maturity involving the genitals, secondary sex characteristics and the skeletal system. Epiphyseal closure may take place early, and the stature may be short although most of these girls grow to a satisfactory height. Although sexual precocity has commonly been attributed to tumors of the pineal, pituitary, adrenal, hypothalamus or floor of the third ventricle, pituitary tumor, granulosa cell tumor of the ovary, ovarian dysgerminoma, and ovarian chorioepithelioma, these lesions have been strikingly absent in almost all of the cases of observed precocious pubertal changes in girls.

The diagnostic investigation involves complete physical examination including pelvic examination under anesthesia, and endocrine study. Comparison of the patient's hormone excretion levels with the normal average chronologic or age basis will indicate whether abnormal hor-monal factors are operating to cause the growth and developmental deviations. Thus, when precocious puberty results from pituitary stimu-lation of the ovaries, the estrogen assay will be within normal limits or not excessive but when due to adrenal or ovarian hyperplasia or tumor, the assay will be high and even as high in a child as in the normal adult.

Treatment. Since in nearly all pediatric cases the precocity is simply a premature physical development in a child otherwise normal, treatment is largely psychotherapeutic in which the patient merits less attention than the family and particularly the mother, who must be reassured that the child's physical developmental condition will shortly be matched by maturation of her age-group companions. Operation is necessary only when definitive endocrinopathy is found.

In the Male. Sexual development and testicular growth is normally manifested in boys between eight and ten years of age, with full puberty between twelve and fourteen years, and in a fifth not until after four-teen. During this four to six year period, growth and genital development progress at variable rates, often with sudden spurts which delight the parents and worry them when the growth is slower; they should be apprised of these facts.

Hypergenital function or *hypergonadism* is extremely rare in the young male, and may result from testicular stimulation by the same brain lesions which cause genital stimulation in the female (q.v.). Con-genital hypertrophy of the testicle has not been observed to cause these changes in our experience but some testicular gonadal tumors and notably the rare interstitial cell adenoma of the testicle may produce excessive androgen secretion. Tumor of an ectopic adrenal rest in the testicle has been known to cause virilism in boys.

Sexual infantilism or *hypogenitalism* is identified by the disproportionate smallness of the testicle and external genitalia in relation to the general somatic development (Figs. 190, 191). It may result from primary testicular hypoplasia, tumor, or other destructive diseases of the anterior pituitary lobe (hypopituitarism) or of the hypothalamus. Collateral thyroid and/or adrenal deficiency as well as disturbances of carbohydrate metabolism often exist.

Diagnosis. When pituitary hyperactivity causes sexual precocity in the young male, the 17-ketosteroid output in the urine will not be above the levels of adolescence or of the normal male, while in hyperplasia or tumor of the adrenal or tumor of the testicle the output levels are excessive, even up to 50, 60 or more milligrams in twenty-four hours. In hypopituitarism with failure of elaboration of pituitary gonadotropins, there is failure of the gonads to mature and to produce their sex hormones; the F.H.S. output in the urine is diminished. On the other hand, in gonadal dysgenesis and hypoplasia the production of sex hormones are scant or none, and in the male the F.S.H. output is increased and notably after castration.

Pituitary infantilism, commonly known as Fröhlich's syndrome after the original describer (1901), has been loosely applied to most fat prepubescent or pubescent boys who do not have the disease Fröhlich described (Fig. 191). He reported a dwarfed rather than an obese boy,

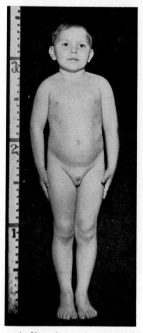

FIGURE 190. Hypogenitalism in a nine-year-old true pituitary dwarf.

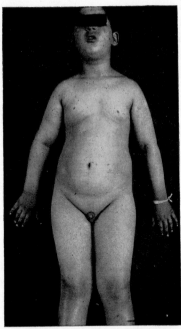

FIGURE 191. Sexual infantilism (Fröhlich's syndrome) in a thirteen-year-old boy in whom the characteristic features of the condition are well demonstrated.

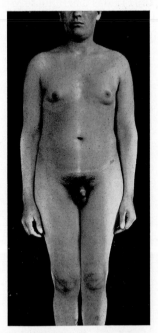

FIGURE 192. Sexual infantilism. Fröhlich's syndrome in a twenty-three-year-old man including gynecomastia, feminine body contour, and abnormally small genitals.

with proportionate genital retardation, and attributed the condition to hypophysial involvement from extension of a suprasellar cyst, there being severe headache, vomiting, marked eye signs and partial blindness, and rapid accumulation of pelvic girdle fat. The genitalia were not undersized but were buried in deep fat. Bartels (1906) called the condition *adiposogenital dystrophy*. Levi-Lorain (1908) infantilism is the same as dwarfism and retarded sexual development in the female. The distinguishing features of these conditions are shown in Table 12. True Fröhlich's syndrome is rare but juvenile obesity is common; it is often hereditary and dietary, and most of these children will develop into normal adults. In some cases, however, the hypogenitalism persists, and even gynecomastia may develop (Fig. 192).

Other *dwarfing syndromes* include cretinism, mongolism, nutritional disorders, cerebral injury, and diabetes mellitus, but none except Laurence-Moon-Biedl syndrome show genital retardation. In adiposogenital dystrophy the sex organs are infantile, marked obesity is prominent over the trunk, breasts, hips, and mons veneris, but skeletal development is frequently retarded. The pubic and axillary hairs are extremely sparse or totally lacking, the patient being asthenic, sluggish, mentally laggard or even a true defective. Retinitis pigmentosa as well as polydactylism has ⱡeen noted in some of these patients.

Diagnosis of hypogenitalism in young males requires precise local examination with pushing back of the suprapubic fat sufficient to feel the penis clearly. The length and size of the penis is measured for comparison with the norm as are the testes which so often are imbedded in a reflexly ·ontracted scrotum, in turn buried deeply by surrounding fatty tissues (Fig. 192).

TABLE 12. COMPARISON OF FRÖHLICH'S SYNDROME, OBESITY OF
ADOLESCENCE AND LAURENCE-MOON-BIEDL SYNDROME*

	FRÖHLICH'S SYNDROME	OBESITY OF ADOLESCENCE	LAURENCE-MOON-BIEDL SYNDROME
Onset of symptoms	Any age	About 8 years	Birth
Obesity	Moderate	Moderate to excessive	Marked
Genital development	Delayed	Boys: slow Girls: normal	Delayed
Development of secondary sex characteristics	Delayed	Boys: slow Girls: normal	Delayed
Skin	Dry, scaly	Moist; perspiration increased	Moist
Skeleton	Slender	Heavy	Heavy; polydactylism
Headaches; vomiting	Present	Absent	Absent
Eyegrounds	Choked disk or optic atrophy often present	Normal	Retinitis pigmentosa; optic atrophy
Mentality	Usually normal	Usually normal	Retarded
Family history	Usually normal	Often familial	Often familial

* Warnaky, in Mitchell-Nelson, 1950.

Abnormally mobile testes must be pushed down into the scrotum to be satisfactorily palpated. With the suprapubic fat retracted upward and the scrotum elevated, an examining finger is pressed deeply forward at the penoscrotal angle. The testes can then be felt if they are in the scrotum. Examination of the testicular biopsy specimen shows an arrest of tubular development, fibrosis of the interstitial tissues, and numerical diminution of Leydig's cells.

When hypogonadism is not caused by pituitary or other tumor requiring surgical treatment, the *prognosis* and future *therapy* will depend fundamentally on the status of the testicle. To determine this, chorionic gonadotropin (A.P.L., antuitrin "S" or follutein, etc.), is given to stimulate pubescence. When the testicle responds by enlarging, it indicates the hormone should be therapeutically employed. When there is no testicular response (primary anorchism or atrophy of interstitial cells) replacement therapy with androgen should be given: testosterone propionate, 10 to 15 mg. intramuscularly thrice weekly or 30 to 40 mg. daily by mouth, or 150 mg. subcutaneous pellet injection every six months. The dose requires adjustment and, when suitably arrived at, must be continued throughout life. Thyroid gland extract must sometimes be coadministered and a slimming diet maintained, high in nourishing proteins to compensate for the caloric restriction, together with accessory panvitamins.

Turner's syndrome in the male is characterized by rudimentary testis, delayed growth and congenital malformation—a web (sphinx) neck and cubitus valgus being characteristic. The penis and prostate are hypoplastic but the testes are of normal size, contour, consistency and sensitivity, yet histologically show arrested development of spermatogenic cells and complete absence of interstitial cells of Leydig with a consequent low 17-ketosteroid output. Usually nevi are scattered over the body.

Klinefelter's syndrome (Klinefelter, Reifenstein and Albright, 1942; Heller and Nelson, 1945) is characterized by small testes showing variable hyalinization of the seminiferous tubules, disappearance of Sertoli's cells and germinal epithelium, with the interstitial cells of Leydig present in large groupings. These patients show azospermia, increased F.S.H. in the urine, variable habitus and libido, and normal or subnormal 17-ketosteroid excretion in the urine and, strikingly, *gynecomastia.*

In **testicular dysgenesis** described by Del Castillo et al., there are small testes, azospermia, absent germinal epithelium, but an excess of Sertoli's cells which form the tubules, and no gynecomastia. Some boys develop gynecomastia during periods of rapid virilization.

In **sexual infantilism** in young males and in many cases of hypospadias, the high estrogenic factor is frequently disclosed by a study of the prostatic utricle which is the homologue of the uterus and a müllerian duct derivative, it being unusually large and sometimes four to six times normal depth or even simulating a uterus and fallopian tube (Figs. 140–142). In short, these sexually infantile males show surprising traces of female anatomic development, particularly of structures of müllerian origin. This is discussed under hypospadias in Chapter 6.

Eunuchoidism, a rare condition, is caused by bilateral congenital absence, hypoplasia or atrophy of the testes with a striking diminution or even total absence of male sex hormone excretion. Eunuchoidism is (1) *primary* when there is no other evidence of endocrinopathy, and (2) *secondary* when it occurs with undescended testicles or in testicular hypoplasia associated with pituitary or adrenal disturbances as in Fröhlich's syndrome.

In *primary eunuchoidism* interference (delay) with epiphyseal union results in disproportionate elongation of the extremities with a short trunk (eunuchoid gigantism). The voice remains high pitched, while pubic, facial and axillary hair is absent or scant; the hips, buttocks, abdomen and breasts become fat, and the genitalia remain small, often buried in pubic fat. The patient may have erections but no ejaculations.

In *secondary eunuchoidism*, the patient is adipose, dwarfed, mentally and physically sluggish (dystrophia adiposogenitalis, Fröhlich's syndrome), with hypogenitalism, sparse growths of body hair (dystrichosis), and high-pitched feminine voice; the growing boy has a disturbing sense of genital inferiority. The output of gonadotropins is high in eunuchoids; the 17-ketosteroid level is that of the female.

Surgical loss of the testicles (eunuchism), bilateral torsion of the spermatic cord, or glandular degeneration consequent to intracranial changes may also occur. The physical manifestations of castration are not fully evident until puberty and after; the normal secondary sex characteristics do not develop, the patient becoming sexually neuter.

Familial (*hereditary*) eunuchoidism (Laurence-Moon-Biedl syndrome) is characterized by short stature, hypotrichosis, primary total gonadal failure due to anterior pituitary failure, mental sluggishness or deficiency, often with polydactylism and retinitis pigmentosa. The distinguishing characteristics are shown in Table 12.

Treatment. This is the administration of testosterone as the propionate methyl ester or subcutaneous pellet, and properly administered will not only improve the boy's psychologic outlook but will stimulate his genital development. Here the treatment is that already indicated under treatment of sexual infantilism (q.v.). In some instances great psychologic help may be achieved by implanting plastic or noncorrosive metal (preferably silver) testicular prostheses in the scrotum to suggest the presence of normal size gonads.

INFERTILITY IN THE MALE

It is now generally accepted that in about half of barren marriages, the fault lies with the husband; determination of the character and degree of his spermatic inadequacy, as well as possible treatment, lies within the province of Urology. Throughout history until perhaps forty years ago, the wife characteristically bore the onus of childlessness. Today in enlightened quarters it is customary to examine the male partner first and determine his degree of fertility because it is far easier than the more extensive examination required of the female. The examination may disclose that the husband is only relatively sterile because of a correctible condition or investigation may show relative infertility on the part of each partner.

The degrees of fertility may be summarized or classified as follows:

1. *Sterility* or *absolute infertility* indicates complete agenesis of spermatozoa.
2. *Relative infertility* indicates there are some spermatozoa present but inadequate for insemination or conception (oligospermia).
3. *Primary infertility;* a barren union; no living children.
4. *Secondary infertility;* couple has one or perhaps two children but unable to produce more.

The functions of the various segments of the male sexual apparatus are as follows:

1. Testes produce spermatozoa and secrete hormones, chiefly androgens.
2. Epididymides and vasa deferentia are concerned with the conduction and storage of spermatozoa.
3. Prostate and seminal vesicles elaborate or secrete the fluid vehicle for the spermatozoa while
4. Urethra and accessory glands deliver the semen.

It is apparent that a small or limited lesion in the epididymis or vas deferens for example may be adequate to block this chain of transportation. The anatomy and physiology of these organs have been discussed in Chapter 4 and need not be repeated here. *Aspermatogenesis* may be congenital as in the Klinefelter syndrome (q.v.), may be due to genetic absence of spermatogenic cells, or to mumps orchitis in which there is commonly total degeneration of the spermatogenic cells. It is believed that liver damage may produce an overbalancing activation of estrogen and, by inadequate nutrition, pituitary gland dysfunction result in an insufficiency or low threshold of gonadotropic hormones (Mulinos and Pomerantz, 1941).

Experimental evidence has demonstrated that *vitamin A deficiency* decreases spermatogenic activity which will respond to adequate replacement therapy; vitamins B, C, and D apparently have no relation to spermatogenesis but lack of vitamin E will cause pronounced and irreparable damage of the spermatogenic cells without affecting the interstitial cells. Physical agents may also induce aspermia; *any condition which impairs the circulation of the testicle damages the germinal epithelium,* and with or without gross changes in the gonad. Aspermatogenesis consequent to x-irradiation has been reflected in the abnormally high incidence of sterility in the pioneers of radiology and has been amply confirmed experimentally. Atomic irradiation spermatogenic damage, as studied after the Japan bombing, is often temporary with recovery after many months. Spermatogenic activity is highly susceptible to increased temperature, even of only 2 to 4 degrees, as evidenced in transplantation experiments of gonads from the cooler confines of the scrotum to the warm abdomen, and recovery with gonadal replacement in the scrotum.

The Pituitary Gland and the Endocrines. Present knowledge of the scope of the function and secretory activity of the pituitary gland is schematically indicated in Figure 193. It is believed that the neural stimulant arises in the hypothalamus from which impulses are passed to the pituitary.

In the problem of infertility we are concerned with the follicle stimulating hormone (F.S.H.), the luteinizing hormone (L.H.), the lactogenic hormone (L.T.H.)—the gonadotropic hormones—and the adrenocorticotrophic hormone (ACTH).

1. F.S.H. stimulates the germinal cells of the testicular tubules and the Sertoli cells.
2. L.H. controls the secretion of androgens by the testicular Leydig cells, and with FSH may stimulate spermatogenesis.
3. L.T.H. *may* influence the Leydig cells.
4. ACTH stimulates the reticular cells of the adrenal cortex to elaborate steroid hormones.

The various target areas influenced by pituitary secretion are indicated in Figure 193 but in the problem of infertility in the male we are concerned with its effect chiefly on the testes, the seminiferous system, prostate, seminal vesicles and the adrenals.

Chapter 13 is devoted to the adrenals. As concerns the present problem of infertility, the adrenals in the male contribute about two thirds of the male androgen excretion, the androgen output in the female by assay estimation of 17-ketosteroids in the urine is approximately two thirds that of the male. The administration of cortisone (compound E) suppresses adrenal activity and decreases the excretion of 17-ketosteroids

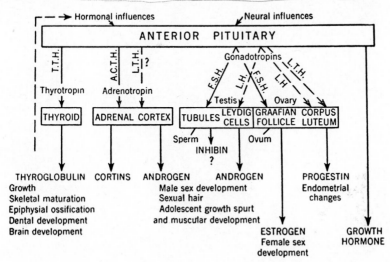

FIGURE 193. Hormones of the anterior pituitary. (From L. Wilkins, The Diagnosis and Treatment of Endocrine Disorders in Childhood and Adolescence, Springfield, Ill., Charles C Thomas, 1950.)

while the administration of ACTH increases the androgenic salt-retaining glyconeogenetic activities of the adrenal functions which are thus mediated through the pituitary.

In the clinical problem of infertility, the most important elements in the structure of the testicle are (1) the germinal epithelium cells from which spermatozoa are derived, (2) the interstitial cells of Leydig and (3) the Sertoli cells (Figs. 36, 194). The cells of Leydig and the cells of the adrenal cortex have a common embryologic origin, and both produce the steroid precursors of the 17-ketosteroids found in the urine. The powerful androgen *testosterone* is today recognized as the male sex hormone, for, although its influence on spermatogenesis is still unclear, it causes the masculine distribution of hair, mobilizes skin pigment, increases muscular growth and development, stimulates development of the male genital accessory organs, and reverses the effects of castration. Its effects are evident not only in the body at large but notably in the prostate, seminal vesicles and, in hypophysectomized animals, testosterone prevents testicular atrophy.

The *Sertoli cells,* anatomically intimately situated among the germinal cells, the spermatogonia (precursors of spermatozoa), contain lipids and afford temporary anchorage for spermatozoa before they start their seminiferous tract journey (Fig. 36). Little is known of Sertoli cell hormone elaboration; some observers believe they throw an estrogenic hormone into the circulation under the influence of F.H.S., or liberate a hormone *inhibin* which is not androgenic and is able to depress or inhibit FSH production by the pituitary. Some believe it stimulates LH production and augments spermatogenesis. In any event, the specific hor-

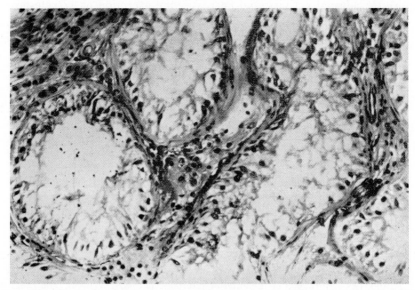

FIGURE 194.   Testicular deficiency. Germinal aplasia of seminiferous tubules. (Hotchkiss, in Campbell's Urology.)

mone has not been isolated and large amounts of testosterone will depress FSH elaboration.

The microscopic anatomy of the normal testicle is shown in Figure 36 and an aspermatogonic one in Figures 194, 195, in various stages of inadequate spermatogenesis.

During their travel from the testicle to emission through the urethra, the spermatozoa pass through the vasa aberrantia into the epididymis where they further mature or ripen. From there they pass up the vas deferens to the seminal vesicles where they may be stored. The more important apparent function of the seminal vesicles is the secretion of the bulk of the seminal vehicle containing considerable fructose together with phosphates, protein, nitrogen and chlorides. By metabolism the spermatozoa gain energy from fructose; in the metabolic process fructose is changed to lactic acid. The prostatic secretion on the other hand is low in fructose but contains large amounts of fibrinogen and fibrinolysin which bring about liquefaction of the semen after its emission from the body.

EXAMINATION OF A MALE FOR FERTILITY

The family physician should be able to carry out with reasonable accuracy the necessary tests for infertility, using only the microscope and laboratory equipment that most doctors have in their offices.

History. The acquisition of certain historic data may be invaluable in the over-all evaluation of fertility or of the patient's infertility. The patient should be questioned regarding (1) occupation, e.g., radiologist

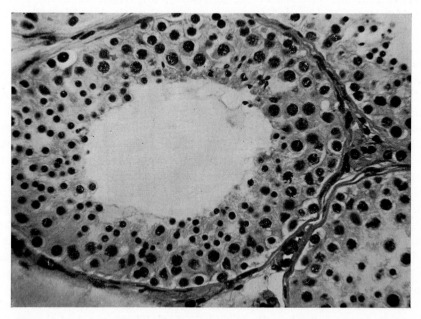

FIGURE 195. Infertility in the male. Spermatogenic arrest; seminiferous tubules (Hotchkiss). Peritubular fibrosis associated with inguinal cryptorchism is shown in Figure 137.

or atomic worker, (2) childhood diseases, e.g., mumps or access to diagnostic irradiation as for fractures, and so forth; improperly descended testicle, trauma of genitalia or operations upon the genitalia; venereal disease, especially gonorrhea with epididymitis. The story in adulthood is concerned largely with prolonged illness, pronounced obesity or hypogenitalism; in the marital history one is concerned with whether there has been previous progeny by the present wife, or, whether previously married to another, children by her.

√ In the study of infertility it is surprising how often one finds that the patient has no conception of the anatomic considerations or mechanics of intercourse. One patient who should have known better thought that by simply parking alongside his wife's thigh something immaculate would happen and they would have a child. It should be ascertained whether intercourse is practiced so frequently as to keep the well nearly dry, or if it occurs with any reasonable relation to the ovulation period.

Data concerning the wife's reproductive record are invaluable, not only as concerns her present condition but in past marriages, for example. Perhaps she has been found gynecologically normal, and/or the husband has had previous examinations for infertility, and if so, reports of the sperm counts and other findings at that time should be known.

In the physical examination inspection of the body will disclose the growth of hair, breast development, adiposity, general body contour, external genital development, and especially penile formation or malformation as in pronounced hypospadias. One also notes the presence, size, texture, and position of the testicle(s), inflammation of the epididymides, status of the vas deferens, prostate and seminal vesicles. Finally, the examination of the semen is performed.

Laboratory Tests. The most important are (1) the urinalysis including culture, (2) examination of the prostatic fluid especially for pus content, and (3) semen analysis. Additional tests which may become indicated by the initial examination findings include a blood Wassermann, basal metabolism study, blood count, postcoital study of spermatic migration, blood sugar tolerance, x-ray of the sella turcica, urine assay for 17-ketosteroids or for gonadotropic and estrogenic hormones or substances.

Semen Analysis. Specimen collection: Preferably this is taken as a fresh masturbation specimen obtained in the office; afford the patient locked-in bathroom privacy. If this does not work, a condom specimen can be obtained if the rubber is first boiled in a sodium bicarbonate solution to get rid of the spermatocidal oils it usually contains. Or the patient may collect the specimen in a large-mouth jar at home by masturbation or by coitus and withdrawal. He should abstain from intercourse for four to five days before the specimen is collected. Guarding against chilling of the specimen is unimportant.

Examination of the specimen thus collected is given in detail in most laboratory manuals such as Todd and Sanford. The amount of the specimen, its pH (I use nitrazine paper), and its viscosity are estimated; the last reflects the fibrinolysin enzyme activity in the prostatic fluid. The rapidity of change from a highly viscous to a watery solution may be an important observation.

A drop of semen is then placed on a slide, covered with a thin coverslip, and thus the motility of the spermatozoa is studied, the chief points of interest being the character of the activity, whether sluggish or aggressive, the percentage of motile cells as well as immotile and abnormal cells, and the duration of activity. In half the cases motility will persist for at least twelve hours.

An accurate spermatic cell count is made by using the Neubauer white blood counting chamber and pipette. The semen is well-mixed by shaking, is then taken in to the zero mark half way up the pipette. The chamber of the pipette is then filled (sucked up) with a mixture of saturated solution of sodium bicarbonate and 1 per cent phenol. The cell count is carried out by the same technique used in counting white blood cells. Five blocks of the sixteen large square units are counted for spermatozoa and six ciphers are added to this number which will give the number of spermatozoa per cubic centimeter of sperm. Cells are also stained and fixed for comparative study of their morphology as to maturity or anomalous formation. This may be done by Harris' hematoxylin or Meyer's hematoxylin stain techniques to be found in laboratory manuals. It must be recognized that the value of the counts is only relative; the normalcy of the morphology of the spermatozoa and their physical aggressiveness are primary considerations.

In carrying out the semen analysis certain data are of prime importance.

Normally the *volume* of seminal output should be between 3 and 4 cc.; less than 2.5 cc. nearly always means a low count, that is, less than 30 to 40 million sperm per cubic centimeter. The data from MacLeod's studies as shown in Table 13 indicate the wide range of count in fertile and infertile males. This table from MacLeod and Gold suggests their evaluation of seminal specimens as based upon an extensive study.

Study and experience have shown that a young adult male with a sperm count of less than 20 million per cubic centimeter is unlikely to bring about conception.

Testicular biopsy is now employed widely by students of infertility as it enables an accurate anatomic and prognostic diagnosis to be made in nearly every case, serving to distinguish congenital aspermia from the

TABLE 13. FERTILITY AS INDICATED BY SPERM COUNT (MACLEOD)

	COUNT/CC. IN MILLIONS	% ACTIVE CELLS	% NORMAL CELLS
Poor	Less than 20	Less than 40	Less than 60
Adequate	20–39	40–59	60–79
Good	40+	60+	80+

failure of delivery of sperm because of anatomic blockage or disease, as in epididymitis. Testicular biopsy also enables evaluation of disturbances of the endocrine system as the testicle is involved. While testicular biopsy is not a reliable guide to therapy, the discovery of a thoroughly hopeless azoospermic or aspermic testicle with absence or hyalinization of the seminiferous tubules as in Klinefelter's syndrome, or of congenital hypoplasia of the testicle, congenital aplasia, arrest of spermatogenic development, or widespread peritubular fibrosis with tubular replacement by connective tissue, for example, will spare the patient extensive, expensive, and fruitless therapeutic tests.

Medical Treatment. Unfortunately the medical treatment of infertility in the male is highly speculative, yet should be pursued except when testicular biopsy and repeated sperm counts indicate the hopelessness of success.

If the patient is completely aspermic (azoospermia), there is scant hope of therapeutic success. Nutritional aid by diet with added vitamins A, B complex, and E is given, as is thyroid whole gland if the basal metabolism shows thyroid deficiency. Although the employment of gonadotropins is in general unsatisfactory for the stimulation of spermatogenesis, in several patients of mine the hormone has apparently been beneficial as witnessed by improved sperm count and the achievement of fertility after months and years of apparent hopeless barrenness. The administration of testosterone to stimulate spermatogenesis is still *sub judice*. It has been observed that with the administration of relatively large amounts of testosterone (25 to 50 mg. testosterone propionate daily intramuscularly), a drop in the sperm count occurs. Yet two to four months later by "rebound," the count rises to a much higher level than it was initially and in some cases conception has occurred under this circumstance (Heckel, 1951). Prediction of the result of this therapy is quite impossible.

Surgical Treatment. This consists chiefly in prophylaxis by placing improperly descended testes in the scrotum by the third or fourth year of age, remembering that testicular maturation begins about the fifth year. Treatment of prostatitis, lower urinary tract obstruction and particularly urethral stricture is sometimes all that is needed.

Vaso-epididymal anastomosis is fruitful in about 25 per cent of the cases in which the epididymis is blocked off by an old inflammatory scar, especially in gonococcus epididymitis. In failure of urogenital union (q.v.), vaso-epididymal anastomosis might conceivably be of help in some cases. The anastomosis procedure is indicated only when testicular biopsy shows that normal spermatogenesis is taking place in the testicle, and urologic examination indicates blockage of the seminiferous tract, this usually being in the epididymis. In successful cases, sperm will usually be found in the ejaculate after eight to ten weeks postoperatively and often increase greatly in numbers as free spermatic drainage is maintained. But they may subsequently disappear should postoperative stricturization occur at the site of anastomosis.

MASTURBATION

This, the so-called secret vice because people don't talk much about it and it is characteristically conducted in private, is common to all animals, races, ages, and both sexes. The studies of Kinsey et al. (1948) suggest that 92 per cent of the population at some time or other has engaged in masturbation to the point of orgasm. Many reputable psychiatrists infer that everybody is or has been at some time a masturbator and do not attach much importance to the act. Certainly its dangers have usually been greatly exaggerated to the child, what with the threat of insanity, weakness, or pimples on the face; too often some local mental incompetent is pointed out as the horrible end result of masturbation. On the other hand, in older children and adults, masturbation even in moderation leaves its imprint of inferiority and in excess, its trail of pathologic changes especially in the urethra, prostate, verumontanum, seminal vesicles in males, and labia and urethra in females.

In infants and young children masturbation is frequently practiced by thigh friction or thigh rubbing, while in older children it is performed by manual manipulation of the genitals, but it is rarely a sex conscious act before the seventh or eighth year. About 90 per cent of infants who masturbate are girls while in later childhood the ratio is reversed, becoming about even in adults.

In general in children, masturbation has been frequently attributed to local irritation of balanitis, phimosis, adherent prepuce, vesical or urethral stones, rectal worms and constipation. Commonly the indulgence is acquired and persisted in because accidentally it was found pleasurable. Sometimes the nurse inaugurates the habit to keep the child quiet and in older children it results from the example of companions. The act is recognized as an antisocial manifestation, precisely as is enuresis, encopresis, truancy, juvenile criminality, reflecting parental neuroticism, excess parental disciplinary compulsion, dislike for another individual, frequently a bossy mother, or as a depreciation of the opposite sex, but in all instances reflecting that the child feels insecure, unwanted or unloved.

As important as are the psychologic aspects of masturbation, the organic changes it may induce by habitual or excessive practice merit grave consideration. The tissue changes induced by habitual masturbation are phases of chronic pelvic congestion and include leathery balanitis, traumatic urethritis, prostatitis, seminal vesiculitis, verumontanitis, orchalgia, varicocele, vaginitis, leathery type of Hottentot labia, congestive salpingitis, oophoritis, pelvic varices and so forth. The clinical picture of lower abdominal pain, backache, urinary frequency, and dysmenorrhea perhaps, reflects the anatomic changes produced by habitual masturbation.

Diagnosis is suggested by these tissue changes as well as by the observation of a child or an adult who is continually arranging his genitalia, but most cases pass unrecognized. Some patients when directly accused will admit the practice.

Treatment of masturbation depends to a large extent upon the age of the patient. In infants no attention need be paid to the practice; in young children the important consideration is diversion of the attention from the genitalia by creation of an interest in games and play and without punishment or parental emotional display toward the habit. In short, in the young, the chief therapeutic effort must be placed on the shoulders of the parents as in the treatment of enuresis (q.v.); in adults the treatment is usually by substitution of normal sexual outlet together with treatment of the congestive damage of the genital tract the habit may have inflicted, that is, treatment of prostatitis, seminal vesiculitis, sterilization of the urine and so on.

Thus, the treatment properly should entail a complete examination to determine any local causes of masturbation which must be eliminated. This may mean circumcision or the removal of urethral or vesical neck obstruction, stones or foreign bodies, correction of constipation, neutralization or alkalinization of highly irritant acid urine, or the elimination of intestinal parasites. The irritation of prostatitis may perpetuate the habit and require local treatment. A clue as to the intelligence and psychologic peculiarities may be the benefit of a mental examination.

In patients of all ages the cure is indirect and with the inculcation of self-reliance, overlooking temporary discouragement, and in children avoiding not only punishment but the giving of rewards, the employment of fear, criticism, a superior attitude, or, above all, a discussion of the child's problem within his hearing. In the case of a child all measures are apt to be fruitless unless the child receives an abundance of parental affection, care, and love and is afforded a sense of security and of being wanted. Unless parents can fulfill these considerations, the child remains under a handicapping emotional strain certain to be manifested by undesirable behavior whether masturbation, enuresis, vandalism, thieving or otherwise. When there is no demonstrable organic cause and conservative medical treatment fails, psychiatric investigation and therapy should be employed but as a final rather than as an initial step.

CHAPTER 9 *Neuromuscular Uropathy*

NEUROMUSCULAR disease of the urinary tract is of far higher incidence than commonly recognized, is always potentially serious, often actually grave, treatment is generally unsatisfactory, and in a discouraging large number of patients there is no hope of cure. In infants and children neuromuscular uropathy results predominantly from anomalies of spinal fusion with (1) failure of neurovertebral development, or (2) secondary involvement of the neural structures of the lumbosacral cord. As indicated on page 345 the condition may be acquired as it usually is in adults, and caused by irritative, degenerative or inflammatory lesions of the spinal cord or peripheral nerves: chiefly cord injuries, tumors, myelitis and syringomyelia. The first group, the traumatic cases, are of ever-increasing incidence not only with more motor vehicle accidents but injuries incurred during work, and falling in large measure within the authority of the Workmen's Compensation Act. The beds of the Veterans Administration hospitals are even today well filled with patients with paraplegia and other grave neurologic conditions incurred in World War II; during the past decade thousands initially in these hospitals have died from these injuries (renal infection and urinary calculous disease) while many others are still hospitalized outside the government domain or are invalid at home.

All of these nerve lesions produce changes in the urinary tract which are recognized as (1) atrophic, or (2) the result of urinary stasis or back pressure (see Chapter 5), and are generally complicated and accelerated by (3) infection. It is axiomatic that in neuromuscular disease of the urinary tract infection can be anticipated in every case and its control or eradication is a fundamental of intelligent treatment. In this chapter we are concerned principally with the clinical considerations of neuromuscular uropathy, recognizing that complicating infection and obstruc-

337

tion (acute or chronic pyelonephritis, stricture, stone or prostatism, for example) are likely to overshadow the basic neural condition and of themselves be serious therapeutic problems.

Neurophysiology of the pelvis and ureter has been discussed in Chapter 4.

Hypertonia of the ureter is reflected by stronger and more frequent peristaltic contractions, occurs in acute ureteral or periureteral inflammation, or in acute obstruction such as produced by calculi or kinks. Disturbances of extrarenal innervation by inflammation, stone, or other irritating agents may, by stimulation of the renal sympathetic nerve supply, induce reflex persistent contraction or spasm of the musculature (1) surrounding the necks of the calyces to cause hydrocalycosis or (2) of the pelvic outlet to engender hydronephrosis.

Atony of the ureter is characterized by localized or generalized, diminished or completely suspended contractility of the duct. It is almost always accompanied by dilatation which may be enormous. Atony may be (1) congenital or primary, or (2) acquired or secondary.

Congenital or **primary atony** is most often bilateral and the renal pelvis may or may not participate in the dilatation (Fig. 196). The ureter achieves its highest degree of dilatation in advanced congenital atony

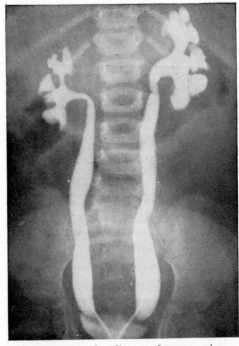

FIGURE 196.   Atonic neuromuscular disease of upper urinary tract associated with bilateral achalasia at the ureterovesical junction. The ureterovesical junction readily accommodated an 11 F. ureteral bulb without difficulty. Mild secondary infection. The lateral ureteral dilatation in the absence of longitudinal dilatation is believed by some to signify an atonic neuromuscular rather than obstructive (ureterovesical junction) condition. The author does not attach great importance to this observation or distinction.

which is commonly designated as *primary megaloureter* to distinguish it from the obstructive variety. Although a large number of these cases has been reported under the title primary megaloureter, few indeed of these bear close scrutiny as in nearly all there is coexisting neuromuscular vesical involvement of which the ureteral manifestations are but a part. The characteristics of congenital ureteral atony are (1) large, rigid, gaping, immobile ureteral orifices, (2) altered ureteral dynamics, (3) free vesico-ureteral reflux, and (4) ureteral dilatation which is predominantly transverse with little or no ureteral lengthening, angulation or kinking. These features are readily demonstrable by cystoscopy (meatoscopy) and cystography. Yet these conditions may be encountered *in toto* in some cases of chronic urinary infection without a neuromuscular background and disappear following eradication of the infection.

Primary megaloureter has been ascribed to dysplasia or functional disturbance of the neuromuscular mechanism of the ureter in a manner analogous to congenital dilatation of the colon (megacolon, Hirschsprung's disease) but in which parasympathetic agangliosis of the spastic segment has been demonstrated (Swenson et al., 1952). We have seen several instances of Hirschsprung's disease in the young with neuromuscular disease of the urinary tract but always including the bladder.

Dysplasia of the ureteral musculature has also been adduced to explain primary megaloureter. Until the third or fourth month of fetal life the ureters are wide in comparison to the rest of the body, and they are devoid of musculature until the second month. Shortly thereafter fibers appear at the vesical end, and by the sixth month the entire ureter and pelvis have acquired their definitive musculature. It is believed *congenital megaloureter* results when (1) the muscular development of the ureter is incompleted, (2) the fibers are hypoplastic, (3) the coating is unusually thin or (4) the enormous dilatation of the early months of fetal life simply fails to disappear. Yet the condition is seldom recognized in the living until changes due to urinary stasis or infection have occurred to complicate the picture.

Acquired ureteral atony is secondary to neuromuscular vesical disease, acute or chronic ureteral obstruction (e.g., ureteral stone), or even an obstruction at the vesical outlet or peripherally. The atonic changes are intensified by infection and urinary stasis, and especially when prolonged.

NEUROMUSCULAR VESICAL UROPATHY

Axiom: In neuromuscular disease of the urinary tract the bladder must always be considered primarily involved until proved otherwise.

Knowledge of the neuro-anatomy and normal physiology of the bladder is fundamental for (1) correct interpretation of the urologic findings and, perhaps even more important, (2) for rational treatment. While treatment in a large portion of patients with neuromuscular uropathy can be only palliative rather than curative, the early recognition of the disease permits the institution of rational therapy which generally promotes improvement; in some instances cure will be achieved before irreparable damage is done and, in nearly all instances, symptomatic relief can be afforded.

Nerve Supply of the Bladder. This is independently bilateral, its components being (1) autonomic (a) sympathetic and (b) parasympathetic), and (2) somatic.

The *autonomic nerve supply* of the bladder and adjacent urethra follows the embryologic formula: the sympathetics supply the structures of wolffian duct origin (trigone, ureteral orifices, seminal vesicles, prostate, and ejaculatory ducts), while the parasympathetics predominantly innervate the detrusor of cloaco-allantoic derivation. Both sympathetic and parasympathetic pathways convey sensations of pain as well as of vesical distention. The sensory and motor nerves of direct spinal origin constitute the *somatic innervation* which is largely confined to the vesical outlet, deep urethra, external vesical sphincter, and accessory perineal muscles. Suprasegmental pathways join these lower systems with higher centers in the cord, cerebral cortex, and especially the lower part of the midbrain—the cortico-vesical center which controls urination and governs bladder tonus having been localized near the leg center. The nerve supply of the bladder is schematically shown in Figure 197.

Sympathetic Innervation. The sympathetic system arises in the

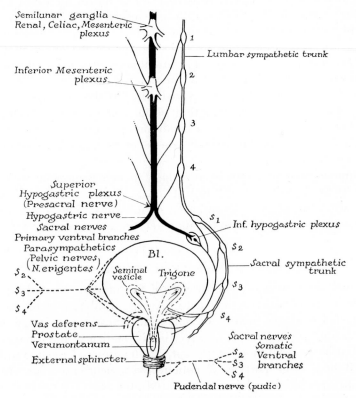

FIGURE 197.   Innervation of the urinary tract. Schematic representation.

lateral horn cells of the gray matter of the spinal cord from which the fibers pass from the cord to the anterior roots in the thoracolumbar region (dorsal 11, 12; lumbar 1, 2). From the first dorsal to the second lumbar region nonmeduled or white rami communicantes pass as preganglionic fibers to the paravertebral, celiac, mesenteric, and renal plexuses. From these plexic ganglia fibers go downward preaortic to the level of the aortic bifurcation to form the superior hypogastric plexus, sometimes known as the *presacral nerve* (Fig. 197). This group of nerves, composed of a variable number of separate small trunks, curves over the sacral promontory to become the hypogastric nerve and shortly the inferior hypogastric plexus on each side. Sympathetic neurons pass with the parasympathetic fibers bilaterally down through the pelvic plexus to give off small branches which are the sympathetic innervation of the bladder, prostate, seminal vesicles, posterior urethra and, in the female, the uterus. Sympathetic fibers accompany the vesical arteries: this probably technically precludes total sympathetic denervation of the bladder.

Section of the sympathetic fibers (resection of the presacral nerve) causes relaxation of the structures just noted with no changes in the bladder wall, the effects being even less notable postoperatively in women. Thus the physiologic activity of the sympathetic vesical innervation is of slight or no importance in urination, being concerned fundamentally with the activity of the trigone and lower ureter, vasomotor control, and ejaculation.

Parasympathetic Innervation. These, the important nerves of micturition, are derived from cells in the lateral gray matter of the cord from which neurons pass out on each side through the ventral roots of the second, third, and fourth sacral segments to form the presacral ganglia (pelvic nerves or *nervi erigentes*). Parasympathetic fibers pass from here to the pelvic plexus from which on each side they are distributed to peripheral ganglia in the bladder wall and vesical outlet (Fig. 197). Complete bilateral severance of the parasympathetic vesical innervation produces urinary retention with overflow, later to be followed by increased tonicity of the bladder wall (autonomous bladder) and a spontaneous reflex evacuation (automatic bladder). Voluntary urination is impossible but can be performed when the parasympathetic interruption is unilateral. With bilateral loss of parasympathetic control and chronic vesical retention, hypertrophy of the bladder wall occurs with a persistence of feeble contraction waves, attributed to the operation of an intrinsic network of nerves in the bladder wall, the unusual change ultimately ending in muscular atony.

Tactile, thermal, and the important sensory elements of the urinary tract pass through the sympathetics, while division of the parasympathetic or pelvic nerves largely deprives the bladder of its normal motility and sensation, converting it into a variably atonic sac. Section of the spinal cord or brain stem at levels up to the pons produces the same results and reflects the maintenance of normal detrusor tone by the brain centers.

Somatic Nerve Supply. This is both sensory and motor to the bladder and is largely through the pudendal (pudic) trunks. Sensory stimuli reaching the central nervous system through the somatic, sympathetic and parasympathetic nerve trunks may, by synaptic overflow, excite motor response in several spinal segments. As demonstrated by tetraethylammonium chloride blocking of the autonomic nerve impulse transmission, the sensory somatic nerves are both anatomically and physiologically apart from the autonomic. Of clinical importance, particularly in spinal fractures and cord tumors, is the observation that *interruption of the spinal tracts at the sixth thoracic level abolishes all visceral sensation and with a similar lesion lower down at the eleventh thoracic level, bladder sensation is abolished.* This places the chief sensory fibers of the inferior hypogastric plexus between the eleventh thoracic and third lumbar cord levels.

The sacral somatic sensory nerves arise bilaterally as posterior primary divisions of the second, third and fourth sacral nerves to form with the motor fibers the *pudendal nerve trunk* which subsequently divides into the perineal nerve and the dorsal nerve of the penis or clitoris. The pudendal nerves carry muscle sense and superficial sensation from the bladder dome together with sensory fibers to the penis, perineum, posterior urethra and trigone. Bilateral injury of these nerves produces saddle anesthesia of the perineum and other structures they innervate although a sense of vesical distention may remain mediated through the autonomics (persistent sensation in the trigone and adjacent bladder). The pudic nerves also transmit proprioceptive sensations from the external sphincter and functional accessory structures, especially the penile corpora, bulbocavernosus and ischiocavernosus muscles.

The somatic system *motor innervation* is derived from anterior branches of the second to fourth sacral nerves which join with the sensory nerves just described to form the pudendal or internal pudic nerve. A division, the perineal nerve, gives off branches to the external sphincter, corpus cavernosum, bulbocavernosus (compressor urethrae) and ischiocavernosus muscles. Although maintaining tonus of the external sphincter muscle, section of these pudic nerves causes slight or no urinary incontinence.

Because of their common embryologic derivation from hind gut, there is intimate segmental relationship of the nerves of the bladder, external genitalia, and rectum. Thus, pain of vesical inflammation and irritation is often referred to the area supplied by the perineal divisions of the pudic and inferior gluteal nerves, or through the inferior hemorrhoidal nerve to the rectum. Similarly, rectal lesions such as fissures, worms and the like may reflexly cause vesical disturbances, notably urinary frequency, occasionally enuresis, and rarely acute retention. Despite experimental evidence suggesting that the pudic nerves can be cut with impunity, in operating by the perineal route due precautions should be observed to preserve these nerves. This is done largely by using a midline incision which begins behind the central point of the perineum and passes backward toward the lateral rectal margin rather than toward the ischial tuberosities.

The *supersegmental tracts* must be considered in vesical dysfunction, for the lesions of the upper neuron segments produce spastic paralysis with hypertonia. In cord lesions involving the posterior column segments with loss of sensory components as in tabes for example, loss of the supersegmental conditioning reflex results in inadequate inhibition of the sensory reflex so that the patient reflexly voids without knowing it. Cortical and upper sensory lesions may, but do not always, cause painful frequency with spasticity of the vesical detrusor, and lower spinal lesions often cause paralysis with atony, vesical retention, and incontinence with overflow. Lower neuron lesions (sacral) produce hypotonia, atony or flaccid paralysis. In acquired neuromuscular vesical disease the clinical picture is usually patchy, depending upon the nature and severity of the onset, as in injury for example, and the prodromal duration. It is seldom that an accurate topical diagnosis can be made until the disease is firmly established.

Physiology of the Bladder and Urination. The desire to urinate is dependent upon intracystic pressure (tension of the vesical wall) rather than upon the fluid-volume content.

The function of the bladder is to receive urine from the ureters, retain it and, under voluntary control, periodically to discharge it. The average *physiologic capacity* is about twice the volume at which the first desire to void is felt, that is, about half the anatomic capacity. In extensive cystometric studies, I (1937) found that children eight to ten years of age have the initial desire to void at an intracystic pressure of 9 to 11 cm. of water, the bladder volume varying between 80 to 100 cc. in comparison to the values of the adult, 15.5 to 16 cm. of water pressure with 140 to 180 cc. of fluid volume.

The vesical capacity and frequency of urination are vastly influenced by reflex, psychic, and local irritative factors.

Normally the bladder wall exhibits wavelike contractions of variable rhythm which increase in intensity and frequency as filling occurs. As the physiologic capacity is approached these contractions become stronger and increase the intracystic pressure sufficient to cause, by stretch reflex, the desire to urinate to be registered in consciousness. Until this point in bladder filling is reached, voiding is prevented by subconscious inhibition through the spinal tract from the brain to the sacral reflex center (lateral horn synapses).

With vesical distention, voluntary cerebral inhibition becomes active causing firm contraction of the external sphincter and perineal muscles. In voluntary urination there is willful relaxation of this cerebral inhibition, and urination occurs with contraction of the detrusor, shortening of the longitudinal fibers of which at the vesical outlet brings about opening of the orifice.

The most widely accepted explanation of the mechanism in voluntary urination is as follows (Denny Brown and Robertson, 1933): The external sphincter (compressor urethrae muscle) is inhibited (relaxed) through cerebral impulses transmitted by the parasympathetic nervi erigentes, aided by voluntary impulses carried through the pudic nerve. Inhibition of the external sphincter through the sympathetics or passively has also been experimentally shown to occur (Gruber). At any rate, without vesical contraction and expulsion of urine into the deep urethra, urination does not normally take place. Urine in the deep urethra is not an essential part of the urinary act, for in many patients following transurethral resection of the bladder neck, for example, urine is constantly in the prostatic canal but the patient remains continent because the external sphincter is competent. Contraction and simultaneous shortening of the trigone or of Bell's muscles (the ureteral ridges) coincident with detrusor contraction depresses the lower segment of the vesical outlet (so-called internal sphincter), flattens the uvula and literally pulls open the internal vesical orifice. Depression of the vesical neck is further added by contraction of the levator ani muscles, and abdominal muscular contraction helps to express the urine. The deep urethra in the male is emptied by the voluntary strong milking stroke brought about by contraction of the accessory urethral and perineal muscles.

Some (Lewis, 1945; Emmett et al., 1948, and others) have described vesical emptying as the concentric opening of the bladder outlet as a result of foreshortening of the longitudinal bladder musculature consequent to general detrusor contraction, the muscular segment of the bladder outlet being composed of (1) the thick edge of the detrusor urinae muscle which exhibits striking concentric contractility, and (2) the concentric contracting muscular components of the prostatic urethra.

Reflex urination occurs *in utero* shortly after the fifth month when urinary secretion begins. Urination in infants is a lower reflex arc phenomenon believed to function through autonomic extraspinal centers so that the bladder empties itself with the first stimulus of the desire to void, and in the neonatal period this may be every twenty to forty minutes or less. Cerebral voluntary control is usually established by the age of thirty months. It is seldom justifiable to consider a child less than four years old as enuretic and in some children normal bladder control may not be established by puberty.

Varieties of Bladder Disturbances. These may be classified according to etiology as congenital, acquired or unknown. Many classifications have been devised on the basis of *tonus* as (1) hypertonic or spastic, (2) hypotonic or atonic. No present classification of neuromuscular disease is adequately comprehensive nor satisfactorily descriptive as, for example, tabetic cord bladder may also be clinically atonic bladder. For practical purposes I prefer to employ the groupings as (1) cord bladder in which demonstrable disease of the central nervous system causes vesical dysfunction, and (2) idiopathic atonic bladder in which there is no somatically demonstrable neurogenic lesion except that the vesical motor activity is reduced without notable change in sensation. Here the etiologic lesion whether congenital, inflammatory, mechanical or unknown is presumably in the motor peripheral nerves or in the terminal vesical intramural nerve network and without striking sensory changes. In this last group it is probable that the enormously dilated atonic thin-walled bladder is not always the result of disease in the intrinsic vesical nerve network, but is due to unrecognized nonneurogenic, or cystoscopically unrecognized obstruction at the vesical outlet. Yet, fortunately and despite difficulties of academic classification, this last group usually responds satisfactorily to treatment by transurethral resection of the vesical outlet.

According to etiology, neuromuscular vesical disorders may be classified as:

A. *Congenital*   I. Malformation or dysplasia of the brain, spinal cord, nerves, or spine. The changes in the peripheral nerves or cord are commonly concomitant with the vertebral condition.
               II. Neuromuscular dysplasia of the bladder wall without demonstrable cause or associated maldevelopment of the cord and nerves.
              III. Infection, as syphilis.

B. *Acquired*   I. Toxic nerve injury produced by
                  a. Infection (e.g., anterior poliomyelitis, syphilis, diphtheria)
                  b. Inflammation
                      1. Spontaneous neuritis, myelitis not due to (a)
                      2. Poisons (lead, arsenic, and the like; very rare)
             II. Trauma (e.g., spinal fracture or other cord injury)
           III. Tumors of or involving the nervous system
          IV. Degenerative lesions (syringomyelia, etc.)

C. *Unknown (idiopathic, a large group)*

Congenital Neuromuscular Vesical Disorders

Spina Bifida. Congenital malformation of the spinal central nervous system is almost always accompanied by vertebral maldevelopment. In normal embryonic closure of the neural tube, the surface epithelium of the lips of the neural groove unites in the midline, and failure of the tube to close properly results in spina bifida, meningocele, myelocele, meningomyelocele, and syringomyelocele (Fig. 198). In meningocele the tube closes but with a bulging at the point last to unite and this corresponds to an anal organ defect in vertebral fusion. With incomplete fusion of the mesodermal vertebral arches, spina bifida results and may occur at any point and involve the anterior as well as the posterior segments of the vertebrae.

Spina bifida occulta, the mildest form of vertebral defect, occurs in approximately a third of all individuals but is rarely of clinical concern.

True spina bifida occurs about once in 1500 individuals, and in these cases is apt to be clinically manifested by functional disturbances of the bladder and rectum and/or of the lower extremities (Figs. 199, 200). While calcification of the vertebral arches may be lacking, there is usually a fibrous layer which bridges over the imperfection. In half the cases there is dimpling at the site of the spina bifida, often with hypertrichiasis, pigmentation, or scarring of the overlying skin and, when present, it is pathognomonic of spina bifida. Occasionally a congenital dermal sinus, with or without epidermoid or dermal cyst (pilonidal) occurs at the point of sacral defect. Lipomatous deposits at the point of neural arch malformation are extremely common in spina bifida as in all congenital defects of the vertebral axis. These fatty inclusions are continuous with the subcutaneous fatty layer of the glutei, nearly always penetrate the dura, and are attached to the conus. Masses of intraspinal lipomatous tissue may also be present, varying in size and in the production of compression symptoms as the patient substantially gains or loses weight.

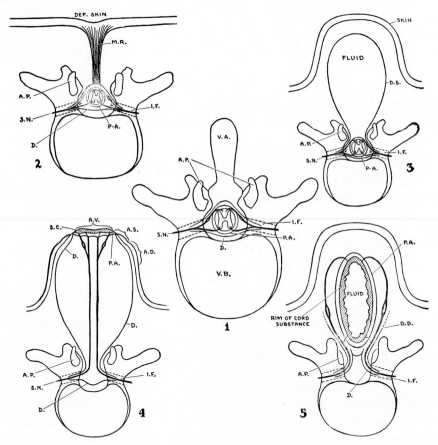

FIGURE 198. Congenital defects of the lumbosacral spine. *1*, normal relationships. *V.B.*, vertebral body; *V.A.*, vertebral arch; *A.P.*, articular processes; *D*, dura mater; *P.A.*, pia mater; *S.N.*, spinal nerve; *I.F.*, intervertebral foramen.

2, spina bifida. The depression of the overlying skin is indicated, also the membrana reuniens (*M.R.*)—fibrous tissue passing from the skin to the dura.

3, meningocele. Bulging of the dural sac (*D.S.*) and of the overlying skin is indicated.

4, myelomeningocele. The spinal cord (*S.C.*) is exposed. *A.V.*, area vasculosa; *A.S.*, area serosa; *A.D.*, area dermatica.

5, syringomyelocele. The spinal cord is distended with fluid; the dural defect (*D.D.*) is one of incompletion (composited after Fraser).

Anomalies of other systems frequently coexist with spina bifida. They are often incompatible with life. Spinal cord tumors such as lipomas, fibromas, angiomas, chondromas, teratomas, dermoids, sacrococcygeal cysts, predominantly congenital, are sometimes found at the point of vertebral defect. Cartilage or aberrant neural elements are often engulfed in the fibrous mass. The vesical and rectal dysfunction is chiefly of the paralytic variety often with paralysis or weakness of the legs and, commonly, clubfoot. Many of these children are subnormal mentally and otherwise in poor health.

The fatty deposits described in the second preceding paragraph, as well as the accompanying perineural fibrosis suggest a protective mechanism of Nature to close over the vertebral gap. On the other hand, by nerve traction, compression and functional interruption, these conditions commonly cause clinical disturbances in the peripheral structures they innervate, notably by inducing irritative lesions of the posterior primary divisions of the sacral roots when the injury is moderate, or complete sensory paralysis when the nerve damage is total.

In the *irritative* variety there may be pain and paresthesia over the distribution of the involved nerves and by reflex mechanism through

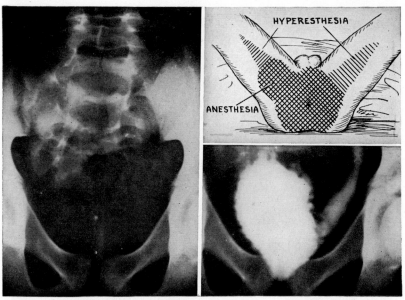

| Fig. 199 | Fig. 200 |

FIGURE 199.   Advanced neuromuscular vesical disease secondary to congenital malformation of the sacrum (lateral deviation and curvature) in an eleven-year-old boy examined because of persistent enuresis and pyuria. The malformation resulted in moderate sensory loss of the five sacral nerves and caused cutaneous sensory changes of the saddle type (diagram)

FIGURE 200.   Advanced neuromuscular vesical disease secondary to congenital malformation of the sacrum. Cystographically is demonstrated relaxation of the vesical outlet with funneling of the posterior urethra, marked trabeculation of the bladder wall with numerous cellules, and vesico-ureteral reflux.

the autonomic nerves, vesical hypertonia with enuresis or even true incontinence. As the lesion progresses, nerve degeneration ensues, there
is variable anesthesia over the sacral nerve distribution, vesical retention
sometimes with overflow, and there may be true paralytic incontinence.

Nerve lesions in spina bifida are attributable to traction, compression
or faulty myelinization. Traction is produced by the vertebral growth
process. The conus in the fetus lies at the fourth lumbar vertebral level,
normally comes to rest at the twelfth dorsal to second lumbar level but,
with fixation of the nerve roots at the site of vertebral defect, traction is
exerted on them by the receding conus. As a result of this traction there
is mechanical compression and stretching of the nerves. At first this
produces an irritative syndrome but with advancing nerve damage,
paralytic manifestations. The fibrolipomatous masses which are nearly
always present at the site of vertebral defect cause further compression
of the nerves, and the removal of these masses alone is sometimes followed by improvement in nerve function.

Meningocele is a more advanced lesion than spina bifida, is characterized by midline protrusion of the dura or the dura and pia arachnoid

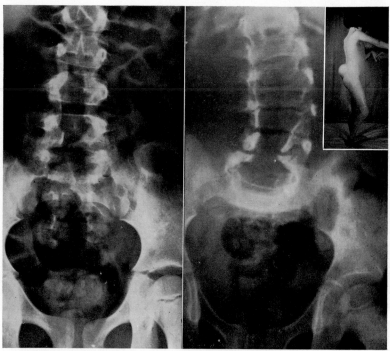

Fig. 201   Fig. 202

FIGURE 201.   Spina bifida occulta. In an eight-year-old boy examined because of
enuresis. There is incomplete spinal fusion from the first sacral vertebra down; the lumbar
vertebra are normally fused.

FIGURE 202.   Neuromuscular vesical disease. Meningocele in a three-year-old girl
with profound neuromuscular vesical disease (chronic complete retention and overflow).
Pressure on this lumbar mass caused headache by increasing the intracranial pressure.

through the vertebral cleft with a collection of spinal fluid in the dural sac, either posterior or anterior to the cord or both and, according to the site of defect, may attain a diameter of 6 or 7 inches (Figs. 201, 202). A thin layer of skin usually covers the dome of the protrusion but sometimes there is leakage of spinal fluid with cutaneous redness, maceration and infection. Bladder disturbances are less common in meningocele above the sacral level than in sacral spina bifida or sacral meningocele.

Myelocele is a more serious malformation than meningocele and as schematically shown in Figure 198, there is protrusion of the pia mater, dura arachnoid, and posterior segments of the spinal cord roots through the posterior vertebral defect.

Syringomyelocele or **myelosyringocele** is the most profound of these neurovertebral malformations and is formed as a protrusion of the spinal membranes and the cord in which the central canal of the cord is greatly distended by fluid to cause compression nerve atrophy. The mass is often smaller than meningocele, is not always in the midline, may be covered with normal skin, and always produces grave neurologic disturbances.

As a result of these neurovertebral malformations, there are commonly produced in neurodependent structures (1) sensory changes (anesthesia, hyperesthesia, paresthesia), (2) motor changes (hypertonia, muscular spasm, hypotonia or paralysis), and (3) atrophic changes. *Edema* in the local area suggests vascular changes while cutaneous ulceration and/or a drainage sinus in the anesthetic area reflect atrophic changes.

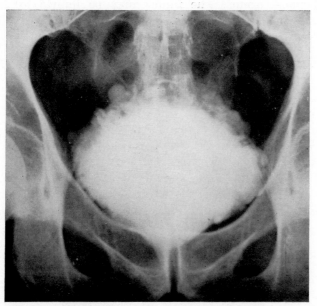

FIGURE 203. Tabetic bladder as cystographically demonstrated in a sixty-year-old man with urinary leakage. Advanced trabeculation of bladder wall and slight paralytic funneling of vesical outlet.

Neuromuscular dysplasia or **primary atony of the bladder** is believed to be etiologic in many cases of vesical disturbances or distention in the absence of demonstrable obstruction or central nervous system disease. It has been likened to primary ureteral atony (q.v.) and the two may coexist. Dysplasia of the terminal neurons and end organs in the bladder wall has been adduced to explain the congenitally thin vesical musculature composed of hypoplastic muscle cells. Vesical amyotonia is frequently observed as a manifestation of amyotonia congenita (Oppenheim's disease) in which the anterior horn cells fail to develop normally and particularly in the lower cord segments. In Werdnig-Hoffmann progressive muscular atrophy, there is progressive degeneration of the anterior horn cells, especially in the lower cord, and simulates Oppenheim's disease.

Congenital syphilis is usually fatal in the early months of life and is rarely a cause of neuromuscular vesical disease. A few instances of juvenile tabes of this genesis have been reported.

In tabes dorsalis and other forms of central nervous system syphilis, usually acquired, the vesical disturbances—chiefly retention and/or incontinence—are the initial symptoms in a fourth of all cases, and death generally results from urinary infection and renal failure (Fig. 203).

ACQUIRED CAUSES OF NEUROMUSCULAR VESICAL DYSFUNCTION

Nontraumatic nerve injuries may be produced by (1) infection, (2) inflammation without bacterial invasion, or (3) neurotoxic damage by virus or chemical agents. The injury may be limited to the central nervous system (multiple sclerosis, syphilis, anterior poliomyelitis, men-

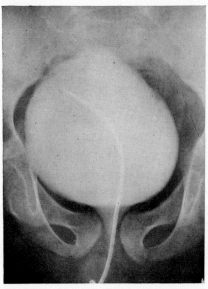

FIGURE 204. Cystogram in a four-year-old boy with vesical paralysis consequent to anterior poliomyelitis. Four ounces residual urine. Paralysis of the vesical outlet is indicated by cystographic funneling. Urinary incontinence.

ingitis, Landry's paralysis, myelitis) or to the peripheral nerves but both may be involved (Figs. 204, 205). With lateral spinal column involvement in the congestive or engorgement stage of poliomyelitis, for example, temporary urinary incontinence often occurs and sometimes the vesical paralysis persists. Myelitis may occur in measles, influenza, pertussis, scarlet fever, pneumonia, vaccinia, varicella, mumps or diphtheria, in toxic chemical poisoning by lead, bismuth, arsenic or alcohol. Neurotoxic vesical disturbances sometimes occur in the primary anemias, diabetes, or even with horse-serum paralysis.

Vesical Spasm. In the absence of acute infection, vesical spasm results from reflex sphincter spasm with inability to void. The exciting agent may be vesical or renal calculi, vesical foreign bodies, highly concentrated irritating urine, inflammation or obstruction of the vesical outlet or peripherally in the urethra, disturbances of the rectum, especially fissures and worms, vulvar, or juxta-vesical disease such as appendicitis. Detrusor spasm may occur with complete spastic emptying, perhaps with only a few drops being passed at a time and often, and accompanied by painful residual vesical spasm.

Treatment of bladder spasm consists of (1) an increased fluid intake, (2) neutralization or change in titer of the urine, (3) hot sitz baths (water temperature 108° to 110° F. for ten minutes), (4) hot compresses over the bladder region, genitals, and/or perineum and, occasionally, (5) medication. Atropine sulfate and barbituric acid derivatives are given in spastic incontinence for sedative effect. Urecholine or other parasympathomimetic drugs (q.v.), or a rectal suppository of papaverine 10 to 25 mg. is administered in spastic retention. Catheterization is seldom indicated but one must be sure that there is no organic blockage such as a small stone jammed in the urethra or an unrecognized contracted bladder neck or adenomatous prostatic hypertrophy. With bed patients not responding satisfactorily to employment of the above procedures, it may be necessary to establish a hydraulic bladder splint which maintains a small quantity of fluid in the bladder to keep the bladder walls at rest, and prevent complete emptying with the accompanying painful spasm.

Traumatic Nerve Injuries. Spinal fracture with partial or complete maceration or section of the spinal cord is of frequent incidence in traffic accidents, falls, industrial accidents, and military activities. With complete transection of the cord there will be total sensory and motor paralysis below when the injury is at the tenth thoracic level or above. With injury below the first lumbar level the sensation of bladder filling and evacuation remains; this reflects a sensory component in the sympathetic supply of the bladder.

Cerebral injuries often cause bladder dysfunction, particularly with basal skull fractures and hypothalamic involvement. *Obstetric* injuries to the infant occur chiefly in breech presentations resulting most often from the excessive traction demanded in difficult deliveries, stretching of the spinal cord rather than compression being the usual trauma. Obstetric cerebral palsy accounts for 1 to 2 per cent of neonatal deaths. The vast majority of traumatic spinal injuries, however, occur in older children and adults and entail a high immediate mortality. They also cause a high morbidity because of the neuromuscular disturbances engendered, and particularly of the bladder with complicating neurospastic obstruction, secondary infection, later stone formation, and ultimately death in urinary sepsis.

Clinical Syndromes in Complete Transverse Spinal Injury. Promptly following receipt of injury there is (1) spinal shock followed later by (2) autonomous vesical paralysis and, still later, by (3) automatic voiding. The gravity of the patient's condition or of the traumatic changes in the central nervous system or later of complicating infection, stone formation, and so forth may terminate this clinical sequence or may kill the patient.

Spinal Shock. With complete transverse section of the spinal cord at any point from the cervical region to the third sacral level acute atonic urinary retention occurs which may persist for one to several days depending upon the gravity of the initial spinal "shock." The bladder becomes enormously distended, often well above the umbilicus, and would seem about to burst. Cerebral control is lost and there is partial or complete paralysis of the detrusor through the interrupted reflex of motor nerve function with relaxation of the bladder wall. Because the suprasegmental sensory nerve tract is divided, the bladder distention causes no pain. Paradoxical or overflow incontinence develops as renal secretion distends the vesical sphincter beyond its spastic retention point. With the development of spinal shock and complete chronic urinary retention, unrelieved, early death from urinary sepsis is likely. Therefore, do not delay indwelling catheterization to relieve the overdistention and to begin antibacterial therapy to combat infection. If the patient cannot void acceptably after a week, establish suprapubic cystostomy drainage.

Following recovery from the initial spinal shock, the bladder usually develops reflex activity which may be (1) autonomous, or (2) automatic, the type depending on the gravity of the traumatic lesion, with the initial recovery varying from twenty-four hours to as long as a year and a half.

The *autonomous bladder* develops in most cases as recovery progresses. The bladder, still cut off from the central nervous system by injury of the spinal reflex centers or by interruption of fibers comprising the reflex arc, slowly develops muscular activity with relatively feeble, irregular, uncoordinated contractions which force out some urine but do not empty the viscus. In this autonomous stage there is no control, there is constant leakage and vesical residuum.

The bladder wall activity is engendered by the stretch reflex, stimulated in turn by the vesical dilatation, and operates through the intrinsic nerve net in the bladder wall which begins to show some hypertrophy while the vesical outlet remains lax. When the destructive lesion is in the cauda equina and sacral segments, the patient may not progress farther than the autonomous bladder stage.

Most patients, depending on (1) the level and degree of cord injury,

(2) the absence of severe infection, and (3) a satisfactory general condition, may be expected to progress to the stage of "automatic" bladder.

Automatic Bladder. This is manifested by periodic involuntary reflex urination in the recovery stage following complete transection of the cord above the sacral segments. Voiding can usually be stimulated by mass reflex upon pricking or stroking stimulation of a trigger point such as the leg, penis, scrotum, tapping the abdomen, or even moving the leg. Automatic bladder reflex does not occur in incomplete transection of the cord nor when there is severe urinary infection or residual shock. Since the automatic bladder does not become distended, rarely over 8 or 10 ounces, and the residual urine after reflex evacuation is seldom over 2 to 4 ounces, the wall of the bladder becomes more or less thickened and coarsely trabeculated with variable relaxation of the vesical outlet.

The trigone and bladder outlet participate in the bladder wall hypertrophy and this may cause variable obstruction, especially with superimposed infection, fibrosis, induration or increasing rigidity of the orifice. This explains not only the rationale of transurethral resection of the vesical outlet in many of these cases, but why good functional results are commonly obtained. Moreover, in these cases as in the more usual type of cord bladder of tabes, myelitis, and the like, a transurethral resection is often performed to remove the obstruction at the bladder outlet and give the detrusor the balance of power. Following this the patient learns vesical control by practicing urination at regular intervals, usually every three hours, and employing both straining and manual abdominal compression, continuing the performance on each occasion until no more urine will come away. This both improves detrusor tone and reduces the urinary residuum.

Spinal Injury Less Than Total Transverse Section of the Spinal Cord. Hemisection or limited crushing commonly occurs but fortunately the vesical and other clinical manifestations are neither so striking, classical, nor prolonged as in complete transection. Following recovery from spinal shock, sufficient voluntary control is usually present to enable the patient to void by conscious straining aided by manual abdominal compression. Secondary bladder neck obstruction may develop as indicated in the preceding paragraph, and for this reason transurethral resection is commonly indicated. Yet in traumatic cord injuries of all varieties, urinary sepsis is outranked only by the initial traumatic shock as the cause of death.

Tumors. New growths of the central nervous system, either benign or malignant, are common enough in adults but extremely rare in children, ependymoma being the commonest primary spinal cord tumor in children. Most spinal cord tumors cause nerve compression with peripheral degeneration. Extradural growths and tumors of the conus medullaris and cauda equina are more likely to cause dysuria than lesions higher in the cord, the compression factor depending on the rate and extent of the growth which in turn is reflected in the mode of onset and in the severity of the symptoms. In slow growing intramedullary tumors, symptomatic manifestations may be delayed six to eight months. With tumor growth, increasing compression and particularly with sacral tumors, disturbances of urination and dysuria increase rapidly. Later bladder paralysis and incontinence occur. If the tumor is higher in the cord, the bladder manifestations are not only delayed but may be limited to urinary frequency and dysuria. Yet incontinence is present in two thirds of all tumors higher in the cord and of more than twelve months' duration. As the cord tumor progresses there is peripheral somatic pain in the extremities, hyperesthesia, spastic rigidity, contraction, and later sensory and motor paralysis according to the segmental distribution affected by the growth. The urologic picture becomes paralysis, incontinence, residuum, and death by urinary sepsis, by the tumor or its metastases, or by intercurrent disease. Cerebral tumors may produce cortical vesical retention or incontinence.

Following successful removal of the central nervous system tumor, gratifying rehabilitation of the bladder has occurred in many cases. Yet one must be sure that the bladder is emptying itself, and that complicating infection is controlled or eradicated.

Nonbacterial degenerative changes of the spinal cord (multiple sclerosis, posterolateral sclerosis, syringomyelia) with posterior lateral column involvement generally cause chronic bladder dysfunction with ultimately incontinence, residuum and renal infection (Fig. 205). Lateral

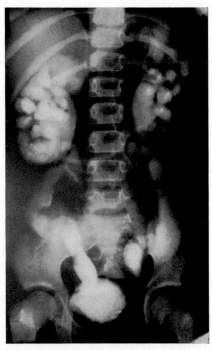

FIGURE 205. Cord bladder of sphincterospastic type due to myelitis in an eight-year-old girl. Urine contained 25 per cent pus by volume. Residuum 6 oz. Cystogram (above) shows extreme dilatation of upper urinary tract. Permanent cystostomy drainage. Uremic death two years later.

column lesions in spastic spinal paralysis induce hypertonia or spasm of the bladder wall and sphincters with urgency, frequency, and difficulty of urination. Here, as in all forms of neuromuscular disease, the fundamental therapeutic considerations are the maintenance of free urinary drainage and eradication of complicating infection.

UNKNOWN ETIOLOGY

There is a large group of patients with unquestionable neuromuscular disease of the urinary tract yet in whom the topical neurologic examination is negative, or the findings are indefinite. There is reduced motor activity of the bladder, the viscus becoming a large dilated, rather thin-walled atonic sac with pale mucosa, fine trabeculations, no vesical outlet relaxation or loss of sensation (Fig. 206). Some of these are diagnosed as atonic bladder or primary neuromuscular vesical dysplasia resulting from motor lesions of the intramural somatic nerve network of the bladder. On the other hand it is possible that some are cases of unrecognized bladder-neck obstruction. In some, the dominant lesion appears to be chronic sphincterospasm at the vesical outlet, a condition to which the term *achalasia* has been applied and thought to be analogous to chronic cardiospasm, pylorospasm, or to the rectosigmoid spasm observed in Hirschsprung's disease. Swenson and his co-workers in the study of Hirschsprung's disease demonstrated an agangliosis or lack of parasympathetic ganglia in the myenteric plexus in the spastic rectosigmoid and, by embryologic analogy, bladder and gut being one, applied their findings to the etiology of "idiopathic" neurogenic bladder disease. Yet the case

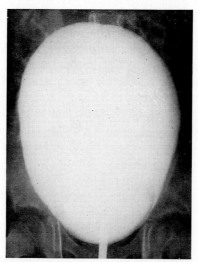

FIGURE 206. Atonic neuromuscular vesical disease in children. Postchoreic asymptomatic atonic dilatation of the bladder in a four-year-old boy. The condition is believed to be but a manifestation of the general muscular atony which characterizes chorea. In this and other similar cases observed following chorea, there have been no somatic changes suggestive of central nervous system disease.

for parasympathetic agangliosis as the cause of atonic bladder with chronic sphincterospasm of the vesical outlet has not been convincingly made.

A large dilated bladder with residual urine and without demonstrable vesical neck obstruction always suggests the likelihood of a neuromuscular basis for the condition (Fig. 206). Many of these patients are relieved or are restored to essentially normal function by transurethral resection even when the cystoscopic examination does not disclose true bladder neck obstruction.

Changes in the Bladder and Upper Urinary Tract in Neuromuscular Uropathy. These will depend on (1) the etiologic nerve lesion, (2) whether the spinal reflex arc is maintained as well as the tonus of the bladder and sphincter, and (3) whether infection exists. To repeat, the musculature of the bladder is characteristically hypertonic or spastic following trauma or other destructive lesions above the fourth lumbar segment of the cord but is hypotonic with complete loss or destruction of the sacral innervation by injury, congenital neurospinal malformation, toxic injury or other process which destroys the sensory limb of the reflex arc. Residual urine appears in increasing amounts to cause the physiologic bladder capacity to be correspondingly reduced, and progressively induces more frequent urination and even incontinence with irritation, distention, or overflow.

With continued urinary back pressure when neuromuscular vesical retention exists, there is progressive injury of the upper urinary tract in which the renal damage is the most important. These changes have been indicated in Chapter 5 and it should be noted that late in the disease the ureters are often dilated to the size of the bowels, either large or small, usually bilaterally, and sometimes longitudinal ureteral dilatation doubles the length of the channel with extreme secondary kinking and angulation with increased urinary stasis (Fig. 205). Infection develops eventually in all of these cases and of itself may be a cause of death.

Vesical symptoms are those of urinary frequency, dysuria, paradoxical overflow, or chronic complete retention with the manifestations of infection added as persistent pyuria. In children the clinical picture commonly causes the erroneous diagnosis of enuresis to be made and the underlying lesion to be overlooked. Similarly with infection, too often the physician is satisfied with the diagnosis pyelitis when a grave pyelonephritis, infected hydronephrosis, secondary stone or diverticulum exists or complicates the picture.

In advanced neuromuscular vesical disease from any cause, the patient is usually continually wet from (1) partial paralysis of the sphincters with incomplete incontinence; (2) paralysis of the detrusor (retention with overflow), or (3) total paralysis. The rectum is apt to be similarly paralyzed so that constipation or fecal incontinence complicates the clinical problem. Occasionally it is the rectal disturbances which take the patient to the doctor.

Diagnosis in Neuromuscular Uropathy

The history is of the utmost value as it discloses whether the clinical manifestations have been present from birth, when they first appeared, if an acute infectious disease or injury preceded their occurrence; whether there have been recurrent attacks of acute urinary retention, chronic vesical distention, complete urinary incontinence, anal incontinence, lower intestinal tract disturbances, leg deformities, especially clubfoot; weakness, atrophy, paralysis of the leg muscles or other symptoms suggestive of central nervous system disease. In spinal cord injuries should be learned the nature of the trauma whether by spinal fracture, stabbing or gunshot.

Physical Examination. This is primarily a careful neurologic investigation with special attention directed to the status of the structures innervated by the individual segments of the lumbosacral cord. Congenital clubfoot, paralysis of the lower extremities, sacromeningocele or a sacral dimple, often pigmented and/or covered by a coarse heavy growth of hair, commonly reflect a lumbosacral neurovertebral defect. Study of the sensory innervation of the saddle area (perineum, buttocks, inner upper thighs) may disclose anesthesia, hyperesthesia or paresthesia (Fig. 199). Anesthesia of the plantar surface of the foot has been noted in more than 80 per cent of clinically important spina bifida occulta. Observation should be made as to paralysis of the perineal muscles, atrophy, and motor disturbances of the lower extremities, contraction of the knee in flexion, congenital dislocation of the hip, trophic ulcers of the feet, diminution or absence of urethral sensation, all of which are suggestive of destructive lesions of the sacral or lumbosacral cord.

A rectal examination should be part of every complete physical examination and is a MUST *when neuromuscular disease is under investigation.* An atonic rectal sphincter with a dilated rectum above is pathognomonic of neuromuscular disease. In general, the anal and vesical sphincters are isotonic, the explanation being their mutual embryologic derivation from the primitive cloaca and their common central innervation.

Examination of the blood and spinal fluid for syphilis should be done as should investigation of the pupillary and deep reflexes, and altered sensory responses in other portions of the body. Determination of the patient's mental capacity sometimes gives a clue especially in the young; many children with congenital neuromuscular disease are mentally deficient. Often, however, the somatic neurologic examination is negative and the diagnosis will be made by urologic study of the bladder and contiguous channels.

Radiologic Examination. The initial x-ray study should be a *plain scout film* of the urinary tract for evidence of spinal malformations, fractures, dislocations and other injuries as well as calculi; spinal defects are best visualized in stereoscopic films.

Contrast intraspinal radiography by the injection of radiopaque medium into the subarachnoid space is often helpful in the diagnosis of lower cord lesions associated with defects of spinal fusion. By this method complete or incomplete transverse blockage is demonstrated, the usual observation in subarachnoid blockage being the presence of small amounts of the radiopaque medium irregularly trickling down the sides of the obstruction in inverted U-formation or perhaps down only one side. Today the method is employed chiefly in combination with laminography.

Cystography. This may demonstrate a spastic hypertonic detrusor or a chronic paralytic dilatation (Figs. 203–206). The cystographic vesical outline is commonly normal in early or mild neuromuscular disease but when pearshaped and often trabeculated, suggests *cord bladder*, particularly in the female.

The *spastic bladder* is small with irregular outline delineating the rugae of trabeculation of the contracted hypertonic wall. There may be expulsive opening or relaxation of the vesical outlet with medium observed in the posterior urethra.

The *atonic bladder* on the other hand may be cystographically enormous, sometimes filling the entire pelvis, and extending well into the abdomen (Fig. 206). The outline is smooth and round and reaches its largest size in the otherwise asymptomatic atony of the postchoreic stage. The outline of the inferior segment of the continent atonic bladder is smoothly regular and resembles that seen in mild contraction of the vesical outlet.

In *paralytic hypotonic* bladder there is some funneling of the prostatic urethra reflecting the relaxation or paralysis of the internal sphincter and is of diagnostic significance. Trophic ulcerations, infection or urinary retention may cause irregularity of the bladder outline as cystographically reflected in trabeculation; cellule formation or even diverticula may be present.

Cystographic reflux is frequently present in neuromuscular vesical disease, especially when the bladder outlet is spastic. The entire upper tract may be cystographically outlined (Fig. 205). Yet the diagnosis of neuromuscular disease should be guarded when based on cystography alone. Cystoscopy and often cystometry must be employed in addition to the foregoing described procedures to establish the diagnosis and even with these aids there may still be doubt.

Cystoscopy. In the cystoscopic diagnosis of neuromuscular vesical disease one observes the type and severity of trabeculation, alteration of sensation, relaxation of the vesical outlet and adjacent urethra, and the integrity of the motor control. Good motor control with diminution of sensation suggests that the important lesion is in the upper cord level. The cystoscopic picture of an atonic bladder resulting from lesions of the peripheral or intramural nerves is different from that in cord bladder caused by demonstrable disease of the central nervous system.

In *cord bladder in males*, cystourethroscopy discloses relaxation of the vesical outlet with sometimes panoramic visualization of the entire verumontanum, vesical outlet, and adjacent bladder floor. In the hypertonic stage of cord bladder there is generalized coarse trabeculation with hypertrophy of the trigone, cellules, saccules, *bas fond* formation and often diverticula. Yet the cystoscopic picture often simulates that seen in mild vesical neck contracture; the two varieties of blockage may coexist.

In *tonic cord bladder* the vesical outlet tends to remain spastic, the thickened hypertrophic bladder orifice with hypertrophy of the trigone may produce variable obstruction; the bladder wall is hypertrophied. Thus, the cystoscopic picture in both cord bladder and the usual type of vesical neck contracture is frequently strikingly similar, a reduction of sensation usually being present in the neurogenic form (see third succeeding paragraph). Cystoscopic evidence of vesical atony without sharply decreased sensation is one of the most important points in differentiating between a lesion of the terminal nerve supply in the bladder wall (atonic bladder) and one involving the central nervous system (cord bladder) in which the sensory changes are the rule. *Atonic paralysis* is the late degenerative stage of cord bladder, commonly with coarse hypertrophy of the bladder wall, and is to this extent cystoscopically distinguishable from the atonic bladder without demonstrable central nervous disease.

In the *female with cord bladder* the vesical changes are less marked than in the male; due in part to the absence of the firm prostatic collar, there is a greater relaxation of the posterior urethra in females. Yet in cord bladder the sensory changes occur precisely as in males, and in advanced cases the bladder wall changes may be cystoscopically indistinguishable from those in the male.

In *atonic bladder of peripheral or intramural nerve origin*, cystoscopically the dilated bladder wall appears smooth, sometimes with fine trabeculation. There is variably reduced expulsive force. The bladder outlet is generally tonic and may simulate the spastic outlet in tonic cord bladder. Dilatation of the atonic posterior urethra in association with atonic bladder suggests a central cord lesion but cystography will often demonstrate vesico-ureteral reflux in atonic bladder.

The *cystoscopic differential diagnosis* between spastic vesical outlet syndrome and the congenitally contracted bladder neck is a frequent problem. In the neurospastic obstruction the margins of the vesical outlet may also project into the visual fields, particularly over the inferior segment of the outlet from which the trigone and vesical floor often fall away to form a broad based *bas fond*. Hypertrophy of the musculature of the hypertonic vesical outlet explains this bladder-neck picture and especially when the cystoscopic view simulates that of median-bar obstruction. In contracted bladder neck, on the other hand, the firm collar-like constriction often grasps the cystoscope as a sclerotic median bar also may do, an observation in striking contrast to the usual relaxation, or at least absence of grasping of the instrument in the neuromuscular syndrome. In contracture of the vesical outlet, the trigone regularly becomes hypertrophied because of the increased effort necessary to open the internal vesical orifice, often an important differential diagnostic observation. Yet it must not be overlooked that both neurogenous and nonneurogenous conditions may simultaneously be obstructive factors; an atonic dilated viscus with a huge residuum may be the result of unrecognized nonneurogenous vesical neck contracture. Here cystometry must be employed in making the complete diagnosis.

Cystometry. This is a useful method of determining the neuromuscular vesical motor balance and sensation in terms of fluid volume and intracystic pressure (Fig. 207). The determinations are made by measur-

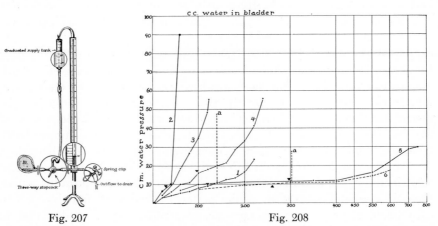

Fig. 207   Fig. 208

FIGURE 207. A readily constructed simple cystometric apparatus contrived and extensively used by the author for nearly twenty-five years. Potassium permanganate solution 1:10,000 is used as the recording medium. As measured units are introduced into the bladder (we observe increments of 20 cc. in children, 50 cc. in adults), the intravesical pressure is recorded. By employing the drip valve in the reservoir system, the introduction of fluid into the bladder is slowly continuous. The factors noted for the graph are the intracystic pressure in centimeters of water (ordinate) and the intracystic volume (abscissa).

FIGURE 208. Cystometrograms, normal and abnormal. The point of first desire to urinate is indicated by a triangle. The vertical dotted line indicates the combined expulsive force of voluntary abdominal contraction and vesical contraction as registered in the bladder. This is notably reduced in the hypotonic cord bladder. *Curve 1* shows average in twelve normal children. *Curve 2.* In this eight-year-old boy with traumatic myelitis of the seventh cervical level with motor and sensory loss below, there was advanced cystitis, fine trabeculation of the bladder wall, with atonic external sphincter and lax vesical outlet. A hypertonic bladder with incontinence existed, in short, an autonomic reflex or undisciplined bladder. *Curve 3* was obtained in a ten-year-old boy with urinary frequency, whose clothes had always been wet since birth. Rectal incontinence occurred at times; there was saddle anesthesia of the perineum (S_{3-5}). Tonic bladder, lax outlet, residuum 125 cc., neuromuscular vesical disease of parasympathetic irritation type. Improvement followed urethral instrumentation (local irritation or psychic?). *Curve 4* was obtained in a six-year-old boy with contracture of the vesical outlet and hypertrophied bladder wall. The point of desire to urinate (15 cm. water pressure) is at a slightly higher level than average for children. The pressure is high at average capacity (myogenic curve). *Curve 5* was obtained in a ten-year-old girl with atonic cord bladder subsequent to spina bifida from S_2 down; the neurologic examination was negative; pronounced cystitis, moderate trabeculation; cystocele, lax bladder outlet, and a tonic external sphincter were observed. The cystogram showed bilateral reflux with massive hydroureter and hydronephrosis. *Curve 6* was obtained in a six-year-old girl with atonic bladder secondary to myelitis of unknown etiology. Bladder sensation was greatly reduced and the capacity under low pressure enormously increased.

ing intracystic pressure as known increments of fluid are slowly but continuously introduced into the bladder, the data obtained being plotted as a curve; the fluid volumes introduced are recorded as abscissas and the intracystic pressure as ordinates. Usually two curves are made in which normally the second curve is higher because of irritation of the deep urethra and bladder wall coincident to the initial examination, but in neurogenic disease the second curve is usually lower than the first.

The cystometric data we are interested in obtaining are the pressure-volume values at which (1) the initial thermal (cold) sensation is noted, (2) the point at which the first desire to urinate is felt, (3) the point of imperative urination (vesical pain), and (4) the total expulsive force of the vesical musculature aided by increased abdominal pressure induced by straining. When the bladder is partially filled, the patient is instructed to void and the recorded pressure indicates the total expulsive force. *The general trend of the cystometric curve is the important thing, and volume-pressure readings at the various levels are of only relative value.* Accurate cystometric studies require satisfactory cooperation on the part of the patient. The determination of thermal sensation, that is, the point at which the patient feels the introduction of cool fluid into the bladder, is often dissociated from pressure sensation.

In cystometric studies we are fundamentally concerned with whether the disease under investigation is of *myogenic* or *neurogenic* origin or is the result of both factors. The myogenic elements are concerned with the expulsive force of the bladder, whether normal or altered by obstruction at the vesical outlet or peripherally, and whether compensatory hypertrophy or decompensation of the bladder wall exists. As indicated four paragraphs back, this is of special value in the differential diagnosis of congenital contracted bladder neck when the picture simulates that of cord bladder. Neurogenic factors are concerned with hypotonia, hypertonia, atonia, hyperirritability, hyperesthesia, or hypesthesia.

In *hypertonic neuromuscular vesical disease* the threshold of sensation is increased or "moved to the left" on the cystometric curve, and the pressure curve is greatly increased with reduced vesical capacity (Fig. 208). In the *hypotonic bladder* the curve is flat with diminished sensation (threshold "moved to the right"), low voluntary pressure, and large volume (Fig. 208). In the *myogenic bladder* the desire to urinate is registered at approximately normal intracystic pressure, the capacity is variably increased, while the filling pressure is characteristically higher than normal. In the absence of infection or inflammation of the urinary tract, vesical hyperirritability as cystometrically demonstrated suggests an irritative lesion of the lower cord (parasympathetic, pudic). A cystometric demonstration of atonic bladder wall with reduced sensation suggests a destructive lesion of the lower cord, cauda equina, or peripheral nerves. In some cases thought to be entirely myogenic, cystometry may reveal unsuspected neuromuscular disease as a partial or even total component. Yet cystometry is not a reliable guide in topical neurologic diagnosis and serves principally to distinguish between myogenic and neurogenic vesical disturbances.

PROGNOSIS

Prognosis in neuromuscular disease depends largely upon the etiology and whether it can be ameliorated or corrected. The outlook in most cases is extremely grave, the institution of free urinary drainage and control of infection being the limits of therapeutic possibility and without which treatment, at least three fourths of the patients will have an untimely death of urinary sepsis and/or uremia.

COMPLICATIONS

Complications are extremely frequent in neuromuscular vesical disease, especially when of central nervous origin. The more important of these complications are infection, stone formation, and upper urinary tract dilatation; urethritis, periurethral abscess, penoscrotal fistula, or epididymitis are often the result of prolonged or improper indwelling urethral catheterization. Trophic ulcers, chiefly decubital, occur in 2 to 5 per cent of these patients and demand special nursing care.

Infection may be expected in every case of neurogenic bladder, the usual organisms include Proteus vulgaris, Aerobacter aerogenes, Pseudomonas aeruginosa (Bacillus pyocyaneus), Esch. coli, Streptococcus hemolyticus, Streptococcus faecalis, Staphylococcus aureus and albus and generally as mixed infections. Unfortunately, the organisms are often of the urea-splitting varieties which cause high urinary alkalinity and predispose to phosphatic stone formation as observed in 10 to 30 per cent of the patients. Stone deposit is about equal in the kidney and bladder and in not more than 10 per cent in the ureter. Upper urinary tract dilatation occurs in a third to a half of the patients.

TREATMENT

The treatment of neuromuscular uropathy depends upon the etiology and, generally even more important, the vesical manifestations, that is, whether there is (1) retention, or (2) incontinence. The prospect of the patient with neuromuscular vesical disease has been vastly improved through greater attention to the general condition with proper hygiene, by prevention of constipation, by scientific dietetics, by liberal fluid intake, by vitamin therapy, and especially by modern antimicrobial therapy. Bedridden patients with cord bladder caused by advanced spinal disease require particularly careful nursing to prevent bed sores which trophic changes in the skin and wet sheets encourage. Yet this may largely be prevented by proper indwelling catheterization or suprapubic cystostomy drainage and help to spare the patient a life on the Bradford frame. By a nourishing diet the resistance of the patient is raised and adequate protein feeding will prevent weight loss through toxic destruction of the body tissue.

Dietetic efforts to achieve high acid or alkaline-ash residue for the prevention of stone is worthwhile if it is not too upsetting to the patient; it is rarely advisable in children.

The administration of vitamins must be adequate to meet the normal needs or a little more, and particularly vitamin A as a prophylactic factor against the formation of phosphatic calculi. The tendency toward urinary alkalinity which with recumbency and infection favors stone formation, may be regulated toward normal by chemotherapy and dietary urinary acidulation (Chapter 11). Excessive urinary acidity is seldom high enough to require alkalinization.

Prevention or control of complicating urinary infection is a cardinal requisite of good treatment and together with other measures just enumerated will do much to prevent stone formation in bed patients long confined. A large fluid intake will reduce the concentration of the crystalloids in the urine, and correspondingly help against stone formation. Prophylactic salicylamide administration in this connection is still *sub judice*. Antibacterial therapy is administered in large doses as outlined under the treatment of chronic urinary infection in Chapter 7.

Drug Therapy. The drugs of the choline series commercially available (acetylcholine, Doryl, Mecholyl and, more recently, Urecholine) are valuable in stimulating bladder emptying. The choline derivatives stimulate the parasympathetic innervation and their action is antagonistic to that of epinephrine. Acetylcholine overdosage is promptly counteracted with atropine. *Yet no acetylcholine derivative should be used to stimulate bladder emptying when organic obstruction at the vesical outlet or peripherally is known to exist.* The drug may be given as acetylcholine hydrochloride or hydrobromide or as we employ clinically, Mecholyl (acetyl-beta-methylcholine chloride 0.2 gm.) or Doryl (carbaminoyl-choline 0.25 mg. or $\frac{1}{120}$ gr.) given in tablet form two to four times daily by mouth according to age and size of the patient and apparent benefit. Urecholine (urethane of beta methylcholine chloride, Merck) is used today in doses of 1 to 3 mg. in children and 3 to 5 mg. in adults given subcutaneously (never intramuscularly or intravenously!) at thirty-minute intervals for three doses, or to stimulate continuous bladder emptying may be given in subcutaneous doses of 0.02 to 0.5 mg. two or three times a day to be reduced or stopped should side effects occur.

Other parasympatheticomimetics to stimulate bladder emptying include Trasentine, Furmethide, Tolserol, and Syntropan. It will be found that by employing these compounds in neuromuscular vesical retention type of disease without organic obstruction, stimulation of vesical emptying will be achieved but only so long as the medication is continued. Let the patient skip the medication for a day or two, and the residuum and previous difficulty recur.

Catheterization. This may be (1) periodic, or (2) indwelling.

Periodic Catheterization. Frequently one catheterization relieves acute retention of postoperative or nontraumatic spontaneous sphinctero-spastic type but in patients with neuromuscular bladder disturbance of the acute traumatic spinal variety or the more commonly observed neuromuscular type so often secondary to lumbosacral spinal malformation, repeated catheterizations, three or more times a day, are necessary if the bladder is to be kept within limits of normal distention. Prolonged intermittent catheterization is inadvisable because (1) it fails to keep the bladder sufficiently decompressed unless performed too often and, no matter how gently performed, it causes important urethral traumatization, (2) prostatitis and epididymitis may follow with variable and unavoidable infection of the deep urethra with, ultimately, infection of the entire urinary tract, (3) leakage of urine frequently occurs between overdue catheterizations and encourages maceration of the skin or the production of bed sores, and (4) urinary leakage and decomposition make the patient and his surroundings foul smelling and socially objectionable. When repeated catheterization is properly carried out aseptically, it requires the constant attention of a skilled instrumenteur which of itself excludes most nurses.

Indwelling catheterization may carry the patient through severe, acute, or prolonged retention, or prepare him for suprapubic drainage or other surgical attack. Once indwelling catheterization is established it should be continuous which means a catheter should never be shut off. Yet indwelling catheterization has no place in the permanent treatment of chronic neuromuscular vesical retention and its use for more than two or three weeks at the longest is usually attended by serious complications which require its discontinuance. Foreign body urethritis due to the catheter, periurethritis, periurethral abscess, urethral fistula, urethrovesical ulceration, trophic changes, and severe urinary infection rule out its permanent employment. The method of fixation and management of the indwelling catheter is discussed in Chapter 5 (Fig. 54); the employment of a balloon catheter (Fig. 55) is preferable to the anchorage of the tube with adhesive strips.

Tidal and other complicated drainage systems involving indwelling catheterization have been widely used, but in our experience simple cystostomy drainage works best when the bladder must be relieved for a long period and does not impede the rehabilitation toward normal vesical function.

When urethral catheterization is employed in the retention type of neuromuscular vesical disease, the existence of urinary infection and the specific bacterial etiology must be determined at once and actively combated by intensive antimicrobial therapy (see Chapter 7). Thus (1) grave urinary infection and its potential disastrous complications are largely controlled or eliminated, (2) the kidneys are spared needless damage, (3) the vitality of the urinary tract is immeasurably protected, and (4) rehabilitation is accelerated and aided. When urinary infection, either acute or chronic, is a complication of neurogenous retention and particularly in spinal injury, employ suprapubic cystostomy rather than indwelling catheterization.

Manual abdominal compression (Credé) has been widely employed in the past in the treatment of acute vesical retention following spinal injury but is contraindicated when the obstruction is not neurogenous. If, following cord injury, the bladder has not already been catheterized and infected, and no voiding has occurred after six to eight hours and the distention is not pronounced, the Credé manipulation may be tried. The ulnar margin of the hand is transversely pressed into the abdomen above the bladder, the main pressure being exerted in the direction of the vesical outlet. It is usually necessary to maintain this pressure for two to three minutes before the flow of urine starts and this at first may be scant. The maneuver is repeated at intervals of one to two hours and the expressed urine may progressively increase, often decreasing the vesical distention down to the level of the pubis. The procedure is more satisfactorily carried out in the female whose short urethra doubtless encourages the opening mechanism. Yet Credé's method is to be countenanced only in the absence of proper equipment for aseptic catheterization or when the physician is hopelessly timorous about performing catheterization.

To sum up, the prevention, control or cure of urinary infection and the maintenance of free urinary drainage are fundamental therapeutic considerations in the treatment of neuromuscular vesical disease and demand particularly rigorous attention in bedridden patients. When vesical retention is not relieved in a week by indwelling catheterization, cystostomy drainage should be established and maintained until it is proved the bladder can function acceptably. Most urinary infections which develop in neuromuscular vesical disease must be considered to be of the ascending or urogenous variety. Other considerations in treatment are (1) orthopedic management of injury to the vertebral column and other structures, (2) removal of central nervous system tumors, and if present (3) the treatment of cerebrospinal syphilis even though its etiologic relationship to the vesical condition may be indefinite.

Technical treatment of neuromuscular uropathy is directed at correction or rehabilitation of the structures at fault in the production of the dysfunction. This entails (1) utilization to the utmost of remaining control or reflex factors, and (2) substitution of factors (transurethral resection, cystostomy, indwelling catheterization, spinal cord injection, rhizotomy, and so forth) which will not only improve drainage or inhibit the neural elements at fault in causing overactivity of the musculature, but will encourage favorable elements which may still be present.

Overdilation of the vesical outlet by instruments, either sounds or Kollman dilator is of only temporary benefit, although for a time it may materially improve the ease of urination and reduce the residuum exactly as favorable results are obtained in similar overdilation of the esophagus in chronic cardiospasm.

Cystostomy Drainage. High suprapubic cystostomy is the treatment of choice in the retention type of vesical disease caused by injury of the spinal cord when automatic micturition is not promptly established, or when prolonged catheterization is contraindicated or seems unwise. With the drainage tube placed high in the bladder dome and well above the pubis, the tip of the tube is more easily kept away from the trigone and bladder floor to prevent pain and irritative reflex manifestations when anesthesia is not present. A simple method of fixing the drainage tube is shown in Figure 59. Employment of the Campbell cystostomy trocar makes establishment of suprapubic drainage an extremely simple procedure which can be done with the patient in his bed or in the office (Fig. 57). Unless the back is broken or there are other contraindications to ambulation, trocar cystostomy permits the patient to be up and about shortly, and it forestalls severe renal impairment and injury of the bladder wall by back pressure. Yet once established it must be continuous. Moreover, it avoids urethral trauma and other urethral complications (periurethritis, periurethral abscess, urethral fistula) prostatitis, seminal vesiculitis and epididymitis so common to repeated catheterization.

Cystostomy drainage is maintained until the bladder is sufficiently rehabilitated to warrant its discontinuance. In evaluating this, the tube is clamped off and the patient is allowed to go a matter of hours or days under simulated closed bladder conditions. When all seems well, the recheck of residual urine is easily made by having the patient empty himself while the suprapubic tube is clamped off and when he has done his best, open the tube and determine how much is left in his bladder—the residuum. Normally it should be zero. If the residuum is more than 50 or 60 cc., the drainage should be continued until examination suggests that more active treatment such as transurethral resection may help. Unless such prospects are good, continue the suprapubic drainage indefinitely.

Thus preliminary cystostomy is often employed for variable periods preparatory to transurethral resection, or while further neurologic and urologic study of the patient is being conducted or orthopedic complications such as a fractured spine, fractured pelvis and the like are being treated or are mending.

Transurethral resection of the vesical outlet is indicated in neuromuscular vesical disease when there is (1) spastic vesical outlet with retention but good detrusor tone, or (2) achalasia with or without complicating bladder-neck fibrosis. The rationale of transurethral resection in these cases lies in the mechanical weakening of the bladder outlet by removal of sufficient tissue to enable the hypotonic or atonic bladder to empty itself aided, when necessary, by abdominal straining or manual (Credé) compression. Thus residual urine is diminished, variable bladder wall tone is regained, there is relief of incontinence and an increase in functioning bladder capacity. Yet following transurethral resection it is sometimes necessary to operate again to remove more tissue. When in doubt as to how much tissue to remove, one should err on the side of removing too little; removal of too much may be followed by incontinence.

Neurosurgical Procedures for the Relief of Neuromuscular Vesical Dysfunction

Laminectomy. Here the neurosurgeon exposes the cauda equina, excises lipomatous, fibrous, or other tissues compressing the underlying nerves and, in the absence of such compressing masses, attempts to free the sacral nerve roots from traction by removing interfering bone as necessary. The procedure has been employed both in vesical retention and in vesical incontinence, chiefly in association with spina bifida vera, and with variable benefit. It is likely that in unsuccessful cases (1) injury or myelodysplasia of the sacral roots has advanced so far that even following the operation the faulty condition of the motor nerve supply prohibits their competition against a spastic vesical outlet and/or external sphincter, or (2) not all the nerve roots are liberated.

Presacral neurectomy has been advocated in cases of sympathetic imbalance but is now largely discarded for this purpose. It is definitely contraindicated when anomalies of lumbosacral fusion or sacral cord disease are demonstrable because the involved parasympathetic innervation is likely to be meager or ineffective. Similarly pudendal neurectomy, blocking of the pudendal nerve, as well as rhizotomy and chordotomy have been employed with variable success and generally unfavorably.

Bladder Re-education. This is required following neurosurgical and/or urosurgical rehabilitation in patients who preoperatively were partially or totally incontinent with or without vesical retention. Fundamentally it consists in the start-stop-start exercises commonly employed in postprostatectomy leakage. Unless the patient is able to retain urine in the bladder, the viscus is filled by catheter with sterile water or saline after which he starts to urinate, passes a few drops, then voluntarily attempts to stop the flow and soon to start to void again; this is repeated until the bladder is empty. Sometimes the cycle is repeated four or five times while the bladder is emptying.

When the patient has been in vesical retention preoperatively, his exercise objective is to empty the bladder to the best of his ability, employing both abdominal straining and, if necessary, suprapubic manual compression. After getting out a variable amount of urine, he waits twenty to thirty seconds, voids again, then waits half a minute or so, and continues as long as any appreciable amount of urine comes. The secondary, tertiary or subsequent voidings often represent dependent drainage from the greatly dilated upper urinary tract. Yet this method, practiced at regular intervals of two and not over three hours, results in strengthening of the bladder wall and reduction of the residuum, assuming that only the neurogenic factor exists, the vesical neck obstruction having been adequately corrected by transurethral resection when indicated.

Treatment of neuromuscular vesical incontinence is a problem only in cases of atonic or paralyzed external sphincter with partial or incomplete incontinence as distinguished from the paradoxical overflow incontinence of retention. The field of possibilities for surgical care of the incontinence is indeed limited because most muscles which might lend themselves anatomically and physiologically have their nerve derivation from the diseased spinal segments and cannot, therefore, be used. Sling operations to elevate or compress the urethra and bladder neck have been employed with a discouraging incidence of failures although now and then a patient has been fortunate. The fascial sling operations employ chiefly the pyramidalis muscles and rectus fascia; the gracilis muscle works well for this procedure. Penis clamps are a nuisance to employ for continuous urinary control because excessive penile edema and excoriation commonly develop; cystostomy drainage is preferable. Ureterosigmoidostomy with transplantation of the ureters to the rectum is usually out of the question because the bowel and bladder are similarly paralyzed.

Fortunately many patients with vesical paralysis and urinary leakage have just sufficient sphincter tonus to retain perhaps 15 or 30 cc. of urine and in these cases the maintenance of free suprapubic drainage alone serves to keep the patient dry. The bladder is kept sufficiently empty so that the small remaining sphincter tonicity successfully resists the hydrostatic pressure of the minimal amount of urine present.

Ligation of the deep urethra and the establishment of permanent suprapubic drainage is advised in the treatment of the totally incontinent patient whose therapeutic outlook is otherwise hopeless. The chief complication of this regimen is the tendency to phosphatic incrustation of the inlying tube with secondary bladder stone formation. This can be largely avoided, however, by frequent changing of the suprapubic tube— every two to three weeks, control of urinary infection, especially the ammoniogenic variety, and the daily irrigation of the tube, bladder and catheter with Suby solution "G" or "M" (Chapter 11).

ENURESIS

Enuresis is the unintentional and usually unconscious voiding of large amounts of urine which occurs predominantly during sleep and in the absence of organic disease, either of the nervous or urogenital systems. It is usually called bed wetting, and is of clinical importance after the age of three years, by which time normal habits of urination and defecation should be established. Although by definition enuresis is a purely functional condition occurring in the absence of neurologic or urologic disease, it is discussed at this point because in the minds of many physicians and of the laity at large, it is commonly thought of as a "nervous" affliction. Day wetting occurs in about 10 per cent of enuretic children, particularly during the afternoon nap, but may occur at other times as well; it may happen when the child is awake. Unfortunately, most children and adults who habitually wet their clothes are treated as victims of a purely functional condition, which it doubtless is in at least 95 per cent of the cases.

When the condition is not cured by medical treatment or psychotherapy intensively administered during a period of three months, a complete urologic examination is indicated. In a series of over 1800 children I have personally examined on the basis of this criterion, more than 60 per cent have shown urologic disease adequate to explain the symptoms and clinical picture, and by the therapeutic test appeared to be the probable etiologic factor. When the patient voids the urine comes in a steady full stream rather than with intermittency, dribbling or the small stream of obstruction or neuromuscular disease.

The correction of enuresis is important (1) for the child as it enables him to develop normally into a substantial adult, and (2) for the parents as it affords them peace of mind which, in turn, encourages a normal wholesome home life. The very occurrence of enuresis in a child should warn the parents that something is wrong with the child's world which does not give him the assurance and security he needs, or that there is a possibility he has true organic urologic disease.

In infancy the act of urination is a lower arc reflex and, with central nervous system maturation, it should become a conscious function with cerebral control by the thirtieth month and, in general, with an inhibitory influence during sleep. We seldom consider children under four years of age as candidates for urologic examination solely because of enuresis. A mentally normal child will ultimately develop control of his bladder and bowels except when a physical condition exists which requires medical or surgical treatment. Normal bladder control may be disrupted by a wide variety of lesions involving not only the urinary tract (meatal stenosis, phimosis, balanitis, ureteral or vesical stone, urinary infections, and the like), but by nervous system disease (spina bifida, cord tumors, hematomyelia, transverse myelitis, cord injury, etc.) or reflexly by diseases of other body systems including rectal fissure, inflammation, fecal masses or worms, gastrointestinal disturbances or even as remote irritations as foreign bodies in the nose.

Etiology and Pathogenesis. Enuresis is one of the commonest disturbances of the young, having a reported incidence varying with different observers from 12 to 26 per cent. I think it is even more than the highest figure given here because parents commonly consider it only as a bad habit, not sufficiently important to merit medical attention. There is no striking difference in sex incidence although more girls are treated for the condition. Most enuretic children are brought for examination between the ages of five and eight years; untreated it usually disappears by puberty but I have seen it in several adult males who became concerned about the condition only as they were about to be married.

Until enuresis came to benefit measurably by the ever increasing general interest in urologic conditions in the young, its fundamental problems stirred the investigative interest chiefly of psychologists and psychiatrists and this, no doubt, explains the wide variety of etiologic hypotheses advanced. Doubtless many of these notions are fundamentally sound if not considered exclusively.

Nationality, illegitimacy, prematurity, abnormally long gestation, economic condition of the patient, heredity, and racial differences are of mild influence, if any, and can be disregarded on the whole. Intelligence, urinary acidity, pollakiuria, disturbances of renal function, diuresis, digestive disturbances, hypertrophy of the tonsils and adenoids and dreams have no particular influence. Deep sleep is not an etiologic factor although it is almost universally offered by parents as a convenient alibi for lack both of proper training of the child and of their affection toward the child. In so many of these cases, the sleeping child with a full bladder consciously or subconsciously resists the urge to get up to urinate because he does not want to be bothered. Nor does enuresis occur during deep sleep in a child whose proper habits of urination have been established.

Unquestionably a *desire for attention* is the fundamental factor in most cases and especially in a child *dethroned* by the arrival of a new baby. The dethroned child reflects his antagonism, insecurity, jealousy, or juvenile delinquency (inferiority complex) in enuresis, masturbation, physical attacks on the new arrival, and other antisocial manifestations. Oddly, such reactions are predominantly against the one who does the most for him, and gives him the most attention—this being most often the mother, but may be a father, stepmother, or indulgent relative or friend of the family. Many believe that this feeling of insecurity is the commonest single etiologic factor in enuresis.

Enuresis is sometimes *imitative* on the part of children who knowingly observe the increased attention heaped upon an enuretic brother or sister. The habit may not begin until the child has inadvertently learned that his father, mother, or an admired relative, or another outside the family circle has been so afflicted. The incidence of enuresis is highest (10 to 20%) in children relegated to institutional life which must be considered the antithesis of normal home life, and this applies but slightly less to foster home life in which the child is unhappy and feels insecure.

In both enuretic and nonenuretic children, dentition, talking, walking, and height-weight factors are identical.

Illness accounts for the onset of enuresis in some children after habits of regular bladder function have been established by the irregularities and relaxations of habit training because of the illness. The total fluid intake is of slight concern; the improvement or disappearance of enuresis following withholding of fluids after four o'clock in the afternoon, an ancient therapy for bed wetting, is chiefly successful pseudosuggestion. A normal child with a full bladder will get up to urinate while the enuretic child will wet the bed even on a limited fluid intake.

Striking, however, is the *persistence of infantile traits* in enuretic children in whom the habit is attributed to a sense of physical inferiority, encouraged in turn by delayed weaning and the prolonged dependence on the mother's breast. This augments the maternal attachment with its resulting babying and lack of early bowel and bladder training, such children often wetting while sitting on their mothers' laps.

Children with persistent infantile traits are recognized by their whining, whimpering, soiling, clinging nature, wanting to suck a nipple —either the mother's or a bottle's, and a desire to continue wearing diapers. These persisting infantile traits are also reflected by the ease with which the child (1) yields to attempts to solve his problems (lack of persistence), (2) is reduced to tears, (3) fails to assume responsibilities suitable to his years, or (4) shows great changes in mood and temperament for trivial reasons. On the other hand his general immaturity may be reflected as he is grouchy, irritable, whining, complaining, moody or restless, fidgety, readily excited or hyperactive. Many are slow, passive, dawdling, avoid rough games for fear of injury and would rather read books or play with girls. Enuresis has been described as a triad of (1) sexual stimulation, (2) fear, and (3) refractoriness coupled with pronounced general infantilism (Weber, 1946).

Heredity has been thought by many observers to be an etiologic factor in a third of the cases of enuresis, but this factor is more generally environmental than genetic. Most psychologists and psychiatrists accept the premise that one neurotic in the family means all are neurotic, and in enuresis a high incidence of identical familial behavior pattern is found, the enuretic child also being neurotic and highly unstable, ill natured, or unreasonable.

There are two types of neurotic parents: (1) those who show no concern, and (2) those who show too much concern towards the child's enuresis. The first group, often because they were bedwetters themselves, commonly minimizes the importance of their child's condition, and not only fails to establish early habits of continence in the child but does not hesitate to convey to him the futility of efforts to correct the incontinence. The second group, the demonstratively overconcerned, is the more important as concerns enuresis because a production number is made of the problem in the atmosphere of the home and among the family members. In the consultation room the parents and usually the mother, commonly monopolize the conversation with a recital of their own vesical disturbances in childhood, all of which has been heard many times by the child.

Defective Habit Training. As important as are the various predisposing factors enumerated here, *the most important single cause of enuresis is defective habit training* of the child, and explains the enormous number of children who fail to become continent until the age of eight or ten years, puberty, or even adulthood. Two thirds of patients with true enuresis have personality and psychoneurotic defects, being considered by some (Menninger, 1948) as an aggressive hostile response to a situation. Certainly more than half of all cases of true enuresis have a psychogenic cause.

Emotionalism ranks first among the psychiatric causes, and is engendered by a wide range of factors but all fundamentally affecting the child's sense of security and of being loved and wanted. Emotionalism engendered by parental maladjustment is the most common situation, existing as an etiologic factor in half to two thirds of the homes of enuretic children who, buffeted between the incompatible parents under continuous tension, seek emotional outlet in undesirable habits such as enuresis, encopresis (defecating in bed or in the clothing), masturbation, stealing, truancy, tantrums, hysterical outbursts, thumb sucking, nail biting, and the like. Parental overemphasis on the enuresis problem generally leads the child to gain his desired end by uncooperative behavior. Similarly, emotional distress among soldiers in the world wars explains the incidence of the recurrence of enuresis with the assumption of military activity; in World War II there were approximately 250,000 enuretics in 10,000,000 draftees. But enuresis among officers was extremely rare.

Masturbation is of slightly greater incidence in enuretic children and generally as an antisocial act, but it may have associated etiologic importance when it causes inflammatory or congestive lesions of the deep urethra, verumontanum, prostate and seminal vesicles in boys, and urethrotrigonitis in girls.

A wide variety of psychoanalytic explanations have also been advanced as causes of enuresis but there has been no conclusive evidence to warrant general acceptance of these for, as Smith states regarding the notion that enuresis is a safety valve for children who are victims of neurotic anxiety, there is no reason to believe that in the great majority of these bed wetting relieves anything but bladder pressure.

Organic Urologic Disease as a Factor in Enuresis. When enuresis is not cured within three months by intensive medical and psychologic therapy, a complete urologic examination is indicated. In my own experience based on examination in over 1800 of these cases, uropathy adequate to explain the symptomatology was demonstrable in over 60 per cent, and one in eight of these children had residual urine, varying from a few cubic centimeters to chronic complete retention and, in most instances, previously unsuspected. Removal of the causes of obstruction whether it be urethral valves, contracture of the bladder neck, hypertrophy of the verumontanum, urethral stenosis or stricture, and the like was commonly followed by cessation of "enuresis." When neuromuscular vesical disease is demonstrated, its treatment is that previously discussed in this chapter. A large number of children with enuresis have spina bifida, a third of all individuals being born with spina bifida occulta, but the malformation is etiologically associated with neuromuscular disturbances in not over 5 per cent. Loss of rectal control is often manifested by encopresis which is noted in 3 per cent of all cases of functional enuresis, an act attributed by psychologists to uncooperative behavior analogous to enuresis. Enuresis consequent to uropathy is not to be recognized as true enuresis; a wide variety of lesions have been demonstrated including ectopic ureteral openings which may cause continuous or intermittent incontinence of urine in half of the cases, but this is not true enuresis. Two patients referred for examination because of enuresis had large urethral diverticula which filled upon urination and by gradual emptying later caused wetting of the clothes. Balanitis, inflammation or local irritation of phimosis, urethritis, prostatitis and excessive urinary acidity or alkalinity may stimulate the urinary reflex as may rectal worms, constipation or lesions of the upper urinary tract.

In a large proportion of children referred for examination because of enuresis, urinary infection was found; in three patients it was renal tuberculosis, the secondary vesical manifestations causing the nocturnal incontinence and day frequency. Stones and hair pins have been found in the bladder. Yet, this is not true enuresis; irrespective of the diagnostic label, the patient is entitled to recognition of the basic uropathy and intelligent treatment.

Symptoms. Enuresis persists from infancy into childhood in 80 per cent of the cases, and in most instances as a result of faulty or no habit training. The appearance and disappearance of the habit may be spotty or periodic, with relapse after several weeks or months of apparent cure. As a rule, enuresis persists longer in boys than in girls, usually ceasing with the onset of menstruation. Day wetting (enuresis diurna) seldom appears until nocturnal enuresis is well established. The diurnal manifestation may be simply frequency, urgency, and other reflection of vesical outlet irritation or dysfunction, symptoms thought by many to be initial in enuresis.

Enuresis usually disappears spontaneously by the tenth year and when beginning after this period the prognosis is less favorable. Enuresis persisting after menstruation is established regularly bespeaks a deep-seated psychogenic problem.

Diagnosis. The first objective is to determine whether the manifestation is a true or functional enuresis or results from organic disease of the urinary tract, particularly of the obstructive or neurogenic variety. As a result of urologic examination in children presumed to have functional enuresis, we have discovered practically every lesion of the urinary tract known to exist in the adult.

A careful history taking reveals that in about half the cases at least one parent has had urinary symptoms, chiefly frequency of urination, and often suffered bedwetting as a child. Those who carry their enuresis into adult life generally have an organic urologic condition, chiefly obstructive in the urethra or at the bladder outlet rather than a simple "nervous" bladder. These lesions usually require urethral dilation with sounds or sometimes transurethral resection of the vesical outlet or other urosurgery.

By careful physical examination one must determine that there are no local irritative lesions such as preputial or clitoric adhesions or calculi, balanitis, stenosed external urethral meatus, fused labia minora, vulvovaginitis, rectal fissures or worms, foreign bodies in the bladder or vagina, constipation, masturbation, or urinary infection.

It is, therefore, necessary to recognize (1) emotional or psychologic abnormalities, (2) endocrine disturbances, (3) irritative lesions, (4) neurologic disease, or (5) uropathology. The history will suggest whether the enuresis is the persistence of an infantile trait, or began after habits of normal urination were established or, perchance, reflects organic urinary tract disease. While most enuretic children appear normal, some are exceedingly nervous, ill behaved, uncooperative, and often show extreme genital consciousness by keeping the legs firmly crossed (the adductor syndrome), or by clutching the genitalia to prevent examination. Excessive genital consciousness is common in enuretics of both sexes; habitual masturbation is generally reflected by prostatitis in boys, and often by a tough leathery labial hypertrophy (Hottentot) in girls.

Should urologic examination be indicated, the procedure is carried out as previously described in Chapter 3, and this should include urography of the urethra, bladder and upper urinary tract, or cystometry in suspected neuromuscular vesical disease (q.v.).

In my urologic studies of enuretic boys, posterior urethritis, verumontanitis, prostatitis, or anterior trigonitis have been most often found, generally attributable to faulty sexual hygiene, infection, or peripheral obstruction, singly or in combination. In enuretic girls, urethritis and urethrotrigonitis have been the most common cystoscopic findings. In both sexes congenital urethral obstruction and particularly stenosis of the external meatus has been most often demonstrated as the fundamental lesion.

Treatment.   Today there is no reliable cure for functional enuresis; more than fifty drugs and methods have been endorsed by a legion of clinicians. It is still largely true that the physician's successes will parallel his enthusiasm for and faith in his particular method. However, spontaneous recovery occurs ultimately in nearly all enuretic children; much can be accomplished by prophylactic, medical, psychologic and, when needed, urologic therapy.

Prophylaxis.   This is summed up in the training of the infant in regular habits of micturition and defecation. Thousands upon thousands of mothers have not the slightest conception of what this means, how fundamentally easy it is to carry out; they do not wish to be bothered, they have no conception of child care or, because of the necessity of having to work on the one hand or of opulence on the other, relegate the care of their children to others at a crucial formative period.

Child training should start when the child is able to sit up, and after nursing he is placed and kept on a suitable size chamber pot until he voids. If this is conscientiously carried out, in a few weeks regular habits of urination and defecation will be established, and subsequently maintained. He should be taken to the toilet to void four or five times a day at regular intervals. This should and can be done without arousing the child's antagonism to the training program. Emotional scenes serve only to give the child the center of the stage which will lead him to wet his bed simply to annoy his parents and thus attain revenge for their unpleasantness or to achieve unwarranted solicitude. The child should be urged to hold his urine thirty to forty minutes longer than usual in the daytime to increase the bladder capacity. After recovery from illness during which established habits of elimination may have been disrupted, resumption of the prophylactic effort should be prompt and the results may be expected to be as satisfactory as they were initially. Failure to subject these recuperating children to retraining accounts for most reappearances of enuresis following incapacitating illness.

In the care and management of an enuretic child it is well that his mother largely has this responsibility until he is two to three years old, her attitude and relationship being friendly, tender and social. By the third year the father should assume responsibility of carrying on this attitude and introducing the child to new interests and social contacts. A child thus ideally started in life can be expected to make his own social relations by the time he is six. A cooperative attitude on the part of the parents and other members of the family towards the child as well as towards each other will foster a normal physical and psychic growth, and establish a foundation on which enuresis will develop only by reason of some outspoken and usually discoverable abnormality of structure or function. Companionship with other children of his age is most important to forestall antisocial manifestations and give him a broad sense of social responsibility. Failure to have or make pleasant relationships fosters a deep feeling of uncertainty and social insecurity in the child from which he may suffer undue teasing and humiliation. As a corollary, during this period, pampering, scholastic overwork, and undue punishment for minor infractions, or artificially setting the child up in an ivory tower are to be avoided.

Medical Therapy. If the child has never had proper habit training this should be instituted at once and conscientiously pursued; in many instances it alone will achieve the desired result. Experience with even a few enuretic children should convince any clinician of the importance of directing his major efforts at the mother who is usually neurotic, emotional, irritable, maladjusted, unsympathetic or egocentric, and in most instances largely to blame for the child's functional disturbance. To the child the importance of enuresis may wisely be minimized; in planning the training program, the child should be given the initiative or at least made to feel that the whole schedule is his idea.

The parents should be told that the fault is primarily theirs, that their attitude towards the child must be unemotional, and by precept and conversation build up by reassurance and encouragement, the child's self-confidence and will to overcome the habit. His sense of security must be increased to the utmost, for until he feels this strongly it will be extremely difficult to cure the enuresis and prevent relapse. Sometimes a change in school and surroundings is desirable, for in the new environment the child develops new social interests, wishes to make a good appearance in keeping up his end, and is removed from the individual (usually the mother) against whom he consciously or subconsciously established the enuretic defense. If he stays dry for a month, the cure is likely to be permanent except as return to former surroundings may lead to recurrence of the habit.

Sharply *restricting the fluids after 4 o'clock* in the afternoon makes little sense as the enuretic bladder will empty itself with only 2 ounces in it as surely as with 6 ounces.

Picking the child up during the night is a widely employed practice to forestall enuresis but does no good unless the child is thoroughly awakened and knows what is going on and why. If the approximate time of the bedwetting is known, the parent tries to anticipate it and puts the child on the toilet until he urinates; this may be as early as 10 o'clock or as late as 4 in the morning. Usually it is best that the father do the picking up particularly if the wetter is a boy. But wake him up when he is picked up even if he has to be made to wash his face or brush his teeth, so that he knows he is being put on the toilet and why. The mere carrying of a drowsy child to the toilet where he consciously or subsconsciously urinates without being fully aroused, only encourages the enuretic habit.

Many alarm devices have been contrived to awaken the child when his voided urine closes an electric circuit to ring a bell or cause a shock. Yet by the time he is awake, he has usually soaked the bed. In older cooperative enuretic children, a schedule can sometimes be arranged using an alarm clock which they set themselves for about thirty minutes prior to the suspected time of wetting, and reset after they have returned to bed following bladder emptying in the bathroom. Eventually they get tired of bothering with the clock and decide it is easier to stay dry than be awakened during the night. Similarly in boys the employment of a penis clamp is frequently effective in habit training, the voiding during sleep causing painful urethral dilatation which awakens the patient. As he successfully persists, he gets tired of fooling with the gadget and develops the will to stop wetting.

When it is determined that the child has no organic disease of the urinary tract, I lean to the "Let them stew in their juices!" treatment which, though extreme, is effective when the psychoneurotic or over-emotional mother can be persuaded to cooperate. The problem is not discussed with the child, fluids are not limited, and he is allowed to sleep throughout the night even though he wets several times. The bed linen and pajamas are changed once a week or whenever it is done for the rest of the family. The roughness and unpleasant odor of the bed and the sleeping garments soon furnish sufficient stimulus to stay dry. The child enjoys the rough linen and odorous urine no more than his mother or the housekeeper who, if they relent, defeat the treatment and the child wins his point.

The management of some highly emotional, irritable, uncooperative, neurotic enuretic children sometimes requires a properly qualified child psychologist or psychiatrist. In most instances the mother rather than the child should receive the treatment. Unfortunately, there are relatively few equipped by training in psychiatric theory to whom I would feel safe in turning over such a child with the hope of a rational and wholesome attack upon his problem. I see no reason why such a child should be exposed to the commonly tendered psychiatric sewage. Acceptable psychiatric assistance is not available in many of the smaller cities and communities and the child's physician must necessarily undertake the child's problem on his own.

Drug Therapy. *Atropine* (belladonna in one form or another) is still the most widely used drug and is usually administered as an antispasmodic. Pharmacologically atropine is indicated only in cases of parasympathetic imbalance (hypertonic bladder), the drug being a parasympathetic inhibitor. Its effect is to relieve the relative tonicity of the vesical outlet and relax the detrusor with corresponding increased vesical capacity. It is, therefore, contraindicated in atonic bladder or in sympathetic imbalance which, cystometrically, comprise a fourth of the cases and in which the administration of small doses of ephedrine is sometimes effective (cf. infra).

Atropine is usually given as the tincture of belladonna (.00003 gm. or 1/2000 gr. of atropine sulfate per minim), the initial dose being one drop per year of age given morning and night, and increased daily by one drop until the physiologic effects (flushing of the face, acceleration of the pulse, dryness of the throat) occur. The dose then is reduced one drop and continued for at least two weeks after wetting has ceased and there is reason to believe the habit has been broken. Resumption of the drug following relapses is commonly ineffective and suggests that much of its value is probably psychotherapeutic. *Ephedrine sulfate* in doses varying from 25 to 50 mg. a day has been employed empirically in the same manner as atropine with reported benefit in many cases. Yet the ephedrine effect in some children has been so pronounced as to induce acute retention and for this reason is not warranted for the treatment of functional enuresis. *Benzedrine* has been employed to promote lighter sleep; *testosterone* in doses of 10 to 20 mg. per day orally has been effective in an encouraging number of enuretic boys and girls, the hormone increasing muscular (detrusor) tonus, the stimulation most enuretics do not need, the good results suggesting successful psychotherapy.

Psychotherapy by suggestion strives to restore the child's confidence in himself through encouragement and optimism. Threats and punishment, humiliation and the like have no place in the treatment of enuresis and every effort should be made to assure the child that his condition is neither serious nor incurable, and with cooperation and help on his part, he will have a dry bed. Encouragement with rewards, gold stars, calendar keeping with dry days and nights appropriately marked thereon makes the psychic treatment a game with many, especially when the slogan, "I will stay dry!" is added. *The child with functional enuresis will be cured as soon as he develops the will to stay dry*. Since it achieves for them the attention they desire on the one hand and a form of revenge on the other, most enuretics have no wish to exert will power and have no desire to awaken. In the therapeutic course every effort must be bent to avoid making the enuretic child feel that there is nothing in life but urine, wet sheets, his bladder, and the toilet seat.

Urologic Treatment. When conservative medical or psychologic treatment has proved fruitless after an intensive trial of three months, urologic examination should be carried out. Further treatment will be that indicated by the demonstrated disease and with the eradication of which the enuresis usually ceases. Only by accepting the broad urologic view-point and affording these children the study to which they are entitled, will unsuspected major uropathy be disclosed. As many of these children grow older, they are able to keep a dry bed by getting up at night but conversion of night wetting to nocturia must not be considered a cure, for in nearly all of these patients some major uropathy will be found, whether congenital obstructive lesions at the vesical outlet, in the urethra, vesical stone, diverticulum or, commonly, persistent infection.

In young girls with enuresis, urethral stricture and urethrotrigonitis involving the posterior urethra and anterior trigone have been the most frequent urologic findings in our series, the inflammatory lesion ranging from mild to extreme. Sometimes large edematous mucosal blebs are seen and in long-standing cases cystic and papillary changes in the mucosa about the vesical outlet appear identical in all respects with those observed in adult women with long-standing urethrotrigonitis. Here adequate urethral dilation and the instillation of one, two, or three drops of silver nitrate 1:1000, or light fulguration of the disease-bearing area is usually rapidly curative and with this the enuresis commonly ceases. Similarly in males, the mere passage of catheters to determine residual urine or of a sound to ensure normal urethral patency has often been followed by cessation of the enuresis and here the benefit may be ascribed to the establishment of free urinary drainage rather than to successful psycho-therapy.

CHAPTER 10   *Injuries of the Urogenital Tract*

Introduction. It is imperative that as physicians we be aware of the increasing importance of urogenital tract trauma; certainly the economic scavengers of the legal profession are! In major accidents of all kinds there is grave likelihood of urogenital injury and, conversely, today's horrible incidence will be reduced only with measures enforced to prevent such tragedies. *Accidents kill more children after infancy than any single disease;* four fifths of these accidents to children over five years of age are ascribable to the errors of adults, notably motor and street accidents. In adults in civilian life, the most common causes of serious injury of the urogenital tract are motor vehicle accidents, followed closely by accidents in industry. In military activities or warfare, gunshot or explosions account for most urologic injuries which, in turn, comprise about 2.5 per cent of all war trauma. Usually these injuries are but part of generalized body trauma involving one or more other systems. With the ever-expanding operation of the Workmen's Compensation Act, industrial trauma has received great attention. Surgical accidents, and here we are thinking particularly of instrumental trauma during urologic examination, are rare indeed at the hands of the properly trained and experienced instrumenteur. Yet in the young, particularly, an inflamed or otherwise diseased ureter may be perforated by a catheter ever so gently passed.

INJURIES OF THE KIDNEYS

These organs are injured more often than any other urinary tract structure and this is particularly striking in children. Although the kidneys are protected by surrounding bony and muscular structures, they may be injured by abdominal, loin or lumbar blows, by falls of the body, by indirect force, by sudden muscular exertion or by penetrating wounds.

Each kidney is somewhat movable normally, the right usually more than the left, moving with changes in position of the body and with respiration, the most secure fixation being that of its vessels to the aorta and vena cava (Fig. 209). Normally a fifth to a fourth of the kidney extends below the costal margin posteriorly and with inspiration as much as a half may extend below the last rib, particularly on the right side. This part is exposed to injury by direct force transmitted through the soft tissues of the loin or abdomen, or may be broken upon the rib while serving as the lower arm of a lever with the rib as a fulcrum. Because of its free natural mobility the kidney is further exposed to injury when great force is applied to exaggerate this motion suddenly. Thus, in the fall of the human body and suddenly checked on landing, the action upon the kidney produces not only a bursting effect but a sudden jerk upon all its attachments, leading to subsequent abnormal mobility or even a snaplike action on the pedicle which tears the vessels, sometimes completely. A mobile, low-lying, ectopic kidney or one enlarged by hyperplasia, hydronephrosis or tumor is more directly exposed to trauma than a normal size, normally placed organ. Usually the spine affords protection yet its transverse processes and especially the lower ribs, may be factors of danger when the blow is received in the lateral loin or over the anterior abdomen to crush or lacerate the kidney against the skeleton. Or, a sharp blow from behind may drive the lower ribs in to contuse or lacerate the kidney, and in costal fractures sharp fragments may penetrate or tear the organ.

It is likely that the normal mobility of the kidneys is a relative protective mechanism but that the comparative fixation of the right kidney by the liver accounts for the somewhat higher incidence of right-sided renal injuries. The perirenal fat is an added protective measure in adults but in the young this layer is extremely scant. The same blow that injures

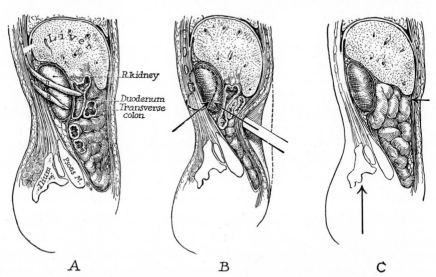

FIGURE 209.   Renal injury. Mechanics involved in the various types. *A, B*, with a blow from in front, the last rib acts as a fulcrum. If the patient is struck from behind, the kidney may be contused against the liver. *C*, renal injuries in falls; the principal injury is often by whiplike action in which the renal vascular attachments may be severed.

the kidney may gravely injure interposed or adjacent abdominal viscera, often with laceration of the overlying peritoneum.

The *mechanics of renal rupture* or fragmentation are based on the fact that the kidney is an encapsulated organ filled with blood and when struck a sudden blow, and by the law of hydrostatics, "force exerted upon any part of the fluid is transmitted equally in all directions throughout the mass" affecting the kidney, therefore, as a bursting force. If mild this may cause only minute lacerations involving the cortex, or the capsule, but with severe injury there is diffuse fragmentation, may be multiple bisections, or even pulpefaction (Fig. 210). With rupture of the kidney the degree and course of hemorrhage or of urinary extravasation will depend upon the extent or location of the wound. This may be about the kidney, upward to the pleura, or by peritoneal laceration, into its cavity.

Etiology. This may be by:

1. Direct Force:	Blows over the kidney area and falls striking upon the back, loin or abdomen, crushing force as in run-over injuries.
2. Indirect Force:	Falls of the body landing upon the head, feet, buttocks or other parts, and without direct trauma over the kidney area.
3. Sudden Muscular Action:	As in lifting heavy objects or cranking a motor.
4. Penetrating Wounds:	Gunshot, shell, stabbing, piercing objects such as fence spike, branch of tree and the like.
5. Surgical Procedures:	Chiefly for diagnostic purpose.

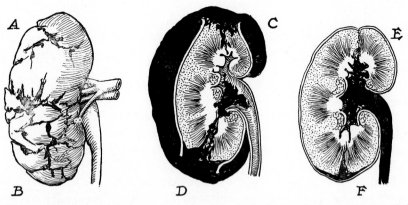

FIGURE 210. Renal injury; various types. *A*, single fissure. *B*, fragmentation of the kidney. *C*, laceration of the renal capsule and parenchyma with perirenal hematoma but without penetration of the pelvis. *D*, same as *C*, except the pelvis is penetrated. *E*, laceration of the parenchyma with profuse bleeding into the pelvis. *F*, parenchymal laceration with subcapsular hematoma.

The renal parenchyma and pelvis have been injured by too forceful injection of radiographic solutions, or the ureter has been penetrated by a diagnostic catheter. In surgical trauma the amount of force exerted and extent of tissue damage are not mutually reciprocal.

Pathology. Direct or indirect violence to the kidney may cause contusion, laceration, rupture, piercing and/or crushing. The various types of injury and their resulting change in the kidney are schematically shown in Figure 210 and the mechanics involved in the different types of injury in Figure 209.

Contusions comprise about two thirds of all renal injury, are usually the result of a relatively mild trauma, and are manifested by ecchymosis with minute subcapsular tears radiating in all directions from the point of impact. A subcapsular hematoma may form and blood in the collecting tubules causes microscopic or macroscopic hematuria. When capsular laceration does not occur, a subcapsular hematoma may dissect extensively between the cortex and the capsule (Fig. 210).

Laceration or *rupture* of the kidney occurs with violent trauma. Ruptures generally follow the distribution of the large arterial trees, may involve the cortex with or without rupture of the capsule, with or without injury of the vessels within the perirenal fat. *Extravasation* does not occur unless there is direct communication between the pelvis or lacerated renal tubules and the perirenal tissues. With cortical laceration and opening of a pelvioperirenal path, extensive extravasation of urine and blood is the rule; it may extend downward to the pelvis, scrotum, or abdominal wall, upward to the subphrenic space or if the peritoneum has been ruptured, into this cavity. Laceration of the larger intrarenal vessels is usually followed by hemorrhagic infarction of the area they supply (Fig. 211). *Hematuria* may promptly cease when the pelvic outlet or the ureter is firmly plugged by clots. Unilateral *anuria* may result from (1) transverse laceration or (2) complete obstruction of the ureter, or (3) extensive laceration of the renal blood supply, and temporary anuria involving both kidneys is often reflex or is secondary to shock. Secondary infection of the perirenal hematoma may be anticipated when renal infection is known to be present. Occasionally, the hematoma becomes converted into a fluid cyst.

Pre-existing disease, particularly of the obstructive variety, predisposes to renal injury, especially high obstruction such as ureteropelvic stricture, ureteropelvic blockage by aberrant vessels, pelvic stone, or pyonephrosis. Simultaneous trauma of other structures such as the lungs, diaphragm, skeleton, or abdominal viscera is common and may outrank in gravity the urinary injury. Shock results from hemorrhage, injury to the local tissues, or neurologic disturbances, and occurs in nearly every case of serious renal trauma although in children especially its onset may be delayed.

Symptoms. Injury of the kidney is manifested by one or more of the following symptoms: Shock, renal pain, tenderness in the loin, inspiratory pain, appearance of a mass in the loin, hematuria, pallor, falling blood pressure, a diminution of circulating red cells and hemoglobin, variable elevation of the white blood cells and occasionally anuria and coma. Signs of external trauma may or may not be present and their absence does not rule out renal injury.

The chief symptoms of shock are pallor, cold and clammy skin, a small, soft rapid pulse, restlessness, thirst, and often disorientation. While this picture frequently develops immediately after trauma, in some patients its appearance is delayed for several hours and this is particularly true in children. Unfortunately the delayed appearance of shock is likely to postpone for many hours urgently needed supportive treatment and sometimes active surgical attack.

Pain is the most constant symptom of kidney injury, is usually manifested by a severe boring or tearing sensation felt in the loin or upper abdomen, and is present in practically every case. The degree of pain and of injury are not necessarily reciprocal. Pain on inspiration is common, is referred to the injured side, abdomen, loin or back. *Tenderness* in the loin is generally most intense and pronounced in the costovertebral angle but may be elicited over the entire abdomen. When the ureter is obstructed by clots, severe colic may ensue. Muscular rigidity in the loin

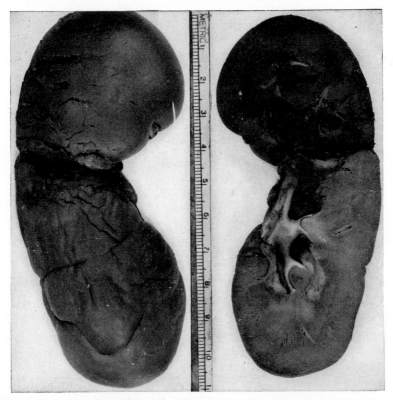

FIGURE 211. Traumatic bisection and partial fragmentation of the kidney in a ten-year-old girl run over by a truck. Nephrectomy. The hemorrhagic infarction of the lower renal pole resulting from interference with the blood supply is noteworthy.

or abdomen of the injured side is nearly always present to such a degree as to interfere with satisfactory palpation of the injured organ and its surroundings. When rigidity does not preclude satisfactory examination, a mass will usually be found in the loin when perirenal hematoma or urinary extravasation follows rupture of the organ. Yet with slow development, this mass may not appear until late. In any event the essential palpation should be extremely gentle lest fresh bleeding be stimulated. With extravasation into the peritoneal cavity, shifting dullness may be elicited, and at once warrants operation and a bad prognosis.

Hematuria is the most characteristic sign of injury of the urinary tract, occurs in more than 90 per cent of renal injuries and may be microscopic or profuse. Its absence from the urine may mean: (1) the collecting tubules have failed to drain the red cells into the pelvis which (2) *a*, is not lacerated, or *b*, is extensively ruptured; (3) complete laceration or transverse section of the ureter; (4) plugging of the ureter by clots, or (5) laceration of the renal pedicle. Stringy blood clots representing casts of the ureter are sometimes passed, and profuse renal bleeding may repeatedly fill the bladder with clots and threaten life. Bleeding may also originate in the lower urinary tract injured at the same time as the kidney; this must be determined by urologic investigation.

Anemia regularly accompanies renal injuries with profuse bleeding, and a complete blood count should be made as early as possible to distinguish clearly between anemia and the pallor of shock as complicating factors, and to establish a basis for comparison as clinical progress is studied. Early after injury the white blood cell count will be normal or slightly increased but with bleeding into the peritoneal cavity; a high leukocyte count, chiefly polymorphonuclear, is regularly observed and also may appear with the development of secondary perinephric abscess. As bleeding continues, the red cell count and blood pressure fall. The blood pressure is often extremely low when the patient is first seen in shock.

Gastrointestinal syptoms are predominantly reflex manifestations caused by trauma to the celiac axis, from extravasation into the peritoneal cavity or perchance from direct injury of intra-abdominal viscera. Nausea, vomiting and distention with rigidity of the abdominal musculature develop, but peritonitis is seldom evident until at least twenty-four hours after injury.

The *clinical course* depends upon the severity of the lesions and the occurrence of infection. With mild injury, shock, local tenderness and rigidity are proportionate and hematuria lasts but a few hours and disappears. In more severe injury, however, internal bleeding may be evident and, later, sepsis originating in or about the urinary tract. In grave injury there is usually initial profound shock, vomiting, and temporary unconsciousness. The clinician must be keenly aware of progressive changes in the clinical picture lest the opportunity to save life be passed, and this usually means by operation with hemostasis, drainage, liberal transfusion of whole blood and intensive antimicrobial therapy.

Diagnosis. A comprehensive examination is not always possible in renal trauma without grave jeopardy to the patient. When it can be obtained the history may indicate the nature and violence of the injury, whether there was shock, collapse, loss of consciousness, bleeding and pain. Some patients are first seen in coma. The physical examination usually discloses contusions, lacerations, or skin perforations in the renal area suggesting renal injury but a rigid abdomen and signs of intraperitoneal trauma commonly cause the urologic injury to be overlooked. If possible the loin should be palpated before rigidity has appeared but most gently because of the danger of inciting fresh bleeding. A blood count must be taken at once to indicate (1) the degree of anemia and leukocytosis, (2) the need for transfusion of whole blood, plasma or saline infusion and (3) to establish a norm or base line for comparison of future blood counts. When the patient voids fresh blood from the beginning of urination, the lower urinary tract should also be examined. If he cannot void he should be catheterized. In renal contusion the hematuria is usually transient. When renal injury follows slight trauma do not overlook the possibility of an underlying antecedent congenital anomaly, hydronephrosis, calculus, cystic or neoplastic disease, or nephritis. Jaundice and bile in the urine suggest hepatic injury. With hepatic or splenic injury there is usually hemorrhage into the peritoneal cavity with shifting dullness and occasionally even a fluid wave.

Differential Diagnosis. Contusion of the loin or abdomen with subcutaneous or subparietal bleeding, rupture of perirenal tissues with hematoma formation, or serious hemorrhage and hematoma in the loin may occur without rupture of the kidney but may demand incision and control of bleeding. Injuries of the peritoneum and other organs especially the intestine, liver, spleen and bladder must always be searched for and appropriately treated. Intraperitoneal hemorrhage is manifested by shock, free fluid in the peritoneal cavity, tympanites, signs of hemorrhage, rigidity of the abdominal wall, tenderness usually most marked over the site of peritoneal injury but commonly diffuse. A mass is rarely palpable and there is high leukocytosis. Peritoneal injury without hemorrhage produces shock, rigidity, tenderness and tympanites.

X-ray study of the urinary tract should be made to determine (1) alterations in the outlines of the kidneys or psoas muscles, (2) that two kidneys are present, and (3) skeletal fractures. Occasionally a stone will be demonstrated; obscuring of the renal outline and isolateral psoas muscle outline together with a concavity of the lumbar spine on the side of the injury are suggestive of perirenal extravasation, inflammation, or suppuration as in perirenal abscess.

Excretory urographic films are of value in about three fourths of the cases of renal injury but should always be made as soon as the condition of the patient warrants, and this is generally within six to twenty-four hours following injury. Yet in some cases the study can be made immediately before shock is manifested, and here the demonstration of a sound functioning kidney on the uninjured side is one of the chief ob-

jectives of the examination lest removal of the injured organ would leave
a diseased, cystic, hypoplastic or no renal mate. In mild renal injury as
suggested by repeated blood counts and maintenance of blood pressure,
the pyelogram is normal but with pelvic laceration, extravasation of the
medium into the parenchyma and externally into the retroperitoneal
space is usually demonstrable (Fig. 212). Pelvic filling defects usually
result from blood clots. In the excretory study, the initial plain film is of
importance when it demonstrates obliteration of the psoas muscle shadow
and often lateral scoliosis isolateral with the injury.

Cystoscopy. When the excretory study is unsatisfactory and the
condition of the patient suggests that the injury is not a minor one, a
cystoscopic investigation is essential.

A rapidly falling red cell count and hemoglobin estimation call for
voluminous transfusion and immediate surgical intervention but when
this can justifiably be delayed, urologic investigation is advisable. At
cystoscopy blood will be seen emerging from the ureteral orifice of the
injured kidney, or by chromocystoscopy with indigo carmine, the uninjured organ will be determined adequate to support life. Bilateral retrograde pyelography will further fortify the diagnosis, the injection of
medium being particularly slow and gentle on the injured side to avoid
inciting fresh hemorrhage. Yet cystoscopy and pyelography should not

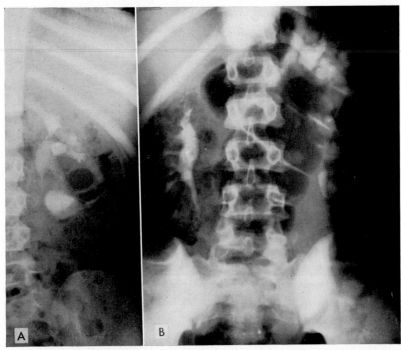

FIGURE 212. Rupture of the upper segment of the left kidney. *A*, there is considerable localized extravasation of the injected urographic medium. *B*, further extravasation of the urographic medium down the left lumbar gutter; normal right pyelogram.
Nephrectomy.

be performed even in severe renal injury unless one is prepared to operate at once. Nevertheless, one should not allow the patient to die of shock or hemorrhage while attempting to make an accurate and inclusive anatomic diagnosis. If he is still bleeding freely and although the precise site and nature of injury is unknown, surgical intervention should be carried out without great delay. The competent surgeon will explore promptly to save the patient's life and will perhaps simultaneously complete the diagnosis. Only abdominal exploration may reveal the true condition. If possible, however, it is best that this surgery be postponed until the period of shock is over except when massive bleeding persists or there is evidence of intraperitoneal rupture or other severe trauma.

The chief dangers from kidney injury are death from hemorrhage or, later, infection and disability.

Treatment. Treatment of renal injury may be (1) conservative, and (2) surgical.

Conservative therapy with supportive measures and the combat of shock should be employed unless there are profuse hematuria and definite signs of continued bleeding. About two thirds of all patients with renal trauma may be successfully treated conservatively, the choice of this therapeutic course being fortified by excretory urographic findings as well. In mild renal injury the patient is put to bed and antimicrobial therapy is prophylactically administered or is given to combat known existing infection; this may forestall grave retroperitoneal phlegmon. Warm blankets and other forms of external heat are applied; morphine is given for pain or restlessness; the body fluids are restored by transfusion of whole blood, or by intravenous infusion or hypodermoclysis of 5 per cent glucose in physiologic saline solution. Hypotension is also combated by the intravenous administration of norepinephrine 4 to 5 mg. per 1000 cc. of 15 per cent glucose and normal saline. Occasionally necrosis occurs at the point of norepinephrine injection or along the injected vessel.

During this period of medical treatment gentle periodic examination of the loin for the appearance or increase in size of a mass, together with repeated blood counts every half hour should be made. In all external penetrating wounds of the urinary tract *tetanus antitoxin* should be given and especially when dirt has been introduced. First make sure the patient is not serum sensitive lest he require desensitization before antitoxin can be safely given.

The conservatively treated patient should be kept quiet until there has been no hematuria for a week. Especially is this important in children in whom delayed bleeding or the recurrence of vigorous bleeding frequently follows premature resumption of activity; I have twice seen death from uncontrollable hemorrhage occur in young patients allowed up and about prematurely.

Surgical Treatment. Continued bleeding, recurrence of hematuria, perirenal extravasation or suppuration, or anuria of twenty-four hours duration indicate that conservative treatment is inadequate and surgical intervention is needed. Operation is urgently indicated for: control of bleeding in severe hemorrhage, persistent anuria, intraperitoneal trauma and the drainage of infection following injury. Even with a good anesthetist, operative speed is desirable. When there is evidence of intraperitoneal injury the abdomen is first explored and the viscera repaired; the peritoneum is drained if indicated. The bleeding is stopped, exploration of the kidney is made and nephrectomy is performed but not until palpation has disclosed a good kidney on the other side or this has been previously demonstrated by intravenous urography, chromocystoscopy or retrograde study. Nephrectomy should not be employed when conservative surgical treatment can be substituted with ligation of small bleeding vessels, suture of lacerations, evacuation of perirenal clots, free drainage through the loin of bloody or urinous extravasation, or of suppuration in the retroperitoneal spaces. Limited mattress suture closure of larger renal rents or partial kidney resection with removal of a hopelessly lost renal segment will conserve some of these organs.

Rapid nephrectomy is indicated when (1) there is extensive bleeding which cannot be controlled without ligation of a considerable portion of the total renal blood supply, (2) when more than a fourth of a kidney has lost its blood supply by injury, or (3) when the patient is in profound shock. When the renal pedicle has been lacerated close to the aorta or vena cava or following nephrectomy, ligation of the pedicle is difficult or the patient is in grave shock, he should be speedily returned to bed with clamps left on the pedicle to be loosened on the third or fourth day, and removed on the fifth day. Postoperative treatment includes adequate blood transfusion, a large fluid intake by mouth, intravenous infusion, hypodermoclysis or proctoclysis with sufficient opiate to keep the patient comfortable. Meanwhile antibacterial therapy is intensively administered.

Complications of Renal Injury. Following conservative surgical treatment of the kidney persistent *urinary fistula* may demand late nephrectomy. Delayed *secondary hemorrhage* is the most important complication, usually appearing about the seventh to tenth day after injury and far more often in patients treated conservatively than surgically. Subphrenic abscess, duodenal fistula, secondary pyonephrosis, or infected hydronephrosis may also develop; the last two especially following *obstruction* by traumatic upper ureteral stricture. Complications may require drainage, ureteropelvioplasty, partial renal resection, renal suture or, most often, nephrectomy.

Prognosis depends not only upon the severity of the renal injury and its associated complications but the promptness and accuracy of the initial diagnosis and therapy. In general the mortality in uncomplicated severe renal injury is 25 to 30 per cent, hemorrhage accounting for most early deaths while sepsis, intraperitoneal and/or pulmonary complications or late hemorrhage cause most late deaths.

RENAL "CRUSH" SYNDROME

In the development of this syndrome there is no direct trauma to the kidney itself, but following severe injury to other parts of the body, especially the extremities and chest, the renal function is gravely impaired or becomes zero, and the condition progresses to terminal uremia. If the patient is to survive, the kidney slowly resumes function in seven to ten days. Crush syndrome initially was recognized in World War I and received deserving attention in World War II, especially in the bombing casualties in England and particularly in those people pinned under rubble for many hours. Yet it also occurs in industrial accidents, notably in mines but also in other civilian accidents.

According to its *clinical manifestations* the crush syndrome has been classified as (1) functional and (2) organic. The *functional* variety results from extrarenal injury, the azotemia being consequent to decreased glomerular filtration, and increased waste products formation as observed in severe hemorrhage and other causes of oligemic shock and accompanied by electrolyte loss, dehydration, vascular stasis, and cardiac tamponade. The *organic* variety is consequent to extensive burns, crushing injury including explosive pneumatic shock, traumatic hepatic necrosis, obstetric shock, intravascular hemolysis, and blockade of renal tubules by sulfonamide crystals or myoglobin.

Pathology. In patients dying in uremia of crush syndrome, the gross appearance of the kidneys on section is normal except that they are unusually heavy, greatly swollen and extremely wet (edema). Microscopic examination shows tubular nephritis similar to that observed in bichloride of mercury poisoning, but the cloudy swelling, acute parenchymatous degeneration or necrosis of the tubules is confined to the ascending limbs of the loop of Henle and the second convoluted tubules to which condition the term *lower nephron nephrosis* has been applied. Uric acid and phosphoric acid, two substances occurring in human metabolism, have been found to produce this lesion and in distinction to the upper nephron (upper segment of first convoluted tubule) lesion caused by the usual experimental renal poisons.

The specific localization in the lower nephrons has been attributed to the normal high acidity of the urine filtrate in these tubular segments which adversely influences the toxic activity of excreted substances and particularly myohemoglobin which is regularly found in the lumina of the lower tubular segments in crush syndrome. The myoglobin is derived from traumatized muscle, is carried through the blood to the kidneys and is precipitated in the highly acid urine of the lower nephron segment which may thereby become occluded.

Trueta Shunt. From experimental work Trueta et al. (1947) concluded that much of the renal failure results from cortical anoxia, the circulatory disturbances being caused by neuromuscular reflexes in consequence of which vascular spasm shunts a large portion of the blood from the cortical nephrons to produce ischemia and diminish glomerular function. As a result of the arteriovenous shunt, the blood is believed to be by-passed through intrarenal circuits including the vasa recta and glomeruli in the corticomedullary zone. This diminished rerouting leads to tubular anoxemia and degeneration with reduction of function. If the kidney function can be maintained for eight to nine days the organs will probably recover and here employment of the artificial kidney has found certain application. Yet the conception of *arteriovenous shunt* is not universally accepted and it must be recognized that all renal factors concerned in the causation of crush syndromes are not known.

Symptoms and Diagnosis. Patients injured by bomb blast, explosion or otherwise and especially those long confined by overlying debris, are found in shock, the severity of which will be influenced by the gravity of the injury and hemorrhage and the lapse of time. When blood transfusion or plasma, normal saline and/or dextrose are administered promptly, most of these patients will revive and for hours or days appear to be progressing satisfactorily. Yet the urinary output diminishes, the blood pressure rises, the blood plasma shows increased urea, potassium and phosphate retention, and acidosis. The retained potassium adversely influences the heart and in the terminal uremic picture appearing in seven to ten days, a failing cardiac action resembles that seen in potassium poisoning.

Treatment is that of toxic anuria, and if the patient can be tided over for seven to ten days by supportive treatment or by the artificial kidney, the tubular units may again begin to function. Yet the delayed mortality has been exceedingly high.

Injury of the Renal Pedicle

This may occur without rupture or laceration of the kidney and most commonly results from crushing injuries including difficult delivery. Yet the patient may fall, landing on the buttocks, and the whiplike snap caused by the momentum of the falling kidney suddenly stopped may completely tear the renal pedicle from the great vessels. In one of our neonatal cases studied post mortem following difficult delivery and birth trauma, the left kidney was found free floating in the abdomen. Occasionally in lesser laceration of the renal pedicle, thrombosis and clotting may prevent fatal hemorrhage but the kidney will probably be lost. With even lesser vascular injury there may be only transient pain and hematuria with great or little renal infarction or thrombosis. The usual symptoms of rupture of the renal pedicle are profound shock, severe anemia, and isolateral anuria. The condition of the patient generally precludes an accurate diagnostic study; nearly all cases require rapid nephrectomy with prompt and complete hemostatis.

Spontaneous perirenal hematoma (perirenal apoplexy) has been observed in a few patients with pronounced hypertensive vascular disease, adrenal apoplexy (spontaneous hemorrhage), aortic or ovarian aneurysm, hemorrhage into the perirenal fat, leukemia, hemophilia, sepsis, periarteritis nodosa, arteriosclerosis, the symptomatic picture suggesting renal injury. The diagnosis is made at operation.

INJURIES OF THE URETER

These are extremely rare and when due to external trauma, it is usually received at the same time as renal injuries or concurrent with severe retroperitoneal injury. The rarity of ureteral injury by external forces is explained by its deep location; through half of its course it is surrounded by pelvic bony walls. Most external injuries of the ureter are due to crushing and almost all caused by motor accidents or by a kick. Ureteral injuries are chiefly external penetrating wounds or surgical accidents, most commonly catheterization trauma, clamping, laceration, ligation, denudation, or division of the ureter during pelvic operations, particularly hysterectomy, and, not infrequently, injury of the terminal ureteral artery branch in the Wertheim operation with resulting gangrene of the terminal ureter. It is unusual to penetrate a normal ureter with a catheter unstiffened by a metal stylet but a diseased ureter can be penetrated with unsuspected ease; periureteral extravasation usually follows and often with subsequent suppuration (Fig. 213). Parenthetically, a catheter stiffened by a wire stylet should never be used for ureteral instrumentation, especially in the young. Great care and gentleness in the catheterization of ureters is the best prophylaxis against instrumental ureteral injury.

The *symptoms* always suggest injury to the kidney but are seldom as extreme and require similar diagnostic investigation. In many cases of renal trauma only the pelvis is lacerated. A force sufficient to injure the ureter almost always injures other abdominal viscera as well. When the initial shock passes off the pain ameliorates, hematuria ceases but after a few days a mass may appear in the loin. A mass caused by peri-

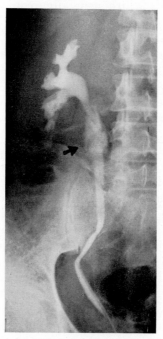

FIGURE 213. Ureteral injury by catheter perforation with periureteral extravasation.

ureteral extravasation and/or phlegmon will be found occasionally with early local gangrene.

A thorough urologic investigation is warranted in all cases. Excretory urography may disclose the site of the injury, urinary leakage, and peri-ureteral extravasation but retrograde ureterography and pyelography may be necessary to obtain a satisfactory urographic demonstration. The dangers of stirring up fresh bleeding or of introducing or disseminating infection by the ureteral catheterization and ureterography are minimal, and may be disregarded if one is prepared to operate at once. In rare instances ureteral injury has led to massive retroperitoneal urinary cyst formation; in Alyea's case—a three-year-old boy—the cyst held six liters.

Treatment. This corresponds in general to the treatment of renal injury. Unless there is a retroperitoneal collection of urine, blood or pus, or there is sepsis, treatment should be conservative with indwelling ureteral catheter, rest in bed and supportive measures as outlined under treatment of renal trauma. When conservative treatment is contraindicated or fails, the ureter should be promptly explored; ureterotomy, pyelotomy or ureteral anastomosis is performed and adequate drainage established. Other surgical procedures which may be needed include deligation, ureteroneocystostomy, ureteroureteral anastomosis, ureteral reconstruction or nephrectomy.

Complete section of the ureter, and especially in its upper segment, usually demands nephrectomy; only rarely is anastomosis of the trau-matized normal-size ureter successful. Subsequent stricture formation produces hydronephrosis which generally requires nephrectomy. When anastomosis of the ureter is attempted it is well to leave a catheter in the duct not only to facilitate suturing and to splint the ureter after repair but to drain the kidney pelvis as well. Small lacerations of the ureter require only drainage, not suture. When the lowermost ureter is severed, employ ureteroneocystostomy, reconstruction of the lower end of the ureter using a vesical flap, or ureterosigmoidostomy. Ligation of the ureter above the point of injury as a substitute for nephrectomy is poor practice.

INJURIES OF THE BLADDER

The bladder may be injured by penetrating wounds (including surgical accidents) and by rupture (Fig. 214). Fundamentally all trau-matic injuries of the bladder receive the same clinical and therapeutic considerations but the etiologic differences merit special consideration. Penetrating wounds of the bladder may be externally caused by sticks, gunshot, pickets, or surgical instruments, and internally by bony spicules, instruments or objects introduced into the bladder such as knitting needles or hairpins. The point of entrance is usually suprapubic but may be through the perineum, vagina, rectum, or obturator foramen; in the last instance the patient usually falls on a picket or pitchfork handle or sits on a nail. Fragments of clothing and dirt are usually carried into the wound by penetrating objects at the time of explosion or other accident. In some instances a spicule of wood has inadvertently been left in the wound. The point of external entry is usually evident and together with the history makes the diagnosis. In several recorded instances, the bladder in a hernial sac has been unwittingly incised at the time of herniotomy. With crushing wounds of the pelvis, bony spicules may perforate the bladder wall and often there are complicating injuries of the abdominal contents, especially the small intestine and rectum.

Symptoms and the clinical picture largely depend upon the gravity of the lesions, whether the peritoneum has been perforated, and whether infection exists.

Perforation. In *intravesical perforation* by a sound, cystoscope, or lithotrite, the instrumenteur is rarely aware of the accident for several days when the unfavorable condition of the patient demands investigation. Similarly darning needles, hairpins and other objects or foreign bodies perforating into the bladder from the vagina establish a urinary fistula which may extend to cause peritonitis on the one hand and vaginal leakage of urine on the other. When the bladder is accidentally incised during herniotomy or other surgical procedure, it should be promptly closed with an inverting suture, avoiding the mucosa, and an indwelling urethral catheter left in the bladder for at least seven days. Today most simple penetrating wounds of the bladder can be treated by indwelling catheter drainage and intensive antibiotic therapy. When there is evidence of pelvic phlegmon or peritonitis, surgical intervention with drainage is required.

Rupture. This is the most frequent major vesical injury, about 10 per cent of bladder ruptures occurring in children. Most bladder ruptures in adults are in males. In the female the bladder rests somewhat lower in the pelvis while the nature of male activities, particularly earning a livelihood, are much more violent. The vulnerability of the bladder to injuries is in direct ratio to its distention and it is a question whether an empty bladder is ever ruptured. The distended bladder is always an abdominal viscus and is therefore exposed to the same external violence as other abdominal organs (Fig. 214). Yet it may be perforated by a bony spicule, sharp instrument, or it may be torn as in pelvic fracture. More-

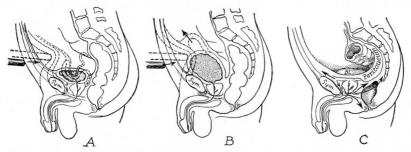

FIGURE 214. Injuries of the bladder. Mechanism of vesical rupture. *A*, in a slightly filled bladder retroperitoneal rupture occurs more frequently. An empty bladder may be lacerated but does not rupture. *B*, when the bladder is full and trauma is in the anterior-posterior position, the rupture is usually intraperitoneal. *C*, course of extravasation in extraperitoneal laceration; perirectal and retroperitoneal infiltration may be extreme.

over, chronic distention, infection or ulceration by weakening the bladder wall predispose to spontaneous rupture. Yet true spontaneous rupture probably never appears, the trauma being no more than a slight misstep or fall, an unnoted suprapubic kick or blow, or even the exertion of getting out of bed or straining at stool. Sometimes the rupture follows a fall or a kick in the abdomen.

In adults a third of all bladder ruptures occur during acute alcoholism when the viscus is greatly overdistended but in children the majority are associated with motor injuries. In motor injuries the victims are sometimes passengers but equally often pedestrians who are crushed against another car or struck down and run over by the vehicle. Associated pelvic or other skeletal fractures commonly occur. In all cases of pelvic fracture, rupture of the bladder should be suspected, and the possibility of rupture of the posterior urethra should not be overlooked. Moreover, in a third of the cases of pelvic fracture without vesical rupture, gross hematuria or disturbances of urination such as acute retention or marked dysuria occur.

The bladder may rupture intraperitoneally or extraperitoneally.

Intraperitoneal ruptures constitute about two thirds of all bladder ruptures, free fluid is found in the abdominal cavity, and the dome of the bladder is most often the site of laceration which is generally transverse but may have a bizarre shape. Rupture may open both into the peritoneal cavity and the extraperitoneal perivesical space. When the rupture occurs at a point where the bladder wall has been crushed or torn, it often forms a thin lacework effect so that the actual urinary leakage is slow and the bladder capacity apparently remains approximately normal; this largely negates the catheter test of bladder rupture (q.v.). A bladder rent may extend down through the vesical outlet well into the posterior urethra (Fig. 215).

In the absence of peripheral obstruction, minor vesical lacerations or ruptures may become walled off and spontaneously heal or the lesion become important only when infection develops.

In *extraperitoneal rupture* the course of extravasation will be guided by the various fascial structures of the deep pelvis as shown in Figure 175. Extensive edematous urinous infiltration of the abdominal musculature and perivesical tissues ensues, these being soggy grayish, or grayish-red, dead looking, and may contain abscesses. Gas bacillus infection, usually other than B. welchii, is sometimes present as well as widespread suppuration. Occasionally the extravasation extends along the spermatic cord to the scrotum.

Symptoms. Following pelvic injury and rupture of the bladder there is usually shock which persists for a variable period. One fourth of all patients brought to the hospital are in shock, comatose or moribund and some die promptly. The appearance of these patients usually suggests internal hemorrhage. There is generally low abdominal pain which may be most excruciating when pelvic fracture coexists. Later the abdominal pain is generalized. The whole abdomen is tender and rigid. Hematuria, dysuria or inability to void, together with exquisite tenderness in the bladder region, suggest severe vesical injury. Yet the dysuria may be due to (1) reflex sphincterospasm, (2) urethral injury, or (3) absence of urine in the bladder because of anuria or of intraperitoneal urinary drainage. With peritonitis, the abdominal tenderness and rigidity spread and intensify, and nausea and vomiting appear; gastrointestinal upsets in vesical rupture are unusual except with complicating peritonitis. In mild cases there may be only pelvic discomfort, slight urinary difficulty perhaps with hematuria, but toxemia and sepsis may be anticipated in every case with urinary extravasation. The mortality is vastly increased by delay in making the diagnosis.

Diagnosis. Here the important considerations in the history are the time, nature, and site of impact, whether consciousness was lost, vomiting occurred, was the patient subsequently able to void or was there hematuria. Yet grossly clear urine does not necessarily indicate an intact bladder. In external vesical penetration the site of entry may be the only clue as, for example, in a comatose patient picked up from the street. Fluid wave or shifting dullness is noted in half the cases with intraperitoneal rupture. Yet abdominal rigidity may preclude satisfactory palpation.

Rectal examination is important to determine if perivesical extravasation and brawny induration of urinary phlegmon exist. An ancient and

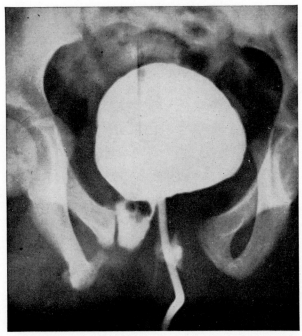

FIGURE 215. Bladder injury. Rupture of the bladder near the vesical outlet in a five-year-old boy run over by a truck. The extravasation is here cystographically indicated near the bladder neck and in the membranous urethra. The last resulted from laceration of the triangular ligament in association with fracture of the pubic bone and separation of the symphysis.

most inaccurate test for ruptured bladder is that of catheterization. No urine and only a small amount of blood may be obtained; clots may plug the catheter. Sometimes an enormous quantity of fluid is returned, far more than usual vesical distention would suggest; this signifies drainage of the peritoneal cavity or perivesical space filled with urine.

In the *catheter mensuration* test, a known amount of fluid is injected and the quantity returned by catheter is measured. Even with a ruptured bladder and especially one with slow leakage, the quantity return may be essentially that injected. The drainage of an abdominal pool of urine is by far the most significant of any of the catheterization tests. Yet a previously uninfected peritoneal cavity may by this test become infected.

With the catheter in the bladder, cystographic injection may be expected to show the site of laceration and relative degree of extravasation. Yet in the absence of shock this information may usually be achieved by excretory urography (cystography) and without subjecting the patient to the introduction of infection.

Excretory urography is the first step and often discloses perivesical or periurethral infiltration, edema or extravasation with or without pelvic fracture. The tear-drop or pear-shaped bladder (Fig. 216, Prather, 1948), so called because of its inverted pear-shape cystographic outline, reflects compression of the lower vesical segment and upward displacement of the upper segment by extensive perivesical edema, infiltration, hematoma or extravasation, and rupture of the bladder or adjacent prostatic urethra; it most often accompanies pelvic fracture. In some instances the cystogram may show the bladder entirely disrupted from the urethra at the bladder neck.

When the vesical rupture is *extraperitoneal* and high, the extravasated contrast medium, blocked by pericystic edema and intact peri-

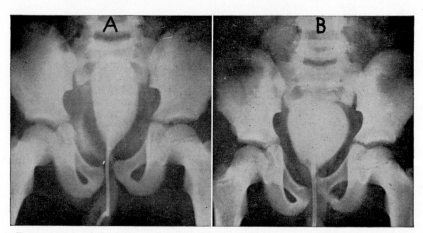

FIGURE 216. Bladder injury. *A*, "tear-drop" cystogram in an eight-year-old boy who had been struck by a truck and suffered pelvic fracture. The peculiar bladder outline results from compression of the viscus by perivesical hemorrhage, edema and/or urine. *B*, weeks later, following absorption of the perivesical hematoma and edema, the cystogram is again normal. (Courtesy Dr. George C. Prather and Journal of Urology.)

toneum, may cystographically suggest a diverticulum of the posterior superior aspect of the bladder wall. With extensive extraperitoneal rupture the cystographic medium diffuses widely about the pelvis, downward toward the bladder base and upward retroperitoneal. In *intraperitoneal* rupture, the medium extends extensively throughout the pelvis, peritoneal cavity and iliac fossa with little medium evident in the bladder itself. Cysto-urethrography may also demonstrate vesical or deep urethral extravasation.

Cystoscopy is the most accurate method of diagnosis in bladder rupture but copious bleeding or inability to distend the bladder because of intraperitoneal rupture may render the method useless. *It should be omitted if the diagnosis can be made without it.* A low and falling red blood cell count and hemoglobin indicative of hemorrhage is the most important laboratory finding. Leukocytosis is pronounced and high, especially with complicating peritonitis. In many cases complete diagnosis requires exploration and particularly when the patient is in poor condition and there is evidence of peritonitis and/or rupture of another abdominal viscus.

Treatment. The initial supportive treatment of bladder rupture is precisely the same as that employed in treatment of renal injury described earlier in this chapter to which the reader is referred. Once the diagnosis is made, hopeful waiting is fruitless because the clinical course is one of rapid decline.

Cystostomy should be performed without delay and the peritoneum explored at once even though intraperitoneal rupture is not suspected. Existing visceral injuries are attended to, the peritoneal rent is hastily closed by the minimum of sutures required to grasp the bladder musculature. The important step is the establishment of free suprapubic bladder drainage, leaving a tube of large caliber anchored in the bladder. With this, bleeding and extravasation will promptly cease and small unsutured bladder wounds will heal. Bony spicules, foreign bodies or other abnormal findings in the bladder should be removed. Many patients with extraperitoneal bladder rupture have been saved by ample bladder drainage alone. Perineal urethrostomy drainage is inadequate.

When pelvic fracture complicates rupture of the bladder, reduction of the fracture and the application of plaster must be deferred until the urologic lesions are adequately treated; free urinary drainage by a well working tube will avoid soaking the cast. The pelvis is immobilized by a firm binder, suspended as a hammock or sling from a Bradford frame. The legs are kept extended and the patient is able to move himself by aid of a pulley.

Complications. Shock and hemorrhage may be immediately fatal as may extravasation and sepsis later, and generally within a week. Although peritonitis develops in about two thirds of intraperitoneal ruptures, in many of these cases the urine is sterile and surgical intervention, establishment of free drainage, and intensive antibacterial therapy may be expected to save the patient. Yet associated injury or rupture of other

intra-abdominal viscera may be fatal, as often is the added shock of
pelvic fracture. The fracture may be complicated by acute osteomyelitis,
or infected bony spicules may lead to persistent urinary fistula (chiefly
vesical) or an acute pelvic suppuration. Stricture at the vesical outlet or
in the posterior urethra is frequent following injuries of these parts and
may cause a suprapubic fistula to persist in the cystostomy wound.

Prophylaxis against or combat of existing infection is by intensive
antimicrobial therapy according to specific bacteriologic indication.

Prognosis and Mortality.   The prognosis is always grave in all cases
of bladder rupture during the first week. This will be favorably influenced
by the rapidity and adequacy of surgical treatment. The establishment of
free drainage of the bladder and sites of extravasation, the liberal employment of whole blood transfusion and the intensive administration of
antimicrobic agents are life saving.

Prior to the introduction of sulfonamide therapy, 68 per cent of all
patients with rupture of the bladder died. This mortality has now been
cut in half, the mortality ratio of the patients with intraperitoneal and
extraperitoneal involvement being approximately three to two.

Prolapse of the Bladder.   This occurs as an eversion of this organ
through the urethral meatus and because it develops only in females, it
is discussed in Chapter 14. It is extremely rare.

Hernia of the bladder is unusual, protruding most commonly through
the inguinal orifice or through the linea alba, but it may be femoral,
obturator, intraperitoneal, extraperitoneal, direct or indirect, interstitial
or interparietal, reducible or irreducible, sliding, complete or incomplete,
single or multiple, inflamed, incarcerated, strangulated, and may accompany hernia of the bowel or omentum. In males the hernia is usually
inguinal and in females femoral.

The causes of bladder hernia are (1) those of hernia in general, (2)
congenital malformation of the bladder, and (3) obstruction at the vesical
outlet encouraging the viscus to herniate through the internal inguinal
ring as a back pressure blowout process. Commonly the condition produces no symptoms but is accidentally discovered at the time of herniotomy when, as in many reported cases, unwittingly it may be incised.
The hernial mass will vary according to vesical distention and completely
disappear with urination. *Pis en deux temps* may occur as in vesical
diverticulum. Alteration of the size of the hernia by urination suggests
the diagnosis. Stereoscopic cystography will confirm it. The treatment is
surgical with reduction of the hernial contents to the pelvic cavity and
closure of the hernial opening. A large extruding vesical mass should be
resected and in all cases etiologic distal obstruction removed and the urine
sterilized.

INJURIES OF THE PENIS

Self-mutilation accounts for most of these. Contusion is the most
common variety and results from pressing, pinching or other severe

trauma of the penis. Grasping, pulling or pinching of a playmate's genitals is a frequent boyhood practice and sometimes inflicts serious penile injury, especially to the urethra. Similarly the organ may be injured by a blow or a kick.

Penile injury by trouser zippers is of increasing incidence. Fracture of the penis occurs when the erect organ is forcefully broken but this is largely confined to boys in their late teens and young adult males. Hematoma results and late scarring frequently produces chordee and variable impotence, and in some instances appears to be the traumatic factor in the development of Peyronie's disease (q.v. Chapter 8). There is subcutaneous hemorrhage with marked discoloration, and often localized or diffuse hematoma. The last frequently follows circumcision. I have seen subtotal penile amputation result from rabbinical circumcision.

In severe penile injury the corpora may also bleed. Rest, a firm bandage, and the application of cold are usually adequate treatment but freely bleeding deep wounds may require packing or suture. Should abscess develop, incise and drain.

Incised wounds or gunshot wounds are comparatively rare; several instances of gunshot or shrapnel amputation of the penis have been reported in military action. The penis, usually the frenum, may be torn during masturbation or intercourse and generally with profuse hemorrhage. Owing to its generous blood supply even a severe incised or traumatized penis will often heal if immediately sutured. When the penile blood supply has been completely divided, amputation must be performed. Conservative treatment by suture may save the organ. In all severe penile injuries late sclerotic distortion of the organ may make erection imperfect, unsatisfactory, or painful.

Dislocation of the penis results only from severe trauma, the organ being torn from beneath its skin and from the mucosal attachment at the glans. It is inverted and disappears into the scrotum, tissues of the groin, or suprapubically, and an enormous hematoma forms. There is acute urinary retention or urine may be passed directly into the tissues. Extravasation rapidly increases the size of the peripenile mass. An immediate attempt should be made to restore the penis to its normal site and the bladder must be drained by urethral catheter, perineal urethrostomy or suprapubic cystostomy.

Avulsion of the penile skin leaves the organ completely denuded. It occurs most often when the trousers in the area are accidentally caught in a machine belt or gears; in severe cases complete emasculation has resulted. A simple method of treatment is to implant the denuded penis beneath the skin of the anterior scrotal wall and when local conditions are satisfactory after a month or two with good healing and absence of infection, the penis is mobilized and covered with scrotal skin.

Penile Strangulation. In the great majority of these cases the constriction is consequent to some masturbatory act such as putting the organ into the neck of a bottle, or through a steel washer, wedding ring or roller

bearing (Fig. 217). Occasionally boys fasten rubber bands, strings, rings
or even tie hair around the base of the penis. Mothers have been known to
tie off the organ to prevent bed wetting, and in a five-year-old boy with
gonorrhea I saw, the mother had tightly tied off the penis at the base to
stop the discharge. In all such pronounced constrictions edema and thrombosis promptly occur, often progressing rapidly to gangrene. Stricture and
fistulae result unless the constriction is promptly relieved, or the penis is
lost by gangrene.

A ring may be filed off with a Gigli saw or a fine jeweler's saw,
followed by the application of hot dressings. Jewett advises making four
equidistant longitudinal incisions through the skin down to Buck's fascia
avoiding vessels as far as possible. The local edema is squeezed out, and
with the penis well lubricated, the ring is drawn forward and removed,
exerting a little extra squeezing of the glans to get rid of the obstructing
edema. The local injection of hyaluronidase might be expected to help as
it does in the reduction of paraphimosis. Multiple aspirations of thrombosed penile corpora may dislodge hematomatous or thrombotic areas. If
the penis is gangrenous, amputation well into healthy tissue is indicated.
Urethral stricture may be anticipated in all severe penile constrictions
and commonly urethral fistulae develop. Periodic progressive dilation of
the stricture is necessary and with this the fistula will almost always close
spontaneously.

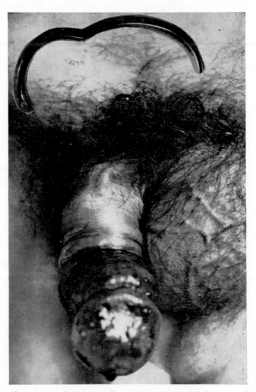

FIGURE 217.   Penile strangulation and gangrene caused by metal ring constriction.

INJURIES OF THE URETHRA

These frequently result from self-introduction of pencils, needles or other foreign bodies for masturbation or are caused by straddle injuries, by the inexpert passage of sounds, catheters, cystoscopes or other instruments. The mucosa may be torn, false passages incited, copious hemorrhage occur, and periurethral abscess or urinary extravasation follow. The urethra may also be lacerated by kicks, accidental explosions or gunshot wounds, may rupture by overdistention of injected fluid as at urethography for example, or from increased urinary pressure behind a urethral stricture or stone. The urethra may also be secondarily injured by the injection of strong chemicals, especially when used for antivenereal prophylaxis. I well remember the urethra of a physician who prophyactically injected himself with a 1 per cent solution of mercury bichloride. The canal came away as a cast; obstinate extensive stricture followed. The canal may be perforated externally by a picket or by wood splinters.

With *urethral rupture* urinary extravasation and periurethral phlegmon usually develop and can be forestalled only by prompt establishment of free urinary drainage, preferably by external urethrostomy.

Extreme gentleness and skill is the prophylaxis against both diagnostic and therapeutic instrumental injury.

Treatment. Rest and the local application of cold should be instituted at once and, when there is bleeding and hemorrhage, a snug elastic bandaging of the penis over a catheter will usually stop the bleeding as well as preserve free urinary drainage. Bleeding from the bulbous and deep urethra will frequently stop promptly if the patient sits astride a large rolled-up bath towel. If bleeding continues despite these measures perform perineal urethrostomy without delay.

Urethral prolapse is a lesser manifestation of the same conditions which foster vesical prolapse (q.v.) and requires essentially the same treatment. Because it is limited to females, it is discussed in Chapter 14.

Rupture of the urethra is the most serious of urethral injuries, most often follows straddle injuries of the perineum, the urethra being crushed against the pubic rami. In the female only the anterior part of the urethra is thus injured. The mechanism of urethral injury is shown in Figure 218. Rupture also complicates pelvic fracture involving the membranous urethra and adjacent prostatic canal in the male. With pelvic rupture bony spicules may cut through or crush the canal, or a kick may cause the trauma. Many grave urethral injuries have resulted from booby trap land mine explosions.

Symptoms of urethral rupture are chiefly urinary difficulty with dysuria, pain, hematuria and local swelling, and usually in a degree proportionate to the gravity of the injury. When the urethra is completely ruptured transversely the patient usually cannot void nor can a catheter be passed, and perineal hematoma with extravasation appears promptly. In posterior urethral rupture the blood may drain back into the bladder rather than from the meatus. The corpora cavernosa are commonly lacerated in pelvic fracture and injury of the pudic nerve or penile blood supply is later evidenced by faulty erections or impotence. A history of local injury—penile or perineal trauma followed by urethral pain, tenderness, hematuria, urinary difficulty, and local swelling—suggest the diagnosis which must be made promptly and treatment instituted. Because of bleeding, urethroscopy is usually of no value but gentle urethrography will demonstrate if urethral rupture has occurred, extravasation of the contrast medium pointing the rupture and extent of extravasation (Fig. 218). In rupture of the membranous urethra the contrast medium is arrested at the site of injury and diffuses through the perineum so that no cystographic outline is obtained. If the rupture is in the prostatic urethra the medium diffuses about the bladder neck and if in the anterior urethra there is localized extravasation of the contrast medium.

Prognosis depends upon immediate treatment of urethral rupture and its complications including infection. It is uniformly good in uncomplicated cases with adequate follow-up dilation over months and years. Periurethral phlegmon, traumatic shock, infection or other grave conditions adversely color the prognosis.

Treatment. If the patient is seen early before extensive extravasation has occurred, a urethral catheter should be passed at once to prevent or limit urinary extravasation. This together with rest, the local application of cold, and the administration of antimicrobic therapy is usually adequate. The catheter is removed after ten days, and two weeks after this sounds are passed and periodically thereafter, often enough to prevent the formation of traumatic stricture.

In less fortunate cases when the patient is not seen until late or

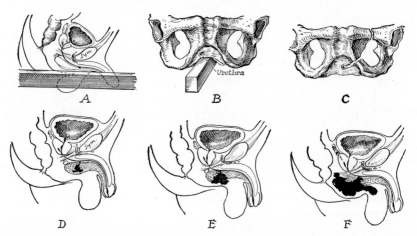

FIGURE 218.   Injury of the urethra. *A*, in straddle injuries the canal is crushed against the pubis. *B*, frontal view of *A; C*, laceration of the urethra in pubic fracture; *D–F*, rupture of the urethra and the development of periurethral hematoma or phlegmon (urinary extravasation) following urethral trauma. *D*, first degree rupture; there is hematoma in the corpus spongiosum; *E*, second degree rupture; tear in the urethral wall with urinary leakage (compare with Fig. 215); *F*, third degree rupture with extravasation of urine through the tear in the urethra, corpus spongiosum and its sheath.

when the initial injury is severe with prompt spread of periurethral phlegmon, the bladder must be drained at once by perineal urethrostomy, or, when this is technically impossible immediately after injury, by suprapubic cystostomy. If the deep urethra has been completely divided it is best to perform immediate suture of the severed ends, excising fragments of tissue which show loss of their blood supply. Here a small indwelling urethral splint catheter together with suprapubic counter-drainage will usually produce a good result providing the urethra is periodically dilated thereafter to prevent traumatic stricture formation.

Unless the treatment just outlined is carried out promptly, skillfully and thoroughly, sclerotic closure of the seriously traumatized canal may be anticipated. This leads not only to grave obstruction but usually to the development of multiple fistulae—perineal and/or suprapubic—discharging stinking urine, advanced pyelonephritis and infected hydronephrosis which, unless relieved, will be shortly fatal. Conscientious *periodic dilation of the traumatic stricture is the most important phase of the postoperative treatment*. Strictures in the bulbous urethra not responding to periodic dilation should be treated by excision of the scar-bearing area with end-to-end anastomosis, but even here follow-up dilation with sounds is demanded.

INJURIES OF THE SCROTUM

The scrotum may be injured by kicks, blows, straddle injuries, explosions, gunshot or other penetrating wounds, or self-mutilation, and even without injury of its contents. Purpura, ecchymosis or scrotal hematoma frequently occurs in breech presentations consequent to excessive compression of the scrotum and testes during labor; sometimes the spermatic veins are ruptured with testicular thrombosis and massive intra-scrotal hematoma as in two cases I have seen in the newborn. Contusions are followed by ecchymosis and hematoma which, owing to the laxity of the tissues, often become extensive. With penetrating injury of the scrotum its contents are also likely to be injured. If the scrotal wound is large, the testicle may protrude—the so-called *hernia testis* (Fig. 180).

The chief concern is the introduction of foreign matter into the scrotum by the penetrating injury. Such wounds should be promptly cleaned, treated with a skin antiseptic, and a surgical dressing applied with the administration of tetanus antitoxin. As a rule, a tight compression bandage will check mild scrotal bleeding but profuse hemorrhage requires ligation of the bleeding points. Unless this is done promptly a large scrotal hematoma is certain to develop. Loss of scrotal skin by partial or complete avulsion is generally followed by prompt regeneration and does not require skin grafting although in the reformation of the scrotum the testicles may be left in a bizarre and unnatural position.

Fortunately the scrotum, like the scalp, has a generous blood supply so that gangrene from trauma alone is extremely rare and almost always is the result of secondary infection.

INJURIES OF THE TUNICA VAGINALIS

Injury of the tunica vaginalis is nearly always a collateral of scrotal injury. Its response by serous effusion produces *traumatic* hydrocele, or if the cavity of the tunica vaginalis is filled with blood it is an *hematocele* (Fig. 179). Spontaneous hematocele has been described in leukemia. Symptomatically hematocele and hydrocele are indistinguishable but the aspirated fluid contains free or clotted blood in the first condition and clear hydrocele fluid in the second. The hematocele may simulate malignant tumor of the testicle but usually does not feel as heavy as tumor; when there is the slightest question the scrotum should be opened as it should be when pain and the size of the scrotal mass increase. Having opened the scrotum, all bleeding points are ligated and the sac is everted behind the cord before the testicle is replaced to prevent subsequent hydrocele formation. Antibacterial therapy is liberally administered.

INJURY OF THE TESTICLE

The organ may be contused, lacerated, punctured or displaced. Although exposed to trauma the free mobility of the testes doubtless explains the rarity of their serious injury.

Contusion may result from falling astride a solid object, kicks, blows, pinching of the clothing, compression at the time of birth delivery or, not infrequently, squeezing by the rough hand of another. A variable orchitis follows, often with epididymitis. There is ecchymosis within the substance of the gland and in severe cases there may be hemorrhagic infarction. The last occasionally occurs in difficult and prolonged breech delivery. Following severe traumatic orchitis, testicular atrophy and isolateral sterility is the rule. In some Oriental countries harem eunuchs are "prepared" in boyhood by severe squeezing of the testes; atrophy of the glands and sterility results. Mild traumatic orchitis in the young may not cause the glands to diminish in size but they may simply fail to grow.

All but mild injuries of the testicle cause severe and sickening pain which is often referred to the epigastrium with nausea and vomiting. The pain results largely from compression of the edematous testicular substance within the firm inelastic tunica albuginea and, by enteric reflex, vascular dilatation of the mesenteric vascular tree occurs and sufficient to produce faintness. There may even be collapse and profound shock, a syndrome frequently observed in testicular injury, especially by kicking. Hematoma of the testicle frequently develops.

If the testicular substance protrudes through the scrotal wall the condition is known as *fungus testis* and generally requires orchiectomy as does secondary infection, pulpefaction or hemorrhagic thrombosis of the gonad. Some degree of atrophy may be anticipated in all traumatized testes not removed.

The *treatment* is rest, support of the scrotum and an ice cap locally in mild cases. Infection is rare except in penetrating injuries and if it does not disappear with intensive antibacterial therapy, orchiectomy is usually required, as it may be in severe complicating hematoma of the testis.

Laceration of the testicle (tunica albuginea) is rapidly followed by hematoma and in other respects symptomatically simulates contusion. The diagnosis is made at operation and when the testicle is not completely bisected, conservative resuture is advocated, with care that extruding margins of the testicle may be clipped away; *under no circumstances should the testicular tubules be pulled out.*

Incised or puncture wounds of the testis are usually caused by nails, sharp sticks, or falling astride a branch, picket or the like. Penetrating injury by a trochar employed for aspiration of hydrocele has often been a factor. Following testicular injury, hematoma usually develops promptly and, infected, becomes abscess. As in all severe accidental penetrations other than surgical, tetanus antitoxin should be given. Usually conservative therapy with rest in bed, suspension of the scrotum (Fig. 186) and an ice cap will suffice unless hematocele develops and demands immediate evacuation, or necrosis or infection of the testicle requires orchiectomy.

Traumatic displacement of the testes occurs largely in males run over by automobiles, trucks, or wagon wheels or as a result of various crushing injuries. The site of displacement will depend on the anatomic factors and notably the size of the inguinal ring and the direction and force of the blow (Fig. 135). The usual sites of displacement are toward the anterior superior spine of the ilium, over the pubis, along the penis or, rarely, even torn from the body. There is profound shock, nausea, vomiting, and local pain, the diagnosis being made by the history and palpation of the displaced testicle unless local acute swelling prohibits. *Treatment* is replacement of the testicle to its normal site by open reduction if the condition of the organ warrants its salvage, otherwise perform orchiectomy. Seldom can the testicle be reduced without open operation, and in any event atrophy will subsequently occur.

Injuries of the epididymis accompany trauma of the testicle, clinically and therapeutically are alike, and the differential diagnosis is made at operation. See also Torsion of the Spermatic Cord in Chapter 8.

INJURIES OF THE SPERMATIC CORD

Injuries of the spermatic cord are usually due to surgical procedures and are evidenced by a large hematocele of the cord. Sometimes the cord is tied off during an improperly performed varicocele operation or is constricted by an inguinal ring sutured too tightly at herniotomy. Yet the injury may result from external violence. When the artery of the vas is spared the nutrition of the testicle may be relatively preserved so that gangrene does not occur although variable atrophy is certain. Mild cord injury responds readily to rest and an ice cap locally, but if there is hemorrhage and an increasing hematoma, the cord must be exposed and the bleeding stopped. Infection is the chief complication and should largely be prevented by antimicrobial therapy.

Laceration, compression or crushing of the vas deferens occludes the duct and produces isolateral sterility. In an increasing number of patients prompt excision of the injured or occluded segment with end-to-end anastomosis will re-establish the lumen.

Injury of the spermatic cord by torsion is discussed in Chapter 8.

INJURIES OF THE PROSTATE AND SEMINAL VESICLES

These are rare except as complications of pelvic fracture. Yet the prostate may be injured by unskillful urethral instrumentation particularly as false passages are made.

Laceration of the prostate is almost certain to be followed by traumatic stricture of the prostatic urethra. I have seen a cystoscope passed straight through the prostate in adults. Grave injuries of the prostate, its capsule and adjacent structures have occurred many times during transurethral resection of the vesical outlet. Laceration of the prostate is generally followed by profuse hemorrhage which is likely to be serious as the periprostatic venous plexus is torn, and extensive as the perivesical and retroperitoneal spaces become filled with blood. The usual symptoms are local pain at the vesical outlet, variable hematuria, dysuria or inability to void. Laceration of the prostate is almost certain to be followed by traumatic stricture of the prostatic urethra.

Treatment may usually be conservative with the insertion of a large freely draining urethral catheter to prevent urinary extravasation. The patient is put to bed and antibacterial therapy is intensively given. During conservative treatment the physician must be alert to the onset of periprostatic and pelvic phlegmon which demands prompt drainage of the bladder and perivesical spaces.

Early prostatic suppuration is best drained through the perineum.

Should periurethral, perivesical or peripelvic phlegmon develop, surgical drainage is required from below, above or by both routes according to the local findings.

In injury of the prostate in pelvic crushing, the condition is essentially that of rupture of the posterior urethra in which prompt urethrostomy is demanded together with adequate drainage of secondary periurethral and peripelvic phlegmon.

CHAPTER 11   *Urinary Calculous Disease*

Introduction. A urinary stone is a concrement composed of crystalline or amorphous elements bound together by a colloidal reticulum and in calculous growth the biophysical and biochemical components pile up on one another in "rhythmic precipitation." The character of a stone is determined by its chemical composition which may show wide variation and cause great differences in appearance, contour, rate of growth and radiopacity, characteristics which enter into both its diagnosis and treatment.

According to architecture, stones are classified as primary or secondary. *Primary* stones have no nucleus but form as pure crystalline structure, precipitate in sterile urine, and on cross section are radially striated rather than laminated. Primary stones occur most often in infants in whom they are generally associated with gastrointestinal disorders, deficient alimentation or faulty elimination. *Secondary* calculus which comprises the vast majority of all stones, may also occur in sterile urine but possesses a nucleus which may be a small primary stone, blood clot, cellular debris, or even a clump of bacteria. These calculi show more or less definite lamination and are nearly always predisposed to by urinary stasis (obstruction) and/or infection.

Lamination results from stratification of crystalline and colloid layers, the colloid being derived from gels normally in suspension in the urine and/or from inflammatory exudate. The colloid is an albuminous material which some believe is fibrin and is most abundant in mixed calculi.

Stones may be hard or soft. *Hard* stones show definite lamination without a demonstrable nucleus and the character of the lamination reflects changes in the colloidal content of the urine during formation of the stone. *Soft* stones are less densely bound together because of excessive

407

crystalline components. These stones characteristically form rapidly and chiefly of phosphatic salts, the stone structure often being so insecure as to permit it to be readily crushed between the fingers when freshly removed from the urinary tract.

COMPOSITION OF STONES

The predominant composition of urinary calculi in their order of frequency in adults and children is shown in Table 14.

Stones of only one composition do not occur but they are spoken of as "pure" when one salt comprises more than 90 per cent of the content. Most stones are mixed and are made up of two or more crystalloids. Calculi are also classified as amorphous or crystalloid.

Phosphatic stones are composed both of crystalloids and amorphous calcium phosphate although ammonium magnesium phosphate is also commonly present. They characteristically form in an alkaline or a neutral urine and only rarely in acid urine. Usually they are small, rounded, smooth, white or yellowish-white, laminated and grossly show their crystalline spectrum. Their rapid growth is favored by ammoniogenic bacterial activity, notably by B. proteus. They are often small yet may grow to enormous size, nearly filling the bladder or completely filling the kidney pelvis. In the body they are often extremely soft and when first removed may even crumble in the fingers.

Calcium carbonate calculi are extremely rare, chalky in appearance and consistency but may be brownish or reddish-brown from old blood.

Uric Acid Stones. Uric acid deposits in the collecting tubules of the medullary papillae during late fetal and early neonatal life are well preserved in the markedly acid urine of high uric acid content of this period and when the urine is allowed to stand overnight, small reddish-brown crystalloid collections precipitate out (cayenne pepper). The passage of a shower of these crystals may engender ureteral colic and in infants this accounts for many attacks thought to be intestinal colic.

Most uric acid stones as observed later in life are hard and brittle, round, highly polished and yellow or yellowish-brown, the color being due to blood pigments derived from traumatic or congestive bleeding consequent to the stone. While the smooth surface and, in general, the small size of uric acid stones encourages their passage through the ureter,

TABLE 14.   COMPOSITION OF URINARY CALCULI

ADULTS	CHILDREN	COMPOSITION
1	4	Phosphates (calcium ammonium magnesium)
2	5	Carbonates (calcium ammonium magnesium)
3	1	Uric acid
4	2	Urates (ammonium sodium potassium)
5	3	Oxalates (calcium ammonium magnesium)
6	6	Cystine
7	7	Xanthine

Fibrin, bacterial, cholesterol, urostealith, carbon and indigo stones have been observed but are most unusual.

when rough or spiculated the calculi may be retained in the pelvis or ureter. Commonly they become nuclei for phosphatic, carbonate, or oxalate stones and particularly in the bladder. Uric acid calculi comprise about 10 per cent of all urinary stones and a third to a half of those found in infancy and childhood. Pure uric acid stone is not radiopaque and may fail to be recognized by plain x-rays alone although even a small amount of calcium in the stone will usually render it faintly opaque. Nonopaque stones are urographically demonstrated as negative shadows in the radiopaque medium (Figs. 223, 224) but if the viscus is distended with air they will generally become faintly visible in the pneumogram (Fig. 236).

Urate calculi are unusual in adults but are the commonest stones found in infancy and childhood. The ammonium and sodium salts are the usual ones, are laminated, moderately hard, and resemble, but are more reddish-brown than, phosphatic calculi.

Oxalate calculi are of high and ever-increasing incidence in adults and rank second to uric acid and urate stones in the young. They are generally less than 2 cm. in diameter, extremely hard, laminated, present a rough surface which may be spiculated (nutmeg, mulberry or jackstones), and are brownish-black from hematin derived from blood liberated by stone trauma. *Calcium oxalate* is the usual form encountered, these rough stones notoriously clinging to the mucosa and passage through the ureter induces intense local agonizing spasm which delays their progress, or they may even become ennested in the ureteral mucosa.

Cystine stones are composed predominantly of this substance, an intermediate sulfur-containing amino acid which, owing to faulty protein metabolism, is excreted into the urine and may be deposited in hexagonal crystal form. The condition is rare as *cystinuria* occurs only once in about 15,000 individuals and only 2 to 3 per cent of these form stones. These stones are usually yellow or light yellowish green and upon exposure to light become definitely greenish, with a smooth or granular surface. As a rule, they are small, ovoid or round with a smooth waxy surface, are frequently multiple and deposited in facet formation, have a soapy appearance and feel and cut like hard soap. They are striated rather than laminated and are nonradiopaque or only faintly radiopaque, depending upon the calcium content. They form only in acid urine and because of this a few have been therapeutically dissolved *in vivo* by alkalinization of the urine.

Xanthine stones are extremely rare, smooth, hard yellowish-brown or cinnamon color, form only in acid urine, and are seldom over 1 cm. in diameter. Xanthine is an intermediate product of purine metabolism and like cystine these stones are nonopaque. They may be the nucleus for uric acid or other calculi in which calcium is admixed.

ETIOLOGY AND PATHOGENESIS OF URINARY STONE

There is today no single causative factor known responsible for stone formation. Present knowledge attributes urinary stone development to one or more of four possible direct causes: (1) vitamin A deficiency; (2) excessive crystalloid excretion including the hypercalciuria of hyperparathyroid disease; (3) infection of type specific bacteria; (4) genesis from calcium plaque formations in the renal pelvic submucosa or in the renal tubules.

Infection, urinary stasis and/or trauma are the usual predisposing factors.

Urinary stone is predominantly a disease of males, and especially of the bladder and urethra. This is largely attributed to the higher incidence of vesical neck obstructions in the male as contrasted to the short patulous urethra in females through which small stones more readily pass. The highest incidence of urinary stone is in the years before ten and after fifty; most young patients found to have stone are examined because of so-called chronic pyelitis in which abdominal pain and persistent pyuria are the dominant symptoms.

Familial influences are of no importance except in cystine stone disease in which hereditary diathesis is recognized. In general, *racial considerations* are of little importance; *dietary considerations* and the variable removal of urinary tract obstruction by circumcision has been advanced to explain the slightly lower incidence in Jews. *Geographic considerations* are important chiefly as to faulty diet and insufficient vitamin intake, particularly in some parts of the Orient and in the tropics. Yet in the United States there is a striking increase in the incidence of phosphatic stone in the citrus areas of Florida and California, attributed to the urinary alkalinization resulting from habitual excessive consumption of citrus fruits or their juices—high in alkaline ash and low in protein and vitamin A (acid ash). It is probable that in tropical countries a faulty diet with protein and water-soluble vitamin deficiency is of greater moment than dehydration and an excessively high crystalline content of the urine.

Diet.   Experimentally it has been shown that calculi may be readily produced in animals placed on a vitamin A deficient diet. (Osborne and Mendel, McCarrison, Higgins.) This diet produces derangement of the normal renal chemical function and a keratosis of the renal epithelium; crystalline deposits in alkaline urine occur about the keratinized cells as a nucleus. Yet in urinary crystalluria most of the stones or a large portion of their content is amorphous deposit. The *hardness of a drinking water plays no part nor does crystalluria per se appear to be an important factor.* In hypercalciuria, however, and whether idiopathic or due to hyperparathyroidism, the urine is generally highly alkaline, often infected with ureolytic organisms, and stone formation is common. Here the treatment with increased fluid intake and the administration of sodium acid phosphate is usually successful because the last (1) moderately reduces the pH of the urine to lessen precipitation of the calcium, (2) decreases urinary calcium by combining with calcium in the upper urinary tract to form insoluble calcium phosphate, (3) supplies added phosphate to the body to aid in maintaining a more normal calcium-phosphorus balance (cf. Cordonnier and Talbot, 1948). Moreover, the administration of ammonium chloride instead of a high acid-ash diet for urinary acidification doubles or trebles the output of calcium in the urine.

Hyperparathyroidism in Calculous Disease. Carefully controlled experiments and clinical observations show that faulty metabolism (hypervitaminosis D, hypercalcemia, hyperphosphatemia) secondary to disease of the parathyroid gland may produce stone formation. The incidence of parathyroid disease in the United States far exceeds its progressively increased recognition.

It is believed to be responsible for 4 to 5 per cent of cases of renal calculi, and when this etiology can be proved in a given patient, removal of the diseased glands (usually four) is the treatment.

In parathyroid tumor which is usually benign, an excess of parathyroid hormone is excreted to cause a hypercalcemia and hyperphosphatemia which induces direct removal of calcium from the bones.

Infection. The importance of urinary infection in calculogenesis has been recognized for a long time. While stones may form in sterile urine, in most stone-bearing patients the urine is infected and most often by urea-splitting organisms; the urea is broken down into ammonia and carbon dioxide with resulting formation of ammonium carbonate which combines with magnesium salts and phosphates to form ammonium magnesium phosphate in the urine. This is insoluble and engenders a urinary alkalinity which results in the precipitation of other earthy phosphates. The chief urea-splitting organisms encountered are the colon bacillus, proteus bacillus, staphylococcus, and streptococcus, essentially in this order of incidence. Yet renal calculi may form in sterile urine.

Urinary Stasis. Urinary stasis together with infection is demonstrable in most cases of urinary calculi and must be considered as an important predisposing cause; primary calculi form in the absence of each of these factors. The stasis may result from obstruction or neuromuscular inertia; frequently it results from immobilization of the patient by prolonged illness or orthopedic conditions. Not only does urinary stagnation occur but in the immobilized patient there is decalcification of the skeleton as well, the great excess of lime being excreted by the kidneys. The precipitation of phosphates and oxalates depends more upon the amount of lime present than any other factor (Joly).

Trauma. As a rule this is of little concern as an etiologic factor except as it may demand immobilization of the patient as in spinal injury or with paralyzing infection such as anterior poliomyelitis. Pugilists with all the renal trauma they receive show no unusual incidence of kidney stone. But patients immobilized for central nervous system disease and particularly of the spinal cord show a 25 per cent incidence of stone formation, predominantly of the calcium phosphatic variety. It is believed that with the patient on his back the renal pelvicalyceal system drains poorly because the ureteropelvic junction is higher than the calyces. The urine flow is too sluggish to wash away crystalline deposits and these become nuclei for stones.

Biochemical Factors in Stone Formation. It has been shown that with excessive urinary colloids such as occur with inflammation of the urinary tract, there is a predisposition to the precipitation of crystalloids. When these salts come in contact with a colloidal gel they are precipitated in a series of rings (Liesegang rings) instead of in a uniform manner. These crystalloids are composed of substances normally found in the urine such as uric acid or calcium oxalate, but may also be products of disorders of metabolism as cystine, or from urea-splitting bacterial action as ammonium magnesium phosphate. *Any factor which disturbs the crystalcolloidic equilibrium is an etiologic agent in stone formation.*

Submucosal calcific plaques formed in the tips of the papilla of the medulla were demonstrated by Randall at autopsy in many instances, and in surgically removed specimens as well. Microscopic calculi in the tubules of the renal pyramid and occasionally in other tubular segments of the organ were also demonstrated and probably form when droplets of calcareous matter coalesce. Randall concluded that calculogenesis reflects renal papillary damage prior to the deposit of crystalline urinary salts. As the calcific formation enlarges in the walls and intratubular spaces of the papillae, its epithelium covering is lost, and the calcific stone passes into the calyx or pelvis to continue growth and enter the ureter to pass unnoted or with intense pain. Entrapped in the renal calyx, pelvis or bladder, for example, these calcific plaques become a nucleus for stone formation and grow.

Renal Calcinosis. This occurs frequently in infants and young children in particular, and for unknown reasons. There may be widespread renal calcinosis of clinical importance because the kidney is variably damaged and its excretory function correspondingly reduced (Figs. 219, 220). Etiologically these cases of calcinosis have been classified as (1) those dependent upon hypercalcemia and excessive calcium excretion in the blood (metastatic calcification and acute hyperparathyroidism); (2) dystrophic calcification with localization of calcium deposit in degenerat-

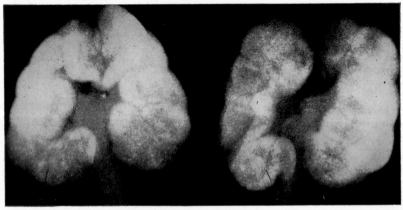

FIGURE 219.   Renal calcinosis. Postmortem roentgenogram of bisected kidneys in a four-month-old infant (Goettsch).

ing or necrotic tissue without hypercalcemia or excess calcium excretion (chemical injury as by mercury bichloride, pronounced acute disturbances of blood acid-base balance and nephrotic changes as in high intestinal obstruction, pyloric stenosis, severe toxemia or infections), and (3) hypercalcemia or hypercalciuria together with renal cellular injury or degeneration (chronic hyperparathyroidism, chronic renal insufficiency, pituitary disturbance, hypervitaminosis D). Yet in urinary calculogenesis, crystalluria is of clinical importance only when urinary infection or obstruction exists; precipitation of the crystalloids may form stones.

Pathogenesis. The rapidity of stone growth is largely dependent upon its site, the reaction and composition of the urine and the presence or absence of infection and urinary stasis. Phosphatic stones in general grow rapidly and even to astounding sizes within four to six weeks, while calcium oxalate or uric acid stones not only grow slowly but seldom to large size. Moreover, urinary acidity retards phosphatic stone growth, while urinary alkalinity delays or may even prevent uric acid calculous formation and growth.

Most urinary calculi originate in the kidney, 90 per cent of these are passed to the bladder and most will leave the body. Wherever the migration of the stone ceases, it will grow in this position, and this is especially striking in the bladder. Yet stones sometimes originate in the bladder, perhaps about a nidus of bacterial or epithelial debris, or a nucleus of phosphatic crystals sometimes broken off from incrustation on

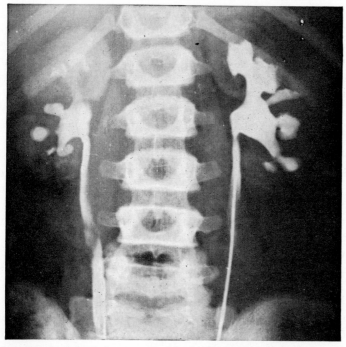

FIGURE 220.   Renal calcinosis in a young girl who developed bilateral renal calculi. Note increased radiographic renal density caused by the intraparenchymal calcific deposit.

an inlying urethral or suprapubic tube. In diffuse renal parenchymal calcinosis, the tissue is peppered with calcific deposits (Fig. 220).

Stones may lie free in the renal pelvis or in a calyx, may become impacted at the ureteropelvic junction, may enlarge to occupy the entire renal pelvis in large dendritic staghorn or coral varieties or may extend into the pelvic outlet to firmly plug this orifice, and in rare instances practically replace the entire kidney. Stones occur slightly more often on the right than on the left; in about 15 per cent of cases, renal calculi are bilateral.

It is axiomatic that any stone in any part of the kidney will damage the organ—to a variable degree and at a variable rate.

By its enlargement in the kidney, stone alone produces congestion at the site of contact with the tissues to produce microscopic hematuria and predispose to infection. The extent of the involvement depends largely upon the site, size, and location of the stone and whether it causes hydronephrosis by pelvic blockage. Additional changes in the kidney will be influenced by hydronephrosis, whether localized calyceal or involving the entire pelvis. These changes are discussed under urinary obstruction in Chapter 5. Ultimately the organ may be reduced to a thin sclerotic shell.

Large smooth stones are more or less firmly fixed; they may be asymptomatic—the so-called *silent* stone—but even here chronic interstitial nephritis develops to a variable degree and frequently appears early. At its point of contact with the pelvis there is desquamation of epithelium often with ulceration and variable sclerotic healing. *Sclerotic contracture* of the kidney about the stone and dense contracting intrarenal and perirenal fibrolipomatosis often develop and by including the renal pedicle may diminish the blood flow, and by periureteral contracture increase the urinary obstruction. In the terminal stage all or nearly all of the kidney is replaced by *liposclerosis*. Secondary infection is usually superimposed and calculous pyelonephritis develops. In complicating acute renal infection the picture is that of acute pyelonephritis, often with the painful syndrome of stone colic added.

In *calculous pyelonephritis* in the advanced cases the organ is riddled with minute focal abscesses which by diffusion and coalescence may become anatomic pyonephrosis. Secondary acute perinephritis or perinephric abscess reflects extension of the infection to the fatty renal envelope; occasionally a stone may rupture through the parenchyma and this commonly leads to extensive urinary extravasation.

Carcinoma of the kidney, notably of the squamous-cell variety, shows a striking correlation with renal calculi. Stone and usually infection are present in nearly half of the cases of squamous-cell carcinoma of the pelvis.

Congestion of the good kidney is frequent, and determination of its anatomic and functional status and whether infected, is one of the most important considerations in the examination of a stone-bearing patient. When both kidneys contain stones, clinical symptoms of urinary toxemia may become alarming as reflected in chronic gastrointestinal disturbances, or toxic central nervous system involvement may promote hyperirritability or depressive manifestations.

SYMPTOMS OF RENAL STONE

Symptoms of renal stone are fundamentally those of coexisting congestion, infection and/or obstruction. Pain localized in the stone-bearing area or along the course of the ureter; disturbances of urination and, with infection, persistent pyuria and hematuria are the usual manifestations of renal stone.

Pain. Nonobstructing calculus in the renal pelvis does not produce acute pain but rather a dull ache in the loin and variable hematuria. An immobile pelvic stone may be "silent." The pain of renal colic, which is most often ureteral colic, may be extreme. Typically it begins in the upper outer loin or in the costovertebral angle as sharply stabbing, cutting or tearing. The patient doubles up, cries out, the face wears an agonized expression, and pallor, sweating and even shock may follow. The colic will last until urinary drainage is established or opiates are effective.

Following cessation of the acute symptoms, sand or gravel or even the offending calculus may appear in the voided urine. Ureteral colic may simulate acute enteric disease especially appendicitis.

In renal ureteral colic the pain is usually referred and generally down to the lower loin, groin, bladder, urethra, spermatic cord, testicle or inner thigh; reflex irritability with frequency, urgency and dysuria appear, or there may be sharp pain in the isolateral testicle with high cremasteric contracture, bladder spasm or extreme hyperesthesia over the anterior and often lateral areas of the thigh supplied by branches of the genitocrural, 2nd and 3rd lumbar nerves respectively. (See syndrome of renal colic in Chapter 5.)

The *subinguinal syndrome of renal colic* (Campbell, 1929) can usually be demonstrated in cooperative older children and adults (Fig. 2). There is marked hyperesthesia over the isolateral upper inner triangle of the thigh, a clinical sign which definitely localizes the lesion to the urinary tract and rules out appendicitis, cholecystitis and other intraabdominal disease. Reno-renal reflex may cause pain localized in the opposite kidney and sometimes anuria occurs. Prolonged reflex anuria of the supposedly good kidney does not occur. If after relief of the shock and pain the "good" kidney does not resume activity, it is because it is gravely diseased.

Upper pain reference may simulate gallbladder colic. Nausea and vomiting reflect synaptic pain reference to the splanchnic nerves; constipation and often abdominal distention are extreme, and vomiting may be alarming. Stimulation of the medulla oblongata by vagus reflex is reflected in marked salivation, clammy sweat, facial pallor, collapse and a small thready pulse. These reflex disturbances will vary with the level of the blockage; the lower the calculus is in the ureter, the more intense will the bladder disturbances be. The clinical course may be recurrent with mild or acute attacks of renal or ureteral colic and particularly when the stone moves and obstruction ensues.

Hematuria may be constant or intermittent and with stone there will always be at least some microscopic blood found. In acute colic the urine is frequently bright red, or if it has been standing in the bladder for some time may be reddish brown or mahogany; stringy blood clots representing casts of the ureter may be passed and themselves cause colic.

Stone is a common complication of renal anomalies, especially in horseshoe kidney, yet any malformation inducing stasis is a potential calcinogenic factor.

Calculous anuria is separately discussed shortly in this chapter.

DIAGNOSIS

A story of pain in or along the urinary tract, hematuria, pyuria, or the passage of gravel or crystals are suggestive but none of these is pathognomonic of calculous disease. There may be a history of previous attacks of colic and the patient may have passed a stone. A history of gout or cystinuria should suggest the possibility of lithiasis. Yet in a third of the cases the history is of relatively little aid except as it calls for adequate urologic examination. Crystalluria and calculous disease are not reciprocal. The crystals of uric acid, urates, oxalates or cystine in crystalluria are usually typical while crystals in stone structure are largely atypical.

The pain of reno-ureteral colic may simulate intestinal colic, appendicitis, or other surgical disease of the abdomen. Yet the cry in enteric colic of infants is spasmodic; there is usually associated diarrhea and no urinary disturbance. During ureteral colic the patient suffers throughout the attack, there is seldom diarrhea, and usually urinary disturbances coexist. The pain of reno-ureteral colic is characteristically in the loin or along the course of the ureter but it may be referred almost entirely to the bladder and lower urogenital tract. In urinary colic the abdomen is frequently soft, fever is absent except when acute infection exists, and there is hematuria, though it may be microscopic.

Abdominal palpation may disclose an enlarged, tender kidney, the degree of mobility depending upon how much the kidney is fixed by perinephritis. There is costovertebral tenderness and deep pressure anteriorly over the kidney causes pain. The differential diagnosis from acute appendicitis, especially when the inflamed organ overlies the ureter and produces hematuria, may be difficult. Yet in appendicitis there is cutaneous hyperesthesia in the area bounded by the umbilicus medially, the anterior superior spine of the ilium laterally, and the crest of the ilium above, while in ureteral colic the cutaneous hyperesthesia is limited to the subinguinal triangle (q.v.). When acute appendicitis is the chief consideration in the differential diagnosis, a normal or nearly normal blood count warrants at least an excretory urographic study, granted that it is better to remove a normal appendix than to overlook an acutely inflamed one. If the diagnosis is still uncertain, perform complete urologic examination. In acute appendicitis the maximum tenderness is usually over McBurney's point and there is muscular spasm, rigidity, and sometimes rebound tenderness. There is no renal tenderness; the white blood count is elevated as is the temperature, the pulse is rapid, and the patient is sick. The differential diagnostic difficulties are increased in retrocecal appendix, especially when it overlies the ureter.

In *biliary colic* the right renal area is not tender and the history suggests antecedent biliary disease. Bile duct colic is referred to the right shoulder or through to the back, there is tenderness over the gallbladder as well as rectus muscle spasm, and the urine shows no blood.

Reflex vagal distention of the abdomen together with failure to pass gas by rectum, and continued vomiting may suggest acute intestinal obstruction, but in kidney stone colic the renal area is the acutely tender spot; blood and usually leukocytes are present in the urine and together with the history and other findings not only suggest calculous disease but demand a prompt diagnostic urologic survey.

A preliminary excretory urographic study may tell the story, establish the diagnosis and give a clue to the relative renal function on each side. When the kidney is blocked off by stone it may exhibit little or no secretion but this does not mean that the kidney cannot be salvaged. In some instances the distended obstructed renal pelvis is protected by pyelovenous backflow (q.v.) and a degree of kidney excretion is maintained.

The urologic examination is carried out as described in Chapter 3. Urine culture commonly shows infection, and albumin will be found in practically every case, as well as scattered leukocytes and epithelial cells. Three fourths of the patients with renal stone will have pus and blood in the urine as will 90 per cent of patients with ureteral calculi and all patients with vesical and urethral calculi.

The albumin is derived not only from inflammatory exudate associated with pelvic irritation but also from accompanying nephritis or pyelonephritis. With ammoniogenic infection the urine may be extremely foul, thickly purulent, and ropy with mucopus. The bacteriologic studies will disclose the invading organism which is attacked on the basis of bacterial-therapy specificity (Chapter 7). Determination of renal function is a helpful guide indicative of therapeutic progress and particularly as the function and condition of the better kidney may become of prime importance.

ROENTGENOGRAPHY

This is indispensable in the diagnosis of urinary calculous disease bearing in mind that in adults about 3 to 5 per cent of urinary stones are predominantly "pure" uric acid and may not be radiopaque.

The plain urogram should include the entire urinary tract and this may be expected to disclose not only stone shadows (Fig. 8) but spinal defects and/or bone changes and especially decalcification or cystic alterations (renal rickets or secondary hyperparathyroidism). Lateral and oblique views, particularly in conjunction with ureteropyelography are invaluable in showing the relation of the shadow to the kidney or ureter.

The radiopacity of the various salt components of urinary calculi depends upon their atomic weights but in the clinical demonstration of stone the total composition and size are factors as well as the thickness of the patient and, extremely important, the perfection of radiographic technique. Shadows of renal calculi are usually smoothly outlined, generally of uniform density, but sometimes with a lighter or darker central portion, and they are not laminated (Figs. 221, 222). Calcified mesenteric and retroperitoneal glands or calcific pyonephrotic debris cast fuzzy shadows of irregular density. The shadows of intestinal gas, feces, enteric coated tablets, biliary calculi (Fig. 225), barium, phlebolith, coprolith, cartilage, teeth or bone of dermoid teratoma, and pigmented molds may confuse; a barium test meal should be withheld until radiographic studies have been completed. About 10 per cent of urinary calculi in children are not radiopaque; these are chiefly pure uric acid stones (Figs. 223, 224).

In short, practically all renal stones are demonstrable by x-rays although the shadow may be faint. They may appear as separate stones in the pelvis or calyces but sometimes as large branching calculi of the staghorn, coral or solid dendritic type (Fig. 221). Yet many apparent

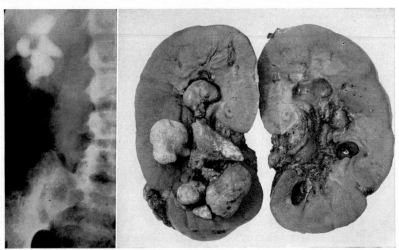

Fig. 221   Fig. 222

FIGURE 221. Renal stone. Massive silent dendritic phosphatic stone which filled the right kidney pelvis in an eight-year-old girl examined because of mild "chronic pyelitis" (pyuria) of three months' duration. No other symptoms. Spontaneous fracture of the lower third of the left femur while running six weeks previously suggested a calcium (parathyroid) metabolic error but neither roentgen skeletal studies nor blood chemistry estimation (serum calcium, serum phosphorus) were confirmatory. Attempted pyelolithotomy. Nephrectomy. Plain urogram.

FIGURE 222. Renal stone specimen in Figure 221.

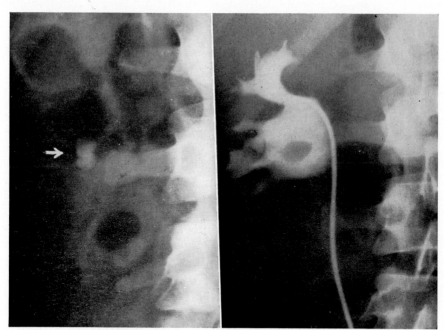

Fig. 223   Fig. 224

FIGURE 223.   Faintly opaque right renal calculus.

FIGURE 224.   Negative shadow in pyelogram caused by renal stone shown in Figure 223.

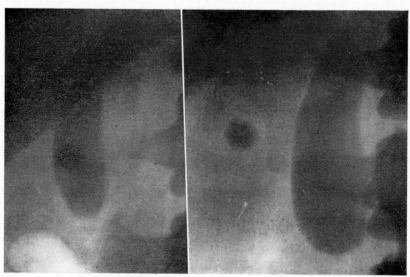

Fig. 225   Fig. 226

FIGURE 225.   Renal stone appearing to be in gallbladder (cholecystogram).

FIGURE 226.   By slightly rotating patient shown in Figure 225 the stone is demonstrated to be in the right kidney and the gallbladder is clear.

dendritic types as urographically demonstrated are simply multiple and faceted.

Cystoscopy in renal calculous disease may be normal but especially with infection there is apt to be congestion about the ureteral orifice of the involved side or purulent ejaculation from this ureteral orifice which, if pyonephrosis exists, is thick, ropy or like toothpaste oozing from the orifice. Without infection, the cystoscopic bladder picture may be normal. Urine ejaculating from the ureteral orifice on the "bad" side may be clear, hazy, bloodtinged, or smoky. Following cystoscopic observation the ureters are catheterized and specimens are collected from each kidney for bacteriologic and cytologic studies, and extremely important is the determination of the function of each kidney should operation be necessary.

The determination of the pH of the renal specimens is stressed by some as a guide to therapy when special diets and/or medications are to be employed. The pH of the bladder urine is not a reliable guide here. In more or less typical cases the pH of the uninvolved kidney will normally be found moderately acid while the pH of the involved kidney will be higher, that is, toward the alkaline side if not actually alkaline.

Pyelography, preferably retrograde, will localize the stone to the kidney pelvis or calyx and will suggest the character of other pathologic changes in the kidney, whether hydronephrotic, hyperplastic, ectopic or suffering other abnormality.

Stereoscopic urograms with the catheter in the ureter will at once localize the calculus shadow to this channel especially if a small amount of radiopaque medium is injected. Lateral and oblique x-ray exposures will localize the stone; biliary calculi lie anterior to the kidney. *A negative x-ray film does not rule out urinary calculus.* Pure uric acid stones are not opaque and cystine and ammonium urate calculi are but faintly visible. Yet these are rare and may be negatively demonstrated as vacuoles in the urographic medium (Fig. 224).

The demonstration of a sound renal mate is a must in the examination and, if the kidney is abnormal or deficient, determine whether or not it may be expected to support life, as these are vital data in the planning and executing of surgical treatment.

Occasionally when an intrarenal calcification is faintly defined or even obscured by the radiographic medium, a pneumopyelogram made by gentle injection of 2 to 4 cc. of air may cause the calculus to stand out sharply against the airgram background (cf. Fig. 236).

TREATMENT

The treatment of renal stone may be prophylactic, expectant, medical or active surgical.

Prophylactic Treatment. This consists chiefly in (1) a large fluid intake to reduce the concentration of urinary crystalloids, (2) a large vegetable intake for its vitamin and anticonstipation factors, especially high vitamins A and B, (3) eradication of urinary stasis, and/or of (4) infection. Gravely injured kidneys do not form primary stones because the crystalloid component of their excretion is relatively or actually extremely low. As a corollary, neither do they excrete chemotherapeutic agents adequate to be effective in the combat of infection and especially with ammoniogenic organisms.

Dissolution of phosphatic calculi and/or prevention of their recurrence by a diet high in vitamin A and B, and an acid-ash (for alkaline urine), or alkaline-ash (for acid urine) has been advocated (Higgins, 1947) but apparently this has not worked too well in the hands of others. Hyperparathyroidism must be ruled out. In bedridden patients early ambulation should be sought and when this is impossible the prophylactic measures should be doubly enforced. The employment of estrogens and aluminum hydroxide gels in the prophylactic management of renal stone is discussed in the sixth succeeding paragraph.

Expectant treatment: When the stone is small, relatively asymptomatic, is situated in the calyx or the renal pelvis, and there is likelihood of its spontaneous passage once it has passed into the ureter, this event may be awaited. Accompanying mild infection should be eradicated with antibacterial therapy and a large fluid intake administered. Recheck plain urograms should be made once in four to six months to note change in size or position of the stone, and the patient re-x-rayed promptly should pain or colic occur.

Medical Treatment. In addition to control or eradication of infection, the dietary treatment may be employed to prevent enlargement of the stone if this is possible, and with the faint hope that the stone may dissolve or disappear.

Diet. The primary objective of *dietary treatment* is adjustment and control of the pH of the urine to a degree that urinary salts are kept in solution and precipitation does not occur. Thus by maintaining urinary alkalinity by employment of the *alkaline-ash* diet, uric acid and cystine crystal is held in solution while by maintenance of an acid urine (pH 5.0–5.2) calcium and magnesium phosphates and carbonates are held in solution. But in the alkaline-ash dietary treatment of uric acid and cystine stones for example, if the urine is rendered *too* alkaline, the earthy carbonates and phosphates will precipitate out. The dietary therapy will be best regulated by analysis of the stone previously obtained from the patient. Although extensively tried by a large number of urologists, the dietary treatment of urinary stone has been largely given up, save by a few enthusiasts such as Higgins. The components of the various diets (high vitamin acid-ash; high vitamin alkaline-ash; low oxalate; low purine diet) are to be found in books on dietetics; Higgins has splendidly outlined them in Campbell's Urology (Vol. I, pp. 797–806). Dietary therapy has proved largely valueless in bilateral renal calculi and in nonobstructive calculi in the presence of urinary stasis and infection. The difficulty here results from impairment of renal function or inability to control the urinary pH as in Proteus bacillus infection, for example; it is practically impossible by dietary means to shift the pH to the acid side.

Hyaluronidase has been employed on the basis of inactivation or dispersion of urinary gels in solution, but to date has failed to achieve the high hopes held for it and the method has been largely discarded. The daily administration of 2 gm. of salicylamide has been held by some to combat phosphatic stone reformation but use of this drug is still under observation.

Calcium stones will often disintegrate in a citric-acid mixture through formation of a complex calcium citrate ion (Albright, Suby and Sulkowitch). The composition of the buffered solutions "G" and "M" developed by Suby is shown in Table 15.

These solutions are prophylactically used in the irrigation of nephrostomy and cystostomy tubes or for continuous irrigation aimed at dissolving renal calcium carbonate or phosphatic pelvic stones, but the disappearance of the stone seldom occurs with this treatment.

The co-administration of estrogens and aluminum hydroxide gel as suggested by Schorr is based on the concept that citric acid, a normal urinary constituent, enhances calcium solubility and estrogenic hormones augment the excretion of citric acid and reduce that of calcium. Employment of estrogen-aluminum hydroxide combination is limited to stones of calcium phosphate, magnesium ammonium phosphate, or calcium magnesium ammonium phosphate. In the intestinal tract the aluminum hydroxide combines with phosphate ions to form insoluble aluminum phosphate which is excreted as such in the stool. Thus the inorganic serum phosphorus is lowered which encourages a more complete resorption of phosphate by the tubules and correspondingly reduces the excretion of phosphate in the urine. As yet this method has not gained wide usage.

To sum up, the medical treatment of urinary calculi including dietary regimens is largely valuable as urinary infection may be eliminated or at least controlled. The dietary methods must be strictly enforced to be effective, are largely impractical in most homes, and are contraindicated in children. In short, by one method or another, most impassable urinary stones must be surgically removed.

Surgical Treatment. The renal damage in simple uncomplicated renal colic is usually transient, and rapid repair ensues with the establishment of free drainage and sterilization of the urine.

Renal stone over 1 centimeter in diameter not quietly ennested in a renal calyx demands surgical treatment and, in general, the earlier the

TABLE 15. COMPOSITION OF SOLUTIONS "G" AND "M" (SUBY)

	G* SOLUTION	M SOLUTION
Citric acid monohydrate	32.5 gm.	32.5 gm.
Magnesium oxide anhydrous	3.84 gm.	3.84 gm.
Sodium carbonate anhydrous	4.37 gm.	8.84 gm.
Distilled water	1000 cc.	1000 cc.

* This solution is adjusted to pH 4.0.
The M solution is less acid and not quite so irritating as solution G.

better. The danger of the stone in the kidney is generally much greater than that of surgical intervention; if calculi remain in the kidney, death of the organ will almost always occur whether by infection, hydronephrosis, pyonephrosis, or by prolonged chronic sclerotic atrophy. The site of the stone and the concomitant obstruction and infection rather than the size of the calculus are the important considerations.

Stones may be removed from the kidney by pyelotomy or ne-

Fig. 227   Fig. 228

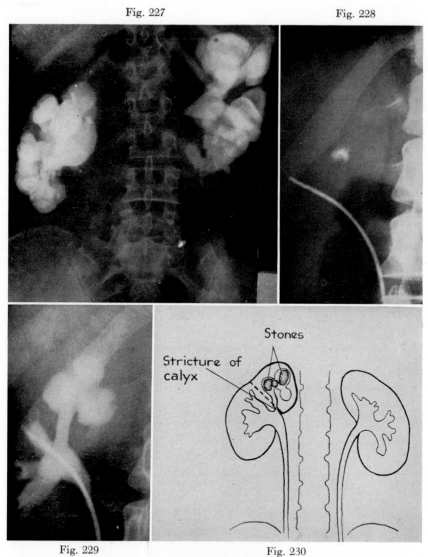

Fig. 229   Fig. 230

FIGURE 227.   Bilateral renal calculosis; advanced, in thirty-year-old woman.
FIGURE 228.   Renal stones in right upper hydrocalyx of forty-year-old woman.
FIGURE 229.   Pyelogram showing local calyceal dilatation (same case as Fig. 228).
FIGURE 230.   Schema of calyceal resection for stone in case shown in Figures 228 and 229.

phrotomy. Renal resection is indicated when the stone is confined to one pole and the rest of the kidney is sound (Figs. 228–230). In the removal of multiple calculi and dendritic stones, radiography at the operating table is of invaluable aid to indicate when all calcareous matter is removed. Nephrectomy is indicated in unilateral calculous disease with a functionally reliable mate, when there is (1) advanced suppurative pyelonephritis, (2) advanced hydronephrosis, usually infected, (3) pyonephrosis, (4) tuberculosis, (5) tumors, (6) large stones which cannot be removed without undue injury to the kidney, (7) multiple stones in inaccessible locations, and (8) repeated stone recurrence with grave renal disease. The seriously diseased ureter should be removed with the kidney.

In *bilateral calculous disease* it is essential to know the type and degree of obstruction and infection, the number and location of the calculi and the separate and combined renal function values. In bilateral calculous disease with large noninfected, nonobstructive, symptomless stag-horn stones or multiple stones simulating stag-horn calculi, operation is seldom urgently indicated. Commonly the surgical damage to the kidney is likely to be much greater than that of the stone, and further stone formation is almost a certainty. With (1) acute infection, (2) infected hydronephrosis from stone blockage, or (3) early pyonephrosis, prompt removal of the stone is necessary if only to establish nephrostomy drainage to maintain life. It is sometimes necessary to perform preliminary bilateral nephrostomy or an initial pelviolithotomy for the removal of an obstructing stone fragment. Occasionally an extremely old or weak patient may be tided over by an indwelling ureteral catheter.

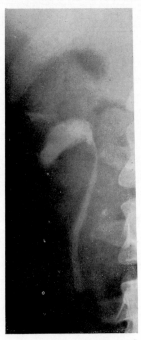

FIGURE 231. Postoperative urogram in case shown in Figure 228.

In bilateral renal calculous disease selection of the kidney to be operated upon first and the procedure to be carried out demands nice surgical judgment. Usually it is best to operate on the better side first, particularly when there are good prospects of removal of the calculi without serious trauma to the kidney and with the thought in mind that the more seriously diseased organ may later have to be removed. Nevertheless, an obstructed kidney causing severe or acute pain should always be operated upon first and at once, as should a calculous pyonephrosis associated with sepsis.

Contraindications to operation are essentially: far-advanced bilateral calculous disease in the presence of other disease with a hopeless outlook as, for example, primary anemia, leukemia, hemophilia, certain forms of central nervous disease, advanced renal or other neoplasia, advanced pulmonary tuberculosis or severe cardiopathy. A tender age, secondary anemia, or malnutrition do not contraindicate removal of renal stone, for with the liberal employment of blood transfusions, fluids and antimicrobial therapy, many apparently hopeless cases can be safely and successfully carried through radical surgery. Acute obstruction or acute renal infection may be combated by prompt employment of a urethral or ureteral catheter, and thus permit conservative rather than radical surgical treatment later to be carried out.

Complications of surgical lithotomy are fistula, infection, hemorrhage, or uremia. Fistula means that peripheral obstruction must be eradicated; infection, hemorrhage and uremia are appropriately treated as described elsewhere in this book. However, postoperative urinary sepsis and pneumonia are often fatal.

Prevention of Recurrent Renal Calculi. The incidence of recurrence of renal calculi following pyelolithotomy or nephrolithotomy is 15 to 25 per cent. By control of infection and dietary regimen, Higgins reported reduction to 3.6 per cent, a figure not even closely achieved by others. Procedures recommended to prevent stone recurrence include (1) a fluid intake of 2500 to 3000 cc. per day, (2) eradication of focal infection (especially teeth, prostate, cervix), (3) elimination of infection by chemotherapy, (4) correction of urinary stasis whether due to urinary tract disease or recumbency, (5) correction and treatment of metabolic diseases such as gout or cystinuria, (6) surgical exploration or excision of parathyroid tumor in established or proved hyperparathyroidism, and (7) stone preventive dietary regimen.

Prognosis in all varieties of urinary calculous disease depends upon (1) the degree of renal damage, (2) the nature and severity of coexisting infection, (3) the size and location of the stone, (4) the promptness and accuracy of diagnosis, and (5) the adequacy of treatment. Prognosis in unilateral calculous disease is nearly always good and in bilateral disease with advanced renal injury is nearly always bad. Fortunately, specific antibacterial therapy and the liberal employment of whole blood transfusion, general fortification by increased protein and vitamin intake, as well as improved technologic therapy, today encourage surgical intervention and save the lives of many patients whose outlook only twenty-five years ago would have been utterly hopeless.

CALCULOUS ANURIA

This may result from blockage of the urinary tract but is seldom bilateral. Usually the ureter of a solitary kidney is obstructed or urethral blockage by stone will involve both kidneys. It has been observed in a three-month-old infant anuric for four days, but is most commonly seen in the fourth and fifth decades. The usual uropathy is that of extreme damage of one kidney by pyonephrosis, advanced hydronephrosis, or sclerotic atrophy with total blockage by stone, and sudden obstruction of the opposite ureter by calculus. An initial bilateral renal colic is generally followed by persistent anuria or the passage of only a small amount of thick bloody urine. The attack may appear painlessly, the patient simply having no urine in the bladder to void.

Calculous anuria is always an emergency condition demanding prompt diagnostic study and the institution of free urinary drainage by indwelling ureteral catheter or open surgical intervention as demanded. There is no medical treatment. The prognosis is always grave with a mortality of about 70 per cent. In the early days of sulfonamide therapy, many cases of calculous anuria occurred consequent to bilateral blockage of both kidneys and/or ureters by acetylated sulfonamide crystal precipitation. Many of these patients have been children, nearly half of whom have died of the condition. It may be the final picture in renal failure in extensive and long-standing renal calculous disease which is generally bilateral and without total obstruction.

In calculous anuria due to obstruction the onset is usually acute with renal colic; the stone is then generally in the upper portion of the ureter but next most frequent in the lower third. The onset of calculous anuria may be gradual and without great disturbance except the patient has no urine in the bladder to pass. But as pelvic pressure or renal congestion increases, there is pain in the kidney region. Prompt roentgenography is called for as well as immediate passage of ureteral catheters to try to bypass the obstruction. If successful, this will give free urinary drainage and the patient will be restored to at least temporary safety while the best subsequent therapy is decided upon. Should the anuria persist following withdrawal of the catheters, immediate surgical drainage is required by ureterostomy or nephrostomy as the case may be.

Treatment of Calculous Anuria. The obstruction must be relieved at once by indwelling catheter, ureteral catheter, nephrostomy, pyelostomy or ureterostomy according to indication. The commonest type of calculous anuria is that in which one ureter is suddenly blocked by ureteral calculus and reflex anuria develops in the other kidney. This phenomenon generally passes off in a few hours although it may last for a few days but in any event the stone blockage must be promptly eliminated by catheter or operation. Occasionally the opposite kidney is congenitally hypoplastic, absent, or totally destroyed by long-standing infection, obstruction, or calculous disease and this may require removal of the stone on one side and later appropriate treatment of the other kidney. In calculous anuria of a solitary kidney or its clinical simulation as just described, when free drainage cannot be promptly established by ureteral catheter, nephrostomy or pyelostomy must be performed at once and with removal of the stone if the condition of the patient permits.

In the *secretory* type of anuria the prognosis is always grave and will depend largely upon the condition of the kidneys before the onset of the anuria. Employment of an artificial kidney if available may afford temporary and occasionally prolonged relief, and encourage at least temporary rehabilitation of the gravely diseased kidney.

Treatment of nephrocalcinosis is employed to (1) relieve acidosis, (2) improve the absorption of calcium, and (3) reduce hyperchloremia and hypercalcinuria. This is best achieved by the administration of a citrate mixture (citric acid 140 gm.; sodium citrate 98 gm.; 1000 cc. of water); this is given as 2 ounces daily of citrate mixture to correct the acidosis and reduce blood chlorides. Space does not permit discussion of the chemical mechanisms and rational of this mixture.

URETERAL CALCULI

Practically all ureteral calculi form in the kidney and more than 90 per cent of these pass to the bladder. The etiology, chemical considerations, and pathogenesis have been discussed under renal stone. More than two thirds occur in the third to fifth decades of life and twice as often in males as in females. Ureteral calculi comprise a fifth of urinary stones in women and children. Right and left sides are involved about equally and bilateral calculi occur in 2 to 4 per cent of the cases. Only rarely do calculi originate in the ureter and when they do, it is nearly always in connection with anomalies such as blind-ending ureters, ureteroceles, ectopic ureters, in dilated segments proximal to a stricture, valves, periureteral fibrosis or adhesions, anomalous vascularization, external ureteral masses, or a neoplasm.

Having left the kidney pelvis the stone will tend to be impeded by the normal ureteral constrictions located (1) at or just below the ureteropelvic junction, (2) where the ureter crosses the iliac vessels, (3) at the base of the broad ligament in women and at the point of crossing of the vas deferens in men, (4) where the ureter enters the bladder, and (5) the ureteral meatus (Fig. 30). About three fourths of ureteral stones will be found in the lower third of the ureter, next most commonly in the upper third, and lastly in the middle spindle. The juxtavesical ureteral segment is the most common site of retention (50–60%). Ureteral calculi show great variation in size from that of a BB shot (2 to 3 mm.) to that of a large cigar. Stones are multiple in 6 to 8 per cent of the cases. Multiple calculi are often faceted together to appear as one large elongated stone. Stones retained in the ureter tend slowly to grow by accretion and, with infection, chiefly by phosphatic deposit.

Stones retained in the ureter will usually produce hydroureter and hydronephrosis according to the degrees of obstruction induced and complicating urinary infection. Flat, grooved or canalized stones may permit sufficient urinary drainage so that little or no urographically demonstrable back-pressure change occurs in the proximal tract. The trauma caused by a stationary stone in the ureter or by a spiculated one whose sharp points dig into the mucosa induce ureteritis, later periureteritis, the deposition of fibrous tissue which commonly become clinical stricture. Peristalsis is interfered with; urinary stasis and inflammatory atony result. With dilatation of the ureter above the site of stone impaction (and generally with local secondary ureteral stricture), the calculus may move up and down above the obstruction like a pea in a pod, and at operation may be found to have moved to the renal pelvis when a low ureterotomy incision was made. The only guide against such surgical embarrassment is a plain x-ray taken immediately before the patient is placed upon the operating table and even this may fail, the stone having moved upward while the patient was being placed in position.

True megaloureter is the result of neuromuscular dysplasia but what is often designated as megaloureter may result from soft tissue obstruction such as stricture and is not uncommonly seen in long-standing impacted ureteral calculus, particularly at the ureterovesical junction. The ureter may become as large as the bowel. Yet by the time examination is made the stone may have passed. The calculus rarely ulcerates through the ureter. The changes in the kidney consequent to ureteral obstruction are described in Chapter 5.

Symptoms of ureteral calculus are characteristically those of renal stone and particularly reno-ureteral colic (q.v.). Intense agonizing colic may suddenly cease and shortly thereafter the patient pass the stone by urethra. The stone may move more slowly with repeated attacks of colic. The severity of the colic does not reflect progress of the stone; usually just the reverse occurs, the stone being firmly grasped by the spastic ureter and moving downward only when the spasm is relieved. Yet the pain may be of a chronic, dull-aching variety and on the right side may suggest cholecystitis or appendicitis, appendectomy being needlessly performed in a fourth to a third of these cases. As a clinical corollary, the virtue of an excretory urographic study prior to any operation for subacute, and especially chronic, appendicitis is apparent.

Reflex disturbances of urination are apt to be particularly striking in ureteral calculous disease; the lower the calculus is in the ureter, the more intense are the bladder disturbances likely to be. Yet only by urologic examination can it be determined to what extent urinary infection with intense inflammation about the vesical outlet is responsible for the vesical symptoms.

More than three fourths of the patients with ureteral stone show blood in the urine. But one in ten has neither pus nor blood cells and the urine is sterile in 40 to 50 per cent, these stones being mostly of the primary variety. Ninety per cent of patients with acute ureteral calculous disease will show leukocytosis; in half of these the white blood cell count will be between 10,000 and 15,000, higher than this in 20 per cent and less in 30 per cent.

Diagnosis will be suggested by the history and simulates that of renal stone which has been previously discussed in this chapter. Occasionally a stone in the lower ureter may be palpated upon rectal or vaginal examination.

Urographic examination must be relied upon to make the diagnosis in most cases. Excretory urographic study alone may establish the diagnosis and reflect the function of both kidneys as well as hydronephrosis. There may be no excretion of radiopaque medium from the kidney above the blocked ureter but nearly always this is a temporary reflex anuria, and function will be satisfactorily resumed with removal of the blockage.

When the excretory urographic findings are definitive, retrograde catheter study can usually be dispensed with except as an aid in establishing prompt renal drainage (Fig. 232). When this examination is not definitive, ureteral catheterization and retrograde ureterography is necessary.

In about 5 per cent of cases the stone will not be detected on the urogram but commonly this is the result of overclouding by gaseous distention of the intestines or by the bony structure of the pelvis which may obscure a relatively nonradiopaque stone. Stereoscopic urograms are

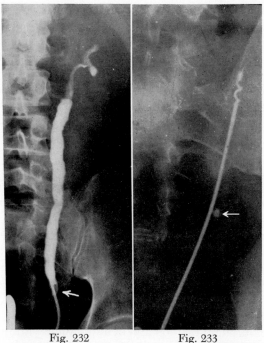

Fig. 232   Fig. 233

FIGURE 232. Ureteral calculus. Mildly radiopaque causing faint negative shadow at point where it is obstructing.

FIGURE 233. Ureteral stone localized by a ureteral spiral tip stone extractor as being within the channel.

most helpful especially when a catheter has been passed up to or beyond the stone (Fig. 233). Anterior, posterior, and oblique exposures should be made. When the suspicious shadow appears at some distance from the ureteral catheter, generous filling of the ureter with radiopaque medium will commonly show the stone to be within the greatly dilated canal or the shadow may be that of a juxta-ureteral phlebolith or calcific lymph gland (Fig. 234). Though now considered an old-fashioned method, I still employ the wax-bulb catheter in cases of suspected ureteral stone not radiographically clear cut; here a stone produces a characteristic clawlike scratch on the wax bulb which is readily distinguishable from the flat shave caused by contact with the instrument. Yet this method is not infallible because the wax may not be scratched if the stone is heavily coated with mucus or mucopus, or a dilated ureter may permit the wax bulb to pass the stone without adequate contact. Still I continue to use the test and with great satisfaction, especially when the stone is non-radiopaque.

Sometimes a calculus may be cystoscopically seen in the ureteral orifice, or to cause a great elevation and local swelling of the overlying vesical mucosa when it is in the intramural portion of the ureter; the orifice frequently is gaping and surrounded by an area of bullous edema.

Treatment. Evaluation of the best treatment for any patient, and it should be distinctly individualized, will depend most importantly on the renal function and the presence or absence of infection. The objective in treatment of ureteral calculi is prevention of loss of function of the kidney and progressive renal damage. When the functional injury of the kidney caused by ureteral calculous obstruction is mild and there is no infection, watchful waiting can usually be safely observed for two to three weeks even if colic recurs. If the stone is not passed in this time, remove it surgically. If the excretory urogram indicates no progress in stone passage, and there is increasing hydronephrosis and, especially when complicated by chronic infection, the calculus should be removed promptly.

When acute or even subacute urinary infection complicates ureteral stone, immediate relief of the obstruction is demanded and preferably by prompt ureterolithotomy. In debilitated patients, a preparatory period of free renal drainage by inlying ureteral catheter will often tide them over until ureterotomy can be more safely performed. The size of the stone is not always a criterion for operation although small stones are more likely to pass spontaneously than large. Yet symptomatically the colics caused by small stones may be most agonizing; "small dogs bark loudest." When an asymptomatic stone becomes impacted and shows no movement within four to six weeks, remove it.

Cystoscopic ureteral dilation and manipulation with the various types of stone extractors (basket, loop, spiral, etc.), should be employed only in calculi in the lower third of the ureter and even here with great care. Introduction or exacerbation of infection may be disastrous; I know of two deaths in one hospital in one year by the injudicious use of this treatment. I prefer the use of single or multiple inlying catheters which are withdrawn within twenty-four hours. If the stone is not removed with a fair trial, operate; repeated instrumentation is likely to lead to catastrophe.

Contraindications to manipulative treatment of ureteral calculi are: when (1) the caliber of the stone exceeds 2 cm., (2) there is considerable periureteritis, (3) the kidney is either hydronephrotic or pyonephrotic, (4) the stone is known to have been present for a long time, (5) several unsuccessful attempts have already been made to remove it, (6) cystoscopy is poorly tolerated, (7) congenital anomalies of the genital organs are present, and (8) severe reaction or acute pyelonephritis follows the first manipulative procedure.

Operation (ureterolithotomy) is demanded when: (1) repeated manipulative attempts fail, (2) the stone cannot be mobilized, (3) renal infection exists (if gravity would be increased by delay), (4) stones are more than 2 cm. in diameter, and (5) ureteral strictures, hypertrophy of the prostate or other conditions cause obstruction, (6) there has been intervening instrumentation, (7) there is intolerance to manipulation or (8) there is disease of the upper urinary tract which itself requires surgery. Here ureterotomy and the establishment of free urinary drainage together with intensive antimicrobial therapy may be expected to rehabilitate the patient promptly and most of them will be returned home in ten to twelve days.

Prognosis. Recurrence of ureteral stone occurs largely as in renal stones, and is noted in about 10 per cent of the cases. Following successful surgery, a check-up excretory urogram after two months is essential to determine the degree of restoration of renal function and to be sure that there is no ureteral stricture. Persisting ureteral obstruction (stricture) should be periodically progressively dilated cystoscopically. Sometimes the kidney does not regain its function; it remains the seat of chronic infection and requires removal. In review, ureteral stones should be recognized and removed early, whether spontaneously, by manipulation or open surgery. Having removed the stone, sterilize the urine and subsequently make sure there is no persisting urinary stasis to predispose to stone recurrence or injure the kidney by urinary back pressure.

VESICAL CALCULI

Most stones found in the bladder originated in the kidney, and in about one in five of these cases renal and vesical stones coexist. Calculi may form in the bladder about foreign bodies, calcareous chips, epithelial or bacterial debris when there is vesical urinary stasis and infection. In children the nucleus of vesical calculi is usually a small uric acid calculus about which urate, oxalate and, in particular, phosphatic deposit has occurred; these constitute about 2 per cent of all vesical calculi in patients of all ages. The chief *predisposing agent* in vesical stone formation is obstruction at the bladder outlet or peripherally which prevents passage of the stone which has usually migrated downward from the kidney, or by creating urinary stasis particularly when infection exists to favor the development of a stone in the bladder. Curiously only 2 to 3 per cent of all vesical calculi occur in women. The high incidence of bladder neck obstruction by contracture or prostatic enlargement, stricture of the urethra, vesical diverticulum, urinary infection and stasis explain the frequency of bladder stones, especially in males between thirty and eighty years of age. The vesical stone causes bladder wall changes similar to those of a foreign body and similar to those noted in the stone-bearing kidney pelvis. With severe infection and inflammation, marked pericystitis develops often with pronounced sclerosis, late contraction of the bladder and diminution of its capacity. The changes in the upper urinary tract are in general those of intravesical obstruction complicated by infection, the rate and degree of damage being influenced in large measure by the intensity of complicating urinary infection.

As the stone moves about in the bladder it causes irritation but may become wedged in the vesical outlet or posterior urethra to cause complete blockage. Vesical calculi not silently trapped in a diverticulum characteristically cause urinary frequency, urgency, dysuria, great straining, tenesmus, strangury, dribbling, enuresis (children), and sometimes chronic complete urinary retention. Pyuria and hematuria are the rule and will be present sometime in every case. When the patient is upright the stone rests on the trigone near the vesical outlet to produce pronounced irritation, often with excruciating tenesmus as the last few drops of urine are passed. The patient grasps his penis and, if a child, screams. This syndrome is known as "fit of the stone." Yet let him recline and the symptoms promptly cease as the calculus rolls away from the bladder outlet to the posterior bladder wall. The patient usually localizes the pain of vesical stone at or near the bladder outlet but it may be referred to the suprapubic, scrotal, perineal, rectal or vaginal region or along the urethra where it is likely to be most intense at the external meatus or frenum. This commonly causes boys to squeeze the penis, particularly the glans, and to pull at the prepuce while girls rub the external urethral meatus, the "hand sign" (Brun) of vesical stone in children. Excessive handling of the genitalia is a frequent indicator of stone or foreign body in the bladder in the young and the reflex irritation may produce priapism. Hemorrhoids, rectal prolapse, inguinal or umbilical hernia often develop when there is marked straining to urinate. When a child shows rectal prolapse, rule out vesical stone. Similarly by somatic reference, the vesical irritation may suggest that of rectal worms. When the vesical outlet irritation is severe enough and especially with ulceration, paradoxical or spastic incontinence may occur or, with an obstructed bladder outlet, overflow or pseudo-incontinence.

In vesical calculous disease urinary infection is commonly of the ammoniogenic variety (Proteus bacillus, urea-splitting staphylococci). Following the experimental introduction of these organisms into the bladder, vesical stone often forms. In early vesical stone disease the bladder mucosal changes are those of mild cystitis with congestion and reddening of the mucosa, but with the advent of infection, pronounced congestion, bullous edema, and ulceration appear. Trabeculation, sacculation and other manifestations of urinary back pressure may be due to urethral stricture or to blockage of the bladder outlet by stone or by antecedent prostatic obstruction.

Diagnosis. Sometimes the patient will give a history of having had renal colic with apparent passage of the stone to the bladder but not from the urethra. There may be a history of vesical pain aggravated or initiated by exercise, irregular or interrupted urination, and terminal hematuria. But other severe vesical lesions such as tumor or foreign bodies may also produce these manifestations. The urine is nearly always abnormal showing albumin, red and white blood cells, often an excess of mucus and epithelium. Infection is usually demonstrable.

Almost all bladder stones are radiographically demonstrable; an enlarged prostate commonly overshadows small stones or those of mild radiopacity (Figs. 8, 235). Stones of low radiodensity may be demonstrated by pneumocystography (Fig. 236). Some stones show lamination.

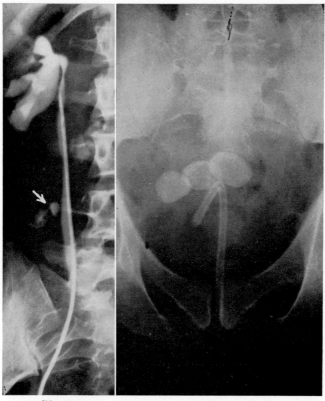

Fig. 234   Fig. 235

FIGURE 234. Juxta-ureteral calcified lymph nodes localized by ureterogram as outside the duct. Note anomalous high ureteral insertion into the renal pelvis.

FIGURE 235. Vesical calculi: in inverted crescent arrangement behind a greatly enlarged prostate.

Bladder stones are predominantly ovoid and lie in the long axis of the horizontal plane. Occasionally jackstones, chiefly of oxalate composition, are found. Yet the diagnosis must be confirmed by cystoscopy which is the most accurate method.

Treatment.   Bladder stones up to 1.0 cm. in diameter in children or not larger than 2 cm. in adults may be removed by crushing (litholapaxy or lithotripsy). Larger stones should be removed by suprapubic cystolithotomy and this is the preferred method for the removal of all bladder stones by general surgeons.

Litholapaxy is contraindicated when (1) the stone is larger than 2 cm. in diameter, (2) is very hard, chiefly oxalate, (3) multiple, (4) the bladder is intolerant, (5) obstruction of the vesical outlet, diverticulum or marked infection exists, or (6) the stone is in a diverticulum. Inability to perform litholapaxy is the absolute contraindication. Obstruction at the vesical outlet, prostatic hypertrophy or other bladder neck blockage is present in over half of the cases and litholapaxy cannot be performed without considerable trauma to the structures in the area. Prostatitis, urethritis, and epididymitis may follow litholapaxy and, even more grave, may be acute pyelonephritis, perforation of the bladder, and septicemia. Additional contraindications to litholapaxy include acute cystitis, contracted bladder neck, tumor, or calculus adherent to the bladder wall and strictures or congenital anomalies of the urethra which do not permit ready instrumentation.

Having removed the bladder stone, treatment is incomplete if peripheral obstruction is not also eradicated and the urine sterilized.

Although the mortality following litholapaxy is considerably less (1–5%) than following cystostomy, most of those treated by open operation were sicker patients to begin with and cystostomy offered their greatest hope. Today with modern antibacterial therapy the mortality from open cystolithotomy alone should not be over 1 per cent.

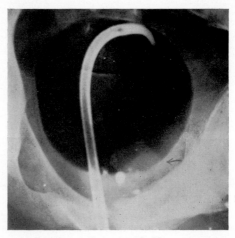

FIGURE 236.   Shadows of faintly radiopaque bladder stones accentuated by pneumocystography.

URETHRAL CALCULI

Urethral stone is predominantly a disease of males and nearly always reflects urethral obstruction. Calculi passing from the bladder to the urethra lodge predominantly in the prostatic segment or in the deep penile portion, especially the bulb or at the fossa navicularis (Fig. 237, *D*). Sometimes they form in rouleau arrangement, becoming multiple and faceted. The development and rate of growth will be influenced by infection and peripheral obstruction. In the female, calculi are usually located in a urethral diverticulum which, in turn, is generally proximal to a congenital or traumatic stricture.

Urethral stones are in general of the same chemical constituency as are those of the bladder and upper urinary tract. Stones which develop entirely in the urethra are nearly always phosphatic. Stones originating in the urethra itself usually do so about a self-introduced foreign body.

Changes in the proximal tract in urethral obstruction have been indicated in Chapter 3 and will be aggravated, intensified and accelerated by infection. The presence of the stone usually produces a urethritis with mucoid or mucopurulent discharge, and even active periurethritis with periurethral abscess or periurethral phlegmon and urinary extravasation may ensue. With complete urethral blockage by the stone, acute urinary retention results.

Symptoms. Urethral stones produce the same symptoms as vesical calculi except they are more localized to the stone-bearing area. Urination or sudden stoppage may occur with inability to pass anything or a mere dribbling. Referred pain may be almost as severe at the tip of the penis in prostatic urethral stone as it is in the perineum or rectum. Stone in a urethral diverticulum may be manifested chiefly by periodic urethral

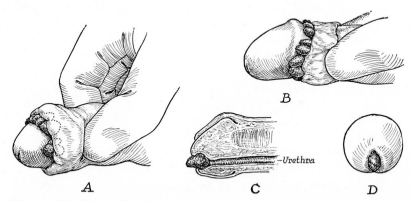

A   *C*   *D*

FIGURE 237. Preputial calculi. Phimosis is essential for the formation of these stones, urinary salts being precipitated in the subpreputial space. Balanitis and purulent discharge from the preputial orifice, often misinterpreted as urethritis, is the most frequent symptom. Treatment: circumcision. Smegmatic calculi are commonly the nidi about which urinary phosphatic crystals and stone are secondarily deposited. *A*, appearance on partial retraction of the prepuce. *B*, condition observed. *C*, urethral calculus blocking the external urethral meatus. Lateral view. *D*, frontal view of *C*. In *C* and *D*, wide meatotomy usually suffices to permit extraction of the stone.

discharge and pyuria; sometimes the patient can palpate the stone in the sac himself.

Diagnosis is made by palpation, urethroscopy and roentgenography (Fig. 236). A grating sensation may be felt when passing a metal instrument such as a sound or a urethroscope.

Treatment. Some urethral stones can be milked forward to the meatus and extracted or pushed back into the bladder and removed by forceps or litholapaxy. Stones jammed in the external meatus will pop out after meatotomy. When these methods fail, urethrolithotomy may be necessary, for with a large calculus in the prostatic urethra suprapubic or perineal cystostomy may be required for its removal. Following recovery of the stone, complicating obstructions along the urethra and at the vesical outlet must be eradicated and subsequently the urine sterilized.

Urethral calculi are unusual in the female because of the short urethra which encourages passage of small vesical calculi and, as a corollary of this, accounts for the relative infrequency of vesical stone in women. Most urethral stones in the female have occurred in diverticula. The symptoms are predominantly those of the diverticulum with lower urinary tract infection, frequency, dysuria, nocturia, pyuria and occasional hematuria. There may be pain during coitus or an occasional purulent discharge may occur with symptomatic relief. The stone can generally be felt by vaginal palpation, is seen by urethroscopy, and demonstrated by urography.

The treatment of a stone in a urethral diverticulum is excision of the sac containing the calculus. Many surgeons find indwelling catheter drainage adequate; I prefer suprapubic trocar cystostomy counterdrainage.

PREPUTIAL CALCULI

The formation of preputial calculi is favored by a tight prepuce behind which primary stones are formed from smegmatic debris in which are incorporated desquamated epithelial cells, fatty substances and bacteria together with a quantity of urinary salts, chiefly calcium (Fig. 237). These stones are soft, yellowish or yellowish-brown, of light weight, and without characteristic shape although they tend to be faceted and molded in the postcoronal sulcus. Soft smegmatic stone deposit in the postcoronal sulcus is often extensive in phimosis and particularly with preputial adhesions (q.v.). Sometimes on breaking down the adhesions in the children, the entire corona is found buttressed with organic calculi which with retention of infected, stagnating urine become nuclei for true phosphatic stone deposits. Stones passed from the urethra may be retained by a tight prepuce.

Preputial calculi may cause no symptoms but usually are responsible for local irritation with inflammation, balanitis, ulceration, discharge, sometimes obstruction of the preputial meatus or even preputial gangrene. Joly reported one such lesion the size of a hen's egg in an eight-year-old boy.

Diagnosis. Preputial calculi should be at least diagnostically thought of in a patient, particularly a boy, who shows unnatural handling of the penis, with squeezing of the glans or tugging at the foreskin. Dense preputial calculi can be palpated through the prepuce, and will be seen when the prepuce is retracted; a dorsal slit may be necessary for this last observation. Some preputial calculi may be demonstrated radiographically but this is generally unnecessary.

The stone may pass from the meatus or ulcerate through the fossa navicularis. There is frequently a discharge from the small preputial edema, and later ulceration. Carcinoma may coexist, perhaps secondary to calculous irritation. Diagnosis is made by palpation of the stone. If associated infection is active when the diagnosis is made, perform liberal dorsal meatotomy and evacuation of the stones; if infection is mild or absent perform circumcision.

CALCULI OF THE PROSTATE AND SEMINAL VESICLES

Here we are concerned with those true prostatic calculi which develop in the acini of the gland itself as a deposit of calcific material on the corpora amylacea. Infection usually plays a part in the calculogenesis in which calcium phosphate and carbonate impregnate the corpora amylacea; prostatic infection is regularly present (Figs. 238, 239). The corpora amylacea are extremely small, round, or ovoid bodies composed of lecithin and a nitrogenous albuminous substance. Although prostatic calculi have been described in boys as young as three years of age they are rarely found before forty. They are observed chiefly in men between fifty and seventy years of age. They may be present as one or two small stones or several hundred ranging in size from 1 to 10 or more millimeters in diameter. They are brownish-gray, smooth, usually of firm consistency but can be crushed.

With acinar obstruction by calculi, debris and desquamated epithelial cells may be retained or variable cystic formation occur, the over-all

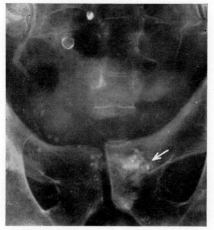

Figure 238. Prostatic calculi causing a "peppering" of densities throughout the glandular area especially on the left.

picture being that of chronic inflammation of the prostate. They do not occur in the adenomatous portion of the hyperplastic prostate but rest in the thinned-out surgical capsule of prostatic tissue about the tumor, and are exposed by enucleation of the adenoma. Associated inflammation is usually low grade but a periprostatitis may occur and even abscess formation with rupture into the urethra. There are no specific symptoms of prostatic calculi, the clinical manifestations being those of coexisting prostatic hyperplasia, chronic prostatitis or urethral stricture, with some-times dull ache in the lower back, perineum or penis. Urinary difficulty is due to obstruction independent of the calculous disease. Hematuria reflects prostatitis. With collateral prostatic abscess the symptoms are of this lesion and not of the calculi.

Diagnosis is most often suggested by rectal examination in which one may feel small calculi over the palpable surface of the gland and especially near the base. There may or may not be stone crepitation. A small cluster of calculi or a large prostatic stone may suggest early car-cinoma, from which it is differentiated by (1) lack of extensive stony hardness with extension to the seminal vesicle(s), (2) absence of crepita-tion, (3) nonfixation of the gland, (4) normal acid phosphatase deter-mination, and (5) roentgenographic study (Figs. 238, 239). In doubtful cases cytologic studies of expressed prostatic secretion may disclose cancer cells to make the diagnosis of malignancy. The palpation of prostatic calculi may suggest tuberculosis but evidence of tuberculous seminal vesiculitis and epididymitis is lacking. Diagnosis will be confirmed by roentgenographic studies in which the shadows of stones may be diffusely evident throughout the gland or may be arranged in horseshoe or ring formation about the urethra. In the horseshoe arrangement the stones are present on both sides of the gland but not in front of the urethra. In pronounced calculosis the entire prostate may appear to be replaced by calcific material (Fig. 239).

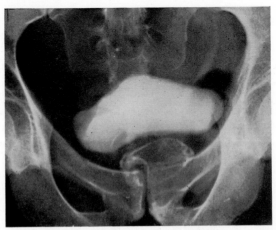

Figure 239. Large calcific stone-like mass in prostate of a thirty-eight-year-old man. No tuberculosis demonstrable nor history suggestive of antecedent prostatic sup-puration or abscess, merely urinary frequency and slight dysuria.

Treatment. None is needed unless urgent symptoms of coexisting disease demand attention. Stones apparently causing continued therapy-resistant prostatitis may be largely removed by transurethral resection. They may also be removed by suprapubic prostatectomy in which, after enucleation of the adenomatous nodules, many calculi can often be scooped away from the surgical capsule of compressed prostatic tissue. Perineal prostatectomy is recommended for removal of large localized stones. If the prostatic calcific involvement is generalized and severe, employ perineal prostatectomy and, if indicated, bilateral seminal vesiculectomy. Open operation, either suprapubic or perineal, gives the best results. Mortality should be nil in transurethral resection for prostatic stone removal and/or in general that of suprapubic or perineal prostatectomy, when either of these methods is used. Stones may be overlooked at operation, or they may variably recur.

Calculi of the seminal vesicles are exceedingly rare, occur chiefly in elderly men, and appear singly or as several in a cluster. The stone nuclei are epithelial cells with a brownish lime-salt covering, the stones being smooth, hard and varying from 1 to 15 mm. in diameter. Chronic inflammation with fibrosis is usually present in the walls of the seminal vesicle whose duct may be completely occluded. As a rule there are no symptoms; hemospermia, painful erections, and perineal discomfort at the time of ejaculation have been present in some cases. The diagnosis must be considered when the symptoms present themselves together. The stony hardness may suggest carcinoma of the seminal vesicle but the radiographic study will show fuzzy or mottled stone shadows in the region of this organ. By rectal palpation one or more hard, tender, smooth nodules are felt in the vesicle. As a rule no treatment is required but if it seems to be demanded, employ perineal seminal vesiculectomy.

FOREIGN BODIES IN THE URINARY TRACT

Most foreign bodies as urologically demonstrated have been introduced into the urinary tract as a masturbatory or an auto-erotic performance by sex perverts, masturbators, malingerers, intoxicated adults, and insane. Practically every known object small enough to pass the meatus has at one time or another been introduced into the urethra and/or bladder. In manipulating the object stuck into the urethra, it slips from grasp, enters the deep urethra of the male or the bladder of the female, and usually ends up in the bladder in the male also although it may stay in the deep urethra. Objects thus introduced include pencils, safety pins, hairpins, bobby pins, rubber tubing, sealing and candle wax, paraffin, gum, straws, plant stems, glass or plastic rod, ice tea sippers, stone, wire, darning needles, toothpicks, grain, seeds, beans, hair balls, shot, buttons, needles, pins, nails, various worms chiefly earthworms, and even a galvanized watch chain, and the round belt from a sewing machine have been reported. Foreign bodies may otherwise appear in the bladder as shell fragments, bullets, splinters of wood, debris, or clothing entering from the outside, pieces of gauze left at the time of operation, or stone may be deposited about cotton swabs, gauze, sutures, thermometers or blood clots. Other foreign bodies that have been left behind after surgery include drains, broken electric light bulbs, or broken off pieces of an instrument, particularly the jaw of a lithotrite. Yet this accident is usually recognized at once and the object removed. Foreign bodies reported entering the bladder after orthopedic surgery include Kirschner wires from pinning the neck of a femur, bone spicules, sequestra, and bone-peg migration to the bladder. In a few instances a dermoid cyst has ruptured into the bladder with discharge of hair (pilimiction), cartilage or other debris. Women, and particularly little girls, may roll up small balls of hair and insert them into the vagina or into the urethra to be recovered from the toilet as manifestations of false pilimiction. The foreign body whether accidentally or intentionally introduced into the bladder, may penetrate the bladder wall and produce pericystic abscess or extend into the peritoneal cavity and cause peritonitis. Darning needles, hair pins, finger nail cleaners and similar metal objects introduced into the bladder have been known to perforate into the vagina or into the peritoneal cavity. Swallowed objects (needles, pins, brooms bristles, etc.) have been alleged to perforate the higher bowel to appear in the upper urinary tract or by rectal perforation to enter the bladder.

With enlargement of the foreign body by calcific deposit in the bladder there is both local irritation and infection. The inflammatory albuminous matrix engendered by the local inflammation holds the crystalloid mass together. The pathologic changes are those characteristic of stone in the bladder or urethra, according to the site of the foreign body. Moreover, the object may jam in the vesical outlet or urethra to cause acute retention. Phosphatic incrustations on inlying catheters (urethral, cystostomy, nephrostomy) often break off to become nuclei for stone formation, and this is particularly notable in the young. The passage of vesical foreign bodies retrograde to the ureter or the kidney pelvis apparently has occurred; toothpicks and blades of grass have been so reported. With extreme infection of the deep urethra, prostatitis and epididymitis may develop.

Symptoms of foreign bodies in the bladder are precisely those of stone as described under calculous disease earlier in this chapter. A urethral foreign body provokes urethritis and often pronounced urinary symptoms. Acute periurethritis may become evident and localized, sometimes with abscess formation or extend as periurethral phlegmon, with both its local and systemic manifestations (q.v.).

The urethral discharge may be mistaken for gonorrhea, as in a five-year-old male patient of mine who had inserted two needles into his deep urethra, the ends of which had become densely encrusted. Low abdominal pain, sepsis, local edema, peritonitis may develop with vesical wall perforation.

As a rule a foreign body is not discovered without a rather complete urologic examination; the patient rarely gives the true history until confronted with the removed foreign body. A foreign body in the urethra or bladder may be identified by passage of a small sound as a searcher. It may be palpated, seen by urethroscopy or cysto-urethroscopy or demonstrated by roentgenography.

Diagnosis. The encrustation of foreign bodies with urinary salts and particularly calcium phosphate or calcium carbonate which occurs in practically every instance aids in the roentgenographic identification and diagnosis (Fig. 240). Paraffin bodies will be seen floating at the bladder dome.

Treatment. This is by removal of the foreign body which often can be accomplished with operating forceps through the tubular endoscope. If instrumental removal is unsuccessful, hazardous or impossible, or there is pronounced pericystitis or vesical perforation, the foreign body should be removed from the bladder by suprapubic cystostomy. Urethral foreign bodies can sometimes be milked forward and recovered but usually the patient has already failed at this (Fig. 241). Often they can be removed with forceps from the bulbous or prostatic urethra or can be pushed into these locations, and removed by external urethrostomy. A simple method for the removal of pins, needles, and similar foreign bodies from the anterior male urethra is shown in Figure 241.

Secondary urethral or periurethral abscess must be incised and drained, and sometimes the foreign body can be removed through the incision. Fistulization will not develop if the distal canal is kept well dilated after removing the foreign body. The incision should be along the ventral aspect of the urethra. Following removal of the foreign body, make certain no obstruction persists and sterilize the urine.

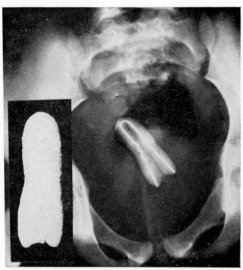

FIGURE 240. Foreign bodies in the urinary tract. Hairpin heavily encrusted with phosphatic crystals in the bladder of a three-year-old girl examined because of "chronic pyelitis." Suprapubic removal. Upon confronting the child with the surgical findings, she admitted having introduced the hairpin herself and obviously as a masturbatory act. Insert: removed specimen.

Paraffin and chewing gum in the bladder will usually dissolve in xylol or benzine but this requires deep anesthesia both to spare the patient pain and permit swishing around the solvent in the bladder. More than one bladder filling with the solvent may be required, the treatment being continued until the cystoscope shows all wax or gum has been washed away, or has been dissolved sufficiently for removal by endoscopic forceps.

Surgical intervention for foreign body of the kidney, especially gunshot, is required only for uncontrollable hemorrhage, increasing urinary extravasation, extensive infarction or thrombosis of the kidney. Usually the surgeon can be conservative with removal of the foreign body, then use suture, packing and perirenal drainage.

Foreign bodies introduced into the vagina sometimes become "lost" and, in turn, are the nuclei for large stones. The clinical considerations are essentially the same as those of vesical or urethral stones with the local irritation, pyuria, discharge, discomfort, and sometimes dysuria with frequency and bleeding. The diagnosis is suggested by the symptoms and confirmed by vaginoscopy. Removal of the object is the treatment. How much good can be achieved by the psychiatric care of psychoses engendering these acts is debatable. This applies also to downgrading sex stimulation with interrupted doses of diethylstilbestrol.

An extremely rare form of genital tract calcification in *fetal or meconium peritonitis* occurs during intra-uterine life as a result of bowel perforation. The escaping meconium works its way through the unobliterated funicular process of the tunica vaginalis to fill the scrotal cavity. Variable calcification of the material in the scrotum occurs and is roentgenographically demonstrable. About a hundred such cases have been reported; Neuhauser states that the x-ray picture is characteristic with intraperitoneal and intrascrotal calcification and cannot be caused by any other condition.

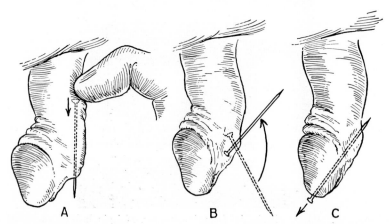

Figure 241. Urethral foreign body. Simple method of removing a pin from the anterior urethra, especially when its point has perforated the canal. When there has been no perforation of the urethra, endoscopic removal is preferred.

LEGAL ASPECTS OF SURGICALLY INTRODUCED FOREIGN BODIES

The employment of red rubber tubing (which contains antimony sulfide) is urged because it is radiographically demonstrable; sponges should have a radiopaque stripe or a metal ring for later identification, as should rubber drains. Yet even marked packs, instruments and catheters have been left in the bladder and particularly in the prostatic fossa after prostatectomy, and gauze sponges and drains have been left in the renal fossa after nephrectomy. Pieces of broken off ureteral catheters or of stone extracting instruments have been left in the ureter. In court the plaintiff must prove his case but usually he can do this if he can gain the removed foreign body. On the other hand, he must prove that its presence was through negligence of the physician and that he, the patient, suffered injury therefrom. The legal attitude entirely favors the patient as courts for the most part take the position that the very leaving of a foreign body in the patient denotes negligence on the part of the surgeon. It is up to the surgeon to produce convincing evidence well corroborated by others that he exercised due care during the operation.

CHAPTER 12

Tumors of the Urogenital Tract

New growths of the genitourinary tract structures comprise about 20 per cent of all tumors in adults and about 25 per cent in infants and children. Ninety-three to 95 per cent of urogenital tract tumors are malignant and all should be so considered until proved otherwise. Especially is this true in every solid mass in an infant or child. The disease is sometimes hopelessly incurable when first symptomatically manifested; with prompt complete investigation upon the appearance of the first symptom—often painless hematuria—and proper radical excision, an otherwise poor prognosis may become good.

TUMORS OF THE KIDNEY

Etiology. The cause of renal tumors is unknown. They occur predominantly in the fifth and sixth decades, an age group average of fifty-six to sixty-eight years, a third more often in males but of no preference as to side, and are most rarely bilateral. An eighth of all renal tumors are found in infants and children.

Symptoms. Renal tumors cause no characteristic symptoms or syndrome. Nearly half of these tumors cause no symptoms until late and are accidentally discovered, perhaps during routine physical examination. Hematuria, tumor and pain are the classical symptomatic triad in adults but in the young, tumor and pain are prominent while hematuria generally appears late or not at all.

A tumor is palpable in 50 to 60 per cent of these patients depending not alone on the size and site of the growth (posterior or upper pole tumors may be missed until large), but on the thickness of the overlying belly wall. Half of these patients have dull or acute *pain*, caused by increased tension of the renal capsule consequent to tumor expansion or have ureteral colic from the passage of blood clots or tumor masses.

Tumors of the renal pelvis *bleed* early, easily and often copiously while those of the parenchyma bleed only when they penetrate the pelvic wall. They may also enter the vascular tree and spread widely by venous transport. *Fever* occurs in 10 to 15 per cent of these cases and shows great variation in character: irregular, high or low, or more or less constant (100–102° F.). Fever is even more prominent in children with renal embryoma or Wilms' tumor. *Gastrointestinal disturbances* are regularly present as the tumor growth continues; this is common to all neoplasia. Doubtless absorption of toxic products from the malignant growth locally or metastatic is an important factor in fever production. General *malaise* develops with loss of strength and appetite, refusal to eat, anemia, constipation, and consequent loss of weight. *Hypertension* is found in over three fourths of patients with Wilms' tumor and warrants a bad prognosis; its cause is unknown.

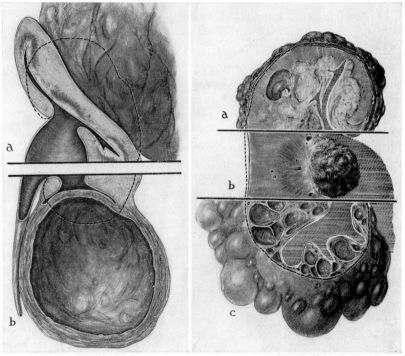

Fig. 242   Fig. 243

FIGURE 242. Renal tumors. Mechanics of pyelographic diagnostic criteria. Pelvic deformity, compression or elongation results from tumors (*a*) compressing the kidney from without, or (*b*) from tumors arising within the kidney as shown here, for example, a cyst.

FIGURE 243. Renal tumors. Schema of urographic diagnosis. Changes in the pelvis in intrarenal tumors: *a*, formation of "spider-leg" pelvis by compression of growing parenchymal tumors; flattening and elongation of the calyces as shown here is usually observed; *b*, pelvic filling defect by a papillomatous growth, *c*, bizarre pelvic irregularity and calyceal rounding as characteristically seen in polycystic renal disease.

The tumor growth may produce a "pot belly" protuberance especially in children, (Fig. 251) or, by pressure of the growth on the spermatic veins, varicocele may appear. The onset of persistent cough, hemoptysis, hemiplegia or other central nervous system syndrome, or pathologic fracture may reflect metastasis from an unsuspected or a known renal tumor.

Diagnosis. The history is often an aid. The tumor may be palpable or even visualized in the renal region and must be presumed to be kidney until proved otherwise. A Papanicolaou stain of the urine may disclose tumor cells.

Excretory urographic study may suggest the diagnosis and, of vast importance, indicate the integrity of the opposite kidney. In the diagnosis of upper urinary tract tumors in particular, retrograde urography is the most reliable method.

Changes in the pelvic outline urographically suggestive of renal tumor are: (1) elongation of the calyces, (2) a filling defect of the pelvis, (3) enlargement of the pelvis with or without alteration of pelvic capacity. All of these are phases of pelvic deformity which is produced by (1) mechanical distortion of the pelvis by the new growth, (2) obstruction of the pelvic outlet and/or upper ureter, and (3) ulceration and necrosis (Figs. 242, 243). As the tumor grows, the involved calyx or calyces are drawn out with and compressed by the neoplasm, eventually becoming a narrow streak—designated urographically as "spider leg" (Fig. 243,A). *Lateral pyelograms* may be expected to rule out tumors of the spleen, gallbladder, liver, intestines, pancreas, omentum or retroperitoneal structures. A gastrointestinal tract study may be needed. Renal arteriography (aortography, see Chapt. 3) will usually demonstrate the tumor-bearing area in the kidney by pooling or puddling of injected radiographic me-

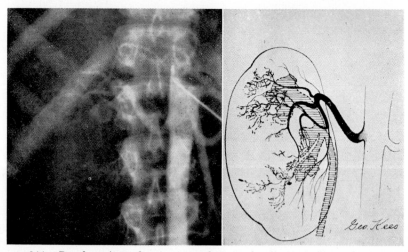

FIGURE 244. Renal angiography (aortography) in the diagnosis of renal tumor. Note "puddling" of medium in the neoplastic mass. (Smith.)

dium (Fig. 244) or, when the tumor is a cyst, by demonstrating the sharply encircled cyst area of nonvascularization (Fig. 245). *Retroperitoneal pneumography* achieved by the presacral injection of 500 or more cubic centimeters of air (Chapter 3) may assist in outlining the kidney and adrenal and if done in conjunction with excretory urography, a striking nephrographic demonstration may be obtained. Occasionally a stone is found in the tumor-bearing kidney.

Roentgenograms of the chest should be made in these cases to rule out pulmonary metastases which, except in hypernephroma or an uncontrollably bleeding tumor of another type, are indications against nephrectomy.

Treatment. This is removal of the tumor-bearing kidney and its surrounding fat as soon as the diagnosis is made. In tumors of the renal pelvis, the kidney, ureter and a cuff of bladder wall should be excised en masse. The usual exposure through the loin suffices for removal of smaller kidney tumors but the thoraco-abdominal or transthoracic approach is enjoying wide vogue now for the removal of large adherent tumor-bearing kidneys as it permits early division of the renal pedicle to mini-

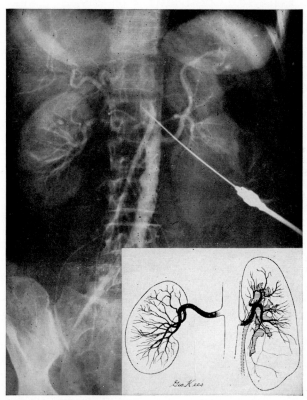

FIGURE 245. Solitary cyst of lower pole of left kidney as demonstrated by renal angiography. Note absence of vascularity and pooling of media in the cyst area. (Drs. Lee Elgin and P. G. Smith.)

mize tumor spread, local bleeding and technical difficulties. The transabdominal route is usually the best for removal of large Wilms' tumors.

Should the tumor prove inoperable, a biopsy specimen should be taken for examination and if the kidney is uninfected, the ureter should be tied off and subsequent radiation therapy employed. Since most of the tumor spread in renal neoplasms is vascular, extensive resection of local lymph nodes is fruitless.

With a well-administered anesthesia, gentle surgical technique, a reasonable operating time and adequate supportive treatment with blood transfusions, maintenance of normal electrolyte balance, and administration of antimicrobial medication as indicated, the operative morbidity and mortality will be low and, in the absence of metastasis, improved prognosis is offered. The operative mortality should not be over 3 per cent.

TUMORS OF AND ABOUT THE KIDNEY

The classification of renal tumors as followed for purposes of presentation are given in Table 16.

TABLE 16. CLASSIFICATION OF RENAL TUMORS

1. *Benign tumors*	5. *Tumors of the renal capsule*
Mixed	Fibroma
Fibroma	Fibrolipoma
Adenomas	Malignant sarcoma
Papillary cystadenoma	Angiosarcoma
Cystic disease:	Chondroma
Solitary cysts	
Endometriosis	6. *Pararenal tumors*
	Solid
2. *Epithelial neoplasms*	Cystic
A. Parenchyma	Malignant
1. Renal cell carcinoma*	Teratoma
Hypernephroma	
Adenocarcinoma	7. *Perirenal cysts*
Alveolar carcinoma	Wolffian
Embryonic carcinoma	Parasitic
2. Nephroma (Wilms')	Lymphatic
B. Pelvis	Dermoid
Papilloma	Hydrocele renalis
Papillary carcinoma	
Squamous cell carcinoma	8. *Malignant perirenal tumors*
3. *Mesothelial neoplasms*	9. *Tumors metastatic to kidney*
Sarcoma	Sarcoma
Neurogenic tumors:	Lymphosarcoma
Neuroblastoma	Thymoma
Sympathicoblastoma	Testicular
Schwannoma	Renal
4. *Renal vascular tumors*	
Hemangioma	

* Mostofi states (personal communication, 1956) "The current (1956) practice among most of the pathologists is to group all epithelial tumors of renal parenchyma as renal cell carcinoma and not to classify them into the various types, e.g., hypernephroma, adenocarcinoma, alveolar carcinoma and embryonic carcinoma. Exclusive of Wilms', if enough sections of a parenchymal carcinoma are studied, more than one histologic type is seen."

BENIGN TUMORS OF THE KIDNEY

These include fibromas, adenomas and mixed tumors. Most of these growths are small and asymptomatic but occasionally they enlarge to be palpable and may even cause pain and/or hematuria.

Adenoma of the kidney is a common enough finding at autopsy but is seldom of clinical dimension before the fourth decade, increasing in importance and incidence as the patient ages. I have urographically seen massive bilateral renal benign adenomas causing great parenchymal damage by compression. Yet this is most unusual, the important consideration being the grave likelihood of simple adenomas becoming cystadenoma, papillary cystadenoma, adenocarcinoma or papillary adenocarcinoma. The urograms suggest tumor but the precise diagnosis will be made at operation or at autopsy. Nephrectomy is the treatment. Resection of the tumor-bearing segment is allowable only when the growth is definitely proved benign.

Papillary cystadenoma which may become as large as a child's head is an uncircumscribed, encapsulated, cystic tumor mass not invading the kidney. Epithelial cells in the cyst wall are potentially neoplastogenic. Tubular structures believed to be of renal origin are sometimes found in these cysts.

Renal cystic tumors. These may assume several forms, most of which are benign but some may become malignant. *Congenital polycystic disease* is discussed in Chapter 6.

Solitary cyst may be congenital (q.v.) but, as experimentally shown by Hepler, commonly results from tubular obstruction and vascular occlusion, conditions frequent enough in adults in whom the lesion is most often seen between the ages of thirty and fifty years. These cysts may contain as little as 10 cc. or as much as 6 liters of clear serous fluid of specific gravity 1.002 to 1.010. In half of the cases the cysts are located at the lower pole and may be readily palpable (Fig. 66); a third are at the upper pole and the others are in the renal midsection. Hyalin, cartilage and bone have been found in the dense cyst wall which may become calcified and radiologically show a clear ring (Fig. 67). At operation the cyst wall is trimmed away to preserve the sound parenchyma of the kidney.

A few instances have been observed of *cystic encapsulated endometrial* tissues in the kidney with no bleeding coincident with menstruation. A palpable mass and pain in the kidney region were the symptoms.

Renal hamartoma is an extremely rare nonmalignant tumor, nonencapsulated, buried in the kidney and containing blood vessels, muscle and fat. It differs from teratoma in the absence of hair, nerve tissue and squamous cells. Hamartomas are believed to originate in a fetal nest of cloacal tissue. They may cause pain in the renal area and microscopic blood in the urine, and on pyelography show a localized pelvic filling defect. If symptoms warrant, nephrectomy is the treatment. Most hamartomas surgically removed have been preoperatively diagnosed as malignant neoplasm.

Malignant Tumors of the Kidney

These are all varieties of cancer, the biologic gravity and prognosis of which will largely depend upon the cellular structure. Yet the clinical picture, symptoms, diagnosis and treatment by nephrectomy are essentially the same in each of the different types: hypernephroma, adenocarcinoma, alveolar carcinoma and embryonic carcinoma including Wilms' tumors (nephroma).

Hypernephromas were so designated by Grawitz (1883) because of their similar appearance to that of the adrenal cortex; he believed them to be adrenal tumors developing in adrenal rests or remnants in the cortex or capsule of the kidney. This notion is not universally accepted, but assay of these hypernephroid growths has shown a cortin content comparable to that of the normal adrenal cortex and which, together with constitutional symptoms, skin pigmentation, and changes in the blood volume often seen with these tumors, lends some support to Grawitz' theory.

Hypernephromas comprise a fourth of all malignant renal tumors. They occur chiefly between the ages of forty-five and sixty, are most rare in children, and are of about equal incidence in each sex and on each side.

Pathology. At first these tumors are localized, firm, rounded and encapsulated, and appear most often at the upper pole. As they grow they usually develop soft spots due to intratumoral hemorrhage or necrosis and the cut surface is adrenal cortex yellow with cystic and hemorrhagic areas, the tumor capsule remaining intact for a long time in slow growing

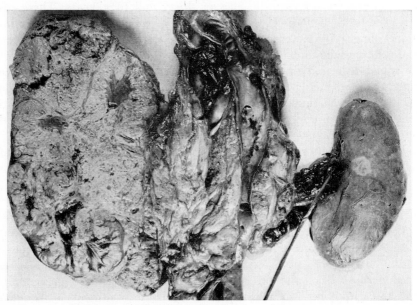

Figure 246.   Hypernephroma removed from a fifty-year-old man. Invasion of the vena cava.

tumors and may even calcify (Fig. 246). I remember two of these tumors at Bellevue Hospital that had to be opened with a saw. *Metastasis* is by (1) blood stream, (2) lymphatics, and (3) direct extension with preference for the lungs and long bones, but no part of the body is exempt; in one patient metastasis to the vagina occurred (Fig. 248). The venous emboli in the lungs give rise to clear-cut, round lesions, roentgenographically designated as "cotton ball" or "cannon ball" (Fig. 253). Unfortunately metastatic lesions may not be apparent for ten to twenty years and may appear locally in the wound scar or elsewhere.

The *microscopic picture* is predominantly that of large cylindrical or cubical cells with clear or slightly granular cytoplasm and resembles cells of the adrenal cortex except for the greater transparency of the tumor cells (Fig. 247). Usually the cells are arranged in cords or sheets but tubular or alveolar patterns are frequent and may cause the diagnosis of adenocarcinoma to be made (q.v.). Yet this tubular arrangement of clear cells in hypernephroma is not seen in the adrenal cortex nor in adrenal cortical tumors, and hypernephroma does not cause sexual disturbances such as virilism. The basement membranes and vascular walls are delicate; intratumoral hemorrhage and necrosis are frequent in highly active tumors when the vascular growth cannot keep up with the tumor-cell extension.

Symptoms. These depend largely upon the rate of tumor growth which may be slow. When rapid, pelvic invasion with hematuria occurs

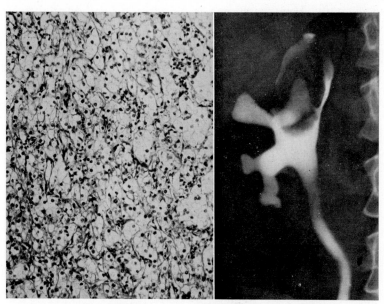

Fig. 247   Fig. 248

FIGURE 247. Hypernephroma histology. The large clear cells commonly simulate those of the adrenal cortex. (Courtesy of Armed Forces Institute of Pathology.)

FIGURE 248. Right hypernephroma in a seventy-year-old woman with vaginal metastases. Note compression and displacement of superior and upper middle calyces.

(75% of the cases). Dull or sharp pain results from capsular distention by the tumor enlargement or ureteral colic may be caused by the passage of clots. Fever occurs in over half of these patients. Symptoms due to metastatic lesions in the lung, brain or bones, in particular, may be much more distressing than the renal lesion.

Diagnosis. In the pyelogram the kidney is enlarged and elongation of the calyces in "spider leg" formation is frequent (Figs. 243*A*, 248, 249).

Treatment. This is by nephrectomy except when metastases are demonstrable. Pulmonary metastases have disappeared in several instances following nephrectomy. Radiation therapy is useless. The average cure rate is not over 10 per cent.

Tuberous Sclerosis. This designates a peculiar and extremely rare clinical triad of hypernephroma, adenoma sebaceum, and tuberous sclerosis of the brain. It is seldom seen after twenty years of age. There are small cutaneous, pinhead size, pointed, yellow-white adenoma-like nodules (adenoma sebaceum), called *epiloia*, and originating in the sebaceous glands. These lesions appear on the face, nose, labionasal folds, cheeks and forehead, and similar nodules may be present in the heart, retina and kidneys.

The nodules in the brain are of smooth grayish-white, hypertrophic glial tissue 2 to 8 mm. in diameter, cover the cerebral cortex and extend downward into the gray matter (tuberous sclerosis). The remainder of the brain is normal but the patient is an idiot, imbecile, or greatly retarded mentally. Hypernephroma is found in nearly all of these cases,

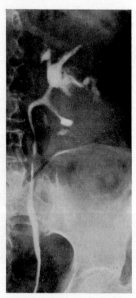

FIGURE 249.   Hypernephroma in a fifty-six-year-old man causing a large filling defect with compression and elongation of the right upper and middle calyces. Nephrectomy with apparent cure ten years later.

yet Mostofi (personal communication) states that in his experience at the American Armed Forces Institute of Pathology, the tuberous sclerosis complex is much more frequently associated with renal hamartoma than with renal carcinoma (hypernephroma). Convulsions and paralysis appear soon after birth with or without muscular contractions. The patient usually dies in early adult life; removal of the renal tumor does no good.

Adenocarcinoma. A third of renal neoplasms are of this type, arising apparently from primarily benign adenoma (q.v.). About two thirds of these tumors occur in males and at any time after twenty years of age, most appearing between fifty and sixty years. These lesions begin as lobulated, hard, cystic masses, vascular, and soon breaking through their capsules to cause hematuria as a prominent symptom. The large vacuolated polyhedral cells of the tumor are often arranged in clear sheets, or in tubular or papillary structure (Fig. 250). *Metastasis* is by the blood stream, lymphatics or direct extension; vascular spread to the skeleton is frequent and especially spinal (osteolytic). Usually the kidney does not become as large as it does in hypernephroma but feels much harder and more solid, and the pyelogram shows pelvic compression without great elongation or "spider leg" formation. The clinical course tends to be rapid with metastasis so that the outlook even after nephrectomy is always grave.

Alveolar Carcinoma. These extremely malignant, highly invasive growths comprise 10 to 15 per cent of renal neoplasms, are made up of rapidly growing tubular structures similar to adult renal parenchyma and, despite nephrectomy, most patients are dead within two years, predominantly from metastases.

Renal Embryoma (embryonal adenomyosarcoma, Wilms' tumor, nephroma, congenital mixed renal tumor). This is the commonest renal tumor of infancy and childhood, comprises 20 per cent of all childhood new growths, has been seen in the fetus and, rarely, in later life up to seventy-five years. Three fourths of these tumors appear before the age

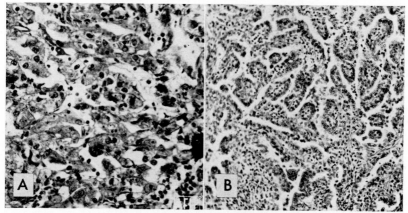

FIGURE 250. Adenocarcinoma of the kidney. (Courtesy Armed Forces Institute of Pathology.)

of five and two thirds before the third year. There is no predilection for right or left side and, in common with other congenital lesions, in paired organs such as the testes, ovaries and eyes, renal embryomas are bilateral in 6 to 8 per cent cent of the cases.

There are many theories of the embryologic origin of these tumors, each notion differing according to the hypothecated time and nature of origin and localization of the anlage of the growths (Ribbert, Busse, Muus, Wilms, Dean and Pack, Geschickter and Widenhorn).

Pathology. Because of its heterogenous histology a wide variety of designations (more than fifty) have been applied to this neoplasm: embryonal sarcoma, adenosarcoma, myxosarcoma, chondromyosarcoma, rhabdomyosarcoma, liposarcoma and others. Because it contains all the elements of the kidney, Deming believes the designation nephroma should be used.

Wilms' tumor enlarges rapidly, sometimes equalling the usual body weight of the child of the age. The tumor surface becomes lobulated or nodular and as tumor growth outruns vascular extension, central necrosis and intratumoral hemorrhage are common, adding softness and fluctuancy to the neoplasm. With tumor enlargement, neighboring viscera are compressed with resulting gastrointestinal disturbances, nutritional failure, constipation or obstipation. Characteristically and in counter distinction to adrenal neuroblastoma which commonly grows backward into the ileocostal space, nephroma growth is forward or lateral and may cause

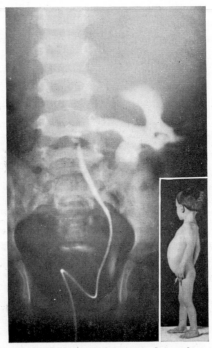

FIGURE 251. Renal embryoma. Pyelogram showing pelvic enlargement, compression and displacement. *Insert:* Pot belly of the patient and his attitude of standing or walking.

abdominal protuberance or "pot belly" (Fig. 251). The tumor-bearing kidney is frequently anomalous—horseshoe, polycystic, solitary or reduplicated.

On gross section these mesodermal tumors present a soft grumous, gelatinous, semi-translucent, edematous tissue of brainlike consistency, gray, grayish-pink or grayish-white or with yellow areas, often with spots of hemorrhage or necrosis (Fig. 252). As a rule fibrous tissue is comparatively scant. There is no true capsule which suggests the fetal displacement of tumor anlagen. The growth spreads chiefly by the blood stream to the liver, lungs, spleen, spine, intestines, diaphragm, scapula, ilium, or skull but may also disseminate by the lymphatics or by direct extension (Fig. 253). No organ in the body is exempt from metastatic invasion in nephroma including even the penile corpora cavernosa. When metastasis exists, the retroperitoneal lymphatics are almost always invaded as well. The metastases are usually composed of round tumor cells but may be as complex as the original growth.

Microscopically these tumors show undifferentiated or partially differentiated epithelium and round cells, often with epithelial tubular and glomeruli-like structure (Fig. 254,*A*), smooth and striated muscle (Fig. 254,*B*), cartilage and connective tissue. The capillaries are most delicate and rupture easily to produce massive intratumoral hemorrhage (Fig. 252). Nephroma must be differentiated from true sarcoma, teratoma, hypernephroma and the neurogenic neoplasms: neuroblastoma, sympathicoblastoma, ganglioma, paraganglioma and schwannoma.

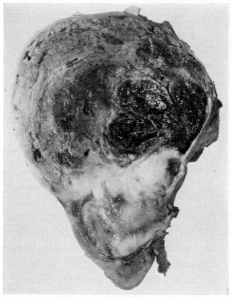

FIGURE 252. Renal embryoma (Wilms' tumor). Specimen showing massive intratumoral hemorrhage. Hemorrhage into the neoplasm caused the sudden appearance of an enormous renal mass in the left loin of an eighteen-month-old boy. Nephrectomy. Death from tumor recurrence. Only a small rim of compressed parenchyma remains (lower pole).

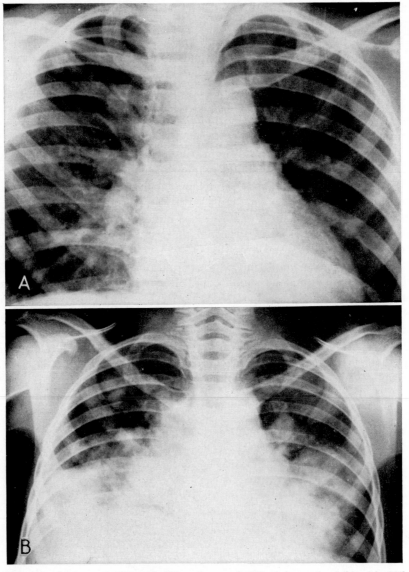

FIGURE 253.   Metastases ("cottonball" or "cannonball") to lungs in child with Wilms'
tumor. *A*, early; *B*, later.

Symptoms.   A mass in the loin is the usual initial manifestation of
Wilms' tumor and in two patients of mine, the child himself first noted
the growth. With tumor enlargement the abdomen may become enormous
and make walking difficult (Fig. 251). With increasing anemia, gastrointestinal compression, and nutritional failure, cachexia, petechiae, jaundice, and cardiac or respiratory embarrassment, the downhill course is
rapid. Pressure on the spermatic veins may produce *varicocele*. *Pain* may
be dull or sharp from renal capsular distention, or from drag or pull of
the tumor mass on the renal pedicle, or colicky with the passage of clots

or tumor debris. *Hematuria* occurs only when the tumor has penetrated into the pelvis and is usually a late symptom. *Fever* occurs in half of the cases and in three fourths there is *hypertension*, these two symptoms being prognostically most grave.

Diagnosis. This is suggested by finding a mass in the renal area and is confirmed by pyelography. *Palpation should be ever so gentle to avoid spreading tumor cells into the circulation.* The renal surface generally feels smooth and at first the kidney is movable, but in the late stages may be nodular, soft and fixed. Although hydronephrosis is the commonest abdominal tumor of childhood, the urogram should at once make the differential diagnosis. Here as with all solid abdominal tumors of childhood, the growth should be considered malignant until proved otherwise.

The Papanicolaou stain of the urine sediment may be positive especially when there has been hematuria.

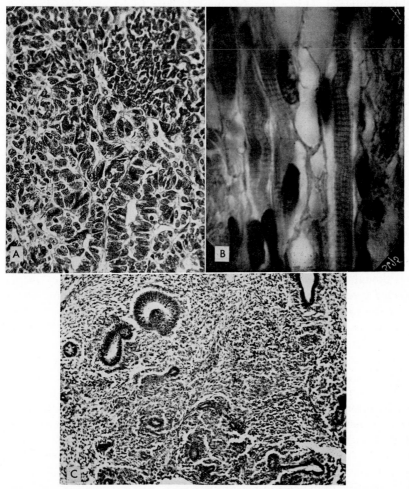

FIGURE 254. Renal embryoma. *A*, spindle-cell type of growth commonly seen. *B*, striated muscle in renal embryoma. *C*, development of renal tubular structure suggestive of earlier fetal life.

Excretory urography will usually demonstrate the tumor and, equally important, the function and status of the renal mate. The possibility of bilateral Wilms' tumor must not be overlooked; the excretory urographic diagnosis had best be confirmed by retrograde pyelography. There is no "characteristic" urogram; in early cases only one segment of the renal pelvis may show compression changes or the whole pelvis may be obliterated and displaced (Fig. 251).

Differential Diagnosis. The rapid growth of Wilms' tumor suggests a highly malignant neoplasm. Yet other conditions may simulate embryoma and must be considered: (1) hydronephrosis is likely to be softer than tumor; (2) polycystic disease is nearly always bilateral and shows "nephritic" changes in the urine and blood chemistry; (3) neurogenic tumors, especially neuroblastoma, tend to extend backwards and be palpable behind and are likely to cause striking renal displacement especially downward. Other less frequent lesions to be considered are (4) adrenal cortical tumors in children which are commonly manifested by sexual changes; (5) pancreatic and hepatic tumors and cysts; (6) retroperitoneal cysts, lymph gland tumors, Hodgkin's disease, perirenal hydronephrosis, perirenal tumor; (7) ovarian tumors, usually bilateral; (8) renal tuberculosis, (9) fecal masses, and even (10) renal or perirenal abscess. In all of these conditions the pyelogram including lateral exposures may be expected to make the differential diagnosis but in rare instances it will be accurately made only at the operating table.

Treatment. This should be by nephrectomy as soon as (1) the diagnosis is made, (2) the child is preoperatively prepared by blood and fluids as needed, and (3) when metastases do not contraindicate. Small tumors may be removed through a loin incision but in general the transabdominal approach is preferred. The transthoracic approach should seldom be necessary in the young.

RADIATION THERAPY. Following nephrectomy, employ immediate roentgen therapy to the operative region, especially the pedicle area, and, when thought needed, to the chest fields. *The remaining kidney must be protected against radiation injury.* Radiation treatment is begun the same day or the next day after operation and continued for a total of 3,000 to 4,500 r units given through anterior, lateral and posterior-anterior portals. Postoperative blood counts, physical examination and repeated chest x-ray studies are required in order to be alert to the child's progress or regression, or for signs of recurrence. If the tumor is to recur, it will usually do so within four to six months and if the patient is apparently tumor free one year after operation, his chance of being cured corresponds to the five year cure period of cancer in adults. The 95 per cent mortality from Wilms' tumor as of forty years ago has been now reduced to about 70 per cent; in infants under one year a cure rate as high as 80 per cent has been achieved by Gross. Neither the smallness of a tumor nor its histology greatly influence the prognosis.

Renal Sarcoma. True sarcoma of the kidney, its capsule or pelvis is most rare, and occurs chiefly in infants or young children but occasionally also in adults and should not be confused with Wilms' tumor, neurogenic or mixed new growths. Renal sarcomas are rapidly growing, highly invasive, metastasize early and widely, and cause a palpable tumor, pain and hematuria. The diagnosis of renal tumor is made by pyelography. Nephrectomy offers the only hope of cure but at least half of these patients will die within two years postoperatively despite intensive irradiation as used in the treatment of Wilms' tumor.

For continuity of presentation, the neurogenic tumors of the adrenal and sympathetic system originating about the kidney are considered in Chapter 13.

Schwannomas are benign, slow growing, excessively rare tumors derived from the nerve sheath of Schwann (Deming).

Vascular renal tumors may be (1) benign, (angioma, hemangioma, telangioma, varix), or (2) malignant (hemangiosarcoma and hemangioblastoma). They are rare, predominantly unilateral, occur at all ages and equally on right and left sides, and in both sexes. They may cause profuse bleeding over many years, according to how long the patient lives and how soon the involved kidney is removed. The pyelogram generally indicates a lesion localized to one major calyx or portion of the pelvis. Nephrectomy rather than renal resection is the treatment.

Tumors of the Renal Capsule

These rare lesions show great variety, lipoma or fibrolipoma being the commonest; myxoma, chondroma, sarcoma, fibrosarcoma and angiosarcoma also occur. They develop chiefly in the female and especially in conjunction with uterine tumors. In general the clinical manifestations reflect the degree of tumor malignancy, some growing rapidly and killing early. The prognosis rests upon the type and extent of growth of the tumor. Treatment is nephrectomy including wide removal of the perirenal fat. Radiation is useless.

Tumors of the Renal Pelvis and Ureter

These comparatively rare growths are chiefly benign papilloma (15%), papillary carcinoma (35 to 40 per cent, Fig. 255), or squamous cell cancer (10%). A few cases of epithelial ureteral tumor have been reported in children as well as mixed cell growths, both benign and malignant. Yet carcinoma of one type or another (papillary squamous, medullary, transitional, epidermoid), comprise nearly three fourths of the primary tumors of the pelvis and ureter (Figs. 256, 257, 258). Neoplasm originating elsewhere may involve the pelvis or ureter by direct extension, by blood stream or by lymphatic metastasis.

The primary cause of these tumors is unknown; conceivably the same factors operate as in the genesis of vesical cancer, namely (1) chronic irritation from infection or the presence of a stone which causes hyperplasia or metaplastic changes in the duct wall, or changes in cell inclusions of inflammatory origin (*vide* pyelitis, ureteritis, cystitis cystica, glandularis or granularis), (2) malignant change in a leukoplakia lesion,

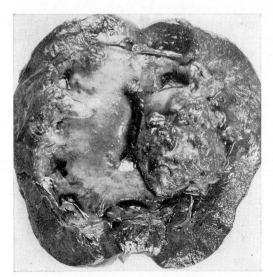

FIGURE 255.   Papillary carcinoma of the renal pelvis.

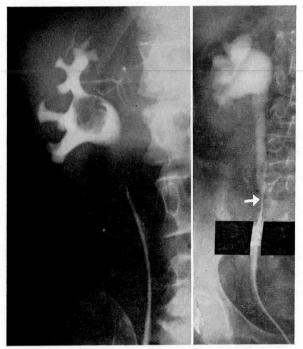

Fig. 256   Fig. 257

FIGURE 256.   Papillary carcinoma of the renal pelvis. Pyelogram showing large filling defect caused by the tumor, also pyelolymphatic backflow which, conceivably, could be
a mode of tumor spread.

FIGURE 257.   Annular carcinoma of the ureter but without complete obstruction.
Metastasis.

or (3) stimulation by an unrecognized carcinogenic agent. Two thirds of these patients are males. More than half of the lesions—both benign and malignant—originate in the lower third of the ureter and more often on the right side. Metastases occur in a third of the cases.

The *symptoms* are those of ureteral or ureteropelvic obstruction, chiefly pain (60%) and hematuria (75%). A papillary pelvic tumor may progress downward to the ureter and bladder, and a ureteral growth may extend upwards to the renal pelvis or both ways. In more than a third of the cases, the ureteral tumor becomes palpable. The *diagnosis* is made by stereoscopic ureteropyelography which shows a tumor filling defect of the pelvis, ureter or both and often proximal dilatation (Figs. 256–258). The Papanicolaou urine stain may be positive for tumor cells but is not reliable as a negative finding. Nephro-ureterectomy with removal of a cuff of bladder wall about and including the ureteral orifice is the treatment and, if done early enough, is curative.

TUMORS ABOUT THE KIDNEY

These growths may simulate renal neoplasms, displace the organ, or cause grave compression or obstruction of the bowels and squeeze other abdominal viscera. When malignant, they are usually fatal. They may be solid benign, cystic or malignant.

Benign Tumors. These perirenal tumors are largely lipomas, fibromas, fibrolipomas, myomas, adenomas, myxomatous or chondro-

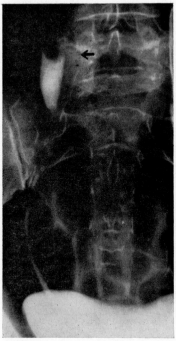

FIGURE 258. Papillary carcinoma of ureter with large round ureterographic filling defect caused by the growth. Ureteronephrectomy. Metastasis.

matous growths of embryonal origin from the neurogenic folds, wolffian remnants, mesonephric (Fig. 259) or urogenital ridges. They may cause local pain, renal compression, dislodgment and/or rotation. *Diagnosis* is made by stereoscopic pyelography including lateral or oblique exposures. *Treatment* is removal of the tumor-bearing area. Yet in the sarcomatous and other highly malignant connective tissue neoplasia the prognosis is generally hopeless.

Perirenal Cysts. These are usually urinous (factitious) and follow traumatic extravasation from the ureter or pelvis or they may develop at the site of a hematoma. True perirenal cysts originate in aberrant mesodermal anlagen (wolffian or müllerian ducts, lymphatic system) and may be single, multiple, multilocular or loculated cystadenomatoma, small or large (100 gm.), and generally unilateral. They have been seen more often in females and on the left side (Fig. 259). These may be urographically simulated by a large aortic aneurysm (Fig. 260). *Mesenteric cysts* form below the kidney. Retroperitoneal parasitic and nonparasitic as well as dermoid cysts (cf. Fig. 259) may simulate renal tumor and cause displacement of the kidney and intraperitoneal compression. The pyelograms, including lateral exposures, will indicate the extrarenal location of the mass; its true nature will be found at exploration. Removal of the benign tumor is curative but, when malignant, the prognosis is always grave. To avoid possible surgical shock of rapid abdominal decompression

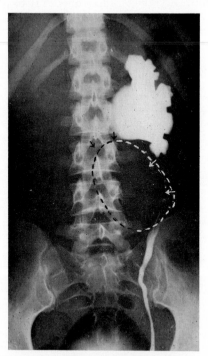

FIGURE 259.   Mesonephric cyst causing hydronephrosis by ureteral blockage in a thirty-year-old woman. Cyst excision with disappearance of hydronephrosis.

upon removal of an enormous cyst, it is generally best to drain the cyst first, with subsequent excision when the patient is surgically stabilized.

Perirenal hydronephrosis (renal hygroma or hydrocele renis) is an unusual cystic envelopment of the kidney in which the capsule forms the parietal cyst wall. By anatomic analogy it has been compared to the testicle within the tunica vaginalis. Perirenal hydronephrosis is practically always unilateral and simulates renal tumor. Its cause is unknown but in the young it is believed to be congenital from nephrogenic anlagen. The cyst fluid is lymphatic exudate and not urine and its presence may be predisposed to by trauma or infection. Large tumors compress and displace the kidney and the intestinal contents as well to cause constipation or more severe bowel obstruction with gastrointestinal disturbances, vomiting and malnutrition. Pain may suggest cholecystitis, ovarian tumor or ureteral colic. On palpation the tumor mass is firm and tense; urography shows pelvic and ureteral dislocation, although the diagnosis of malignant renal tumor is likely to be made. Removal of the cyst, preferably by a two-step procedure when the mass is large (first drainage and decompression with excision later), is the treatment. The prognosis is good.

Malignant Perirenal Teratomas. These growths are derived from totipotent cells originating in the embryonal germinal ridge and give rise to tridermal structure (all germ layers) in the same tumor—skin, teeth, bone, hair, testicle, ovary, liver, pancreas, brain and others. They

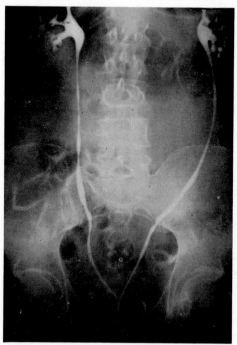

FIGURE 260.   Aortic aneurysm with calcified walls causing abdominal mass and, by compression, ureteral colic. Subsequent fatal rupture.

grow slowly, cause pain, metastasize chiefly to the chest, may compress the intestines or obstruct the upper ureter and induce hydronephrosis. The presence of peculiar calcific shadows (teeth, bone, etc.) in the perirenal area in the plain urogram suggests the diagnosis. The perirenal nature of the tumor as well as its compressing and/or dislocating effect on the kidney is easily demonstrable by stereoscopic pyelography in which lateral or oblique exposures should also be made. The treatment is excision. A six-month-old boy I operated upon for perirenal teratoma twenty-five years ago was well fifteen years later.

Congenital Mixed Tumors of the Kidney. These growths which are situated adjacent to but are not connected with the kidney are derived from renal anlagen, simulate true renal neoplasm, may metastasize, and are treated by excision. Some are biologically benign but many are sarcomatous (fibrosarcoma, liposarcoma or lymphosarcoma), or lymphoblastomas (Hodgkin's), or may simulate neuroblastoma. Excision is the treatment but the prognosis is always grave.

Secondary Renal Tumors. These are largely the acute lymphatic, leukemic or myeloid variety with massive lymphocytic or myelocytic infiltration of the interstitial spaces of the organ. This produces pronounced enlargement, sometimes to three or four times normal size with comparable compression of the pelvis. It occurs in leukemia, lymphosarcoma, lymphoblastoma, is characteristically found in early life and with extensive involvement of all lymph nodes, some of which may compress the ureter or pelvic outlet to cause hydronephrosis. The urine may be normal, show red blood cells or suggest nephritis. The pyelogram shows pronounced pelvic compression, perhaps almost obliteration, and the blood studies suggest the cause. Metastatic thymoma or other dispersed tumors may also involve the kidney. Treatment is ineffective and the prognosis is hopeless.

Tumors of the ureter have been previously discussed in this chapter together with tumors of the kidney pelvis.

TUMORS OF THE BLADDER

These are the most frequent and important malignant tumors of the urinary tract (considering prostatic carcinoma a genital tract lesion) in patients over sixty years of age and account for 3 per cent of all deaths from all types of malignant disease. Vesical tumors attack twice as many males as females and three fourths of those dying with the disease are between sixty-five and eighty-five years of age.

The cause of bladder cancer is unknown. Chronic irritation and inflammation have usually been present for some time before the growth became apparent. Infravesical obstruction, chiefly at the bladder neck, has persisted for years in many of the cases, sometimes with an irritant bladder stone present (cf. tumors of ureter and renal pelvis). Experimentally bladder carcinoma is easily produced by the administration of the coal-tar derivative beta-naphthylamine, and it is probable other unknown or unrecognized carcinogens are inhaled, imbibed, or ingested and become urine-borne irritative agents. Vesical carcinoma is said to develop in 4 per cent of patients with bilharziosis (schistosomiasis); here there is long-continued irritation by the extrusion of ova or worms through the bladder wall.

Pathology. Nearly all bladder tumors are epithelial and occur chiefly in adults; a few mesodermal growths (myxoma, myoma, rhabdoma, dermoid) and various forms of sarcomas have been reported, predominantly in infants and children (Fig. 268). The *malignancy* of bladder tumors is evaluated on their rate of growth and invasiveness. *Prognosis* is based upon (1) the extent of the invasion, whether into or through the bladder muscle wall, (2) the character of the surgical treatment—whether by local coagulation, segmental resection with or without the surrounding tissues and overlying peritoneum, and (3) the comparative degree of

Fig. 261   Fig. 262

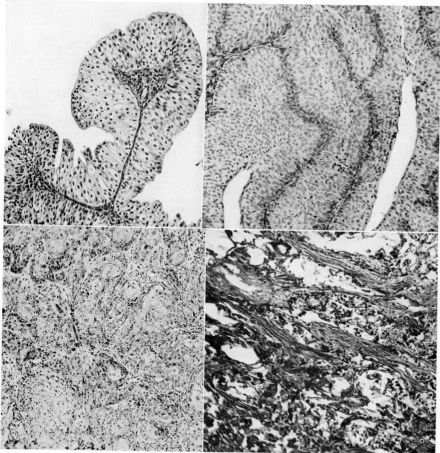

Fig. 263   Fig. 264

FIGURE 261.   Nonpenetrating polyp of the bladder. There is no invasiveness; the basement membrane remains intact.

FIGURE 262.   Papillary carcinoma of the bladder with tumor invasiveness.

FIGURE 263.   Epidermoid carcinoma of the bladder.

FIGURE 264.   Adenocarcinoma of the bladder.

(Courtesy Armed Forces Institute of Pathology.)

differentiation of the bladder cells. Thus, in *"noninfiltrating"* growths, the tumor cells have not penetrated the basement membrane on which they lie (Fig. 261); these comprise a third of the tumors of the Bladder Tumor Registry of the Armed Forces Institute of Pathology. In *infiltrating tumors* on the contrary, the malignant cells have broken through the basement membrane and have entered the submucosal muscle or deeper structures (Figs. 262–264).

Classification of Malignancy. In 1922 Broders introduced gradation of tumor malignancy on the basis of cell structure differentiation. The least malignant (Grade I) carcinoma is composed of well differentiated epithelial cells, that is, they are fully matured. The *criteria of cell differentiation in malignancy* are: (1) variation in size and development of cells (anaplasia) and nuclei (polynucleosis, abnormal size, shape and staining); (2) the number and abnormality of mitotic figures, (3) the nuclear chromatin content (hyperchromatosis), and (4) the disordered arrangement of the cell structure.

The most malignant cells, Grade IV, show complete anaplasia (immaturity or undifferentiation). Grades II and III are intermediate in anaplasia. The Armed Forces Institute of Pathology tumor gradation (since 1951) which is accepted by the American Urological Association has been found generally accurate for prognosis (Mostofi):

    I. Papilloma—if epithelium is indistinguishable from normal bladder.
    II. Papillary carcinoma I, II, and III depending on histology alone.
    III. Papillary and infiltrating grades II and III.
    IV. Infiltrating grades II and III.
    V. Squamous carcinoma.
    VI. Adenocarcinoma—almost all are mucus producing.

NONINFILTRATING TUMORS

Benign papilloma rated Grade I by the Armed Forces Institute of Pathology is the least serious of bladder tumors, the epithelial cells of which resemble the normal bladder epithelium (Fig. 261). Many histologically benign tumors by persistent recurrence are clinically malignant. These tumors may also become histologically malignant. Most benign papillomas cause no symptoms or are accidentally discovered and are cystoscopically destroyed by electrocoagulation. Other benign tumors, but which are extremely rare, include fibroma and myxoma.

Carcinoma in situ or pre-invasive carcinoma shows some degree of epithelial cell anaplasia. This term is used to denote cases in which there may be more than one layer of surface epithelium which shows malignant change without much papillation and without invasion.

INFILTRATING TUMORS

Whether a bladder tumor is papillary or sessile (flat), the presence of malignant cells in the pedicle or bladder wall or both stamps it as an infiltrating neoplasm. Malignant bladder tumors may be grouped as:

I. Epithelial
  1. Papillary carcinoma
  2. Epidermoid carcinoma
  3. Adenocarcinoma
  4. Mucous adenocarcinoma
  5. Undifferentiated

II. Nonepithelial
  1. Mesenchymal: leiomyosarcoma, rhabdomyosarcoma, myxosarcoma, and so forth.

III. Secondary tumors
  1. Metastatic
  2. Direct invasion

Papillary Carcinoma. This is a neoplastic progression from the malignant papilloma (q.v.), the growth being more solid, larger, firmer, and fixed. There may be ulceration owing to neoplastic interference with the blood supply of the tumor and sometimes calcific deposits are found on the surface of the growth. The bladder wall surrounding the tumor base is reddened and granular, and may or may not be edematous. As the growth extends, ulceration progresses, and commonly with heavy phosphatic encrustation. In the late stages a fungating, bleeding, ulcerated and crusted, angry-looking growth increases its base diameter and variably projects filling-wise into the bladder cavity.

Microscopically, the papillary pattern is found to persist, a central blood vessel being surrounded by strands and layers of malignant epithelial cells which may fuse with adjacent papillae (Fig. 262). As the tumor grows and infiltrates the muscle wall, the papillary structure may largely disappear, the picture becoming that of a broad base, ulcerated, sessile, infiltrating neoplasm, or one producing an intravesical space-filling lesion, or an ulcerative excavation.

Epidermoid (skin-like) carcinoma may originate in a papillomatous carcinoma, in a leukoplakia, or from bladder mucosa. It may appear flat, lumpy, sessile, or as a granular patch, later to undergo necrosis and calcific deposit. The bladder wall at this stage is deeply invaded. The microscopic pattern is that common to squamous epithelioma elsewhere with epithelial pearls of keratin and large sheets of sharply defined polygonal epithelial cells (Fig. 263).

Undifferentiated carcinoma is so designated because of the extreme anaplasia or immaturity of its cells and their irregular arrangement with cells well separated from one another; it may be pedunculated or non-pedunculated, the most malignant cells being found in the mural invading portion of the growth.

Adenocarcinoma is a rare deeply infiltrating, sessile, ulcerating vesical neoplasm; it may protrude into the bladder cavity. The histologic picture with its acinar formation strongly resembles that of prostatic carcinoma (Fig. 264).

Mucous adenocarcinoma of the bladder is an extremely rare, firm, sessile and deeply infiltrating tumor. Histologically it shows acinar formation, lined by mucus-secreting columnar epithelium, sometimes presenting in papillary formations, but in any case resembling the mucoid carcinoma of the stomach and intestines from which these neoplasms may appear to be metastatic but are not. They probably arise in urachal or intestinal tissue remnants in the bladder rather than from cystitis glandularis (q.v.) produced by the irritation of chronic inflammation. This is seen particularly in the long-irritated bladder wall in vesical exstrophy.

Metastasis in bladder cancer occurs to the regional nodes in about two thirds of the cases, to the liver in a half, to the lungs in a third, to the spine and pelvis in a fifth, and to other sites alone in less than 10 per cent. The curability of vesical carcinoma depends primarily on the degree of bladder wall infiltration as well as the presence of metastases. Jewett's studies show that the likelihood of metastasis increases and the therapeutic prognosis rapidly depreciates as invasion of the musculature (detrusor) occurs and proportionately to the depth of the invasion. This is well shown in Figure 265.

Mesodermal Tumors. Vesical neoplasms of mesodermal origin usually arise in bladder tissue normally present but may be atherotopic from abnormally present tissue. The *benign growths* are chiefly fibroma, lipoma, myxoma, leiomyoma, hemangioma, or heterotopic growths such as teratoma, dermoid, chondroma and rhabdomyoma. Their removal is curative. Yet *at least* half of the mesodermal tumors are sarcomatous, are seen chiefly in young children, grow rapidly in sessile, polypoid or papillary formation, invade deeply, and metastasize early. They usually obstruct the bladder outlet as in four of my cases, and even with early cystectomy and ureterosigmoidostomy or bilateral cutaneous ureterostomy, the outlook is almost always hopeless.

Metastatic and Other Secondary Tumors of the Bladder. These may be metastatic from distant neoplasms but generally the secondary involvement is by direct extension from an adjacent malignancy in the intestines, rectum, prostate, ovary, uterus, retrovesical areas and/or by downward spread from a new growth in the renal pelvis or ureter. Since the outlook is almost always hopeless, one can only try to relieve pain and make the patient more comfortable; this may mean indwelling catheterization or permanent cystostomy.

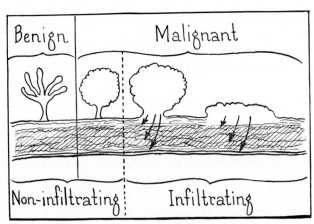

Figure 265.   Schema of bladder tumors indicating the progressive degrees of invasiveness (Jewett).

Tumors of the urachus are rare, appear and behave much as do bladder tumors, tend to become mucus-forming growths (adenocarcinoma), and metastasize early, chiefly to the abdomen and liver.

Endometriosis of the bladder may reach this destination (1) by transurethral transplantation (instruments, etc., Sampson), (2) through the lymphatics, or (3) through the bladder wall itself. It appears as a dark cystic, somewhat bluish, and elevated mass. Aggravation of symptoms as well as urinary frequency and vesical irritation is "monthly" recurrent with menstruation although there may be no hematuria. Castration (bilateral oophorectomy) cures.

Symptoms. *Hematuria* is the earliest symptom in over three fourths of bladder tumors and can be anticipated in every case. It may be *initial* at the beginning of urination or *terminal* at the end, diffuse during entire urination and may stain the clothing. With new growth at or about the vesical outlet, terminal hematuria may be produced as the tumor is squeezed by the final emptying contraction of the bladder wall. Hematuria offers no clue as to the size, location or degree of malignancy of the cancer.

Vesical irritability is a prominent symptom in one third of the cases with frequency, dysuria, burning, urgency and usually pyuria. The tumor may block the bladder outlet to cause obstruction, complete or partial. Pain appears late, locally in or about the bladder area, or distant as in the legs and thighs. With secondary vascular obstruction by tumor, leg edema appears; later there is urinary toxemia, sepsis, and terminal uremia.

Diagnosis. The history may suggest the probable diagnosis, particularly in aniline-dye workers. In adults with pronounced hematuria there is at least a one in four chance that the patient has a bladder tumor. The Papanicolaou stain of the urine may disclose tumor cells. Cystoscopy establishes the diagnosis, however, and reveals the number of tumors, their location, size, general type (papillary or infiltrating, ulcerating or nonulcerating, and so forth), their relation to the ureteral orifices or the bladder outlet, the probable best treatment and the likely prognosis. The cystoscopic picture has been suggested under Pathology. Examination of a specimen taken by cystoscopic biopsy will disclose the type of tumor although several histologic pictures are often found in the same growth. For this reason, one or two biopsy specimens are taken from the periphery of the tumor and one or two from the depth of the growth, including muscle if possible. These specimens should each be separately identified as to their source for the microscopic study.

By *rectal examination* a well-developed infiltrating tumor of the bladder base may be palpated as an indurated, thickened mass, a finding which warrants a hopeless prognosis. Bimanual rectal examination under anesthesia (sodium pentothal intravenously together with curare intramuscularly for abdominal relaxation) will enable the examiner to palpate the prostate, seminal vesicles, bladder floor, lateral pelvic walls, posterior wall, and especially the inferior lateral vesical ligaments extending posteriorly on each side of the rectum. Induration of these ligaments denotes extravesical tumor extension (Fig. 266). For this examination the bladder must be empty of urine. A vesical stone, Foley bag balloon, nonmalignant bladder wall infiltration and induration and thickening may confuse as may adjacent masses such as carcinoma of the colon, ovary or cervix.

Excretory urography will usually indicate the status of the upper urinary tract and cystographically show the bladder wall irregularity, a filling defect caused by tumor, ulceration of the lesion, or the flat fixation of an infiltrating ulcerating growth (Figs. 267, 268). Stereoscopic anterior, posterior and lateral urograms should be made.

Treatment. NONINFILTRATING TUMORS. Benign or malignant papilloma may be destroyed by electrocoagulation, radon seed implantation, or excision by transurethral resection (Fig. 269). Follow-up examination every three months for at least a year is imperative, and thereafter at progressively lengthening intervals for at least five years should there be no apparent recurrence.

Multiple papillomas (papillomatosis) variably respond to the treatment outlined in the preceding paragraph but eventually the tumor may be expected to get the upper hand and here cystectomy with ureterosigmoidostomy is nearly always required.

INFILTRATING TUMORS. (1) Known extravesical spread of the cancer, (2) advanced renal damage by infection or hydronephrosis, or (3) other grave complicating disease such as cardiorenal or neurologic disease

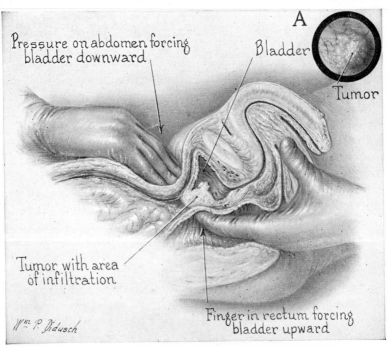

FIGURE 266. Bimanual recto-abdominal examination of the anesthetized patient to determine presence and nature of extravesical spread of known bladder tumor (Jewett).

is a contraindication to radical treatment of infiltrating bladder cancer; palliative therapy must be employed if no more than permanent cystostomy. When conditions and prospects are favorable, however, the tumor should be promptly and vigorously attacked. External radiation, even when massively applied through the open bladder, has been disappointing. Electrocoagulation through the open bladder will cure only when the tumor is relatively superficial, and in large infiltrating tumors must be considered only a palliative measure.

Transurethral resection of small tumors of the trigone and bladder wall and transvesical electro-excision of less accessible tumors have enjoyed some enthusiasm and success, but it is decidedly an operation only for the most expert instrumenteur (Fig. 269) lest the patient suffer grave damage by bladder wall perforation, extravesical penetration, extravasation, peritonitis and sepsis. A great many unreported instances of peritonitis have resulted from perforation of the posterior wall bladder and peritoneum by the cutting electrode. It is a method fraught with great danger.

Bladder resection is one of the oldest urologic operations and is still the method of choice of most urologists when the tumor does not extend beyond the bladder; Jewett further limits this procedure to tumors infiltrating only half way through the musculature. When removal of the tumor compromises the ureter, the duct should be transplanted (ureteroneocystostomy or cutaneous ureterostomy). Yet the operation is ill advised when (1) the patient is a poor surgical risk, (2) the tumor spread is indefinite or wide, (3) a bladder too small for comfort will be left, or (4) there are multiple tumors covering a wide area, and (5) the growth involves the female trigone or bladder outlet. Yet I have seen some apparent cures following resection of externally infiltrating tumors in the upper half of the bladder but in which not only the bladder wall but

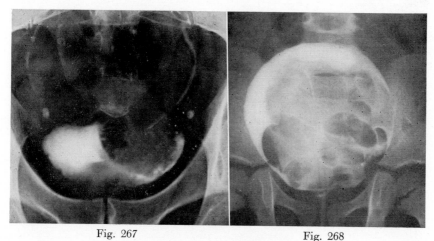

| Fig. 267 | Fig. 268 |

FIGURE 267.   Carcinoma of the bladder. Cystogram showing filling defect caused by tumor.
FIGURE 268.   Sarcoma of the bladder nearly filling the viscus in a four-year-old boy. Cystogram. Metastases.

pericystic fat and overlying peritoneum were widely excised en masse. One such patient with extensive, deeply infiltrating, highly malignant tumor, and in whom the operation was decidedly a gamble, lived twenty-five years tumor free and died of angina pectoris.

Simple Cystectomy. This is indicated by tumors unfit for segmental resection as described in the preceding paragraph and especially with trigonal or bladder neck involvement. *Cystectomy should not be undertaken as a palliative measure.* In this operation, the ureters are transplanted to the sigmoid (ureterosigmoidostomy) and the bladder, prostate, seminal vesicles, and in the female the urethra, are removed but without pelvic lymphadenectomy. To date the late mortality results of treatment of deeply infiltrating tumors favors cystectomy while segmental resection is favored for the superficially infiltrating tumors. The operative mortality is less in segmental resection and more patients are apparently cured after five years. A digest of reported series treated by the two methods suggests about 12 per cent cured by cystectomy and 18 per cent are cured by segmental resection.

Radical cystectomy adds pelvic lymphadenectomy to simple cystectomy, the likelihood of removing all cancer cell-containing nodes being zero, following which apparently no five-year cures have as yet been achieved. *Cystectomy with exenteration* is a huge step beyond radical cystectomy. The rectum, peritoneum, pelvic and retroperitoneal lymph nodes are removed after establishing bilateral cutaneous ureterostomy and colostomy. It is a slaughter-house procedure and I gravely question any

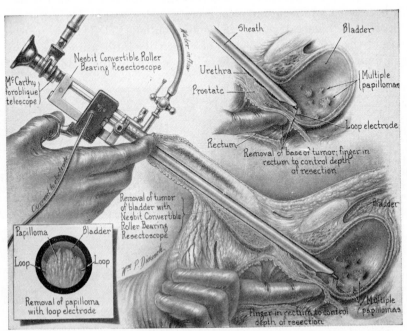

FIGURE 269. Treatment of vesical polyps and superficial papillary carcinoma by transurethral excision and deep electrocoagulation. (American Cystoscope Makers, Inc.)

of those performing the operation would permit it to be done on themselves even with the 20 per cent hope of favorable results it offers for two year survival.

Estrogenic therapy, chiefly by the administration of diethylstilbestrol, has produced no cures but in rare instances has achieved some symptomatic palliation as it often does in prostatic carcinoma. It can do little harm. In less than five cases of advanced and recurrent adenocarcinoma of the bladder, bilateral orchiectomy has been followed by symptomatic improvement.

Treatment of nonmalignant mesodermal tumors such as fibroma, lipoma, and the like, is by electrocoagulation, excision or resection. *Malignant mesenchymal* tumors of the bladder—the sarcomas—are practically all fatal; the only and extremely faint hope of cure lies in wide cystectomy and intensive postoperative irradiation therapy.

Complications of Bladder Tumors. These are principally (1) infection, commonly by the urea-splitting organisms (staphylococcus, Proteus bacillus and Esch. coli), (2) ulceration and necrosis of the tumor, (3) extensive calcific deposits on the tumor in alkaline urine consequent to (1); (4) hemorrhage, (5) ureteral blockage by the bladder tumor and consequent hydronephrosis, (6) urinary sepsis, (7) contracted bladder, (8) tumor recurrence and, most vital, (9) metastasis.

TUMORS OF THE PROSTATE GLAND

Prostatism is the term applied to the urinary difficulties consequent to obstruction caused by lesions at the bladder neck; the intensity of the symptoms may be aggravated by inflammation or infection. The basic lesion, however, is usually benign hyperplasia, median bar, contracture of the bladder neck, or malignant neoplasm, usually prostatic carcinoma. Tumors of the prostate gland are (1) benign, or (2) malignant.

Benign Prostatic Tumors. Excepting benign prostatic hyperplasia, nonmalignant growths of the prostate are extremely rare. Those reported have been fibroma, leiomyoma, leioma and chondroma. Clinically these growths resemble benign hyperplasia and usually are differentiated only with the microscope; they require the same treatment.

Benign prostatic hyperplasia is the commonest tumor of the gland, being present in variable degree in more than two thirds of all males over fifty years of age. Since the exact nature and etiology of prostatic enlargement are unknown (whether it is a myomatous nodule like uterine fibroids or a local hypoplasia as in nodular goiter), the term hyperplasia is justifiably employed as a cover-all designation. In some instances the structure is a pure adenoma and in others the term hypertrophy is correct on a histologic basis.

Etiology. An advanced age of the patient is the only constant factor in prostatic hyperplasia. Neither celibacy nor sexual excesses have exhibited a constant influence. The time-worn and still prevalent fear among many males that gonorrhea leads to prostatic enlargement "later on" has no basis in fact. Among the several theories that have been advanced concerning the pathogenesis of the condition are:

1. That it is a neoplastic growth initiated or excited by hormonal factors but persisting or only mildly regressing with castration or estrogen administration. This is decidedly *sub judice*.

2. The arteriosclerotic theory is concerned with the notion that central portions of the gland suffer diminished blood supply as the vascular bed is reduced by arteriosclerosis. Yet there is no confirmatory evidence of this in other organs of patients with extensive arteriosclerosis.

3. Inflammation of the gland. This leads to fibrotic contracture rather than enlargement.

4. Constitutional, racial, social, metabolic and nutritional factors have been advanced as provocative of prostatic hyperplasia but the evidence is largely inferential.

5. Hormonal disturbance. This notion, differing somewhat from 1 is bolstered by knowledge of the quantitative sex hormone changes occurring in males in late life and senility, the estrogen component of the androgen-estrogen ratio then having the ascendancy. Although clinical observations and some laboratory studies have shown this doubtless occurs, it is quite impossible to offer definitive confirmatory evidence. Still, this is the dominant explanation of prostatic hyperplasia today.

Pathology. The important lesion in prostatic hyperplasia is the formation of multicentric aglandular nodules of tissue (true neoplasia or focal hyperplasia?) which arise in the estrogen sensitive, submucosal, periurethral fibromuscular tissues in the area between the vesical outlet and the verumontanum (Fig. 270). As a collateral observation, the specimen enucleated at operation normally does not include the verumontanum which the tumor growth has pushed downward and forward toward the prostatic apex. Comparably, the seminal ducts have been pushed backward against the "false" or surgical capsule (cf. infra). There is secondary invasion of the aglandular nodules by epithelial elements from the

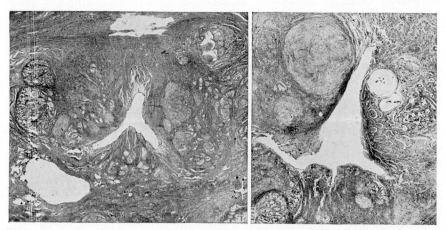

FIGURE 270. Prostatic hyperplasia. Cross section showing nodules of growth beginning in the juxta-urethral tissues. (See text.)

adjacent periurethral glands to give the stromoglandular or acinar structure. In the absence of glandular element invasion, the nodule remains a leiomyoma.

Thus begun, the lesion enlarges along any of at least eight different lines as Randall has demonstrated:

1. Lateral lobes causing urethral compression but not protruding into the bladder.

2. Posterior commissural or median lobe growth causing vesical neck and trigonal elevation by its enlargement.

3. Lateral and median lobe enlargement combination.

4. Subcervical lobe—at lower segment of vesical neck and protruding into the bladder, sometimes pedunculated.

5. Lateral and subcervical lobes.

6. Lateral, median and subcervical lobe.

7. Anterior commissural lobe.

8. Subtrigonal lobe.

Randall indicated varieties 1 to 5 in the foregoing tabulation as the five "fundamental" types; these eight define the prostatic hyperplastic enlargements clinically encountered.

As the prostate enlarges, its shape changes from pyramidal to rounded and generally with backward protrusion or bulging into the rectum. The surface is smoothly elastic.

With lateral lobe compression, the prostatic urethra is narrowed in the central groove and elongated. With upward growth of the tumor, the bladder is entered with pushing aside and often stretching of the muscular "internal sphincter." If the vesical neck encroachment is not completed by anterior commissural hyperplasia, the tumor is commonly described as horse collar, thick on the sides and below, but thin above.

Most pathologists prefer the term hyperplasia rather than hypertrophy because of the qualitative increase in histologically normal prostatic tissue in the lesion. As the hyperplastic nodule(s) increases in size, the remaining prostatic tissue and its glandular structures are compressed centripetally to become the surgical capsule of the gland as distinguished from the true anatomic fibrous capsule. Thus in "shelling out" a hyperplastic prostate when the operation is properly performed, the line of cleavage is along the inner side of the surgical capsule.

With increasing bladder-neck obstruction, hypertrophy of the trigone including Bell's muscles (q.v.) develops because of the increased work required of this structure to contract and help draw open the vesical orifice. The usual changes in the bladder wall and upper urinary tract consequent to vesical neck obstruction and urinary back pressure ensue; this phase of the disease is shown in Figure 43, and is discussed in Chapter 5.

Prostatic Median Bars. *False bars* may result from isolated prostatic hyperplasia, hypertrophic muscular contracture, or periurethral scarring. *True bars* are due to muscular or fibroglandular formations beneath the vesical neck and outside the prostatic capsule, and give rise to a damlike formation across the lower segment of the bladder outlet (Fig. 128). The lesions may be (1) fibrous, dense and unresilient, or (2) glandular, composed of hyperplastic prostatic tissue originating in the subcervical glands of Albarran or from commissural thickening outside the prostatic capsule as part of the general hyperplasia process.

Prostatic fibrosis and **sclerosis of the bladder neck** result from antecedent periurethral infection generally associated with prostatitis and seminal vesiculitis. Initially there is soft inflammatory infiltration at which stage it is readily amenable to treatment chiefly by dilation, but treated unsuccessfully or not at all, scarring progressively occurs with contracture of the bladder outlet, elevation of its inferior segment, the "internal" sphincteric mechanism is interfered with and the symptoms of prostatism appear. Also appearing are residual urine, hypertrophy of the trigone and Bell's muscles, and the upper urinary tract back pressure changes common to all bladder-neck obstruction (see Chapter 5).

Prostatic sclerosis is generally seen at an earlier age (thirty to fifty

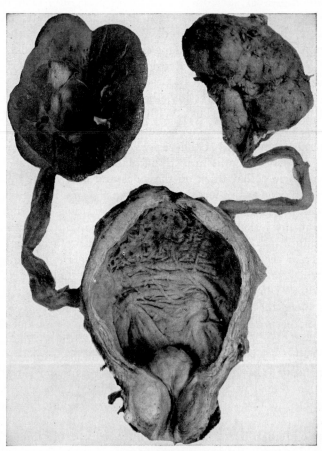

FIGURE 271. Prostatic hyperplasia. Advanced proximal urinary tract back pressure damage consequent to the bladder neck obstruction. (Courtesy Armed Forces Institute of Pathology.)

years) than hyperplasia (fifty to seventy years) and a clinically similar condition—congenital contracture of the bladder outlet—is seen in infants and children but occasionally persists unrecognized even into the third and fourth decades (Figs. 128–130).

Symptoms of Prostatism. These are fundamentally due to obstruction which may be augmented by local congestion and which in turn may be intensified by complicating infection, ulceration or bladder stone.

Increased frequency of urination is the usual earliest symptom, particularly *nocturia*. At first the patient starts getting up about four in the morning to void, later voiding twice and even three or more times during the night, and more frequently than normal during the day. Thus the day frequency increases until eventually he is urinating every hour or two or oftener both day and night. In part, the frequency results from increased irritability of the congested bladder outlet, but, as the residual urine in the bladder mounts, the "working" vesical capacity decreases and the patient must therefore void more often, passing only 3 or 4 ounces at a time but every forty to sixty minutes. Some of the frequency and especially the nocturia may also result from nephritic renal changes with the characteristic low specific gravity of polyuria. This excessive frequency prohibits adequate sleep and rest and of itself wears down the patient. Yet it is surprising how many of these men complain simply of "weak kidneys" or "weak bladder."

Urgency of urination reflects the intensive congestion of the bladder outlet, infection, complicating neoplasm or stone, or perhaps even all four conditions.

Difficult urination (dysuria) results from the diminished caliber of the bladder outlet and from inflammation (infection). The voided stream starts sluggishly, becomes progressively smaller in caliber, the expulsive force diminishes in strength, and it takes longer and longer to empty the bladder to the point of comfort. *Intermittent urination* occurs when extreme contraction of the abdominal musculature or added manual compression are needed to help expel the urine; between squeezes no urine flows.

Finally, the patient becomes unable to void and retention occurs. Unrelieved, overflow or paradoxical incontinence occurs; as more urine enters the fully distended bladder from the ureters, a comparable amount periodically spills over through the urethra to wet the clothing.

Acute retention may occur suddenly in prostatism because of local prostatic edema induced by chilling, alcoholism, sexual excesses, constipation or even appears spontaneously in the aged bedridden. Acute retention appearing early in prostatism may be relieved by catheterization and, because the bladder tone is still good, may not reappear for weeks, months or years, but the obstruction progressively continues. When one or two catheterizations fail to relieve the acute retention, the obstruction should be surgically removed without further delay as it should be in known chronic retention. Until such time as surgery can be safely performed, indwelling rather than intermittent catheterization should be relied upon.

Chronic urinary retention may follow an acute onset but most often develops insidiously as the residuum equals the bladder capacity.

Hematuria is usually the result of intense congestion at the vesical outlet and deep urethra, augmented sometimes by infection, and is more often an early symptom in benign hyperplasia than in prostatic carcinoma. The bleeding is usually mild, intermittent, or terminal, but may be profuse and clots fill the bladder. Often in the last instance, a distended varicose vein has ruptured or a mucosal ulceration caused by complicating infection, calculus or neoplasm has opened a good size blood vessel.

Pyuria nearly always denotes infection; the bulk of the pus may originate in the kidneys (pyelonephritis) but passage of a quantity of foul stinking, purulent urine suggests that an infected vesical diverticulum has been emptied.

Pain may persist as low grade in the bladder, back, perineum or rectal region, aggravated by frequency, stone or neoplasm. Yet it is not as bad as in prostatic carcinoma.

Rectal disturbance or pain results from bulging of the enlarged prostate into the rectum and by compression of the hemorrhoidal circulation. The pain appears as prostatism advances, first as a vague ache, but later as a fullness or even notable pain after urination or defecation. Constipation and hemorrhoids sometimes appear with rectal prolapse, and even pronounced rectal obstruction may develop.

Sexual stimulation occasionally occurs in the early congestive stages of prostatism but as the obstruction advances, sexual interest and ability abate or disappear completely. Yet both interest and ability may reappear after prostatectomy and even, as I have heard wives complain, make the man postoperatively a domestic annoyance with his sexual demands.

As in all types of urinary obstruction, and especially as infection may coexist, the resulting urinary toxemia is reflected in gastrointestinal disturbances which may be sufficiently severe to misdirect attention from the underlying uropathy. A large portion of these patients are treated for months or years for indigestion, gastric or duodenal ulcer, cholecystitis, "liver trouble," constipation, and the like. Anemia may be pronounced; weakness and wasting occur. Myocarditis and cardiovascular disease, often with hypertension, is frequently noted and, as a therapeutic corollary, is likely to show marked improvement following removal of the obstruction and sterilization of the urine. Neurologic manifestations include irritability, loss of interest, moroseness, argumentation, change of personality, periodic loss of consciousness and general nervous deterioration, all of which commonly disappear with improvement in renal function after removal of the blockage. Muscle and joint aches and pains, too often treated as "rheumatism" or "arthritis," reflect the urinary toxemia. The clinical conception and survey, therefore, must be on a broad base because all body systems are likely to mirror the urinary toxemia of prostatism. Unrelieved, the patient may be expected to die in urinary sepsis, uremic coma or terminal exhaustion unless a kindly fatal pneumonia intervenes.

Examination and Diagnosis.   The history will suggest bladder neck obstruction. Careful complete physical and laboratory examinations including blood count, blood pressure, blood chemistry and renal function estimations will disclose coexisting or resultant disease of other body systems. The findings are those common to infravesical obstruction (q.v. Chapter 5).

Radiographic study of the chest and electrocardiography should be part of the examination, and the cooperation of an internist is essential and should be sought if possible.

Abdominal Palpation.   A distended bladder may be felt; a bladder containing 6 oz. in an adult will be outlined by percussion two fingers breadth above the symphysis pubis, or with greater distention may even reach above the umbilicus. The kidneys, liver or other organs or masses may be palpable when pathologically enlarged (hydronephrosis, neoplasm, hydrops of the gallbladder, etc.). Examine for hernia, either enteric or vesical, epididymitis, thickened vas deferens and hemorrhoids.

Rectal Examination.   The proper technique of this investigation is given in Chapter 3. An atonic rectal sphincter may be the first suggestion of central nervous system disease. The *gentle*(!) rectal examination should be done when the bladder is empty. The smoothly elastic, enlarged prostate will be palpated whereas a middle lobe, median bar obstruction or contracted bladder neck will not be evident by rectal examination alone. In contracted bladder neck the prostate is generally sclerotic, firm and often shrunken. The gland is not tender except as acute or subacute inflammation exists.

As the prostate enlarges, the seminal vesicles are pushed upward or laterally and may get out of reach of the examining finger. The median furrow normally palpable on the rectal aspect of the prostate is obliterated or bulges roundly toward the rectum. The width and length of the gland increase; normally it is about the size and shape of a chestnut. Inflammatory induration may give rise to irregular, firm areas or nodules in the gland which to the examining finger may suggest carcinoma; there is an even chance that they may be malignant. Prostatic calculosis, benign neoplasm, sarcoma, tuberculosis and neuromuscular vesical disease symptomatically resemble prostatic hyperplasia in many ways but there should not be great difficulty in making the differential diagnosis. Here it is most important to rule out central nervous system disease such as tabes or cerebral spinal lues; test the pupillary reflexes, ankle jerks and the knee reflexes. Not infrequently disease of the spinal cord and prostatic obstructive disease coexist.

Test for Residual Urine.   With the diagnostic data suggestive of bladder neck obstruction as thus far obtained, the next step is to learn if the patient can empty his bladder completely. He voids until he thinks he is empty. A soft catheter is then gently passed at once and any urine thus obtained represents the residuum. It is a reliable index of the degree of bladder wall decompensation caused by the urinary back pressure, i.e., the relative inability of the bladder musculature to overcome the obstruction. The residuum may vary from 10 to 15 cc. to twice this many ounces.

Catheterization in pronounced prostatic hyperplasia may be disturbing when an unusual length of tube is required to traverse the elongated prostatic urethra to reach the bladder. A soft rubber catheter is the best to use if it will go in gently. Should such a catheter be impassable, pass a 14 or 16 F. modified natural curve silk catheter. *Do not use metal catheters;* these easily perforate the friable inflamed, hyperplastic gland. In median bar, in contracted bladder neck, prostatic fibrosis or in mild hyperplasia, the urethral lengthening is none or negligible but the residuum is often considerable. Yet a diverticulum may account for an apparent large residuum and thus be misleading in the diagnostic study. In early prostatism determination of the residual urine is unlikely to engender renal functional disturbances or incite infection. But in pronounced obstructing prostatic hyperplasia, one hesitates to introduce any instrument into the bladder until operation can be done promptly, or at least until continuous free bladder drainage can be established.

Fortunately by excretory urography both the renal function and, by postvoiding cystography, the residuum can be approximately estimated. After the usual last urographic exposure has been made in the excretory urographic series, the patient empties his bladder as best he can; another x-ray exposure or two is then made. The residuum (radiopaque medium containing urine) is estimated from the size of the postvoiding vesical shadow. This method of estimation can be used with a good accuracy and obviates instrumentation. Thus it neither introduces nor exacerbates infection; it demonstrates the shape and degree of the prostatic hyperplasia, stone, diverticulum, or even papillomatous neoplasm as well as disease elsewhere in the upper urinary tract and notably in the kidneys.

Cystography performed by injection of radiopaque medium through a catheter will afford even better visualization of the outline of the bladder wall and outlet than excretory cystography and may even show vesico-ureteral reflux (Fig. 272). Sometimes the entire upper urinary tract is demonstrated by this method (see Chapter 3).

Urethrography or urethrocystography will demonstrate the pronounced lengthening of the prostatic urethra as well as urethral sacculation, diverticula, strictures and so forth (Fig. 282). Here lateral or lateral oblique exposures tell the story best.

Cystoscopy had best be deferred if possible until the patient is in the hospital and can be operated upon without delay or at least have free cystostomy bladder drainage established should complications arise or conditions demand. This is particularly true in the aged who stand cystoscopy poorly under these circumstances. The principal contraindications to cystoscopy in prostatism are:

1. Acute urinary infection (cystitis, pyelonephritis, epididymitis, prostatitis).
2. Advanced renal dysfunction not responding to preliminary drainage.

3. Instrumental difficulty because of stricture, hemorrhage.
4. Large residual urine.
5. Extra-urinary disease or urinary tract complications contraindicating vesical surgery, usually in a sick or feeble patient.

Cystoscopic study reveals (1) the form of the prostatic obstruction (lateral, median or anterior lobe enlargement, singly or in any combination, contracted bladder neck, prostatic fibrosis, median bar obstruction), (2) trigonal hypertrophy, (3) vesical tonicity, (4) trabeculation, sacculation, cellulation, (5) inflammation, infection, (6) ulceration of the bladder wall, and (7) complicating lesions such as diverticula, calculi or neoplasm. Sometimes there is associated neuromuscular disease; this calls for cystometric study as well (Chapter 9). The length of the hyperplastic gland is urethroscopically estimated and finally, if necessary, the integrity of the ureters and kidneys is determined by catheterization, divided renal function tests, and retrograde pyelography, when preliminary excretory urographic study has been unsatisfactory or perchance omitted.

Median Bar Obstruction at the Bladder Neck. Here the obstructive factor is that of the diminution of the true caliber of the vesical outlet; comparatively it takes a greater degree of median bar formation to produce the same bladder neck narrowing or constriction as that caused by moderate contracture, the effect of the last being concentric and that of the bar semi-concentric. Practically, it is unnecessary to differentiate sharply between the various types of median bar for they all cause essentially the same (1) back pressure changes, (2) symptoms, and (3) fundamentally require the same treatment, viz: transurethral resection.

Symptoms will depend upon the degree of bladder neck constriction (obstruction) and local inflammation due either to congestion or infection. In general, the clinical manifestations are those of prostatic hyperplasia with nocturia first, then day frequency and so on. The *diagnosis* is made by evaluation of the symptomatic picture, the rectal examination dis-

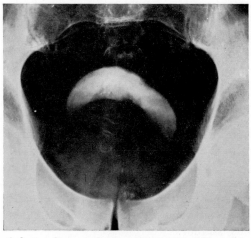

FIGURE 272.   Prostatic hyperplasia producing cystographic filling defect at bladder outlet.

closure of an unenlarged prostate, fibrous, and seldom tender. The cystoscopic study shows the bar formation over the lower segment of the bladder outlet with a sharp upward declivity of the postverumontanum urethra and variably deep *bas fond* behind. Trigonal hypertrophy generally reflects the gradation of obstruction.

Contracture of the Bladder Outlet. Here the entire circumference of the vesical outlet shows intrusion in annular formation, most marked below; the elevation of the inferior lip of the vesical outlet simulates but is to be distinguished from median bar. Local muscular hypertrophy is generally prominent in congenital vesical neck contracture, and there is usually added sclerosis and some glandular hypertrophy in median bar formation and even in some cases of contracture. Yet, fundamentally congenital contracture is a narrowing (Fig. 128) like stenosis of the meatus, ureter or intestine, while in the acquired lesion there is added muscular hypertrophy, sclerosis and often glandular hyperplasia to help bring about the constriction. It is to be distinguished from the usual forms of lobular prostatic hyperplasia, and even of prostatic carcinoma, the last giving an abnormal rigidity to the bladder neck as encountered by the passage and manipulation of and study with the cysto-urethroscope.

The symptoms of vesical neck contracture are the same as in median bar obstruction. In both conditions the usually preferred treatment is by transurethral resection; prostatic massage, urethral dilation, electrocoagulation of the posterior urethra, bladder neck, or verumontanum have no place here. However, in some of these patients seen early, relief over many months or even years may be achieved by conservative bladder neck dilation with an instrument such as the Kollman dilator. Nevertheless, eventually all need operation and commonly by transurethral resection.

Contracted bladder neck with median bar obstruction in the female has become recognized as a fairly frequent lesion in this sex at all ages. In the young the condition is congenital and in many adults develops on the congenital basis of muscular hypertrophy and narrowing of the orifice analogous to meatal stenosis. In older women with this lesion there is commonly considerable posterior urethral glandular hyperplasia in addition to fibrosis and muscular hypertrophy, the symptoms being like those of prostatism and the cystoscopic picture that of median bar or contracture with variable and often large residuum. As a sixty-three year old woman told me, "If I was a man, I'd say I had an enlarged prostate!"—and so she would, what with concentric contraction, large residuum, trabeculated bladder, moderate secondary infection, frequency, nocturia, a constant sense of vesical fullness and never feeling quite empty after voiding. Treatment, as in her case, is careful transurethral resection of the vesical outlet and may be expected to give a most gratifying result. The tissue removed from some of these women looks much like the glandular tissue removed in median bar obstruction in adult males. The symptoms and findings in these obstructions in children are clinically, pathologically and therapeutically similar.

Treatment. Catheterization is employed once or twice to relieve acute retention but when not properly successful in helping the patient to resume free voiding, the catheter should be fastened indwelling or cystostomy drainage instituted until the condition of the patient makes it safe to operate. Discussion of this phase of treatment is continued in the second succeeding paragraph.

Operation. The hyperplastic prostatic obstruction may be removed by suprapubic, retropubic, perineal or transurethral prostatectomy. Yet the only true prostatectomy is the radical procedure as performed for carcinoma in which the entire gland and its true capsule are excised. The usual "prostatectomy" is an adenectomy, the line of cleavage being between the hyperplastic elements of the tumor and the surgical capsule which is the compressed nonhyperplastic prostatic tissue surrounding the "adenoma."

PREPARATION FOR OPERATION. When there is a large residuum, pronounced infection, renal dysfunction, hypertension or general debility, an initial period of free drainage should be observed and especially when acute retention is superimposed on a pronounced long-standing chronic retention. Here the bladder should be gradually decompressed (slowly emptied). Yet the dangers of rapid decompression are generally attributable to complicating acute urinary infection rather than renal shut down per se. In performing this gradual decompression, increments of 100 cc. can be released every thirty minutes or so, making sure that the renal output does not exceed this amount.

If the renal function deficit is not over 50 per cent, employ indwelling catheterization with preliminary vasectomy for a few days or weeks as needed to achieve physiologic stabilization of the patient. For simple catheterization a 14 or 16 F. two-eye soft rubber (latex) catheter serves well. For indwelling catheterization use a 14 F. balloon catheter with a 5 cc. bag capacity, but inflate it with only 2 or 3 cc. of sterile water at the most (Fig. 55, Chapter 5). The alternative, indwelling fixation of the usual two-eye catheter is shown in Figure 54, Chapter 5. When the renal damage, general physical condition or other grave factors present from onset of treatment show no striking improvement from treatment or the patient cannot tolerate an indwelling catheter, establish free counter-drainage by suprapubic cystostomy or trocar cystostomy until such time as the patient is stabilized and ready for operation. The criteria for stabilization are: normal or relatively normal blood chemistry (nonprotein nitrogen less than 50 mg. per 100 cc. of blood, urea, carbon dioxide combining power, sodium and chloride estimations normal or nearly normal and phenolsulfonpthalein output over 50% in two hours). If the patient can also walk briskly fifty feet without dyspnea or cardiac pain, is in fair state of nutrition, and is edema free and on a normal fluid intake, operation may be performed. Unfortunately, many of these patients with prostatism are old, debilitated, poorly nourished and suffer cardiac, pulmonary, arteriosclerotic and especially cardiovascular disease, and require special medical attention not only in their preparation for prostatectomy but during the postoperative course. With this careful preparation of the patient, operation can hopefully be carried out in nearly all, and for those not considered operable, or likely ever to be operable, permanent suprapubic cystostomy drainage must be maintained rather than permanent indwelling catheter drainage.

Profuse bleeding after catheterization or decompression of a chronically distended bladder demands removal of the clots by aspiration and thorough washing out. If the bleeding gets beyond control, open the bladder suprapubically, wash out the clots and leave in a large drainage tube—½ inch or more in diameter. With the institution of free bladder drainage, practically every vesical hemorrhage will spontaneously and promptly cease; this is an axiom in the stoppage of profuse bladder hemorrhage. When the hemorrhage from the congested copiously bleeding prostate does not then cease, promptly enucleate the gland suprapubically, but this emergency prostatectomy is rarely called for.

Yet present-day improvements in surgical technique, anesthesia, availability of blood transfusion, and antimicrobial therapy have thrown safeguards about the patient not enjoyed only twenty-five years ago. For this reason many better risk patients may be operated upon by one-stage prostatectomy with a greatly curtailed period of preoperative catheter drainage and in some instances indwelling catheterization may not even be necessary.

The choice of operation should be the procedure the surgeon is most

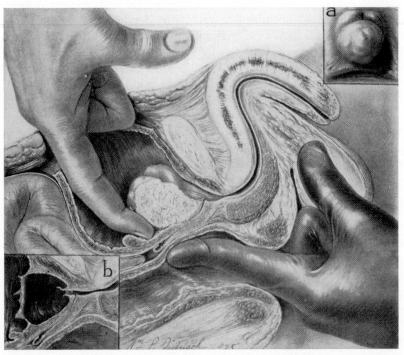

FIGURE 273. Suprapubic prostatectomy aided by a finger in the rectum to elevate the gland (Young).

capable of performing; suprapubic prostatectomy is the safest and most foolproof for general surgeons.

Bilateral vasectomy (division of the vas deferens between ligatures on each side), if performed before any instrumentation is undertaken, will essentially eliminate complicating epididymitis associated with prostatectomy. If it is done after instrumentation, epididymitis will occur in about 5 per cent of these cases and, if not done at all, occurs in 15 to 20 per cent of the patients during or after prostatectomy. This figure used to be much higher, the reduction being attributable to present-day chemotherapy, especially the antibiotics.

Suprapubic prostatectomy is indicated for the removal of a prostate estimated to weigh over 50 mg.—about twice the normal size (Fig. 273). Pronounced intravesical prostatic enlargement should be removed suprapubically. Removal of complicating vesical stone, diverticulum, papillary or infiltrating carcinoma often calls for suprapubic prostatectomy in addition although the mortality is much higher when diverticulectomy or bladder resection is done at the same sitting. When this is contraindicated, do the diverticulectomy or bladder resection first, maintain suprapubic drainage and when the patient is again fit for operation, enucleate the prostate through the enlarged suprapubic sinus tract. To leave the diverticulum is to invite trouble from continued infection, residual urine, and symptoms of prostatism as are regularly found when a diverticulum is left after transurethral prostatic resection.

A *two-stage prostatectomy* must be performed when the patient is a poor risk, a status which of itself today engenders a poorer prognosis than a one-stage operation in the "fair risk" patient. In "good risk" patients the average mortality in one-stage suprapubic, retropubic, transurethral resection and perineal prostatectomy is about equal (1 to 4%) although the complications and morbidity are likely to be highest in the transurethral procedure except when it is done by an expert.

Retropubic Prostatectomy. Millin advises the retropubic approach for: simple benign hyperplasia ("adenoma"), sclerosis of the vesical neck

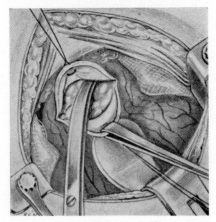

FIGURE 274. Retropubic prostatectomy (Millin).

(median bar), contracture of the vesical neck, calculous prostatitis, prostatic carcinoma, trigonal carcinoma, infected prostatitis, prostatic abscess, congenital valves of the prostatic urethra (Fig. 274). He also recommends the approach for a one-sitting combined surgical treatment by retropubic prostatectomy with (a) diverticulectomy, (b) excision of vesical tumor, (c) vesical calculus, and (d) the radical removal in early cases of a carcinomatous prostate and even partial cystectomy ("inferior cystectomy") in which the prostate and the lower third or half of the adjacent bladder is resected en masse from the vesical outlet, the ureters being disposed of by ureteroneocystostomy.

Perineal Prostatectomy. This is performed for the treatment of the same varieties of prostatic obstruciton as may be relieved by suprapubic or retropubic prostatectomy (Fig. 275). In addition, it includes radical total prostatectomy for carcinoma or other malignancy as well as for dense fibrotic contracture of the prostate. In the total or radical operation, the true prostatic capsule is excised, and in carcinoma, in addition, the adjacent bladder segment (mostly trigone) and seminal vesicles. It demands precision of anatomic knowledge and surgical technique lest the rectum be perforated or sphincteric control be damaged and prostato-rectal fistula or urinary incontinence result respectively. Moreover, with perineal prostatectomy, the patient stands a good chance of losing his sexual powers and, for this reason, the operation should not be advised in young or middle-aged sexually active males unless dire necessity, chiefly malignancy, demands. In general the surgical complications and mortality are those encountered in suprapubic prostatectomy, but today

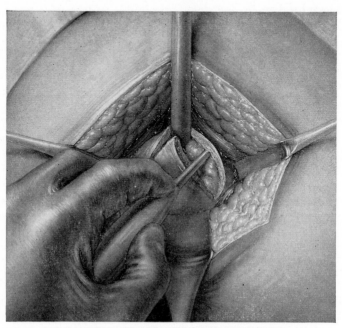

FIGURE 275.   Perineal prostatectomy (Colston).

they occur much less often. Yet as Keyes put it, "Fewer perineals die but fewer suprapubics wish they were dead."

Transurethral Resection. Removal of the prostate by this method is indicated in the treatment of median bars, vesical neck contractures, and for palliative relief in prostatic carcinoma in conjunction with estrogen therapy (Fig. 276). Transurethral resection is employed in benign prostatic hyperplasia when the operation can be completed in a reasonable operating time (sixty minutes or so), and in some cases of retention type of neuromuscular vesical disease. Some experts will remove much more tissue in a given time than others and correspondingly widen the scope of the size gland they will attack. Usually the large glands require transurethral resection in two or three sittings, a double or treble surgical siege and exposure to shock. To me this seems unwarranted when the same gland can be enucleated suprapubically at one sitting in ten minutes.

Despite the extensive salesmanship with which transurethral resection was promoted in the early 1930's as a simple successful operation without important danger, the procedure has suffered greatly at the hands of both trained and untrained blunderers with an over-all mortality and morbidity in excess of open operation. Yet today in the hands of the competent, the mortality is not over 2 to 4 per cent in all cases, hemorrhage and infection being the grave and relatively frequent complications. Bleeding may occur weeks or even months postoperatively. Transurethral resection is decidedly an operation only for expert experienced hands.

Prognosis in Prostatectomy. The outlook for the patients whose condition is too poor (old age, cardiac, renal, pulmonary or enteric dys-

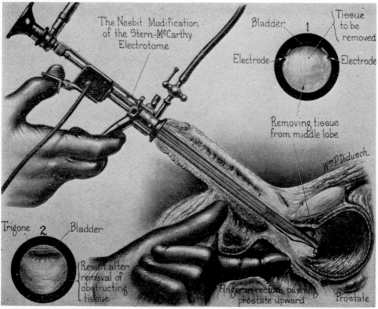

FIGURE 276. Transurethral prostatectomy using Nesbit modification of the Stern-McCarthy resectoscope. (American Cystoscope Makers, Inc.)

function) to permit operation, is maintenance on continuous suprapubic bladder drainage. Continuous wearing of an indwelling catheter is out of the question. On periodic or intermittent catheterization, that is, three or four times in twenty-four hours, the average outlook for life is less than one year although a few live two, or occasionally for several years, death being practically always due to urinary infection. Fortunately, with present-day aids many patients, who twenty-five years ago would have been considered inoperable, can today be prepared for and successfully undergo operation.

Complications and Morbidity. The reason for the higher postoperative mortality rate in octogenarians is obvious; advanced arteriosclerosis is present in more than half of them, hypertension exists in a third, and pronounced myocardial damage in two thirds. In this group embolism and coronary thrombosis are frequent causes of death; terminal pneumonia occurs less often than formerly. Renal failure accounts for more than a third of the postprostatectomy deaths, and cardiac and pulmonary disease for about a fourth each.

Recurrence of Prostatism. The chances of recurrence of clinically evident hyperplasia of remaining prostatic tissue following prostatectomy is about 1 per cent, but following transurethral resection is about 5 per cent and usually in the last instance because the resection was incomplete. Postoperative sclerosis of the vesical neck may occur in any form of prostatectomy and in some instances requires removal by transurethral resection.

Postoperative suprapubic *fistulae* almost always mean that there is obstruction still remaining at the vesical neck or peripherally and needs removal, or that a urethral stricture—new or old—demands dilation. Yet infection, neoplasm, calculus, diverticulosis, tuberculosis, or neuromuscular vesical disease may be the underlying cause and require appropriate treatment. With the establishment of free vesical drainage below, the fistula will close unless it is completely epithelialized or is encrusted with phosphatic material. Deep curettement of the fistula tract may suffice to encourage its closure but failing in this, resect the entire tract. If there is no obstruction, look for a foreign body deep in the wound or at the bladder outlet, especially a gauze sponge; poor nutrition with avitaminosis (A, B, C, E), a low plasma protein content or localized abscess may deter healing.

Postprostatectomy urinary *incontinence* may result from surgical injury of the external sphincter, the membranous urethra having been torn away with the prostatic growth, or the nerve supply having been severely traumatized. There may be a remaining nodule of tissue, scar, or prolapsed mucosa which interferes with sphincteric closure, or neuromuscular vesical disease may have been previously overlooked. Temporary incontinence occurs in about 5 per cent of patients following open prostatectomy, is of somewhat higher incidence after perineal prostatectomy and transurethral resection, and complete incontinence is of highest incidence following total perineal prostatectomy.

Prostatic Cysts. These rare lesions attached to the prostatic surface usually result from congenital occlusion of one or more prostatic ducts, but the condition may be acquired through inflammation or progressively caused by prostatic hyperplasia. The cysts may be single or multiple and vary from 0.5 to as much as 8 to 10 cm. in diameter. The cyst may cause no symptoms or those of irritation, inflammation or obstruction, with urinary frequency and dysuria which, when persistent, prompts the diagnostic urologic examination. The thin-walled, usually shiny cysts, are clearly visualized by cysto-urethroscopy in the prostatic urethra or protruding into the bladder neck, or even into the viscus itself, and will cause a cystographic filling defect. *Treatment* consists of transurethral electroexcision; first the cyst is punctured and then resected at its base.

In females, small cysts may surround the chronically inflamed bladder neck, cause the same symptoms as in the male, and require the same treatment as outlined in the preceding paragraph.

CARCINOMA OF THE PROSTATE GLAND

Carcinoma of the prostate is found at autopsy in about 15 per cent of all men over fifty years of age, although an incidence as high as 46 per cent has been reported. Whether coincident or not, half of the cases seen clinically occur in association with benign prostatic hyperplasia and generally begin in the lobules of the posterior lobe of the gland (the rectal side) which is seldom the site of benign hyperplasia. The growth invades upward, into the hyperplastic tissue, into the seminal vesicles, bladder floor, and to surround the prostatic urethra. Rarely does the cancer begin in the body of the hyperplasia. Structurally the type is adenocarcinoma but may show variations, even in the same tumor: (1) alveolar (Fig. 277), (2) scirrhous (Fig. 278), or (3) medullary (Fig. 279), depending upon the cellular and stromal proportions and arrangements.

All prostatic cancers have a dominant tendency to metastasize by the lymphatics, blood vessels, and by direct extension, the metastatic lesions sometimes being the initial manifestations. One encounters widespread metastases with large nodules in the skull, neck, liver and elsewhere, but the primary prostatic lesions 6 mm. or so in diameter are discovered only at autopsy, yet the metastatic lesions are "characteristically" those of prostatic carcinoma. In addition to lymphatic spread to the internal and external inguinal nodes, extension also occurs along the larger nerve sheaths and doubtless this explains some pelvic pains and especially the "sciatica," lumbago or rheumatism from which so many of these patients suffer early or late. By lymphatic spread upward, tumor masses may compress the larger venous vessels to cause edema of the legs and other regions they drain, may invade the mediastinum and, in the neck, enlargement of the left supraclavicular node (Virchow's node) may be an early harbinger of the disease.

Batson has shown how hematogenous spread through the vertebral vessels explains the extensive spinal involvement which so commonly causes excruciating backache as well as referred pains in isosomatic structures. The lungs and liver are apt to show early metastases, as may almost any portion of the skeleton, especially the pelvis, spine, skull, long bones, and ribs (Fig. 280). These lesions can be radiologically demonstrated; those of the bones in particular may simulate Paget's disease or, in the vertebral bodies, spinal caries.

So early and widespread does extraprostatic carcinoma extend that, as initially observed clinically, the disease is confined to the gland in not over 5 per cent of the cases which represents the small group of patients in whom radical prostatectomy may hold substantial prospect for cure.

Symptoms. Initially the symptoms may be those of benign prostatic hyperplasia or other bladder neck obstruction, or the discomfort of *pain* caused by metastases directly or by pain reference may appear first (back, perineum, groin, thighs, sciatica). *Hematuria* rarely occurs until late

Fig. 277

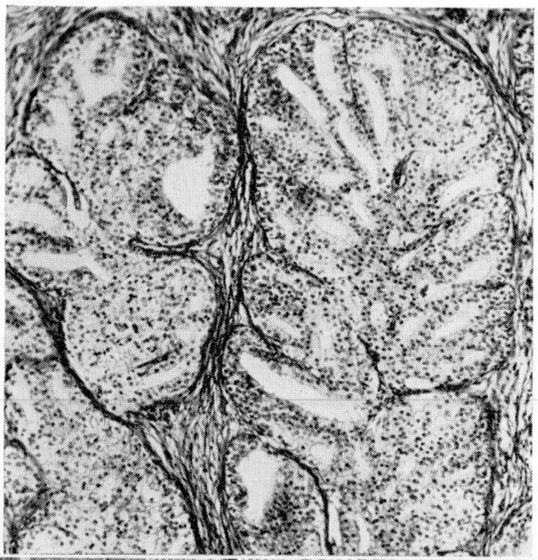

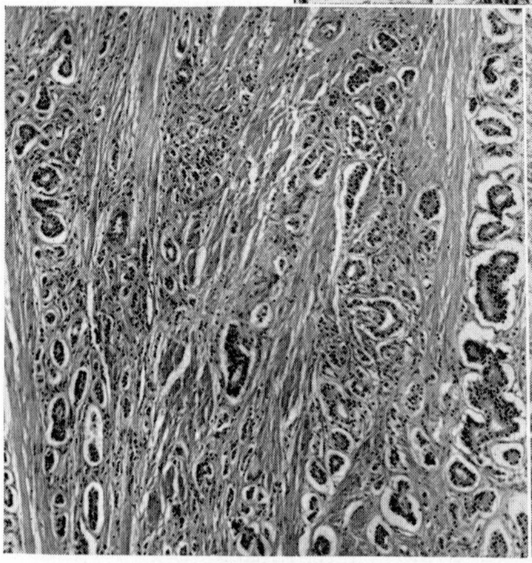

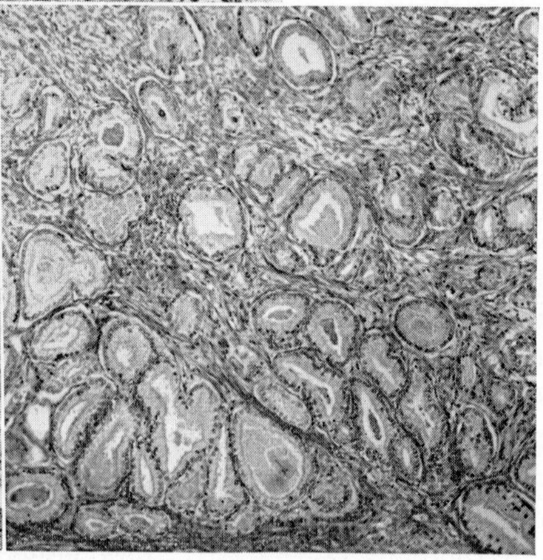

Fig. 278   Fig. 279

FIGURE 277. Alveolar carcinoma of the prostate.
FIGURE 278. Scirrhous carcinoma of the prostate.
FIGURE 279. Medullary carcinoma of the prostate.
(Courtesy Armed Forces Institute of Pathology.)

when the deep urethra or bladder neck are invaded by the cancer; thereafter bleeding may be frequent, distressing and profuse.

Diagnosis. Think of carcinoma of the prostate in any patient over
fifty years of age with a constant low backache or "sciatica"! Think of
carcinoma of the prostate in any patient over sixty-five years of age with
symptoms of prostatism.

Rectal Examination. In prostatic carcinoma the gland may be enlarged, especially if benign prostatic hypertrophy coexists. It may be of
normal size but one or more densely indurated or even stony hard masses
may be felt. The nodules may or may not be tender. For scores of years
textbooks and other medical literature have taught that a stony hard
nodule in the prostate was practically pathognomonic of prostatic cancer,
excluding prostatic calculi readily demonstrated by x-ray. Yet a careful
investigation of this by Jewett and frequent observations by many urologists have shown that this is a discouragingly unreliable guide. For
example, in a histologic study of 211 such stony-hard prostatic nodules,
108 were found to be benign and only slightly less than half, 103, were
malignant. Chronic prostatitis was the commonest cause of the stony hard
induration; all cases of prostatic calculi were excluded from the study.

Of serious prognostic significance is the finding of hard induration
of the base of the seminal vesicles; the greater the distance the hard
prostatic nodules are from the base of vesicles the less the likelihood of
vesicular involvement.

Cancer may be found in nonmalignant prostatic hyperplasia or in
chronic indurated prostatitis. Yet the clues must be followed up.

In well-developed carcinoma of the prostate the gland is variably and
importantly enlarged, indurated and *fixed*—it cannot be budged by the
examining finger as can the normal structure. The lateral sulci may be

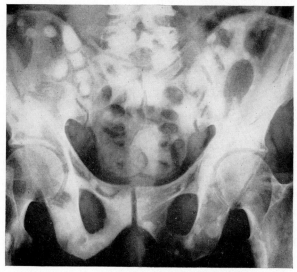

FIGURE 280.   Prostatic carcinoma. Metastases to pelvic bones and lower lumbar vertebrae.

indurated and obliterated. The bases of the seminal vesicles and often the intervesicular plateau—the area of tissue between the seminal vesicles— are indurated or the hard mass may occupy the entire area—according to its degree of extension. If there are several small stony hard nodules, suspect prostatic calculi and especially if there is suggestion of crepitation; the x-ray should demonstrate prostatic stone (Figs. 237, 238).

Cystoscopy will demonstrate the type and extent of bladder neck compression, inflammation and alteration, whether neoplastic or other ulceration has occurred in the carcinomatous segment, and if stone, neo- plasm, diverticulosis or other conditions are present in the bladder. When the excretory urographic study has not been satisfactory, ureteral cath- eterization, divided renal function test and retrograde pyelography are done at the cystoscopic sitting.

Cytologic Studies. Examination of stained centrifuged urine speci- mens by the Papanicolaou technique has shown suspicious abnormal cells in a high percentage of clinically evident prostatic cancers but in some of these cases false negative reports have been made; the results of this method are less reliable than when prostatic fluid is examined.

Cytologic examination of prostatic fluid expressed by massage (to avoid dilution with fluid from the seminal vesicles) has disclosed *cancer in situ* or early growing cancer not clinically evident in about 10 per cent of reported studies, and in more than three fourths (86%; Peters and Young, 1951) of clinically suspected or evident prostatic cancer. Yet to be reliable, the cytologic study must be made by pathologists experienced in this work; it adds another method in the diagnosis of prostatic cancer.

Blood Studies. In disseminated prostatic cancer the *acid phosphatase* of the blood serum is usually elevated and it may be increased in cancer limited to the gland itself. Normally a small amount of acid phosphatase enzyme is present in the blood stream. Two basic analytic methods have been employed for its determination, (1) the King-Armstrong is the most frequently used, and (2) the Bodansky method, details of which will be found in most modern laboratory manuals. In a study of 1150 pooled cases of carcinoma of the prostate from fourteen clinics, Nesbit and Baum found that two thirds (65.5%) of the patients had elevated acid phos- phatase when first seen as did a fifth (20.5%) who had no evidence of metastasis, an over-all group average of 39.9 per cent or two out of five cases. Transient elevation of the acid phosphatase in the blood serum for twenty-four to forty-eight hours has been observed following prostatic instrumentation and massage but for practical purposes this may be dis- regarded. It may be considered that there is no acid phosphatase elevation in benign prostatic hyperplasia. In short, *an elevated acid phosphatase signifies metastatic prostatic carcinoma and may also reflect localized car- cinoma in the gland.*

Alkaline phosphatase enzyme has been found in one-half of the cases (56.7% in the Nesbit and Baum studies) of prostatic carcinoma with or without metastases when first seen, but it is also elevated in Paget's dis- ease, primary bone tumors, metastases to bones, hepatic disease and intestinal obstruction. Therefore, an elevated alkaline phosphatase is not pathognomonic of disseminated prostatic carcinoma while an elevated acid phosphatase is pathognomonic.

When the diagnosis is still in doubt, histologic examination of suspected tissue should be performed. This may be by (1) needle aspiration biopsy, (2) transurethral resection, or (3) surgical perineal biopsy.

Needle Biopsy. Under local or low spinal anesthesia and with a guiding finger in the rectum, a special needle for the purpose (Huffman, Silverman, or even a large spinal puncture needle) is introduced through the perineum into the midst of the suspected tumor in the prostate and by suction or otherwise according to the different mechanisms, one or more pieces of tissue are removed for study. Sometimes examination shows normal tissue even though an early tumor has been overlooked.

Surgical Biopsy. This is much more certain:

A. TRANSURETHRAL RESECTION. Removal of several pieces of the suspected gland by this method may obtain tissue showing carcinoma. Yet the urethral aspect of the gland is generally the last portion to be invaded so the test may be falsely negative unless the gland is well cut into. When the results of other methods have left the examiner in doubt, the transurethral biopsy technique may be used but perineal biopsy is far more certain.

B. PERINEAL BIOPSY. The prostate is exposed as for perineal prostatectomy and one or more deep wedges of suspected tissue are removed for histologic study; the wound is closed. The findings by both frozen section and routine histologic preparation with hematoxylin eosin stain should be known within seventy-two hours and if cancer is found, the perineal biopsy wound is reopened and radical perineal excision of the prostate is performed unless contraindicated by local extraprostatic extension, skeletal or other metastases.

Differential Diagnosis. In the gland itself the "stony hard" nodulation, fixation and irregular enlargement so often found are unlikely to be mistaken for tuberculosis; in the last condition there are other evidences of the infection in the seminal vesicles, epididymides and urinary tract. Subcapsular prostatic calculi may feel stony hard but the x-ray will demonstrate them. Intraprostatic and periprostatic inflammatory induration is more commonly found in a younger age group than those having carcinoma, and the indurated gland is seldom so dense and fixed as it is in prostatic carcinoma. In metastatic prostatic carcinoma, the roentgenograms may suggest Paget's disease (osteitis deformans) which involves chiefly the skull, pelvis and femurs; it appears by x-ray as a greatly increased bone density, trabeculated rather than nodular as in osteoblastic prostatic carcinoma metastases. In the skull in Paget's disease there is pronounced thickening of the tables together with areas of great thickening or of thinning (decalcification). On the other hand, the metastases in prostatic cancer are predominantly osteoblastic with increased density although osteolytic metastatic lesions are occasionally found and may, in the roentgenogram, even suggest bone cyst formation.

Treatment of Prostatic Cancer. Over thirty-five years ago Keyes used to tell us, his residents and house officers, "The man with a cancer of the prostate isn't worth the powder to blow him to hell," (therapeutically speaking, of course). In the interim and despite the introduction of bilateral orchiectomy, estrogen administration, the newer modalities in radiation (radioactive gold, cobalt[60], multimillion volt x-ray machines) and excepting early radical total perineal prostatectomy, the cure rate is scarcely better than zero. Hormonal (estrogen) therapy frequently brings about striking temporary symptomatic relief but no cures.

Subtotal prostatectomy has unwittingly eradicated an occasional cancer—small, early, or *in situ*—in a removed hyperplastic "adenoma." Today radical total prostatectomy—preferably perineal—offers the only hope of cure of prostatic cancer but its field of usefulness properly is limited to the 3 to 5 per cent of patients with no pericapsular or extraprostatic cancer, a comparatively small field for potential cure. A few urologists have applied this operation even though periprostatic induration, especially of the bases of the seminal vesicles, was initially present but "cleared" under estrogenic therapy. As surmised, only a very few of these are apparently cured. Yet only by treating the many do we cure the few.

In a recent review of the cases of prostatic cancer treated by radical perineal prostatectomy at the Johns Hopkins Hospital, Jewett found 39 per cent of 132 cases were apparently cancer-free after five years, and after ten years 49 per cent of the survivors who had only intraprostatic cancer were alive, and 25 per cent of all cases—intraprostatic and extraprostatic cancer—were living. The normal statistical death rate in this age group is 53 per cent.

Radiation treatment of prostatic carcinoma by x-ray does no good, except occasionally as palliation. Interstitial irradiation by implantation of gold seeds has been largely abandoned.

Hormone Treatment. It has been known for many years that castration of men with benign prostatic hypertrophy is frequently followed by variable diminution in size of the gland and in the severity of the symptoms. Harem eunuchs "prepared" in childhood have small prostates. Huggins demonstrated the frequent regression of prostatic carcinoma and its metastases following castration (to eliminate secretion of testicular androgens) and the administration of estrogen. The study Nesbit and Baum made upon 1818 pooled cases showed that the greatest five-year survival (44%) was obtained when combined castration and estrogen therapy (diethylstilbestrol, 5 mg. per day or less) were employed in patients with evident metastases when first seen. This is in contrast to a "control" series (Nesbit and Plumb, 1946) of patients with prostatic carcinoma not so treated, only 10 per cent of whom survived five years. Castration alone was next in effectiveness, but distinctly less valuable than combined castration and estrogen administration, while estrogen therapy alone rated third.

When metastases were present upon first examination, a fifth of these patients lived five years with castration and estrogen therapy, or only castration. Ten per cent lived five years on estrogen alone while

6 per cent lived that long without hormonal therapy. Yet many patients fail to respond to either castration or estrogen, singly or combined, and in relapses these treatments are largely ineffective. This failure is believed due to increased androgenic activity of the adrenals but added bilateral adrenalectomy has to date failed to solve the problem.

In summarizing the treatment of prostatic cancer, it may be said:

(1) When the tumor is limited to the gland, employ radical prostatectomy, preferably perineal, removing the gland, its capsule, the seminal vesicles, and adjacent bladder outlet.

(2) When the tumor growth exceeds the indications for radical perineal prostatectomy, perform castration at once and begin continuous estrogen therapy, 5 mg. or less of diethylstilbestrol according to response.

(3) When the tumor causes grave bladder neck obstruction and does not respond to indwelling catheterization plus castration and estrogen therapy, perform limited transurethral resection to reestablish drainage, or institute permanent suprapubic cystostomy.

While taking estrogens, many men develop tender enlargement of the breasts and nipples, frequently to the size seen in prepubertal girls. It is then necessary to discontinue the estrogen for a week or two or sometimes longer until the exquisite sensitiveness has disappeared with which the breasts will diminish slightly in size.

SARCOMA OF THE PROSTATE

This rare condition is found chiefly in the young, more than half of the 225 cases reported to date being under ten years of age; I have seen it in five young boys. These mesoblastic tumors are histologically identi-

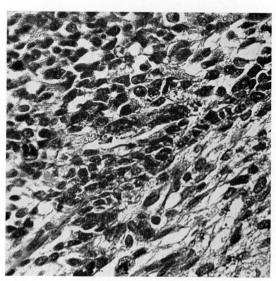

FIGURE 281.   Sarcoma of the prostate in a young boy. Metastases.

fied as adenosarcoma, myosarcoma, cystic myxoma, fibromyoma, round-cell sarcoma, spindle-cell sarcoma, lymphosarcoma, angiosarcoma, fibrosarcoma or rhabdosarcoma. The round-cell tumor is the commonest; it is vascular, spongy, often cystic and characteristically rapid growing. In children the spindle-cell growth is the usual type, invades rapidly, fills the pelvic cavity, and may even cause perineal bulging (Figs. 281, 282). Muscle fibers can be demonstrated in rhabdomyosarcoma, the tumor being derived chiefly from the anterior prostatic commissure containing fibrous tissue and striated muscle cells but may arise elsewhere.

These sarcomas spring from the region of the prostate or bladder neck and I suspect that some of the reported cases may have been of mesodermal trigonal or bladder neck origin rather than prostatic. Yet the hopeless clinical problem is the same. These sarcomas grow rapidly to fill the prostatic area, usually as a soft spongy mass extending up into the bladder and because of their texture have often been misdiagnosed by rectal examination as prostatic abscess. Fibrosarcoma, however, is firm or hard, and may even simulate carcinoma. The soft tumors are grayish or grayish-red on section, often grumous and of brainlike consistency, while the hard, firm tumors are yellowish white and resemble prostatic "adenoma." Carcinoma of the prostate has not been demonstrated under seventeen years of age.

Vascular metastases often occur early in prostatic sarcoma and may be expected in every instance, chiefly to the lungs, liver and skeleton with local spread to the bladder, urethra and rectum. Sometimes the pelvic mass occludes the lower ends of the ureters.

Symptoms of prostatic sarcoma are those of rapidly increasing blad-

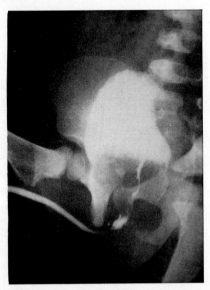

FIGURE 282.   Sarcoma of the prostate. Cystographic demonstration of the great elongation
of the posterior urethra caused by the tumor.

der neck obstruction with vesical overdistention, often with compression closure of the rectum, and terminal uremia, urinary sepsis and exhaustion. The diagnostic clue is the rapidity of the increasing bladder neck obstruction, usually in a young boy. By rectal examination the enlarged gland is usually firm but may suggest abscess. The perineum may bulge or a suprapubic tumor mass may be felt after the bladder has been emptied by catheter. A cysto-urethrogram will show the great filling defect at the vesical outlet as well as compression and elongation of the prostatic urethra (Fig. 282). A specimen for biopsy examination may be obtained by needle aspiration or preferably by transurethral resection.

Treatment. This is usually hopeless because the tumor is so well developed when first recognized. Bilateral cutaneous ureteral transplantation or ureterosigmoidostomy and radical cystoprostatectomy offer the only hope but have apparently succeeded in only two cases, as far as personal perusal of the literature indicates. Radical perineal prostatectomy was once curative in an adult (Young). Radiation therapy accomplishes nothing except temporary palliation with variable but inadequate shrinkage of the tumor. The establishment of permanent cystostomy drainage in the most humane treatment at present for most of these patients who will usually be dead in uremia, toxemia and/or urinary sepsis in two to six months.

TUMORS OF THE SEMINAL VESICLES

These are most rare, are predominantly secondary to prostatic, verumontanum, rectal or adjacent neoplasms, but primary growths may develop in cysts or as benign tumors of the vesicles. Primary malignancy of the seminal vesicles is exceedingly rare. *Cysts* are of müllerian (utricle) or seminal vesicle origin, are predominantly solitary, may grow extremely large and are manifested by pain and/or secondary bladder neck obstruction. The seminal vesicle cyst usually is laterally situated and sometimes contains spermatozoa while the müllerian cyst (utricular) is in the midline and contains no spermatozoa; in each instance the prostate usually feels normal. Some cysts have been demonstrated by radiographic injection. *Treatment* is by perineal excision of small or moderate size cysts, and suprapubic extraperitoneal removal of large cysts.

Benign tumors of the seminal vesicles include myomas, fibromas, and cystadenomas while malignant tumors are chiefly carcinoma in older patients and sarcoma in the younger group. Doubtless some of these tumors actually originate in adjacent tissue.

Symptoms are those of bladder outlet compression and inflammation, even to the point of complete vesical retention.

The diagnosis is suggested by rectal palpation of a mass in the seminal vesicle region—hard or soft according to the nature of the tissue growth. Benign tumors are cured by perineal excision. Malignancy offers a nearly hopeless outlook. Perineal excision of the mass is indicated in the absence of local spread or metastases.

TUMORS OF THE PENIS

Benign. The commonest of these are papilloma (Fig. 283) and condyloma acuminatum or venereal wart; the last is discussed in Chapter 8. Fibroma, adenoma, hemangioma, lipoma, and dermoid cyst have been reported. Excision is the treatment.

Malignant. *Carcinoma* is the usual malignancy of the penis yet comprises only 1 per cent of all urologic cancers. The usual cause is chronic bacterial irritation consequent to phimosis or persistent balanoposthitis. Penile cancer is almost never seen in men who have been circumcised in infancy; a few instances have been observed in Mohammedans who are not circumcised until puberty. A few cases have originated at the site of improper circumcision with infolding of the skin margins. Most patients are between forty and sixty years of age, yet I have seen it in three patients under forty and it has been reported in a two-year-old boy (Creté).

Pathology. The majority of penile cancers are of the papillary carcinoma type originating in a fungating verruca or papilloma. These spread rapidly locally with secondary ulceration of the warty vegetation,

Fig. 283

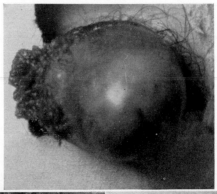

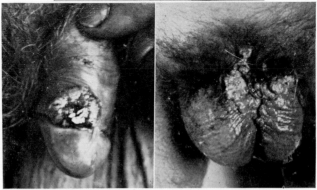

Fig. 284   Fig. 285

FIGURE 283.   Papilloma of the penis.
FIGURE 284.   Epithelioma of the penis.
FIGURE 285.   Cancerous destruction of the penis.

often ulcerating into the urethra, and with metastases to the lymphatics of the groin. The entire glans or the penile body may be ulcerated away, and in extreme cases even to the suspensory ligament (Fig. 285).

Many penile cancers are epidermoid beginning in the margin of a patch of leukoplakia or independent as an ulceration with irregular, raised, hard margins. Commonly these lesions begin at the meatal margin or at the under side of the phimotic prepuce near or at the coronal sulcus (Fig. 284). Histologically these tumors show squamous carcinoma with keratinization and pearly bodies.

Metastases occur primarily to the inguinal and deep femoral nodes or even to the pelvic nodes. This glandular enlargement is prominent in three fourths of the patients when they are first seen. Yet in about half of the cases of penile cancer the inguinal node enlargement is inflammatory adenitis without tumor cells and the swelling disappears following conservative excision of the primary growth.

Symptoms and Diagnosis. As the tumor grows, ulceration is progressive, the part becomes highly sensitive and even painful. With phimosis a purulent, foul, often bloody discharge is noted and there is dysuria with frequency. Untreated, the flat neoplasm progressively extends with ulcerating, ragged, irregular, indurated areas, while the cauliflower type tends to grow to immense size, destroying the phimotic prepuce by gangrene. Eventually penile erosion and necrosis wears it away to the base, including the urethra (Fig. 285). Pyogenic adenitis is prominent and may overshadow underlying inguinal metastases. The suspected lesion should always be widely exposed to sight and palpation employing generous dorsal slit if necessary.

In the *differential diagnosis,* chancroid or soft chancre should cause little confusion with a history of recent intercourse, pronounced inguinal adenitis, demonstration of the Ducrey organisms in the lesion and rapid cure with antibiotics, especially Aureomycin. In luetic chancre, the Wassermann test is positive, the darkfield examination may be, and the lesion is universally indurated. If doubt still exists, the biopsy examination of the removed skin margin is definitive, cancer being found when it is present. Tuberculous ulceration is most rare and there are coexisting tuberculous urogenital lesions.

It is a good rule to consider all penile growths as malignant until proved otherwise.

Treatment. Lesions at the glans not over 2 cm. in diameter and without inguinal metastases may be treated by interstitial radon implantation or by external radon pack or plaque application and some will be cured. In lesions not over this size, conservative penile amputation is a better choice, removing the organ well into healthy tissue, at least an inch proximal to the growth. When large fungating, infected or ulcerating growths are primarily removed, the lymphatic adenitis (especially pelvic) commonly disappears but leaving enlarged hard nodules when they are cancerous.

When the lesion is large and there are histologically demonstrated metastases in the groin, perform radical penectomy with dissection of the inguinal lymphatics, not overlooking the node(s) in the femoral canal (Cloquet's nodes). The urethra is transplanted to the perineum to open anterior to the anus. It is unnecessary to castrate these patients; it is sufficient to split the scrotum widely and preserve it and its contents.

Prognosis. The cure rate after conservative partial penile amputation or radon therapy is about 40 per cent after five years (Dean). In advanced cases requiring extensive inguinal lymph node excision, the apparent cure rate is not over 10 per cent.

Sarcoma of the penis is most rare, about forty cases having been reported, and these showed a great variety of histology: fibrosarcoma, spindle, mixed or round cell sarcoma, endothelioma and even melanosarcoma. In most instances these tumors originated in the tissues of the corpora cavernosa although in infants and children, of which there have been a dozen cases, the site of origin is usually undetermined. The growth forms a palpable tumor mass which on histologic examination shows sarcoma. The symptoms are those of the mass plus the urethral obstruction it causes. Amputation, preferably radical, is the treatment and the outlook is always unfavorable.

TUMORS OF THE URETHRA

Small benign urethral polyps or papillomas are frequently encountered but other new growths are rare. Of the benign tumors, the vascular growths—angioma, hemangioma or varices—may cause pronounced urethral bleeding and may require electrocoagulation or transurethral excision. Fibroma, myoma and fibromyoma have been observed, cause urethral obstruction in some cases and must be excised, usually by the transurethral procedure.

Polyps form as hyperplasias consequent to continuous irritation by infection of the urethral mucous membranes. They often give rise to a chronic urethral gleety discharge but rarely cause obstruction and seldom bleed except with instrumental trauma. Polyps sometimes spring from the verumontanum. These growths have a tendency to be pedunculated and especially in the anterior urethra. I removed one from a ten month old boy; it protruded from the meatus on voiding, was more than 2 cm. long and arose on the urethral roof about 1.5 cm. from the meatus. The diagnosis is usually made by cysto-urethroscopy and the treatment is electrocoagulation or electroexcision.

Papillomas are usually of delicate structure but may develop in mass formation; they bleed readily, may cause obstruction, urinary frequency and dysuria and even undergo malignant change.

In the *female* the urethral growth may protrude from the meatus or back into the bladder outlet. The treatment is electrocoagulation through a urethroscope or transurethral resection. Urethral polyps in the female are clinically similar to papillomas but are of somewhat denser structure, the fibrovascular center of the polyp being covered with urethral urothelium and occasionally showing some gland formations.

Caruncle is a variety of benign highly vascular tumor frequently appearing in the meatus of the female urethra. Usually the growth is a collection of blood vessels covered by squamous epithelium, sometimes making a polypoid mass whose character will depend greatly upon the density of the squamous covering. Its appearance is bright reddish when the covering is thin and dark bluish or gray when thick (vascular granuloma, papillary angioma or telangiectatic polyp). Occasionally the lesion bleeds and there is always the possibility that neoplastic change may occur.

The *etiology* of caruncle is uncertain; chronic irritation or inflammation has been advanced as an explanation. Urethral stricture or urethral angulation consequent to cystocele or vesical prolapse has been thought to interfere with the urethral circulation to promote vascular stasis and the development of varicosities distal to the site of vascular interference and chiefly at the meatus.

Symptoms attributable to caruncle are absent in about half of the cases while in the others the lesion may be exquisitely sensitive to touch, cause persistent pain, reflex urinary frequency and dysuria, hematuria if there is ulceration and, if large enough, cause variable urinary obstruction.

The *diagnosis* is made by inspection but before attempting excision of the growth, a urethroscopic examination is advised that the extent of the lesion into the urethra be determined for complete excision. Electroloop excision of the tumor with coagulation of the base is the preferred treatment as it does a more complete removal than by cutting with a scalpel after which recurrence is much more frequent.

If the caruncle extends deeply into the urethra, use the resectoscope until complete removal has been achieved. Always send an "uncooked" piece of the excised tumor for microscopic examination lest an early malignancy be overlooked.

Carcinoma of the Urethra. Primary carcinoma of the male urethra is extremely rare, usually develops at the site of a stricture but has been known to begin in a papilloma, or in a fistula or in an area of leukoplakia. Most of these tumors begin in the bulbous urethra, seldom in the anterior or prostatic segments. Half of the reported cases have been of the squamous-cell variety, a sixth were adenocarcinoma, and only a small number have been of the columnar-cell type. The tumor may grow slow or fast, with metastases to the deep pelvic glands and sometimes to the inguinal nodes. The youngest reported patient was twenty-two years of age, most being between forty and sixty-five years.

Secondary urethral cancer is an extension from neighboring lesions in the penis, prostate, bladder or rectum.

Urethral cancers usually spread rapidly, causing at first a blood-tinged mucoid discharge but later frank bleeding, urethral blockage with frequency, burning, pain and dysuria. The stony hard lesion may be palpable and may be seen by urethroscopy. Examination of a biopsy specimen should clinch the diagnosis. The Papanicolaou stain of urinary sediment may be further confirmatory.

Treatment. Partial penile amputation 2.5 cm. proximal to the tumor may suffice when the lesion is near the urethral meatus but in most instances radical excision is demanded, shunting the uninvaded deep urethral segment to drain into the posterior perineum. Some small lesions have apparently been cured by interstitial radon irradiation but this is an even more uncertain method than excision. In general the prognosis is always grave and in over half the cases is hopeless when the patient is first seen. Yet a slow growing basal cell epithelioma offers better hope of cure than a young, rapidly growing, prickle-cell epithelioma.

Carcinoma of the female urethra is less frequent than that in the male, dense stricture and urethral fistulization being comparatively less common in women. Occasionally carcinoma develops at the site of leukoplakia or in a polyp; most are squamous cell type, the adenocarcinoma variety being thought to originate in periurethral gland structures. These growths must be sharply differentiated from tumors originating in the introitus, vulva or other adjacent tissues. The *symptoms* are those observed in the male with cancer of the urethra—hematuria, pain, dysuria, frequency and, when the growth is large enough, urinary obstruction. While the condition may suggest tuberculosis, urethral calculus, stricture or benign growth, urethroscopy may give a clue and examination of a biopsy specimen will disclose neoplasm.

Treatment. In early cases limited resection of the urethral tumor and radon implantation have been curative while in more advanced growths radical removal with establishment of permanent cystostomy may be indicated. When the growth exceeds this indication, the prognosis is hopeless and only palliative drainage by suprapubic or urethral catheter is warranted.

Sarcoma of the Urethra. These extremely rare tumors afflict men and women about equally, the histology usually being that of round-cell sarcoma, fibrosarcoma, myxosarcoma or lymphosarcoma, most often in a patient under twenty-five years of age. Some of the reported cases have been infants. In a thirty-year-old patient of mine, the fatal tumor was a melanosarcoma which comprises about a fourth of all urethral sarcomas. The differential diagnosis is made by microscopic examination of removed tissue. Radical excision, often including the bladder, (with ureterosigmoidostomy) is the treatment. Irradiation offers little help, but no aid, even though only palliative, should be overlooked.

TUMORS OF THE SCROTUM

Benign. Polyps, fibromas, adenomas, lipomas of the scrotum are most rare. Hemangiomas, usually congenital, are observed slightly more often; I have seen two instances in young boys. Excision is the treatment.

Malignant. The cancer, known in older days as the "chimney sweep's cancer," results from constant and prolonged irritation—chemical, bacterial or friction of clothing—the tumor beginning, appearing and spreading like penile carcinoma (q.v.). The growth may be cauliflower-like but is usually ulcerative. Basal cell growths, fibrosarcoma and other variations of malignant scrotal tumors have been reported. The symptoms are largely pain, bleeding ulceration, and a foul odor. The diagnosis is suspected upon seeing and feeling the hard margins and base of the growth, and a biopsy examination is confirmatory. Radical excision is the usual treatment removing the regional inguinal lymph nodes as well. Radiation therapy by radon plaque or gold seed interstitial implantation is unreliable but x-ray radiation is sometimes applied following surgery with due care to protect the testicles.

TUMORS OF THE TUNICA VAGINALIS

These are extremely rare. Benign growths include fibroma, myoma, lipoma, adenoma and angioma. Cysts, spermatoceles, hematoceles and hydroceles may simulate malignant intrascrotal tumors and are identified at operation. The *malignant* growths are chiefly rapidly growing sarcomas. There is scrotal enlargement, the overlying skin becomes tense, shiny, and the vessels engorged. The scrotum feels heavier than with hydrocele of comparable size yet the testis and epididymis are uninvolved. Wide excision is the treatment and a poor prognosis is warranted.

TUMORS OF THE TESTICLE

These comprise about 1.0 per cent of all malignant neoplasms in males, accounting for at least one in every thousand male hospital admissions. At least 95 per cent of testicular tumors are malignant (Fig. 286). Most of these growths appear in the prime of life, chiefly between twenty-five and forty-five years of age, although they have been found in the seventh decade; true sarcoma as well as carcinoma and embryoma have been found in infants and young children, nearly all of these tumors in this age group being congenital and derived from totipotent sex cells. They may be bilateral, present even at birth, and the majority are teratomatous.

The wide range of descriptive designation indicates the histologic patterns observed in these testicular tumors, the benign variety are given in the following paragraph: the malignant growths include embryonal carcinoma, chorio-epithelioma or choriocarcinoma, seminoma, sarcoma, interstitial cell tumors, and a wide variety of mixed sarcomatous tissues.

Benign Tumors. These rare growths are chiefly fibroma, leioma, leiomyoma, adenoma, lipoma, lymphangioma, hemangioma, dermoid and rhabdomyoma. If large enough, they cause scrotal swelling but seldom pain. There may be a dull ache from mass weight and drag on the spermatic cord. Excision is the treatment.

Malignant Tumors. Most cancerous tumors of the testicle originate in the organ itself, are highly malignant and, for purposes of classification, these growths have been recently and satisfactorily grouped by Dixon and Moore as given in Table 17.

Testicular tumors apparently of a single structure are believed by

Ewing to represent a one-sided development of a tridermal teratoma (embryonal carcinoma, sarcoma, or mixed), while Chevassu and others have noted that a large portion of these solid medullary growths are comprised of large cells whose morphology and staining reactions correspond to cells of spermatoblastic origin, hence the name *seminoma*. In children tumors of the testicle are usually mixed cell or embryomatous; seminomas are exceedingly rare in the young and occur only in older boys. Seminoma and embryonal carcinoma comprise more than two thirds of all malignant testicular tumors and are believed by many to originate in the lining epithelium of the spermatic tubules. Yet this is not always true, for in some cases teratomatous elements are found. These cancers often begin in the region of the rete testis and spread to the testicle or sometimes to the epididymis.

Seminomas are composed of rounded, clear, sharp-bordered polyhedral cells and are believed to originate from primordial germinal cells (Figs. 286, 287). The structure of the soft, highly cellular seminoma is made up of innumerable larger cells and scant reticulum. The average age of their victims is five or six years older than that for other testicular neoplasms, their growth being slower and less invasive. They rarely give a positive Aschheim-Zondek test (Mostofi), and are highly sensitive to irradiation. As a rule 1500–2000 r (roentgen units) destroy the tumor and correspondingly improve the prognosis, a 50 to 60 per cent cure rate having been achieved in some clinics which is higher than for any of the other malignant testicular tumors.

Embryonal carcinoma (embryonal adenocarcinoma, papillary adenocarcinoma) has been found at all ages, as young as four months. The origin of these growths from totipotent cells is generally accepted by most authorities, the growth showing tridermal structure with predominantly embryonal anaplastic cells but some adult cell types may also be seen (Fig. 288). The presence of chorionic gonadotropins in the urine in some

TABLE 17.   CLASSIFICATION OF TUMORS OF THE TESTIS
(Dixon and Moore, 1952)

A. *Germinal Tumors* (96.5 per cent of testis tumors)
    I. Seminoma, pure
   II. Embryonal carcinoma, pure or with seminoma.
  III. Teratoma, pure or with seminoma
  IV. Teratoma and either embryonal carcinoma or choriocarcinoma or both and with or without seminoma.
   V. Choriocarcinoma, pure or with either seminoma or embryonal carcinoma or both.

B. *Nongerminal Tumors* (3.5 per cent of testis tumors)
    I. Gonadal (strictly)
      a. Interstitial cell tumors
      b. Androblastomas
      c. Rete carcinomas
   II. Tumors similar to counterparts elsewhere in the body: fibroma, angioma, neurofibroma, adenomatoid tumors and fibrosarcoma.
    Other nongonadal tumors (rhabdomyoma, rhabdomyosarcoma, chondroma, chondrosarcoma) probably represent a one-sided development of teratomas.

of these cases indicates the trophoblastic origin of the tumors. They commonly give a strong Aschheim-Zondek reaction.

Embryonal carcinomas of the testicle grow rapidly and spread through the lymphatics to involve the spermatic cord. They will be fatal unless conquered promptly by excision. They are radioresistant and their prognosis is always poor.

Chorioepitheliomas or **choriocarcinomas** are derived from trophoblastic cells, present a rapidly growing, soft, red hemorrhagic tumor which elaborates a feminizing hormone to cause gynecomastia and kindred manifestations (Fig. 289). These tumors grow and spread most rapidly, chiefly through the veins, and are practically always fatal.

The **interstitial cell tumor** of the testis is composed chiefly of Leydig cells. In addition to its local growth, it secretes a virilizing hormone causing *pubertas praecox;* several instances have been reported in recent years. This tumor should be ruled out when sexual prematurity appears in a young boy. Interstitial-cell tumors occurring in adults are seldom hormone producing (Mostofi). *Alveolar carcinoma* of the testis has been observed to behave similar to interstitial-cell cancer in young boys.

Fig. 287

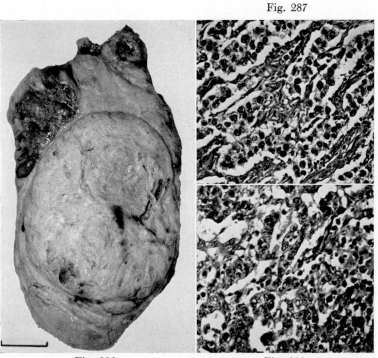

Fig. 286   Fig. 288

FIGURE 286.   Seminoma of the testis. The cystic changes in the lower segment of the gland suggest a teratomatous lesion but microscopically only seminoma tissue was found.

FIGURE 287.   Seminoma of the testicle. Histology. (Courtesy Armed Forces Institute of Pathology.)

FIGURE 288.   Embryonal carcinoma of the testicle. (Courtesy Armed Forces Institute of Pathology.)

Teratomas. These neoplasms usually contain structures derived from all three germ layers in great mixture—cysts, epithelial derivatives, glands, cartilage and other mesenchymal derivatives (Fig. 290). Rarely the teratoma is "adult" or histologically nonmalignant. Teratomas are likely to be more solid than a seminoma, are lumpy depending upon the structure with hyaline, cartilage and cystic masses; there may be chorionic villi present and chorio-epithelioma may develop. As a rule teratomas grow slowly, metastasize late, the metastatic lesion being monocellular in half the cases. They neither give a positive Aschheim-Zondek reaction nor are they radiosensitive. Yet if recognized early and removed promptly, the prognosis is generally good.

Teratocarcinoma. Friedman and Moore use this designation for a large group of tumors composed of nonmalignant and malignant structures, mixtures of teratoma, carcinoma, choriocarcinoma, neurocarcinoma, epithelioma and sarcoma. These growths usually give a strongly positive Aschheim-Zondek test and are largely radioresistant. Their prognosis lies between the poor outlook of embryonal carcinoma and the fair prospects in seminoma.

Etiology. Trauma has long been held to be an accessory factor in testicular tumor development. Such a history is given in at least two thirds of the cases but the injury only directs attention to the small previously unrecognized nodule.

Testicular ectopia, particularly in the abdomen, has been noted in about one in eight cases of testicular neoplasm at Memorial Hospital

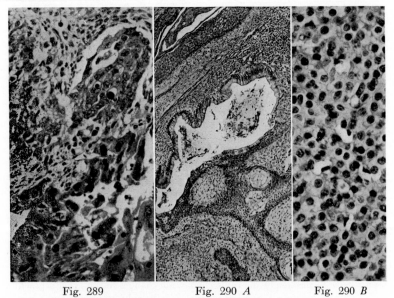

Fig. 289   Fig. 290 *A*   Fig. 290 *B*

FIGURE 289. Choriocarcinoma of the testis.
FIGURE 290.   *A* and *B*, teratoma testis.
(Courtesy Armed Forces Institute of Pathology.)

in New York, occurring in 15 per cent of teratomas in Dean's series at this institution. Yet neoplasm has developed in testicles, previously cryptorchid, properly placed surgically in the scrotum. This emphasizes the congenital faulty testicular structure which may predispose to malignant change.

Tumor Spread. Lymphatic extension from testicular neoplasms occurs along the spermatic cord to the deep iliac lymphatic chain, thence upward along the preaortic retroperitoneal nodes to the epigastrium, mediastinum and via the thoracic duct to the left subclavian vein, with numerous lymphatic tributaries and connections along the way. In the left supraclavicular region the signal node of Virchow is the evil sign of hopeless metastases. The paralumbar metastatic lymphatic mass may cause isolateral backache which in a young male merits special investigation. Blood-borne metastases are predominantly to, and are radiographically demonstrable in, the lungs (Fig. 253). Such metastases are the patient's death warrant.

Tumors of the testicle are seldom bilateral except when congenital in infancy.

Symptoms. Testicular enlargement and increased density or hardness, appearing slowly and painlessly at first, yet maintaining the smooth proportions of the organ, are the initial manifestations. Later the enlarging growth becomes irregular and nodular. The weight of the testicular mass dragging on the spermatic cord causes an ache in the groin and over the hip. The patient may attribute his symptoms to some recent trauma. Intestinal compression by metastatic tumor masses, especially in the epigastrium, may cause constipation and nutritional disturbances. Gynecomastia and other evidence of feminization suddenly appearing reflects chorionic gonadotropin secretion by the trophoblastic tumor. Under these conditions, in some reported cases, a previously cryptorchid testicular mate has descended to the scrotum. Rapid enlargement of an inguinal testicle should suggest neoplasm; when the testicle is intra-abdominal backache is apt to be the first symptom, and later the mass itself causes distress. Yet by this time metastases have usually been recognized.

As in prostatic carcinomas, the size of the primary growth bears little relation to the extent and complexity of its metastases. Hydrocele commonly develops locally and may make the testicle and epididymis undistinguishable from each other unless the fluid is aspirated. Tumor of an intra-abdominal testicle may present a palpable mass or may compress the bladder or adjacent intestine.

Diagnosis. More than four fifths of patients with testicular neoplasm have metastasis when they are first examined; metastases may be palpable in the abdomen, especially epigastric nodes. The signal node of Virchow may be palpable in the supraclavicular fossa or the patient may have an isolateral backache. In any event the scrotum should be examined. The patient should be undressed and varicocele, scrotal enlargement or visible metastases noted. The scrotal skin is loose and of normal color until stretched by the enlarged tumor mass which makes it tense, red, and shiny. The large scrotal mass may seem to cause penile shortening.

Palpation of the testicular mass must be most gentle to avoid squeezing tumor cells into the circulation. Distinguish between the testicle and the epididymis. Aspirate hydrocele fluid if necessary for accurate palpation. Papanicolaou stain of cells in the hydrocele fluid may disclose malignant ones. The tumor-bearing testis feels harder and heavier than normal. Lumpiness in the tumor may be due to cystic masses, a mass of soft medullary tissue, or a piece of cartilage, for example. Usually the spermatic cord feels tumor free. A negative Wassermann rules out gumma.

Excretory urograms may demonstrate low lumbar metastases with dislocation of the ureter or even the kidney. Chest roentgenograms must be made to demonstrate metastases, which are generally of the "cotton ball" type (Fig. 253). Gynecomastia may be present. The Aschheim-Zondek test is positive only in tumors containing trophoblastic tissue, readings of less than 500 mouse units per liter being of no significance. Yet once positive, a continuously negative Aschheim-Zondek test following surgical treatment augurs a good prognosis, but becoming first negative then later positive signifies tumor recurrence.

Differential Diagnosis. The majority of true testicular enlargements are tumors. The *differential diagnosis* includes hydrocele, spermatocele, tuberculous epididymitis, syphilis, orchitis (gummatous type) or, most rarely, neoplasm of the epididymis, cord or tunica vaginalis. When the testicular tumor elaborates a gonadotropic hormone (prolan) as many of them do, it appears in the urine and offers a laboratory test which, when positive in the presence of testicular swelling, points to malignancy. The concentration of prolan is even higher in the hydrocele fluid accompanying testicular neoplasm. Injected into young virgin rats or mice, prolan causes (1) graafian follicle maturation, (2) graafian follicular hemorrhage, (3) follicular luteinization, (4) engorgement of the uterus and cornua similar in all respects to the positive pregnancy test (Aschheim-Zondek, Friedman, and others). A positive test is normal in teratoma and embryonal carcinoma but may be negative in pure seminoma.

Treatment. Removal of the testicular tumor and spermatic cord up to the external inguinal ring is the treatment in growths without evident involvement of the spermatic cord or distant structures. To prevent surgical dissemination of tumor, the cord should be clamped and ligated first at the point of its division at the external inguinal ring and the cord stump anchored with the ligating suture to the adjacent fascia. The distal cord and scrotal contents including the tunica vaginalis are removed by simple gentle blunt dissection. To incise the tumor at any point loses all hope of cure for the patient.

When initially there is reason to believe the tumor has spread upward but not hopelessly, a radical orchidectomy is performed removing the tumor, cord and the continuous lymphatic chain as high as the renal pedicle and some more radical surgeons even enter the mediastinum. The operative mortality of the radical procedure ranges from 2 per cent (Lewis) to 12 per cent (Hinman).

Examination of the conservatively removed specimen may show there is tumor spread up the lymphatics and presumably to the iliac and lumbar nodes, to form large masses along the aorta and vena cava extending to the renal pelvis or still higher to the mediastinum, and even to the skull and brain. This presents a surgically hopeless problem.

Radiation Therapy. The value of radiation will depend primarily on the radiosensitivity of the tumor and secondarily on the extent of extratesticular spread. The probable response may be estimated by a preoperative radiation dose of 1500 r; a week later the tumor is removed and histologically examined.

Seminomas are among the most radiosensitive of all neoplasms and may be expected to be cured by application of 1500 r to all portions of the growth to a total of at least 3000 r each. Yet even a small amount of nonsensitive tumor tissue in the growth makes the outlook bad. Embryonal carcinoma, for example, requires a minimum of 5000 to 6000 r to kill the tumor cell but this mammoth dose is hazardous to use because of great tissue injuries: cutaneous and intestinal gangrene, intestinal perforation or other late grave irradiation effects. In short, in seminoma employ intensive preoperative irradiation, remove the tumor, and follow with postoperative irradiation, even though extratesticular tumor is present. Irradiation of metastases in the chest, neck, skull or a palpable metastatic mass elsewhere is fruitless. In embryonal carcinoma or malignant teratomatous tumors, the outlook even with intensive irradiation is bad. Radiation has no place in the treatment of choriocarcinoma.

The results of *radiation plus surgery* are much better than with surgery alone. The prospects of cure under the best of conditions are indicated by the results obtained in 364 patients at Memorial Hospital as reported by Dean.

Prognosis. This should always be guarded in testicular neoplasms. In Dean's series of 322 testicular tumors of all varieties treated by orchiectomy and irradiation, 199 or 37 per cent were apparently cured five years or more postoperative.

TUMORS OF THE EPIDIDYMIS

These are rare, are in general like those of the testicle (q.v.), occur during the period of greatest sexual activity, and may be benign or malignant.

Benign tumors include angioma, myoma, lipoma, cystadenoma, adenomyoma, and dermoid, the first two being the most often encountered. There is an intrascrotal mass, often with nontransilluminating hydrocele, but the precise diagnosis will seldom be made without microscopic examination. Epididymectomy is the treatment of benign tumors.

Malignant tumors of the epididymis are chiefly adenocarcinomatous; sarcoma, predominantly fibrosarcoma, occurs a third as often. Usually these tumors enlarge rapidly to encompass the testicle in the growth so that the two structures cannot be clearly differentiated by palpation. The treatment is that of testicular neoplasm with removal of the testis, epididymis and cord at least to the external inguinal ring and with post-operative radiation therapy. The prognosis in general is bad.

TUMORS OF THE VAS DEFERENS AND SPERMATIC CORD

These are generally secondary to testicular growths, yet primary tumors, though rare, have been observed, sometimes originating in embryonal cell rests. In many instances the growth has involved the lower cord and epididymis so that the origin could not be determined. Three fourths of these rare tumors are *benign;* fibrolipoma is the most frequent; others include lipoma, fibroma, myxolipoma, myxofibroma, neurofibroma, cystadenoma, myoma, angioma, hemangioma, chondroma, lymphangioma, teratoma, dermoids, and even tumors originating in adrenal rests. The *malignant* tumors are predominantly sarcomatous—fibrosarcoma, leiosarcoma, myosarcoma, rhabdomyosarcoma, sarcoma, reticulosarcoma, myxochondrosarcoma—but even carcinoma has been found. As these tumors grow they may suggest hernia or even hydrocele or cysts of the cord. Benign tumors may be dissected free but when there is any question of malignancy, remove the cord high and the scrotal contents as in seminoma. This must be done when the growth is definitely malignant and, if possible, without opening the tunica vaginalis. Radiation therapy is unreliable but is usually indicated following surgery with due care to protect the opposite testicle.

CHAPTER 13 *The Adrenals*

THE ADRENAL glands, the hormones of which are essential to life, are an integral part of the urogenital system. This is because of (1) the common embryonic origin of the adrenal cortex in conjunction with the urogenital tract, (2) the dominant hormonal influence of the adrenals in the development and function of the gonads and genitalia and, (3) their frequently associated disease processes. Histologically, embryologically and functionally the adrenals consist of two distinct glands: (1) the *cortex* whose hormones in addition to the androgenic content are largely concerned with the maintenance of electrolyte and nutritional balance in the body, and (2) the *medulla* whose hormones (epinephrine and norepinephrine) are concerned chiefly with circulatory and neuromuscular balance (Fig. 291).

Anatomy. The adrenals, one on each side, lie just above the kidneys as flattened, irregular surfaced, encapsulated, rather triangular structures, encased in the perirenal fascia and loosely joined to the kidney on each side by connective tissue. The adrenal blood supply is generous, and often anomalous, from the superior adrenal branch of the inferior phrenic artery and from the inferior adrenal branches of the renal artery and aorta.

The adrenal cortex which comprises 90 per cent of the gland weight (3–5 gm. in adults) is yellow because of lipid filled cells, and has three zones (Fig. 291):

1. *Zona glomerulosa* or outer zone, in alveolar arrangement of irregularly clustered, rapidly dividing cells which are believed to be the youngest or the generative cells in cortical growth.
2. *Zona fasciculata.* This, the widest zone, is composed of radially arranged columns of large clear cells. Medially to this zone is the
3. *Zona reticularis* composed of the older cells in the cortex. It lies

511

next to the medulla as a thin network of fuchsinophilic granule-containing cells believed to be the dominant androgenic cells of the adrenal.

The *medulla* is composed of an extremely rich cluster of vascular sinuses surrounding which are strands of irregularly shaped chromophilic (chromate-staining) cells.

Embryology.   *Cortex.*   About the sixth week of fetal life the cortex is derived as a chain of cell buds from mesodermal cells of the ventral portion of the celomic epithelium. As they grow, they extend between the mesonephros and mesentery into the celomic cavity, later fusing into a cell mass lateral to the aorta on each side to become the cortex. Adrenal

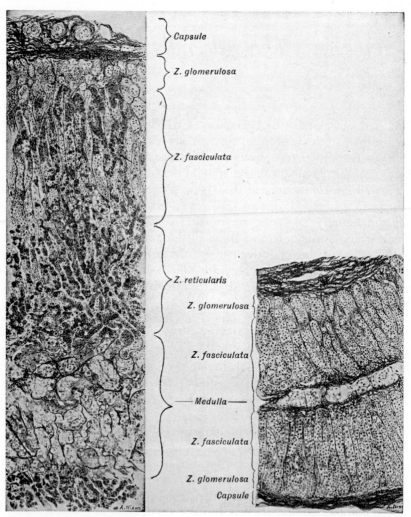

FIGURE 291.   Section of an adrenal (left) of a man and (right) of a six month infant. Mallory-azan stain. About 105 ×. (From Maximow and Bloom, Textbook of Histology, ed. 7.)

buds which do not become incorporated in the cortex disappear, or are found as *interrenal* or *accessory bodies* (Marchand) near the adrenals, kidneys, testes, ovaries, along the retroperitoneal fascia, spermatic vessels or broad ligaments, and are believed by some to be the true cells of hypernephroma (q.v.).

Medulla. This originates in sympathogonia, the ectoblastic formative sympathetic nervous system cells, some of which later develop as sympathoblasts, and from which the sympathetic nervous system is derived. Other sympathogonia become the primative chromaffin cells—the pheochromoblasts. Maturing, these become the pheochromocytes and chromaffin cells of the adrenal and the accessory chromophilic retroperitoneal paraganglia along the aorta, at the bifurcation of the carotid, in Zuckerkandl's body at the bifurcation of the aorta and at the sacrococcygeal body. *These extra-adrenal bodies may become the site of tumors like those of the adrenal.*

By the seventh week the large sympathochromaffin cell body invaginates into or becomes completely engulfed by the developing cortex to complete formation of the fetal adrenal. Adrenal growth is then rapid so that by the fourth month the glands are larger than the kidneys, but, with increased renal growth, at birth the adrenals are only one third renal size. In this relative decrease in adrenal size, involution of the middle and inner cortical zones occurs, but with a fetal cortical layer remaining at birth between the zona reticularis and the medulla. This intermediary layer normally disappears by the end of the first year but, persisting and androgenic, is believed to be a factor in the genesis of the adrenogenital syndrome (q.v.).

Anomalies of the adrenals are frequently seen: *Agenesis* in monsters; *unilateral absence* or *hypoplasia* in a third of the cases of isolateral renal agenesis or hypoplasia, respectively; *ectopic* or *cystic; heterotopia,* the inclusion of the entire gland beneath the renal capsule, occurs more often in males and the gland may thus unwittingly be removed by nephrectomy.

Physiology. About thirty steroid compounds have been isolated from the adrenal cortex, six of which will support life in the adrenalectomized animal and for many months in man. These six are: 11-dehydrocorticosterone (compound A); corticosterone (compound B); cortisone (17-dehydroxy-11-dehydrocorticosterone, compound E); hydrocortisone (17-hydrocorticosterone, compound F, the chief natural product); desoxycorticosterone (compound DOC); and progesterone.

Following total adrenalectomy and unless adequate replacement therapy is properly instituted, there occurs: thirst, nausea, vomiting, muscular weakness, falling blood pressure, tachycardia, coma and death. Deficiency symptoms can be temporarily alleviated with sodium chloride and carbohydrates plus proper corticosteroid replacement.

The adrenocortical hormones mainly regulate:

1. *Electrolyte imbalance,* via desoxycorticosterone (DOC) with re-

tention of sodium, chloride and water; elimination of potassium and phosphorus, maintenance of blood pressure, and capillary permeability.

2. *Carbohydrate metabolism* is regulated chiefly by hydrocortisone (compound F), cortisone (compound E), corticosterone (compound B), and dehydrocorticosterone (compound A). These glycogenetic compounds cause the deaminization of the protein intake and its conversion to carbohydrate which in excess hormonal activity, overloads the liver and becomes deposited in the tissues as fat as in Cushing's syndrome (q.v.).

Excess hydrocorticosterone and cortisone may increase sodium excretion and lead to a negative sodium balance—the opposite of the action of desoxycorticosterone acetate (DOCA). Excess of this group (E, F) decreases uric acid, renal clearance, causes a reduction of circulating lymphocytes and fixed lymphoid tissues, and almost complete elimination of circulating eosinophiles. This effect of excess adrenal corticosteroids on fixed and circulating defensive tissues, appreciably lowers resistance to trauma and particularly to infection.

Protein anabolism and growth is largely controlled by steroids of the androgen structure (androadrenosterone, dehydroisoandrosterone) which in excess cause pronounced masculinization, muscular development and growth, but are not as androgenic as testosterone. Yet these adrenal androgens cause a retention of phosphorus, potassium, nitrogen, and sulfate and are concerned with body growth, development of the external genitalia, axillary and pubic hair. In hypersecretion with sexual masculine precocity in either sex, an increase of fuchsinophilic granules in the cells of the zona reticularis has been noted.

Estrogenic steroids (chiefly estrone and progesterone) are normally produced by the adrenal cortex and are estimated by urinary assay. In excess they may influence development to produce, among other things, gynecomastia.

The administration of the pituitary *adrenocorticotrophic hormone* (ACTH) causes increased production of all varieties of adrenal hormones and was formerly widely used in the treatment of rheumatic arthritides in particular. It has now been largely replaced by synthetic hydrocortisone.

The 17-ketosteroids. As found in the urine they represent metabolized corticoid (androgenic) hormones. In the female they represent the entire androgenic output, and in the male the combined adrenal (two thirds) and testicular (one third) output. The normal total 17-ketosteroid output in males in twenty-four hours is 8 to 20 mg. with an average of 15 mg., and in the female 6 to 16 mg. with an average of 10 mg. This is *increased* in adrenal hyperplasia as in the adrenogenital syndrome, cortical hormonal tumors, especially carcinoma, interstitial cell tumors of the testicle, precocious puberty caused by a hypothalamic lesion and to a less degree after major surgery, injury (trauma), exercise, or high fever. The 17-ketosteroid output is *reduced* in Addison's disease, eunuchoidism, hypopituitarism, starvation, or prolonged illness. In adrenocortical deficiency, melanin pigment deposit regularly occurs in the skin as in Addison's disease.

Adrenal exhaustion. This results from prolonged excessive demands on the two glands as it occurs in severe toxemia, burns, crush injuries, excessive surgery or with unrecognized adrenal hypoplasia, for example. Selye (1947) designated this as the *General Adaptation Syndrome* in which, with progressive corticoid depletion, there is progressively: (1) alarm reaction with a large output of corticoid hormones; (2) stage of resistance; (3) an exhaustion stage. During this sequence, the gland undergoes histologic changes in turn: (1) compensatory hypertrophy with loss of histochemical granules, (2) later increase in granular cells and, finally, (3) cellular degeneration with hemolysis, round cell infiltration and corticonecrosis. Special interest has focused on the preoperative preparation and continued support with adrenocorticosteroids (chiefly hydrocortisone and cortisone) in addition to the usual therapeutic care during surgical treatment in feeble, elderly and/or gravely ill patients.

The medulla secretes *epinephrine* and *norepinephrine* which represents 80 and 20 per cent respectively of its total hormonal output. *The medulla is not essential to life.* The physiologic effects of epinephrine and norepinephrine are comparatively shown in Table 18.

Hyperactivity of the medulla is manifested by paroxysmal hypertension while hypoactivity results in hypotension, lassitude, muscular weakness and in chronic adrenal deficiency, Addison's disease syndrome.

Under resting conditions, the sympathetic system activity largely represents norepinephrine influence while under medullary stimulation epinephrine is the dominant factor. Hormonal tumors of the medulla produce both epinephrine and norepinephrine, the symptoms largely reflecting the composition of the abnormally elaborated hormone mixture.

TABLE 18.   EFFECTS OF EPINEPHRINE AND NOREPINEPHRINE

	EPINEPHRINE	NOREPINEPHRINE
Cardiac output (increased strength of contraction)	+	±
Peripheral resistance (arteriolar contraction)	−	+
Systolic blood pressure	+	+
Diastolic blood pressure	±	+
Renal blood flow	−	−
Oxygen consumption	+	±
Hyperglycemia	+	±
Central nervous system stimulation	+	±
Eosinopenia	+	±

+ = increase;   − = decrease;   ± = equivocal in physiologic dosage.

ADRENOCORTICAL INSUFFICIENCY

Acute. This occurs as a crisis associated with or consequent to:

1. *Adrenal injury* from hemorrhage, infection or exhaustion of the gland following compensatory overactivity induced by burns, trauma, prolonged shock or, notably in infants under one year of age, from spontaneous hemorrhage into the adrenal without infection. It is also seen in children with meningococcemia (Waterhouse-Friderichsen syndrome, purpura fulminans); fulminating septicemia or bacteremia with pneumococci, staphylococci or streptococci; in scarlet fever, diphtheria and other overwhelming infections. The traumatic variety is most often seen following breech presentations but also in adults with severe traumatic injury to the gland. Yet the condition may occur without hemorrhage, there being simply a massive cortical necrosis.

Symptoms of acute adrenocortical insufficiency appear with sudden onset, nausea, vomiting, high fever, cyanosis, abdominal pain, shock, cold and clammy skin, rapid thready pulse, labored respirations, and falling blood pressure. Terminally in the bacteremia varieties, there are usually petechial and purpuric eruptions which may form large ecchymoses as the patient fails.

2. *Adrenal crisis* may occur in patients with chronic Addison's disease and exhaustion of their remaining functioning cortex. The symptoms, except for bacterial rash, are in general those listed in the preceding paragraph. *The patient is always an acute medical emergency and no time should be lost.* There is hypoglycemia, azotemia, hyponatremia and hyperkalemia.

Crisis consequent to congenital adrenal hypoplasia is physiologically similar to that occurring in late Addison's disease. It appears chiefly in female pseudohermaphrodites or in macrogenitosomia praecox in males in whom, despite cortical hyperplasia (dyscorticism) there is often adrenal insufficiency with salt and water loss and circulatory collapse. Several instances in early infancy have been reported.

3. Surgery of the adrenal gland may precipitate crisis when a hyperfunctioning tumor or a mass of cortex is removed and the remaining adrenocortical tissue, through inadequate compensation, is insufficient, atrophic, or there is none. This can sometimes be foreseen by careful preoperative study and dealt with prophylactically by adequate preoperative substitution therapy.

4. Crisis may be consequent to *latent cortical insufficiency*—a low adrenal reserve and usually unsuspected but wholly inadequate to the stress demands of a rigorous surgical ordeal. Vascular collapse is usually the first sign, appearing twelve to twenty-four hours or slightly later postoperative. Other clinical evidence soon appears and the patient's condition rapidly becomes desperate; only prompt medicinal substitution therapy (cf. infra) will save him.

Diagnosis and Laboratory Findings. Observation of the clinical picture as described in the immediate preceding paragraphs should suggest the probable diagnosis. Laboratory diagnostic assistance is usually essential. As a rule, the eosinophile count is high, 100 cells per cubic millimeter being highly suggestive but not pathognomonic of adrenal failure. When there is unexpected postoperative circulatory collapse, high fever, cyanosis and a high eosinophile count, suspect adrenal insufficiency.

Treatment. This aims to replace deficient adrenocorticosteroids, electrolytes, support the circulatory system and combat infection. The patient must be treated for shock with bodily warmth, fluids, oxygen if necessary, whole blood transfusion but *no morphine derivatives or substitutes.*

The *hormonal treatment* of acute adrenal crisis (deficiency) here outlined is for an adult of average weight; the dose requisites in infants and children are proportional:

If *hydrocortisone* is available, give at once intravenously 100 to 200 mg. in 1000 cc. of normal saline-5 per cent dextrose solution over a period of eight to twelve hours. In emergency, give 200 mg. of *cortisone* intramuscularly divided in two separate injections for better absorption, together with 50 to 100 mg. of *cortisone acetate* intravenously followed by 250 cc. infusion of normal saline and 5 per cent glucose solution. Thereafter cortisone 25 mg. is given every six hours until the patient eats normally when a maintenance dose of 25 to 50 mg. is given orally daily. Shortly the true daily requisite will be determined.

Infection is combated with Erythromycin orally and Aureomycin intramuscularly, 1.0 gm. of each daily in divided doses every six or eight hours. Circulatory hypotension is combated with whole blood transfusion and fluids (normal saline) intravenously with 5 to 10 mg. of neosynephrine added as needed. Desoxycorticosterone acetate (DOCA) is used only in refractory severe dehydration, 5 to 10 mg. begin given daily, with dose reduction as the patient improves.

Chronic Cortical Insufficiency. This may occur in (1) Addison's disease (primary adrenal failure), (2) hypopituitarism (secondary adrenal failure), and (3) following partial adrenalectomy.

Addison's Disease. This is rare, occurs chiefly between twenty-five and fifty years of age, and results from adrenal cortical failure. This may be due to chronic tuberculosis of the cortex as in half the cases or a congenital hypoplasia or atrophy, or cortical atrophy of unknown origin. In 2 per cent of the cases the cortical damage is due to amyloid degeneration, tumor metastasis, leukemia, leukemic infiltration, hemachromatosis or histoplasmosis. Usually the gland is replaced with scar, fat and leukocytic infiltration but some medullary remnants are generally found. In some patients a familial tendency has been noted.

Adrenocortical insufficiency due to *hypopituitarism* or *pituitary failure* generally manifests milder systemic symptoms than in Addison's disease, with less disturbance of electrolyte balance, little or no pigmentation, and clear evidence of gonadal and thyroid deficiencies. In addition to the treatment of adrenal deficiency, these patients require thyroid extract and testosterone as such.

Symptoms of Adrenocortical Insufficiency. In Addison's disease or other similar condition due to chronic cortical insufficiency, the clinical picture has certain general features which appear in appropriate sequence: Asthenia with easy fatigability, muscular weakness, hypotension, loss of weight, evidence of hypoglycemia, pigmentation especially about the nipple areola, genitalia, perineum and/or mucous membranes (first sign in 10 per cent of cases), anorexia, nausea, vomiting, diarrhea often alternating with constipation, abdominal pain (chronic appendicitis, cholecystitis), nervousness, irritability, emotional instability with depression, and often reduction of axillary and pubic hair.

Diagnosis. The history and appearance of these patients should suggest the diagnosis. The usual laboratory findings in chronic adrenal cortical insufficiency are given in Table 19.

Tests of Adrenocortical Function. The demonstration of adrenal insufficiency requires certain tests of adrenal function of which the following are the most important:

I. ACTH TEST (Thorn). *A.* In the initial *four-hour screening test,* the eosinophile count is made first and 25 to 50 U.S.P. units of ACTH are injected intramuscularly. Four hours later the eosinophile count is repeated; normally this cell count falls 50 per cent or more; in adrenal insufficiency there is no fall, the count being 100 or more cells per cubic millimeter. Yet only an eosinopenia caused by ACTH is diagnostically significant of adrenocortical activation.

B. In the *definitive test of adrenocortical function,* the basic eosinophile count is made and 80 commercial units U.S.P. of ACTH are then injected intramuscularly and the count is repeated in eight to ten hours. Normally an eosinophile fall of 85 to 100 per cent occurs.

C. The twenty-four hour urine specimen of the day preceding the test is collected for steroid assay as is the twenty-four hour specimen following ACTH injection. Normally the urinary 17-ketosteroids and the 17-hydroxycorticosteroids double or treble in quantity but in adrenal deficiency, fail to do so.

TABLE 19. LABORATORY FINDINGS IN CHRONIC ADRENAL INSUFFICIENCY

1. Increased urinary sodium and chloride excretion.
2. Decreased serum sodium* and chloride concentration.
3. Increased serum potassium* concentration.
4. Decreased urinary 17-ketosteroid and 17-hydroxicorticoid excretion.
5. Hypoglycemia.
6. Small heart size (x-ray demonstration).
7. Adrenal calcification (x-ray demonstration; present in 25 per cent).
8. Abnormal electro-encephalogram (decreased frequency).
9. Abnormal electrocardiogram (low voltage; prolonged PR and QT intervals; nonspecific T-wave changes).
10. Basal metabolism moderately diminished (minus 10 or greater in 25 per cent of the cases).
11. Anemia (accentuated by dehydration).
12. Evidence of active or inactive tuberculosis.
    * Usually.

II. WATER TEST (Robinson-Kepler-Power). In adrenocortical insufficiency there is delayed diuretic response to an acute water overload.

III. WATER DEPRIVATION TEST (Cutler-Power-Wilder). On a low salt, high potassium diet, there is deficient renal regulation of electrolyte excretion as manifested by continued urinary sodium loss with hyponatremia, dehydration, hypotension, hemoconcentration, weight loss and, if severe enough, adrenal crisis.

IV. PROLONGED FAST of twenty-four to thirty-six hours (Thorn et al., 1942) produces hypoglycemia by diminished glyconeogenesis in cortical insufficiency.

V. STANDARD INTRAVENOUS INSULIN TOLERANCE TEST (Frazier et al., 1941) in adrenal cortical insufficiency shows insulin hypersensitivity and an unresponsive hypoglycemia.

Because Tests III and V may induce adrenal crisis, they should be carried out only in the hospital under most strict medical supervision.

Treatment. Mild Addison's disease may often be controlled with increased oral intake of sodium chloride, 5 to 25 gm. and half this amount of sodium bicarbonate daily together with low potassium and high carbohydrate diet.

Fortunately by the administration of crystalline adrenocorticosteroid hormones the cortical deficiency can be rectified and the patient loses all of his symptoms and clinical manifestations except pigmentation, but even this often becomes less marked.

The treatment of *acute adrenal crisis* has been given previously. Having saved the patient from his grave emergency, further treatment is that of chronic adrenocortical insufficiency of whatever cause.

Treatment of Chronic Adrenal Cortical Insufficiency. Cortisone orally in daily doses of 15 to 25 mg. will usually suffice for maintenance. If the patient is overstimulated by the cortisone, it is omitted on alternate days when *hydrocortisone* 5 to 10 mg. is given. When cortisone fails to maintain electrolyte balance, blood pressure and body weight, *desoxycorticosterone acetate* (DOCA) is also given, the maintenance dose of which must be determined by therapeutic trial beginning with a small dose of 2 to 3 mg. in oil and increasing or decreasing as necessary. Once determined, the maintenance dose may be given as microcrystalline suspension of *desoxycorticosterone trimethylacetate* injected intramuscularly once a month, 25 mg. (1 cc.) for every milligram of DOCA required as a daily dosage.

Pellets of desoxycorticosterone trimethylacetate are conveniently used for long-acting maintenance, being implanted subcutaneously under local anesthesia in the axillary, subscapular, or posterolateral abdominal wall. A 125 mg. pellet is used for every 0.5 mg. of DOCA in oil required, the pellets being renewed at intervals of eight to twelve months as needed.

Buccal linguets of desoxycorticosterone acetate in doses of three to five times the intramuscular requirements may suffice when only a small dose is needed but in contrast to cortisone, they must not be swallowed as the hormone is inactivated in the stomach. They are kept under the tongue or upper lip where they will absorb through the mucosa in fifteen to twenty minutes.

In résumé: when adequate, the oral ingestion of cortisone is the simplest therapy with, when necessary, monthly injections of desoxycorticosterone trimethylacetate. When these patients face major surgery, have serious infections or illness which cause physical stress, the oral dose of cortisone must be increased to 50 to 100 mg. per day, or to half this amount when given intramuscularly as aqueous suspension of cortisone acetate.

The preparation for and care of patients during and after partial or total adrenalectomy, and so often bilateral, demands special care, for which the reader is referred to Harrison and Jenkins (1954), Priestley et al., Cahill et al.

HYPERFUNCTION OF THE ADRENAL CORTEX

Hyperadrenocorticism may result from diffuse hyperplasia (Fig. 292), benign adenoma or neoplasm of the adrenal cortex, the bodily changes and manifestations of which will depend upon the type and quantity of hormone elaborated and the age and sex of the patient. *There is no characteristic syndrome of hyperadrenocorticism.* Rather, there is a symptomatic overlapping, ranging from the cortical sexual or adrenogenital syndrome at one extreme to the cortical metabolic Cushing's syndrome at the other, and with a large in-between group of clinical mixtures caused by a dominant hormone which may be masculinizing, feminizing or metabolic. Precise recognition of this middle group is highly dependent on urinary hormonal assay, blood and urine chemistry, x-rays, and some-

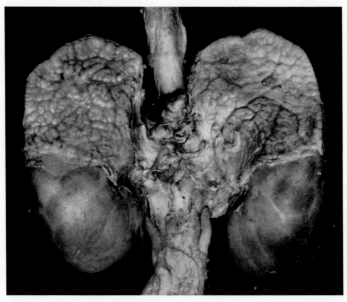

FIGURE 292.   Diffuse cortical hyperplasia of the adrenals in a nine-week-old pseudohermaphroditic girl. (Babies Hospital.)

times even surgical exploration. When there is overproduction of adrenogenic (masculinizing) hormone, the sex organs show pronounced alterations with early secondary sexual bodily changes, and in both sexes toward the adult male type. Excess estrogenic hormone production occurs much less often and causes striking feminization in each sex.

ADRENOGENITAL SYNDROME

This adrenal virilizing syndrome results from overproduction of masculinizing hormone (a) by the adrenal cortex directly, or (b) indirectly through pituitary stimulation of the adrenal cortex (rarely), or (c) by the gonads (also rare).

Overproduction of the masculinizing hormone (1) in utero causes

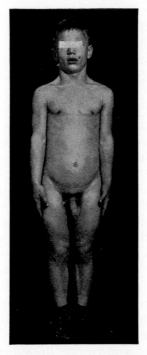

FIGURE 293. Sexual precocity in a four-and-a-half-year-old boy otherwise normal except for an increased output of urinary 17-ketosteroids (9.2 mg. in 24 hours rather than the normal 5.0 mg.). Apparently normal at birth, at one year of age the genitalia were slightly enlarged, and at eighteen months x-rays of the skull demonstrated it to be somewhat large for the stated age. The sella turcica was normal in size and shape and there was no evidence of intracranial tumor. X-rays of the bones disclosed a markedly advanced bone age. One year later exploration of the adrenals disclosed no abnormality nor did biopsy of the rib, testes and epididymides. At four and a half years, he weighed 75½ pounds, was 4 feet 3¾ inches tall (twice the normal size for this age), was well-developed, muscular, presented adult genitalia but without prostatic enlargement. Facial acne, deep voice and pubic hair were present. His mental development was advanced. The metabolic rate was plus 8. He adjusted well to the classroom and has shown no abnormal interest in the opposite sex, being in this respect somewhat different from most "little Hercules" who generally have an abnormal sex drive. (Endocrinology Clinic, University Hospital, and courtesy Dr. Beatrice Bergman and Journal of Pediatrics.)

pseudohermaphrodism in females and macrogenitosomia in males, and (2) after birth causes *virilism* in females and macrogenitosomia praecox in males. Feminizing tumors produce feminism in males.

In the Male. The adrenogenital syndrome is here evidenced by isosexual prematurity and precocious sexual development with pronounced penile, scrotal and prostatic growth, hirsutism, deep masculine voice, and acne (Fig. 293). It may be evident at birth or shortly thereafter and by the second year is often far advanced. The boy grows large but not obese, and the skeleton is chronologically advanced. At first the testicular growth is not remarkable and there is no spermatogenesis except in highly androgenic adrenocortical or pituitary tumors. Yet these boys, many of whom are mentally retarded, commonly become sexually aggressive. By the third or fourth year when macrogenitosomia praecox is most often recognized, the prostate is well developed, its fluid may contain spermatids, erections and nocturnal emissions occur, a beard and moustache generally grow. Such striking masculinization always suggests pronounced adrenocortical hyperplasia or neoplasm; it has also been observed in a few cases of hypothalamic tumors and granulosa cell ovarian tumors in females.

Later, as adrenal hyperactivity continues and the disease progresses, the organ exhausts itself and terminal Addison's syndrome appears (q.v.) or if it does not, the patient stops growing because of premature epiphyseal closure, and fails to mature further sexually. Hypoglycemia, hypotension, and Addisonian pigmentation may develop.

In the Female. The congenital adrenogenital syndrome in this sex is largely a heterosexual pseudoprecocity and may be so marked as to cause the girl to be raised as a boy (Figs. 294, 295). The breasts fail to develop and menstruation is absent. The bifid scrotum-like labia contain no testes, the clitoris is penile and ventrally grooved, the urethral opening far back is mistaken for hypospadias and the vagina may open into the urethra and be endoscopically visualized (Fig. 295). In short there is no normal separation of urethral and vaginal orifices but rather a single urogenital sinus. Hirsutism may appear. When virilism in the female occurs after birth, the clinical picture is the same but there is no urogenital sinus formation. In prepubertal virilism in both sexes, the patient presents a rather characteristic body type: short, muscular, rarely reaches 5 feet in height, shoulders broad relative to hip width, deep chest, legs short relative to body, often with lumbar lordosis and pot belly.

In the past many of these patients have died of adrenal insufficiency but, recognized today, may be successfully treated (see treatment of chronic adrenal cortical insufficiency). Yet sexual prematurity is more often idiopathic or constitutional than due to adrenocortical hyperplasia or tumor (cf. Chapter 6).

Diagnosis. Here it is essential to distinguish between heterosexual development due to (1) congenital malformation, and (2) hermaphrodites with gonads of each sex present (male pseudohermaphrodism with female type external genitalia and genital ducts), and (3) genital maldevelopment consequent to excessive adrenocortical hormonal elaboration as described in the preceding paragraph. In item (1) the secondary sexual development is unpredictable but does not occur before puberty and may not be isosexual while in item (2), the true sex having genetically been determined, it is fundamentally maintained but with heterosexual abnormalities and sexual prematurity.

Adrenocortical hyperplasia occurs at birth or in infancy, the sex ratio is female 3: male 1, a family history of the condition is sometimes obtained and adrenal insufficiency may appear. On the other hand, in adrenocortical tumor, the condition may appear in infancy or childhood, a negative family history is obtained, the sex ratio is female to male 4:1, and adrenal insufficiency is absent. In both hyperplasia and tumor, the 17-ketosteroid urinary excretion is elevated but the administration of cortisone makes the *differential diagnosis* causing amelioration of symptoms and reduction of 17-ketosteroid output in adrenogenital hyperplasia but with no change in tumor. Other conditions to be distinguished from adrenogenital syndrome are true sexual precocity, true hermaphrodism, hypophyseal and pineal tumors.

When in doubt as to the sex of the patient (a) the administration of cortisone will inhibit the steroid output of adrenocortical hyperplasia, (b) biopsy studies of epithelial nuclei may make the distinction between congenital adrenogenital syndrome and male pseudohermaphrodism (Fig.

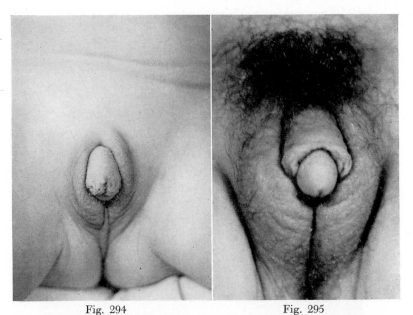

Fig. 294   Fig. 295

FIGURE 294. Adrenogenital syndrome. Genitalia in a three-month-old girl.
FIGURE 295. Adrenogenital syndrome in a four-year-old girl (sister of patient in Figure 294).

120), and (c) laparotomy will disclose the true sex which should be determined in any event by the age of two years and preferably in earlier infancy.

Cortical adrenal tumors and ovarian arrhenoblastomas producing virilism in females must not be overlooked in the diagnostic evaluation.

Treatment. The grave question of how to raise the hormonal pseudo-hermaphrodite girl presents a different problem than in true hermaphrod-ism.

In the adrenogenital syndrome cortisone therapy should be started early and intensively and, if definitive, demands that the child be raised as a girl; clitoric amputation should be deferred until after puberty and in any event until the true sex is determined beyond question. In several instances the amputated "clitoris" has in truth been the penis of an unrecognized male. In my experience, young children of borderline sex differentiation adjust better as boys than as girls; in older children raised as of one sex, for psychologic and social considerations, a change over may be unwarranted or even tragic (cf. Chapter 6).

To date the only *treatment of adrenogenital syndrome* proved ac-ceptable is the administration of cortisone or hydrocortisone which, by causing suppression of the pituitary-adrenal mechanism, results in striking reduction in adrenal androgen output (cf. Wilkins, 1950, 1952). The dose is guided by urinary 17-ketosteroid assays. Treatment begins with small amounts: usually 25 mg. of cortisone acetate intramuscularly every day to infants and children, and 50 mg. per day to older patients. In six to ten days the maximum 17-ketosteroid suppression is achieved and

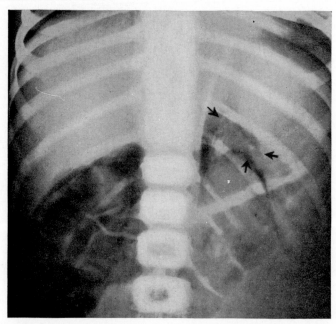

FIGURE 296.   Perirenal pneumography for demonstration of renal and especially the adrenal outlines; in this film the triangular left adrenal is well shown.

maintenance doses of half these "test" amounts (5 to 12.5 mg. for infants and children, and 25 mg. for adults) are continued. Oral administration requires three to five times the intramuscular dose and has been less satisfactory than when injected.

Successful therapy is evidenced by retardation of body growth and of masculinization, and in older females by the beginning or resumption of menstruation, development of the breasts, and sometimes even repression of hirsutism.

In the past, partial adrenalectomy, unilateral or bilateral, and intensive administration of large doses of estrogens have been employed but without success. Moreover, and this is important, large continued doses of estrogens are likely to cause premature epiphyseal closure to stunt the child's growth.

When adrenogenital syndrome is due to adrenocortical tumor, the former surgical mortality of 25 to 30 per cent has fortunately now been sharply reduced. In the surgical cases great care is necessary to maintain the adrenal hormone requirements preoperatively, during operation, and postoperatively.

Adrenal virilism occurring in postpubertal females is nearly always due to adrenocortical tumor; the first genital change is enlargement of the clitoris, accompanied by rapid body growth, and often hirsutism and hypertension. The picture may suggest Cushing's disease (q.v.); the 17-ketosteroid excretion is high. The diagnostic study includes perirenal pneumography and pyelography which may suggest the presence of a tumor (Fig. 296). The neoplasm is not suppressed with ACTH.

The adrenogenital syndrome may also appear in older women, usually before the menopause, with suppression of feminine manifestations, a tendency towards masculinization, hair on the face, development of a male type pubic hair line, thinning of the hair of the scalp or even baldness, loss of libido, and cessation or near cessation of menstruation. The voice deepens, the body configuration becomes mannish, the clitoris hypertrophies and the female sex organs (breasts, vagina, ovaries, uterus) shrink. When not due to cancer of the adrenal cortex, the hypercorticism may continue for a long time without striking change, the 17-ketosteroid assay being elevated, sometimes to thirty or more milligrams in twenty-four hours.

CUSHING'S SYNDROME OR ADRENAL OBESITY

This is caused by metabolic disturbances consequent to excessive elaboration of 11-17 oxygenated adrenal corticoids (e.g., hydrocortisone, cortisone) and not solely from pituitary basophilism as Cushing thought in 1932 when he first described the syndrome. Yet basophile tumors of the anterior pituitary, often microscopic, have been found in a third to a half of the many cases of Cushing's disease thus examined, as have instances of eosinophilic, chromophobic or undifferentiated pituitary masses. Most generally adrenocortical tumors or cortical hyperplasia exist. While dysfunction of basophile cells of the anterior pituitary may stimulate abnormal adrenocortical activity, pituitary disease is not found in all cases, the preponderance of present opinion being that Cushing's syndrome results from adrenocortical hyperfunction, either *sui generis* or by the mechanism of anterior pituitary activation.

Other changes in the anterior pituitary almost regularly found in Cushing's disease include basophilic hyalinization, degranulation and vacuolization (Crooke, 1935) but it is believed these changes are the result rather than the cause of adrenal overactivity. Curiously, pancreatic or thymus carcinoma occurs in 5 per cent of the cases of Cushing's disease and often one or more of the following coexist: pancreatic cysts, pancreatic infarction, pancreatitis, fatty infiltration of the liver, a high incidence of nephrosclerosis, renal calcinosis, and/or calculi. Eighty per cent of these patients show osteoporosis, generalized arteriosclerosis, hypertension, cardiac hypertrophy; cutaneous infections are frequent and the gonads are often decreased in size or are fibroid.

Symptoms. The clinical picture is that of "moon face" and "buffalo neck" type of obesity, with insulin resistant mild diabetes (because of impairment of carbohydrate metabolism), hirsutism, acne, keratosis, plethora, hypertension, muscular weakness, erythremia, edema, negative

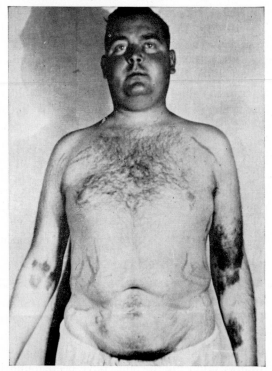

FIGURE 297. Cushing's syndrome. Characteristic are the facial and trunk obesity, plethora, easy bruisability and abdominal striae. Patient also suffered hypertension, osteoporosis with rib fractures, elevated urinary corticosteroid excretion and decreased carbohydrate tolerance. Bilateral adrenal cortical hyperplasia with subtotal bilateral adrenalectomy. (Harrison and Laidlaw.)

nitrogen balance, purplish cutaneous striations, pigmentation, easy bruis-ability, hypochloremia, hypokalemia, hypokalemic acidosis, osteoporosis, mental disturbances predominantly depressive or paranoid, and the geni-talia are generally normal but may show variable precocious puberty (Figs. 297, 298). Several cases of Cushing's disease have been described in children. In the differential diagnosis, obesity, disturbed carbohydrate metabolism, and osteoporosis without voice change or clitoric hypertrophy distinguishes Cushing's disease from adrenogenital syndrome. *In short, Cushing's disease is the diametric opposite of Addison's disease.* When excess estrogenic secretion is present in a male, gynecomastia results, but this should make one first suspect choriocarcinoma of the testicle (q.v.).

The *excess fat formation* in Cushing's disease results from increased carbohydrate anabolism consequent to the greater glycogenic activity; hyperglycemia, glycosuria, and reduced response to insulin occur. Con-version of amino acids to carbohydrate and later to fat rather than into body protein accounts for capillary friability and ecchymoses, striae formation and muscular weakness. Similarly the deficient bony matrix, especially of the spine, and inadequate repair consequent to protein anabolic deficiency explains the skeletal changes (osteoporosis) which

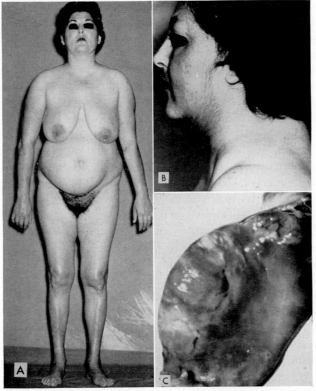

FIGURE 298. Cushing's syndrome in a 30-year-old female showing typical buffalo neck, facial hirsuitism and acne (*B*). Abdominal striations less marked than in Figure 297. *C*, Carcinoma of right adrenal cortex. Adrenalectomy.

occur in three fourths of these cases. Bony weakening, atrophy, demineralization and vertebral crushing and collapse occur with pain in the back, increasing as the patient gets fatter. With skeletal demineralization and calcium loss, urinary calculi—especially renal—are common. There is usually evidence of excess (1) androgen, and/or (2) estrogen secretion. With androgen excess the voice deepens, becomes coarse, facial acne appears with hypertrichosis over the trunk, pelvic areas, and face. There is erythremia, plethora and cutaneous cyanosis together with great susceptibility to skin infections particularly staphylococcic. Bilateral retinal and cerebral hemorrhages occur in many hypertensive polycythemic patients. Such patients make hazardous surgical risks.

In the female with Cushing's disease, the breasts, vagina and the secondary sex characteristics are below normal and menstruation is scant or absent, while in adrenocortical tumor with excess estrogen elaboration, the feminism may be exaggerated and/or precocious.

Diagnosis. Inspection of most of these patients suggests the diagnosis of Cushing's disease, the important laboratory findings of which are:

1. Decreased glucose tolerance; hyperglycemia; glycosuria.
2. Eosinopenia and lymphopenia.
3. Leukocytosis and erythremia.
4. Increased urinary corticosteroid excretion; 17-ketosteroid excretion usually within normal range.
5. Decreased serum chloride and potassium concentration.
6. Increased serum CO_2 content.
7. Osteoporosis (x-ray demonstration).
8. Albuminuria.
9. Hypercholesterolemia.

Perirenal pneumography and pyelography are invaluable diagnostic aids (Fig. 296) but often bilateral exploration of the adrenals will be required to make the definitive diagnosis. Body section roentgenography (tomography) with its elimination of intestinal gas shadows by sharp focus on specific organs may be of help. Thus, to demonstrate the kidney or adrenal tumors, the point of focus is about two thirds of the anteroposterior depth; this is usually 8 or 9 cm. deep from the overlying anterior abdominal skin surface. In summary: when there is any doubt, explore.

In the *differential diagnosis* in Cushing's disease as between adrenocortical hyperplasia and carcinoma, estimation of the urinary 17-ketosteroid excretion is helpful but not entirely reliable. It is elevated highest with tumor (30 to 40 mg. or more per twenty-four hours) and especially with a high beta fraction (40 to 50%); in cortical hyperplasia the 17-ketosteroid output is about half that in tumor (15 to 20 mg. per twenty-four hours), and is lowest with simple adenoma of the cortex (2 to 6 mg. per twenty-four hours). Yet following the intravenous injection of ACTH (20 units, U.S.P.), there is little or no increased urinary corticosteroid output response in cortical carcinoma but good response (increase) in bilateral cortical hyperplasia. By this test adrenocortical carcinoma and bilateral cortical hyperplasia may be distinguished reasonably well.

In the diagnostic study it is most important to recognize that cortical hyperplasia or tumor of one adrenal, especially when heavily secreting hormone, may cause atrophy of disuse of the opposite adrenal. This other adrenal may also be congenitally absent, hypoplastic or itself otherwise diseased and nonfunctioning. Surgery upon the tumor-bearing adrenal is unjustifiable until the status of its mate is determined. In many of these cases, removal of the superhormonal adrenal is followed by crisis of acute adrenal insufficiency in which—if life is to be saved—the patient must be immediately treated intensively as an acute medical emergency.

Treatment. This is hopeless unless a removable nonmetastasized tumor exists; absence, atrophy, or hypofunction of the opposite adrenal is an increased surgical hazard as is the medical condition itself of most of these patients.

Today partial adrenal resection or adrenalectomy, unilateral or bilateral, is the treatment of Cushing's disease and adrenal tumors. The patient must be properly prepared for, and treated through the operative session and later, by adrenal replacement therapy as in Addison's disease. When an adrenal lesion, presumably tumor, is diagnostically identified by x-ray, and apparently confirmed by laboratory studies, the gland is explored and, if malignant, is removed.

If a *benign tumor* is found, it may be resected as is often done with hyperplasia, but the opposite adrenal should also be explored to be sure that there is not a tumor, atrophy or hyperplasia existing there. When both glands are *atrophic*, the existence of an actively secreting ectopic adrenal mass is most likely and should be identified before removing the deficient gland.

In Cushing's disease, subtotal bilateral adrenalectomy has been found most effective, coupled with adrenocortical hormone supportive therapy as indicated. Yet half of these patients will eventually suffer adrenal insufficiency later postoperatively. Additional liberal doses of androgen are necessary to stimulate bone repair of the osteoporosis and to build better muscle structure.

Following successful removal of the tumor, the obesity, hypertension, hirsutism, acne and abdominal striae usually disappear. The *surgical mortality is higher in Cushing's disease than in adrenal hyperfunction.*

Following bilateral partial adrenalectomy some patients carried on postoperative cortisone therapy show the signs of adrenal hypofunction and the symptoms of adrenal insufficiency, with depression, anorexia, headache, nausea, vomiting, diarrhea, debility, weakness and joint pains. The therapeutic indication is prompt adrenohormonal substitution therapy.

Mixed Adrenal Syndromes. These present certain features of Cushing's syndrome (metabolic disturbances, often mild) and adrenogenital syndrome in which masculinization is outstanding with, almost always, hirsutism, hypertrophy of the clitoris, and hypertension. Half of the cases show an abnormal high glucose tolerance curve and osteoporosis, while slightly fewer show the typical obesity, moon face, buffalo neck, plethora, and cutaneous striae of Cushing's disease. The incidence of tumor is somewhat higher in the mixed group than in the Cushing's disease group.

Differential Diagnosis. Arrhenoblastoma of the ovary is rare, occurs after fifteen years of age, and causes virilization like that of adrenal virilization, but the physical findings of Cushing's disease are usually absent. The rare masculinizing tumors of the ovarian hilus (Sternberg) cause changes like those of ovarian arrhenoblastoma but also without the symptoms of Cushing's disease. Bilateral polycystic and sclerotic ovaries may cause hirsutism, amenorrhea, and sometimes virilism in young adult females. Yet all of these ovarian tumors are apt to be found as pelvic masses bimanually palpable. Adrenal rest tumors retroperitoneally along the spermatic cord, or in the scrotum or ovary may show cortical hyperplasia and even carcinoma and behave like the lesions in the more usual adrenocortical hyperfunction.

The differential diagnosis between bilateral adrenocortical hyperplasia and carcinoma has been previously indicated.

Treatment. Exploration of the adrenals is necessary whether adrenalectomy (carcinoma) or partial resection (hyperplasia) is to be done, according to the local pathology and with due attention to the preparation and postoperative care as previously discussed. On the whole, patients with the mixed tumors and manifestations, especially the virilizing tumors, stand operation well in contrast with the high risk of adrenalectomy in Cushing's disease.

Feminizing adrenal tumors in adult males are rare; all but one of the reported cases have been malignant. Symptoms of Cushing's disease are absent. The 17-ketosteroids and androgens are elevated. Adrenalectomy is the treatment.

TUMORS OF THE ADRENAL

Tumors of the adrenal cortex may be nonhormonal (nonfunctioning) or hormonal (functioning). The hormonal group may be found with various manifestations in (1) adrenogenital syndrome, (2) Cushing's syndrome, (3) mixed syndrome, (4) feminizing syndrome, and (5) miscellaneous group including recurrent hypoglycemia episodes (Thannhauser, 1949), and gynecomastia with high urinary secretion of chorionic gonadotropin (Chambers, 1949). Groups 1 to 4 have been discussed previously in this chapter.

Adrenal tumors classified as to their structural derivation are:

I. Connective tissue and vascular tumors (predominantly benign)

II. Cortical tumors

    (a) hyperplasia

    (b) adenoma (benign)

    (c) carcinoma (malignant)

III. Medullary tumors

    (a) ganglioneuroma (benign)

    (b) sympathoblastoma (sympathogonioma, neuroblastoma, neurocytoma)

(c) pheochromocytoma (or paraganglioma)

In general, cortical growths are less malignant than medullary growths.

CONNECTIVE TISSUE AND VASCULAR TUMORS

These include fibroma, lipoma, myoma, neurofibroma, neuroma, hemangioma and lymphangioma which may cause a tumor mass but are nonhormonal. The diagnosis is made as in other types of enlarging retroperitoneal tumors (perirenal pneumography, urography, exploration), and excision is the treatment.

TUMORS OF THE ADRENAL CORTEX

(a) **Hyperplasia.** The cortex becomes two to six or more times normal thickness and is commonly pathologically hormonal. Often the medulla is severely compressed or even degenerated. The clinical manifestations and treatment of cortical hyperplasia have been previously discussed in this chapter.

Small localized nodular light yellow areas of hyperplasia (struma suprarenalis of Virchow) varying from 1 to 10 mm. in diameter are sometimes found but are seldom significant.

(b) **Benign Cortical Tumors.** These are predominantly small benign adenoma which are found at autopsy in a third of all adults. Rarely do they grow to become clinically important by tumor mass or visceral compression. Yet a few of these are hormone producing, depending upon the character of the cells involved, the chief manifestations being masculinization or virilization in girls and older women, or pubertas praecox in boys. With dyscorticism, fatal adrenal failure with crisis may develop (q.v.).

(c) **Malignant Tumors.** These are carcinoma or true hypernephroma; nearly all are hormonal, encapsulated, nodular or irregular in shape and are composed of canary yellow tissue. The cell structure is

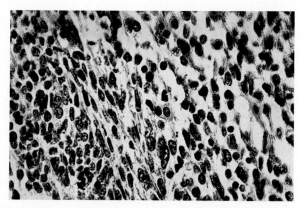

FIGURE 299. Malignant cortical adenoma showing considerable pleomorphism of cells and multinucleated cells. Highly vascular. A similar pleomorphism may occur in benign adenomas. × 225. (Courtesy Armed Forces Institute of Pathology.)

of variable size, often large and square shaped, sometimes arranged in acinar formation with loss of normal adrenal architecture. They may also develop in active adrenal tissue in the juxta interrenal tissue along the spermatic cord, in the broad ligament, ovary or testes. On section they may be firm, soft, or necrotic and even in the same tumor. Characteristically they metastasize early and widely through the lymphatics and veins, preponderantly to the liver, lungs and brain, by direct extension to the kidney, opposite adrenal, or vena cava but seldom to the skeleton. They entail a high mortality, even when treated surgically. About seventy-five cases in children have been reported.

Symptoms. When nonhormonal, as comparatively few of these tumors are, the manifestations are eventually those of renal tumor without hematuria (q.v.).

The symptoms of functioning tumors will depend upon the hormonal activity and time of development. In the young they may cause precocious puberty, Addisonian pigmentation, adrenogenital syndrome, or even the adrenal obesity syndrome of Cushing, and in adults cause predominantly Cushing's syndrome, the clinical and therapeutic considerations of which have been presented earlier in this chapter.

TUMORS OF THE ADRENAL MEDULLA

These are derived from cells of the sympathetic nervous system, the primitive ectodermal cells of which are the *sympathogonia.* Two types of cells are derived from these, the *sympathoblast* which becomes (1) the nonhormonal sympathetic ganglion cell, and (2) the *pheochromoblast* which matures into the *pheochromocyte,* a hormonal secreting cell (epinephrine, norepinephrine). Thus in tumors of the adrenal medulla are evidenced the origin, type and maturity of the component cells, benign growths being composed of mature sympathetic ganglion cells (ganglioneuroma, neuroganglioma) or the extremely immature sympathogonia (sympathogonioma, neuroblastoma) or the chromophilic cell tumors (pheochromocytoma, paraganglioma).

Benign Tumors. Ganglioneuroma. This rare nonhormonal tumor is derived from mature or highly differentiated sympathetic system cells which become large unipolar or multipolar ganglion cells with masses of surrounding nerve fibrils. Rarely immature malignant cells (neuroblastoma) are found in the tumor which grows adjacent to the kidney and/or along the sympathetic chain. Two thirds of these tumors appear before twenty years of age. *Symptoms* are those of the tumor mass and/or visceral compression and the pain it may cause. The *diagnosis* may be suspected at operation but requires microscopic confirmation. Removal of the growth is the treatment.

Nonhormonal Malignant Tumors. Sympathogoniomas are most rare tumors of infancy and childhood and are composed of highly malignant, wholly undifferentiated primitive sympathetic nerve system cells, the sympathogonia. They grow, invade and metastasize rapidly and widely; the prognosis is generally hopeless.

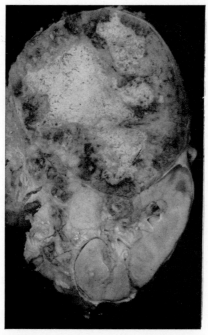

FIGURE 300. Neuroblastoma of the adrenal showing renal invasion by the tumor.

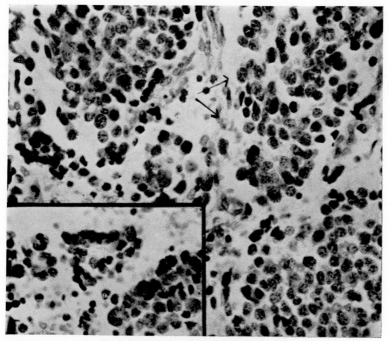

FIGURE 301. Sympathoblastoma (neuroblastoma) of adrenal in a five-month-old child. Arrows indicate alveolation. The cells are large with abundant cytoplasm, vesicular nuclei, scanty fibrils. Few multinucleated forms. *Insert:* One pseudo-rosette is shown. (Courtesy Armed Forces Institute of Pathology.)

Sympathoblastoma or **neuroblastoma** (ganglioma embryonale) is, as the designation implies, a nonhormonal tumor derived from sympathoblasts and sympathogonia in the medulla or, in about half the cases, in other sympathetic ganglion structures. These last include the retroperitoneal, retropleural and cervical sympathetic chain, the celiac ganglion, organ of Zuckerkandl, or even from cells of the central nervous system itself. In general, these neoplasms are extremely malignant (Figs. 297, 298, 300, 301), equaling the Wilms' tumor in this respect.

Neuroblastoma is almost exclusively a malignancy of infancy and childhood, is usually manifest within the first year and has even been found in the fetus. It occurs about as often as Wilms' renal tumor in the young, is of about equal sex and side incidence but, not being congenital, is seldom bilateral. A third occur during the first year, a fourth appear by the fifth year, and a fourth after this time, but almost never in adults.

Neuroblastomas grow so fast that the outlook is usually hopeless when the patient is first examined for the condition. Neuroblastomas vary in degree of maturity; in the same tumor a wide variety of cell malignancy will be found, varying from highly malignant sympathogonia to mature and comparatively harmless cells such as neuroma or glioma. Moreover, cell maturation from immaturity (malignant) to maturity (benignity) has been observed to occur in about 2 per cent of neuroblastomas. As in Wilms' embryoma, the rapidly growing tumors have a tendency to central hemorrhage and central necrosis.

Adrenal neuroblastomas are usually encapsulated, lobular, firmly or loosely adherent to the kidney and on cut section present a dark red, reddish-gray or grayish appearance, depending upon the vascular supply and extent of tumor necrosis. Rarely the growth occurs in an adrenal rest in the kidney itself. By direct tumor growth it may spread down the retrolumbar gutter or up through the diaphragm or, following nerve routes, may reach the central nervous system and vertebrae.

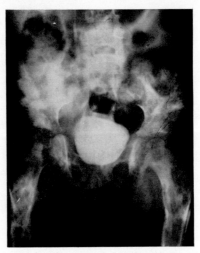

FIGURE 302.   Neuroblastoma of the adrenal. Bony metastases.

Metastasis generally occurs early, chiefly by the blood stream to the skeleton, liver, lungs, brain and other vital structures (Fig. 302). The syndrome and type designation based upon metastatic manifestations (Pepper: liver chiefly; Hutchinson: largely orbital and cranial) should not be used as they are without meaning.

Structurally these tumors show sympathogonia, sympathoblasts, and sympathetic system-like nerve fibrils; pseudo-rosettes of sympathoblasts, hemorrhage and cell necrosis, often with areas of more mature sympathetic nervous system cells with little or no mitosis (Fig. 301).

Symptoms. In most cases the premonitory symptom is a painless mass high in the lateral abdomen in an anemic, sickly looking child. As the tumor grows there is weight loss, increasing pallor and weakness, pain in the side from the tumor itself and in the back or elsewhere from metastases. The toxic cachexia of malignancy soon appears with fever, diarrhea or constipation, respiratory, cerebral or ocular disturbances, pronounced progressive anemia, jaundice, drowsiness and, commonly, increasing to death which in half of the cases occurs within eight months from the initial recognition of the disease and in four-fifths within the first year. Metastases may cause enormous liver enlargement, the appearance of "cannon ball" or "cotton ball" round metastases in the lung (Fig. 251), lumps in the skull, or exophthalmos from retro-ocular tumor spread. Rarely the growth remains relatively localized as a mass between the two kidneys but it is still malignant and not to be confused with benign ganglioneuroma.

Diagnosis. Recognition of the tumor mass and the metastatic spread together with urography should suggest the diagnosis although at first in most instances the lesion is thought to be renal tumor. Radiography demonstrates skeletal or pulmonary metastases. Sometimes aspiration

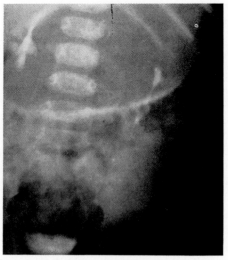

FIGURE 303.   Neuroblastoma of the adrenal. Urographic demonstration of the left kidney
as displaced downward by the tumor.

bone marrow studies disclose osseous metastases before the x-ray does. Urography shows the renal dislocation downward, upward or outward according to the location of the neuroblastoma (Fig. 303), and usually without pronounced changes in the pelvic outline. Yet with neuroblastomatous invasion of the kidney the pyelogram may be that of renal embryoma. When excretory urography leaves doubt, bilateral retrograde pyelography should be carried out. Occasionally ureteral compression by tumor mass causes hydronephrosis or even reduced isolateral renal function. Lumbar perirenal pneumography is unusually dangerous in these cases (puncture into tumor; air embolism) and should not be used but presacral air injection may give a satisfactory perirenal pneumogram.

In the differential diagnosis, Wilms' tumor is the chief consideration and in nephroma there is regularly urographic pelvic change. There is seldom metastatic skeletal invasion except pelvic in Wilms' tumor and, as a rule, it is less rapidly growing than neuroblastoma. Moreover, and an important point, neuroblastoma commonly grows backward into the posterior loin while Wilms' tumor does not. Nonhormonal adrenal tumors grow slowly and may or may not be palpable; hormonal cortical growths produce striking general physical changes as in Cushing's disease, and the hormonal adrenal medullary tumor—pheochromocytoma—induces pronounced hypertensive phenomena (q.v.). Skull metastases of neuroblastoma have been known to simulate the subperiosteal hemorrhage of scurvy; lymphoblastoma produces ascites and widespread lymph node enlargement in which biopsy examination gives the diagnosis as does the blood study in leukemia. Large ovarian dysgerminoma in a girl has simulated neuroblastoma. A rare malignant hemangioma of the renal hilum in a four year old girl grew about the pancreas as a flattened dull red mass resembling lymph glands, and metastasized to the lungs, liver, pancreas, intestines, fat and skin (Campbell, 1937). In most cases the correct diagnosis will be made at operation or autopsy.

Treatment. Combined radiation therapy and early surgical removal of neuroblastoma offer the best, though discouraging, outlook for the patient, some cures having been achieved even when metastases were present. Because of the magnitude of the operation required in many of these cases, the prevention and treatment of shock and other surgical complications demand most strict attention to the patient. The transabdominal or thoraco-abdominal approach is usually indicated. Half of those patients without demonstrated metastases and treated by surgery alone may enjoy cure or long remission. Surgery combined with radiation, and even with hepatic metastases, have apparently cured as in instances in Wittenborg's series. This treatment has produced an apparent cure rate of 60 per cent in children with nonskeletal metastases (Wittenborg).

When bone metastasis is present in neuroblastoma, the outlook is hopeless. In radiation therapy great care must be taken to spare bone marrow injury but often this is unavoidable; fatal pancytopenia is likely to develop. Finally, as in the treatment of Wilms' tumor, ill directed and poorly controlled radiation therapy may be a greater menace than the tumor itself, especially when a sound opposite kidney is gravely and irreversibly injured by x-ray.

Hormonal Tumors of the Adrenal Medulla

There are no hypofunctioning hormonal tumors of the adrenal medulla.

Pheochromocytoma (chromaffin tumor, paraganglioma). The type-cell of these extremely hormonal (epinephrine) neoplasms is the chromophilic pheochromocyte (Fig. 304). In its incipiency, recurrent release by the tumor of excess pressor hormone (epinephrine; norepinephrine) causes concurrent attacks of hypertension (Table 19). As the disease progresses, the hypertension tends to become permanent, a fact noted in 1922 (Labbe and Doumer) but generally recognized only comparatively recently. Yet it should be considered in the study and management of any patient with hypertension, not only the labile and intermittent type but the persistent variety as well. Occasionally asymptomatic pheochromocytoma is an accidental finding by unrelated x-ray study, at surgery or postmortem, while in still another group the lesion is found in cases of sudden death, sometimes by trauma, accident, surgery or stress. Pheochromocytoma is predominantly a tumor of middle age, only a few having been observed in children and in the aged. They occur more often (1) on the right side, and (2) in males; about 10 per cent are bilateral and about the same proportion are malignant.

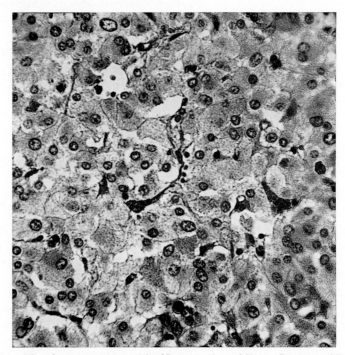

FIGURE 304.   Pheochromocytoma. × 250. (Courtesy Armed Forces Institute of Pathology.)

The tumors first appear in the medulla as brownish nodular hyperplasia of chromaffin epinephrine-secreting cells, the malignant cells showing granules of chromaffin pigment, mitoses, dark-staining cytoplasm, arranged about the blood vessels in lacuna formation suggesting somewhat a glandular structure (Fig. 304). These pigmented cells are also found in the paraganglia cells (hence the term paraganglioma) of the sympathetic nervous system including the carotid body at the bifurcation of the carotid arteries, the Zuckerkandl body at the aortic bifurcation, and in the sympathetic ganglion cells along the retropleural and retroperitoneal sympathetic chain. Also they are found as the enterochromaffin cells of the intestinal epithelium in adults where they give rise to "carcinoid" tumors which are more common than adrenal pheochromocytomas. The comparatively wide distribution of pheochrome cells explains the multiple and extra-adrenal occurrence of these hormonal tumors; sometimes two or more may exist in the same patient. As a corollary, failure of hypertension to disappear following removal of the adrenal tumor indicates a similar tumor doubtless exists elsewhere in the sympathetic system.

Symptoms. Small benign pheochromocytomas are rarely hormonal but as the tumor grows or becomes malignant, it elaborates an excess of epinephrine or norepinephrine which induces acute attacks of hypertension. Epinephrine in excess causes generalized vasoconstriction with hypertension while norepinephrine in excess may induce glycosuria and central nervous system stimulation (Goldenberg, 1951). Yet in tumors with excessive norepinephrine the manifestations are predominantly hypertensive while those of excess epinephrine are predominantly those with hypermetabolism, hyperglycemia and glycosuria.

The *hypertensive attack* may be induced by emotional disturbance, fear, pressure on the tumor, physical overexertion, anesthesia, or may even appear spontaneously. In a third to a half of these patients there are typical attacks which may be transient for a few minutes, last several hours or even days, with headache, trembling of the hands and feet, pallor, palpitation, sweating, epigastric distress or pain, nausea, sometimes vomiting, precordial pain with arm radiation (coronary spasm), cardiac and hepatic enlargement and, in severe cases, pulmonary edema may be fatal.

While the blood pressure may be normal between attacks, with the onset of one, the systolic pressure may rise to 250 mm. Hg or higher and the diastolic pressure to as much as 150 mm. Hg or even higher. The blood urea nitrogen and serum potassium levels are usually raised. Following the attack the patient is left exhausted, often with hyperpyrexia, drenching sweats, hypotension and collapse or even in shock.

Progressively the attacks become more frequent and severe, the basal metabolic rate often rises to +50 or more, there is mental depression, pronounced headache, cardiac palpitation, sweats, visual blurring and in some instances, skin pigmentation or neurofibrolipomatosis has appeared. Because of the extreme hypertension, even over 300 mm. Hg, cerebral hemorrhage occurs in a sixth of the cases.

In a small group of cases there is hypermetabolism, pronounced hyperglycemia with glycosuria together with or without periodic or chronic hypertension and there may even be true diabetes.

Diagnosis. Pheochromocytoma should be considered in all cases of "essential" hypertension in adults or children and in those patients with recurrent acute attacks of hypertension as previously described. Certainly these patients should not be subjected to sympathectomy operations until pheochromocytoma tumor has been ruled out.

Sometimes the adrenal tumor is palpable and gently squeezing it may precipitate an attack. Don't! The basal metabolism is usually increased as may be the blood serum potassium and blood urea nitrogen; renal injury is reflected by albuminuria, casts, and elevated specific gravity. The eyegrounds may show papilledema, retinal hemorrhages, albuminuric exudate and arterial constriction, ophthalmic conditions said to be specific (Bruce). Excretory urography, retrograde pyelography, aortography and perirenal pneumography may satisfactorily delineate the tumor and show coexisting renal displacement and/or compression (Fig. 302). Quantitative studies of urinary catechol (catecholamine) to determine the excretion of epinephrine and norepinephrine (normal 20 to 40 mg. in twenty-four hours) will show increased output in pheochromocytoma.

CHEMICAL TESTS FOR PHEOCHROMOCYTOMA. These have been devised to: (1) induce an attack of hypertension (histamine base, Roth and Kvale, 1945, tetra-ethyl-ammonium chloride, La Due et al., 1948; and mecholyl, Guarneri and Evans, 1948), and (2) to reduce an already existing hormonal hypertension (benzodioxane, Goldenberg et al., 1947; Dibenamine, Spear and Griswold, 1948; piperoxan; Regitine, Emlet et al., 1951). The administration of drugs of the first group, (for example, histamine phosphate 0.025 mg. intravenously) to induce an attack of hypertension is often actually dangerous in functioning pheochromocytoma and for this reason the employment of Regitine and benzodioxane (Benodaine) to reduce hypertension is the adrenolytic of choice. Regitine should be used when the systolic pressure is above 170 mm. Hg and the diastolic over 100 mm. Hg, a positive result being manifested by a fall of more than 30 mm. systolic and 20 mm. diastolic. Benodaine causes a similar fall lasting not over fifteen minutes. Regitine may be given intravenously in the office in a dose of 5 mg., the diagnostic response being a sustained fall of blood pressure of 30 mm. systolic and 20 mm. diastolic for fifteen minutes or more. Similarly, but it should be used only in the hospital, benzodioxane (10 mg. per square meter of body surface) is given intravenously and when the test is positive, produces a sustained systolic blood pressure fall of 15 mm. or more for fifteen minutes. Although it is slightly more risky to use than regitine, benzodioxane almost never produces false positive results but occasionally may give a false negative response. It should not be used for patients with advanced cardiac, cerebral, or renal damage. Dibenamine is not recommended because its effects may last for hours. Piperoxan, 5 mg. intravenously, is used similar to benzodioxane. In case of any doubt collateral tests by the other drugs just enumerated must be employed.

Treatment. The presumptive diagnosis of pheochromocytoma having been established, removal of the tumor is the treatment. By proper use of adrenolytic agents to combat the extremely high blood pressure commonly occurring with surgical manipulation of the gland and pressor agents administered immediately after its removal, and continued to combat progressive blood pressure fall, the previously high surgical mortality of removal of these tumors has been greatly reduced. The entire surgical program demands both expert surgical and medical care, the preoperative and anesthetic preparation being comparable to that observed in extreme hyperthyroidism. Following surgical removal of the tumor, the blood pressure usually promptly falls; its failure to do so suggests the presence of another similar hormonal functioning tumor or of hormonal functioning metastases. This should be confirmed by repeated adrenolytic (Regitine) tests. A secondary tumor may be removed at the same sitting if it is recognized and the condition of the patient permits. Otherwise remove it later. Metastases are generally fatal. In rare instances the blood pressure may gradually decline over a period of several weeks rather than at once, but in these cases the Regitine test is negative. Either the transabdominal or the thoraco-abdominal approach is recommended; the former usually permits better study of the other adrenal.

CHAPTER 14

Urology in the Female

THIS CHAPTER is concerned with some of the special urologic problems in the female. The fundamentals of uropathy—obstruction, infection, hydronephrosis, calculus, tumor and other conditions—discussed in previous chapters are the same as in the male. Yet in the clinical work of the general practitioner, the obstetrician, and the gynecologist, as well as the urologist, there is a vast number of females whose complaint, as they state it, is "weak bladder," "bladder trouble," "weak kidneys" or backache. Most of these patients have one or more of the following symptoms: pain in the bladder or renal areas, urinary frequency, urgency or incontinence, either with leakage on exertion (stress incontinence) or continuous. Sometimes the condition has existed since birth (congenital, e.g., urethral stricture, epispadias, ureteral ectopia) or has developed on the basis of anomalous extra-urinary malformation as in neuromuscular vesical disease consequent to spina bifida or other neurovertebral defects. Yet, only half a dozen women with these complaints will keep a well-qualified urologist most humble, such are the symptomatic vagaries, the varieties of potential etiologic uropathies, often treated with less than therapeutic success. In most of these cases urethrotrigonitis is the usual finding with or without urethral stricture, vesical stone, pyelonephritis, or upper urinary tract obstruction. The symptoms may be cyclic with menstruation (hormonal influence, pelvic congestion), periodic with emotional disturbance, induced by coitus or at times developed as an excuse for avoiding it. In most cases in which the condition is due to local uropathy as apart from infected hydronephrosis, pyelonephritis, ureteral stricture and so forth, local treatment with adequate urethral dilation, endoscopic treatment and urinary sterilization as described in Chapter 7 may be expected to correct the condition rather promptly. Particularly has this been so since the anatomy (Fig. 305) and pathology of the urethra have been more fully studied and appreciated, and the importance of urethral stricture, diver-

541

ticulum, periurethritis, vesical sagging, or vesical neck contracture are more fully understood.

A third of the women I have seen with continuous symptoms of bladder irritation have had some gynecologic operation performed—sometimes for cystocele with perineal repair but more often uterine suspension or even hysterectomy "because the uterus was pressing on the bladder." Yet the vesical symptoms continued, often aggravated by postoperative urinary retention, chronic vesical overdistention and repeated catheterization, but in most instances they were promptly relieved and later cured by adequate periodic progressive dilation of the urethra with local instillation of mild silver nitrate (1:100).

The problem of urinary infection is considered in Chapter 7.

Backache of urologic origin is not uncommon and should be so recognized and correspondingly treated. Backache in women may be due to faulty posture, obstetric strain, gynecologic disease (endocervicitis, prolapse, retroversion, anteversion and so forth), obesity, orthopedic, neurologic or urologic disease. Urologic backache which may be due to hydronephrosis or ureteral disease differs from the other varieties just enumerated in that it is usually unilateral in the posterior flank, may radiate to the ovarian or iliac regions and *is not increased by stooping or bending over.* Yet hydronephrosis, obstructive nephroptosis, ureteral stricture, chronic pyelonephritis or even perinephritis may, by pain reference, simulate orthopedic, enteric, neurologic, cholecystic or hepatic disease or even vesical inflammation. A thorough urologic examination should suggest the correct diagnosis as far as the urinary tract is concerned and rational treatment may be undertaken.

In the evaluation of symptoms in terms of urologic conditions it must be remembered that lesions in organs or structures adjacent to or con-

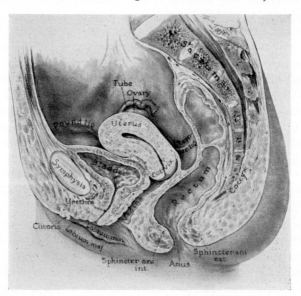

FIGURE 305.   Anatomy of the female urethra and pelvic structures (Anson).

tiguous with the urinary tract may be the site of the fundamental disease and no amount of urologic treatment will satisfy or cure the patient. Yet the adjacent disease may be no more complicated than a chronic cervicitis or endocervicitis serving to feed by congestion, or bacteriologically, an annoying urethrotrigonitis.

When gynecologic disease is suspected as the cause of urinary disturbances or pain in the pelvis, abdomen or loin, at least do an excretory urographic study to be certain the upper urinary tract is normal. In many of these patients the intravenous urographic study will be unsatisfactory or will leave doubt as to the diagnosis; this calls for complete urologic examination with urethrocystoscopy, divided renal function studies and bilateral retrograde pyelography. Commonly this will disclose a urologic cause for the pain—ureteral stricture, hydronephrosis, urethral stricture, urethrotrigonitis, interstitial cystitis, all remediable by local conservative instrumental treatment—and spares the patient the needless "look see" laparotomy, hysterectomy, salpingectomy or even sterilization. As a corollary, the vast number of needless appendectomies annually performed for "chronic appendicitis" would be greatly reduced if all patients about to undergo such operations were first given the benefit of at least satisfactory intravenous urographic study which often discloses ureteral stricture, calculus, hydronephrosis, or obstruction by aberrant vessels, peri-ureteral fibrous bands or masses as the cause of the symptoms.

MALFORMATION OF THE FEMALE UROGENITAL TRACT

Persistent cloaca and its associated lesions have been discussed in Chapter 6.

Congenital fissure of the clitoris is analogous to cleft of the glans penis and suggests the presence of other urogenital tract anomalies. **Absence of the clitoris** is similar to absence of the penis (q.v.).

Congenital hypertrophy of the clitoris is usually a manifestation in the adrenogenital syndrome and its accompanying pseudohermaphrodism (q.v. Chapter 13).

Hypospadias in the female is comparatively rare and is similar to hypospadias in the male in that the urethra opens obliquely on the anterior vaginal roof and proximal to the normal meatal site. When the opening is at or near the bladder neck there is total incontinence and the condition is essentially a vesico-urethrovaginal fistula with incontinence. Associated urologic and nonurologic anomalies are not uncommon. In this condition the vagina is likely to be smaller than normal and have a common outlet with the urethra so that intra-urethral intercourse is sometimes practiced. Incontinence is the dominant symptom and the diagnosis is made both by inspection and urethrocystoscopy. When there is urethral obstruction it should be overcome by dilation with sounds but when leakage is present, a urethral reconstruction with building up of a satisfactory vesical outlet, as in the operation of epispadias (q.v.), is necessary. In constructing the urethra, sufficiently large and long flaps of vaginal mucosa can often be brought together in the midline below over a catheter and control established by the Kelly, Kennedy or other method. Suprapubic cystostomy counterdrainage is most essential during the post-operative and convalescent period.

Fusion of the labia minora is an important though commonly unrecognized anomaly of infants and young girls, is characterized by a midline sealing together of the labia minora, usually leaving a minute unfused area just below the clitoris through which the child urinates and later menstruates (Figs. 306 to 308). The cause is unsettled, some observers believing it to be an acquired inflammatory adhesion rather than a congenital malformation. But the many cases I have seen seemed definitely of the congenital variety.

Vulvar fusion is seldom recognized until the child is four to six years of age, but in a spinster patient it was not discovered until she was sixty-nine. Pyuria is the usual *symptom*, resulting from vaginal collection of

Fig. 306

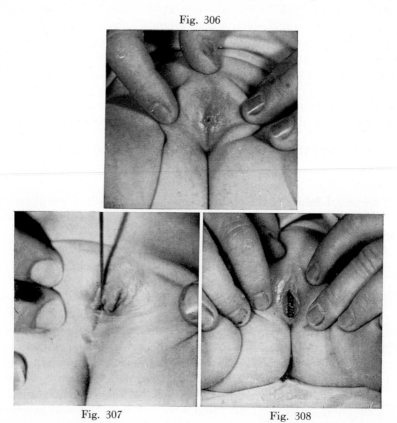

Fig. 307   Fig. 308

FIGURE 306. Fusion of the labia minora. Extremely small orifice in fused labia minora through which patient must void and in later life menstruate. An even smaller orifice was found in a sixty-nine-year-old woman with fused labia minora and through the minute opening she had menstruated.

FIGURE 307. Fusion of the labia minora. Instrument introduced into introitus preparatory to breaking down the labial adhesions.

FIGURE 308. Fusion of the labia minora. Adhesions broken down leaving a normal introitus presenting.

decomposed urine and the collateral inflammatory cellular exudate. Some of the patients I had seen were thought by others to be hermaphrodites. The condition is readily recognized by inspection, the fused labia minora appearing as a smooth, regular, reddish or reddish-blue surface which extends well anteriorly and sometimes the clitoris is completely covered by the midline fusion (Fig. 306). With lateral retraction of the labia majora, the perineum appears as a flat solid surface up to the subpubic level with a minute opening at or near the under side of the clitoris. Local vulvar inflammatory changes may be present. Urethrovesical disturbances with frequency and smarting on urination may be secondary to vulvar infection and urinary decomposition.

Treatment consists in separation of the labia minora by cleavage of the midline fusion and can be readily performed in the office without anesthesia. For this maneuver, I use a hemostat or a grooved director forcefully to make the division down to the deep perineum (Fig. 307). When the fusion is unusually dense, incision under local infiltration anesthesia may be needed, but this is rare. After dividing the fusion, a finger introduced into the introitus will break down any remaining adherence and will insure that the orifice is widely patent, a normal pouting hymen and urethral orifice appearing (Fig. 308). A small pledget of cotton may be left in the introitus for a day to keep the divided labia widely separated, and the patient should be re-examined in a month to make sure that refusion has not occurred.

Atresia of the hymen, fortunately, is rare but may produce grave secondary back pressure damage of the upper urinary tract. The enormous vaginal fluid distention the atresia produces is called *hydrometrocolpos* (secreted liquid from vaginal and uterine glands) before puberty and *hematometrocolpos* after menstruation has begun. The enormously distended vagina compresses the urethra to interfere with urination and to cause pronounced vesical retention, subsequently with widespread dilatation of the entire upper urinary tract and often grave complicating infection (Figs. 309, 311). The *diagnosis* is suggested by palpation of a suprapubic mass in an infant or young girl following emptying of the bladder. Most often a diagnosis of congenital cystic ovary is made. By compression of the mass with one hand and separation of the labia by the fingers of the other, the imperforate hymen will be seen to bulge out like a chewing-gum bubble (Fig. 309). By aspiration through the hymen, a fluid somewhat milky with desquamated epithelial cells is obtained and by injection with a radiopaque medium the enormously distended vagina can be demonstrated (Fig. 311).

Treatment is cruciate incision of the imperforate hymen with subsequent attention to be sure it remains well perforated.

Congenital absence of the vagina is extremely rare, and is often noted as an associated condition in grave anomalies of the urinary tract, particularly renal agenesis. When the patient's prospects are favorable, plastic construction of a vagina may be undertaken.

Hypoplasia of the vagina results from improper fusion of the mül-

Fig. 309

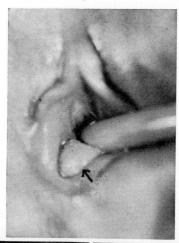

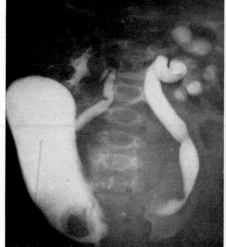
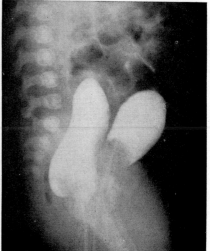

Fig. 310   Fig. 311

FIGURE 309. Atresia of the hymen. Pronounced urinary obstruction in infancy consequent to pressure on the urethra by a large hydrocolpos. This eight-week-old girl presented a rounded firm suprapubic mass 10 cm. in diameter. Various intra-abdominal cystic malformations had been diagnostically suggested by the several surgeons who examined the child. Yet urologic investigation disclosed imperforate hymen with a massive hydrocolpos. Suprapubic pressure caused the hymen to bulge for 1 cm. or more as a grayish ballooning (arrow).

FIGURE 310. Atresia of the hymen. Cystogram; anterior posterior view showing wide vesical displacement to the right by the central distended vagina, with extreme dilatation and lateral deviation of the ureters.

FIGURE 311. Atresia of the hymen. Lateral vaginogram and cystogram indicating the relation of the two structures. Treatment: cruciate incision of the hymen. A similar case in a girl ten hours old was also seen at Bellevue Hospital and radiographically demonstrated.

lerian ducts, making the canal short and narrow. *Other anomalies of the female reproductive tract* associated with urinary tract malformations include bicornuate, unicornuate or infantile uterus, duplication or even absence of the vagina, uterus and rectum, in all of which grave anomalies co-exist in the upper urinary tract; the child may be stillborn.

Vaginal hypoplasia is constantly found in external female hermaphrodism, and in many cases of male pseudohermaphrodism. The hypoplastic vagina may be enlarged, excised, or forgotten.

INFECTIONS AND INFLAMMATIONS OF THE VULVA

These are here considered in their urologic aspects as frequent predisposing or actual causative factors in the development of urethritis and urinary infection. It is realized that in the strictest sense they are in the province of gynecology.

Herpetic vulvitis is similar to penile herpes, beginning as many small vesicles which break down, become confluent superficial ulcers, involve both the mucosa and cutaneous surfaces, and may extend to the perigenital skin. The lesions cause itching, pain and, occasionally, vaginal discharge; local cleanliness and the administration of Aureomycin is the treatment.

Diphtheric vulvitis has occurred in the young as a complication of nasopharyngeal diphtheria. The infection usually invades the vagina with the formation of a pseudomembrane and causes pronounced toxemia. Diphtheria antitoxin is the specific treatment.

Mycotic vulvitis as commonly seen results from infection with *Candida albicans*, the cause of thrush, and appears as white elevated patches of varying size up to 1.5 cm. or more in diameter. The Monilia infection invades the vagina and often the urethra and bladder where the symptoms of cystitis, urethrotrigonitis or persistent pyuria develop. The organism readily grows in brownish-black colonies on Nickerson's medium. *Treatment* consists of painting the involved areas with 1 per cent aqueous gentian violet solution and the administration of suitable antibiotics, chiefly the tetracyclines. The vaginal insertion of mycostatin suppositories (250 mg. once daily) is said to be specific.

Gangrenous vulvitis may follow herpetic vulvitis, syphilis, measles, severe trauma, malnutrition, debility, and is seen chiefly in infants. The acutely swollen tissues are tense, red or reddish purple, rapidly progress to gangrene in a manner similar to that observed in streptococcic penile and scrotal gangrene as described in Chapter 8. The systemic toxemia is usually overwhelming and fatal. Penicillin and Aureomycin must be liberally and promptly administered.

Phlegmonous vulvitis, also known as noma pudendi, is analogous to buccal noma, and is caused by the spirochetes and fusiform bacilli as observed in Vincent's angina. It is a disease of the severely undernourished, is observed chiefly in infants and often as a complication of measles or erysipelas. First, one vulvar lip is involved and then the other, the tissues becoming intensely red, tense, painful, and later gangrenous. Local cleanliness plus the intensive administration of penicillin and mapharsen are specific.

THE FEMALE URETHRA

The female urethra is the homologue of the prostatic urethra in the male (Fig. 305). It is short and relatively wide, at birth being 1.5 cm. long, at puberty 3.0 to 3.5 cm., and in adults 3.5 to 4.5 cm., and 4.0 mm., 8.0 to 10.0 mm. and 9.0 to 12.0 mm. in diameter, respectively. The brevity of the urethra in female infants, bathed in fecal contamination, and with rich lymphatic supply communicating directly with that of the bladder and indirectly with the upper urinary tract accounts in some measure at least for the higher (three to five times) greater incidence of acute urinary infection in girl babies after the neonatal period. The urethral lining is stratified squamous epithelium, there are numerous mucous glands analogous to those of Littre in the male, and Skene's glands, one on each side, open just within the external meatus. In these many glands gonococci in particular find a favorable habitat. Glandlike structures in the posterior urethra, suggesting prostatic homologues, have been reported in many females, the tissue having been removed because of continual urethral infection or bladder-neck obstruction.

The *internal sphincter* in the female is composed of intertwining and circular muscle fibers as anterior extensions of the bladder wall in conjunction with those of the trigone. The external sphincter is comprised of compressor urethrae fibers between the layers of the triangular ligament. The innervation is by the pudic nerves (see physiology of urination). The arterial supply is from the inferior vesical, uterine, internal pudic for the upper, middle, and lower thirds of the canal respectively. The venous return is largely by the vesical, vaginal, and pudendal plexuses while the lymphatics of the posterior urethra drain to the inner group of inguinal nodes and the remainder of the urethra drains through the inguinal glands.

In addition to infections both venereal and nonvenereal, the urethra is subject to mild or violent trauma during coitus and labor, the common late result of which is stricture. During delivery, the urethra may be crushed against the pubis by the child's head or by forceps and this injury is commonly followed by stricture, perhaps not appearing clinically until ten or fifteen years later.

Prolapse of the Urethral Mucosa. This eversion or rolling out of the urethral mucosa through the external urethral meatus in rosette formation occurs only in women and to the inexperienced may be confused with caruncle or urethral prolapse (q.v.). While the eversion is usually mild and limited, it may be pronounced as a reddish-purple, bleeding, highly sensitive mass and suggest eversion of the bladder, prolapsed ureterocele (q.v.), or a gangrenous carcinoma. Pain, dysuria, frequency and/or hematuria with incontinence or retention are the prominent symptoms. The eversion can seldom be examined or catheterized without an anesthetic, so painful is it. Treatment is radial cauterization or, better, if the mucosal mass is large, ligation of it about a large catheter (Fig. 312) as described under treatment of urethral prolapse. Periodically dilate the urethra postoperatively to be sure stricture neither develops nor persists.

Prolapse of the female urethra is an eversion of the urethra (rather than just mucosa) through the meatus and may be complete or incomplete. In the *incomplete* variety only a small portion of the urethra is everted, while in the *complete* variety the prolapse involves up to the bladder outlet. Incomplete prolapse occurs most often in infancy and between the ages of eight and twelve, two thirds appearing under fifteen years of age. Complete prolapse is seen more often in older females and in a few instances the bladder has prolapsed as well (Fig. 312).

Urethral prolapse, like prolapse of the urethral mucosa, is predisposed to by abnormal mucosal redundancy and congenitally poor tissue structure locally but is fundamentally the result of excessive straining

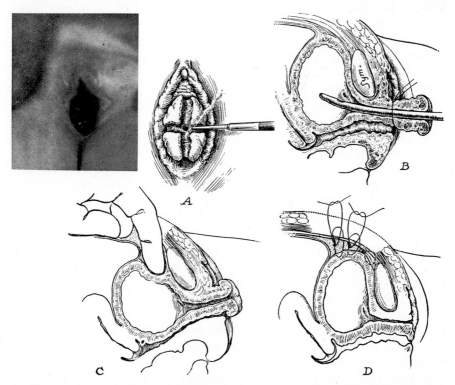

FIGURE 312. Urethral prolapse in a six-year-old girl (insert). This condition is not to be confounded with prolapse of a large ureterocele or vesical prolapse. Treatment. *A*, deep cruciate cauterization; this often suffices. *B*, a large silk or semirigid catheter is introduced into the bladder and is withdrawn a few centimeters thus pulling the prolapsed portion of the canal well forward. A suture is now tightly tied as indicated and, by pressure necrosis, excises the prolapsed segment. This has been successfully employed by the author in several females, the youngest being five years of age, the oldest seventy-eight years. *C*, Hepburn's method by suspension of the bladder. The viscus is freed anteriorly for some distance beneath the pubis and is then elevated well upward, thus reducing the urethral prolapse. The bladder is now sutured to the anterior abdominal and subpubic fascia (*D*).

such as accompanies constipation, during the strain of whooping cough, vesical stone, or severe urethrocystitis. The everted, prolapsed, strangulated mucosa appears in the vulva as a reddish or reddish-blue meatal tumor 0.5 to 4.5 cm. or more in diameter, bleeds freely, is excessively sensitive, and the accompanying edema often occludes the meatal orifice to cause urinary retention. With strangulation, degenerative changes produce fissures or ulceration of the urethra to differentiate the older lesions from the more recent, and in pronounced prolapse and strangulation, thrombotic gangrene may ensue.

Symptoms are those of urethral irritation with frequency, burning on urination, an exquisitely tender mass at the external urethral meatus and, in about half of the cases, hematuria. The severity of the condition should readily differentiate it from caruncle, simple eversion of the meatus, or a protruded polyp, or even prolapsed ureterocele which presents a much smoother reddish globular mass and is readily pushed back into the bladder.

Treatment. The simplest is tying off of the redundant mucosa. A large silk catheter is first passed to the bladder and then slightly withdrawn, thus pulling forward the prolapsed urethral meatus and about the base of the mass a silk ligature is tightly tied (Fig. 312). This strangulation causes sloughing of the evaginated mucosa in about three days and the wound heals kindly. Electrocauterization, making four to five equidistant cruciate coagulations, may effect a cure. More drastic, the redundant mucosa may be excised. In severe or recurrent prolapse, surgical treatment involves suprapubic mobilization of the anterior bladder wall and urethra and reduction of the prolapse following which the bladder is anchored high by sutures to the inner abdominal wall (Fig. 312).

Diverticulum of the female urethra is a relatively frequent finding in older women in whom it occurs more often than in males; it is most rare in the young. In some cases it is congenital but is more commonly an acquired "blow-out" development behind urethral stricture or at the site of trauma (including instrumental), calculi or periurethral abscess. Some of these diverticula in women are multiple, may become cystic or harbor stones. Symptoms are those of urethral irritation and urinary infection with pain, burning, frequency of urination, urgency, dysuria, strangury or hematuria, dyspareunia or even urinary retention. The symptoms usually cause the diagnosis of "cystitis" to be made. There may be installment emptying (pis en deux temps); the patient voids, waits a moment, then voids again. With this further straining the contents of the diverticulum, often thick, purulent and foul, may be passed. Distended by urine or purulent debris, the diverticulum may occlude the urethra. The *diagnosis* is made by urethroscopy, and urethrography will outline the sac. Sometimes a diverticulum can be palpated. *Treatment* is excision which in mild cases can be performed transurethrally by simply enlarging the roof of the diverticulum opening. In large or multiple diverticula, open surgical excision is necessary.

Urethritis in the Female. Nongonorrheal or simple acute urethritis is usually secondary to vulvitis or vaginitis and commonly results from uncleanliness. The condition is frequently seen in females of all ages and follows contamination by feces or infected linens, toilet seats, unclean hands, or the introduction of infection with foreign bodies such as hair pins. The most frequent invading organisms are colon bacilli, staphylococci, streptococci, and pseudodiphtheroids, although many other strains of bacteria have been identified. *Traumatic urethritis* is a frequent result of masturbation in young girls.

The inflammation usually involves only the mucosa and submucosa but with virulent infection it may extend deep, even to cause suppurative periurethritis. Infection may lodge in the small scattered glands of the anterior third of the urethra or in tubuloglandular structures in the posterior third of the urethra and about the vesical outlet. Considerable attention has been directed to these last structures thought by some to be homologues of the prostate gland and to function as foci for infection spread as a lymphatic extension to cause chronic urethrocystitis in girls and "pyelitis" in older females. All observers are not in agreement with this view.

In females the urethral inflammation regularly extends to the anterior trigone and may even involve the entire structure, producing a *urethrotrigonitis* (Fig. 313). These inflammatory changes in the trigone and at the bladder outlet explain the disturbances of urination which are so pronounced when the process is acute, and may be distressing even when the inflammation is mild. *Chronic urethrotrigonitis is the commonest single finding in persistent enuresis in girls.*

Symptoms. There may be no symptoms or extremely mild ones, with variable frequency, urgency, dysuria, burning, or terminal hematuria. In acute cases there is a reddened, pouting meatus, often with a purulent or muco-purulent discharge, by the microscopic examination of which the etiologic organism can usually be demonstrated.

Chronic urethritis may follow an acute urethritis or may insidiously appear as a result of mild inflammation, and frequently predisposed to by a previously unrecognized tight external urethral meatus. The mucosal

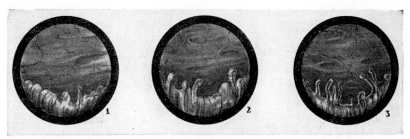

FIGURE 313. Chronic urethrotrigonitis in the young female; cystoscopic view of the vesical outlet. 1, mild edema. 2, elongated fronts. 3, coarse pseudopapillomatosis due to persistent inflammation. This picture is somewhat less commonly seen in males. It is frequently observed in young girls with enuresis and particularly when congenital stricture of the urethra coexists.

changes vary from mild granular urethritis to advanced edema of the
bladder outlet and often with hyperplastic tissue formations, small papillary pedunculated masses, or projecting cystic bodies (Fig. 313). Edema
is usually commensurate with the intensity of the inflammation, the
inflammatory process always extending into the posterior urethra and
onto the anterior trigone at least.

Treatment. Cleanliness of the genitals is the best prophylaxis
against nongonorrheal urethritis in females and especially in young girls.
The removal of the cause of the condition is the first step in treatment and
this may mean removal of a foreign body, cessation of repeated catheterization or of masturbation, or the treatment of vulvovaginitis. Sulfonamide
or antibiotic therapy is administered according to bacteriologic indications.

In chronic urethrotrigonitis make sure there is no accompanying
urethral stricture, with or without periurethritis. Thus, the urethra should
be gently but adequately dilated with steel sounds or bougies in a girl of
eight years to 22 to 24 F., and in the average adult female to 34 or 36 F.
Following the dilation, the urethral instillation of a small quantity (0.5
to 1 cc.), of silver nitrate 0.1 to 1.0 per cent or even stronger is usually
advantageous. As a rule three or four treatments at intervals of ten to
fourteen days will suffice, the most common site of obstruction being at
the meatus.

This treatment will establish free urethral drainage and encourage
absorption of periurethral infiltration. Antimicrobial therapy is coadministered as bacteriologically indicated. Treatment ceases only when the
urine remains sterile and the canal stays dilated. Excrescences about the
vesical outlet will frequently disappear spontaneously following this
therapy and seldom need electrocoagulation.

Excessive frequency of urination, the so-called **irritable bladder of
women,** is one of the commoner symptomatic complexes with which the
physician must deal. In the majority of cases the condition results from a
chronic urethrotrigonitis in which low-grade urinary infection is generally
maintained by an unrecognized urethral stricture and with or without
complicating cystocele. The administration of antimicrobials may bring
temporary relief by ameliorating the infection but it alone cannot strike
at the fundamental problem of urinary stasis, and prompt recurrence of
symptoms upon cessation of medication is almost certain. In short, urethral dilation is also needed. The mere lavaging of the bladder and the
instillation of silver proteinate or whatever solution the physician employs
is of no lasting value except as the catheter dilates the urethra. There are
patients without number who have been subjected to all sorts of perineal
repairs, and abdominal uterine suspensions and other gynecologic mal-
treatment performed as the patient is told, "because the uterus is pressing
on the bladder." I have seen dozens of such women who have gone
through these multiple gynecologic surgical attacks and without relief
until, finally, someone adequately dilated the urethra! This experience is
common to urologists.

Gonococcus Urethritis. Infants and young girls often acquire gonorrheal vaginitis and complicating urethritis by contact with infected bed pans, toilet seats, thermometers, and the like. In older girls and adult women gonorrhea is almost invariably consequent to sexual contact. The stratified squamous epithelial lining of the female urethra corresponds to that of the prostatic urethra in the male and is moderately resistant to the gonococcus. Gonococci may attack, lodge in, and even cause variable abscess formation in the small mucosal glands of the anterior urethra or the para-urethral glands of Skene.

The *pathologic changes* in the female urethra are, in general, similar to those occurring in gonorrheal urethritis in the male with periurethritis, periurethral abscess, or sclerotic healing with stricture formation as the disease or its after effects persist. In general, however, the condition is much less severe in the female urethra than in the male.

Symptoms are those of acute urethral inflammation accompanied by redness, swelling, pouting, or sticking together of the urethral meatus, and a purulent or mucopurulent greenish yellow discharge in which the gonococci can be demonstrated. Vulvitis with edematous swelling and superficial ulceration may develop and cause pain, and sometimes is the manifestation which directs attention to the infection.

Treatment. Having established the microscopic diagnosis, antimicrobial therapy is rigorously administered as in the treatment of gonococcus urethritis in the male as outlined in Chapter 8. Painful and extremely frequent urination can be controlled by urethral anodynes in the early stages; the composition of a satisfactory one is given on page 247. With intensive antimicrobial therapy, not only will the gonorrheal urethral lesion heal but also the vaginitis, cervicitis, bartholinitis, and other lesions falling in the province of gynecology. During treatment, hygienic considerations merit attention with gentle cleansing of the genitals two or three times daily, avoiding trauma or rough handling of the parts. Should periurethral abscess develop at or near the meatus, it may be incised externally; with prompt intensive medical treatment such complications should not arise. The late development of stricture requires periodic dilation with sounds.

Stricture of the Female Urethra. This is extremely common, often congenital but may be due to infection, trauma of instrumentation, coitus, pregnancy or childbirth. Most strictures seen in young girls are congenital and located at or near the external meatus (Fig. 110). Congenital stricture may also occur at the proximal end of the urethra where it is generally designated as contracture of the vesical outlet or bladder neck. In the young as well as in older women with acquired urethral stricture, the condition has most often followed infection—gonorrheal or nongonorrheal —or trauma. Periurethritis and periurethral abscess heal by scarring to produce stricture.

Difficult or prolonged second-stage of labor is one of the commonest causes of urethral stricture observed in middle-aged and older women. The soft urethra of the young mother is mashed against the bony pubis by the oncoming head, and during delayed delivery at this time, the compression of the urethra may cause pronounced vascular anoxemia of the tissues with important injury from this source alone. In some instances stricture has resulted from urethral injury during intercourse in which there is conflict between a small tight vagina and a comparatively large penis. Here the initial manifestations following injury are those of acute urethritis with subsequent clinical stricture in three to five years or earlier. The injury may have been caused by the introduction of foreign bodies employed in masturbation or by rough digital masturbatory trauma as a child, but may also result from straddle injuries or as a complication of pelvic fracture. The period between cause and result in the pathogenesis of stricture is most variable, the traumatic strictures frequently being manifest within three months while most other strictures require three to five years and even longer to form.

Urethral stricture in the female is commonly an associated etiologic factor in the genesis and perpetuation of urinary infection. Especially is this so in little girls. Urinary stasis is produced, infection gains access via the urethral meatus or hematogenously through the kidneys and the bacteria, wherever they may be in the urinary tract, multiply to induce clinically evident infection with fever, chills, often vesical disturbances and pyuria. To what extent the urethral and periurethral glands serve as foci harboring bacteria is unknown, but clinical experience suggests they often play an important part in the perpetuation of infection. Establishment of free drainage from these glands by adequate dilation of the urethra probably does most to help them eliminate their own infection.

Infection retained in the periurethral glands leads to localized leukocytic infiltration with fibrosis and constriction of the urethral lumen. Untreated, the urethral narrowing causes urinary frequency and may lead to retention, partial or complete, even with overflow incontinence which often gives rise to the "weak bladder" or "weak kidney" complaints. In some females with periurethral gland infection and contracture of the bladder neck, histologic examination discloses distinctly glandular structure in removed specimens, sometimes even strongly resembling the histology in infected tubuloglandular tissue in the male prostate.

In urethral stricture congestive inflammation of the proximal urethra, bladder neck and anterior trigone develops which, persisting, causes granular, edematous and polypoid changes in the mucosa, all of which are easily seen through the urethroscope (Fig. 313).

Symptoms of urethral stricture are those of urethral irritability with frequency, nocturia, dysuria, urgency or incontinence, difficulty in starting the stream, passage of a small stream, burning on urination, tenesmus, hematuria especially terminal, urethral, suprapubic, groin, low back, flank or rectal pain. In the young, frequency and nocturia—sometimes with wetting and usually designated as enuresis—is the commonest manifestation.

Diagnosis is made by the passage of bougies or sounds which are grasped, and by urethroscopic visualization; the last is the most satisfactory diagnostic method. Sometimes the white scar of the stricture is recognized. In urethral stricture in the female, urethrotrigonitis is regularly seen with variable chronic inflammatory changes such as cystic bodies, villi, papillary fonds, polypoid excrescences, and occasionally small areas of superficial ulceration about the vesical outlet, even extending into the posterior urethra. With significant obstruction there is variable trabeculation of the bladder wall and there may even be residual urine; the urethra may be dilated proximal to the blockage and in some cases the upper urinary tract is also dilated (Fig. 110). Traumatic urethral stricture is differentiated from the gonorrheal or nongonorrheal variety by the history, its rapid appearance, greater density of the scar, and its stubborn resistance to dilation.

Treatment of stricture of the female urethra is fundamentally the same as in the male with periodic progressive dilation with sounds. Following the dilation, the deep urethral instillation of two or three drops of 1:1000 silver nitrate is helpful in the treatment of chronic inflammatory lesions. As a rule, therapeutic dilation to 16 F. is adequate for a one-year-old girl, to 20 F. for one of five years, to 24 F. for a ten-year-old girl, and 34 to 36 F. for the average adult female. Urethral strictures in the female seldom require cutting, not even meatotomy. Usually not many dilations are required; they are given at lengthening intervals of one, two and three months apart until the urethra stays dilated. Recheck examination should be made in three to six months and dilation repeated. Concurrent with the treatment, the urine should be sterilized by bacteriologically indicated antimicrobials.

THE BLADDER

Inflammation of the bladder, most commonly due to infection and generally designated cystitis, is fundamentally the same condition in each sex, the considerations in the male having been given in Chapter 7 which it is suggested the reader review at this point. Also as in the male, the vesical infection is nearly always secondary to bacterial disease in the urethra or adjacent structures or in the upper urinary tract, especially the kidneys. In the female with "cystitis," urethrotrigonitis is the commonest lesion. In turn it is usually associated with or is secondary to urethral stricture, the treatment of which is the treatment of the "cystitis." This has been described in the immediate preceding paragraph. In short, treatment of "cystitis" is that of the primary cause whether it be stricture, pyelonephritis, pelvic inflammatory gynecologic disease (salpingitis, cervicitis, endocervicitis, pelvic abscess or necrotizing uterine fibroids) or simply cystocele with residual urine and infection. The diagnosis and treatment may require the combined efforts of the gynecologist and urologist.

Interstitial Cystitis. This variety of chronic, patchy submucous cystitis is also known as elusive ulcer, Hunner's ulcer, and interstitial panmural cystitis. The clocklike day and night regularity of frequent urination induced by diminishing vesical capacity and increased irritability still lacks adequate recognition by physicians in general and urologists in particular. Peculiarly, the condition is found chiefly in women (95 per cent); its cause is unknown although Hunner attributed most of his many cases to focal infection, especially in the teeth, tonsils, ears and sinuses, often in association with ureteral stricture and coccic infection, especially streptococcus and staphylococcus. In many of the reported cases the condition has disappeared following removal of an active focus of infection by tonsillectomy, dental extraction, sinus drainage, and so forth, but this is rarely effective as sole therapy.

Pathology. Chronic interstitial cystitis is unusual in that it (1) occurs chiefly in females and over the bladder dome, (2) is found frequently in the absence of associated urologic lesions, (3) is highly resistant to treatment, and (4) is often scarcely less troublesome and

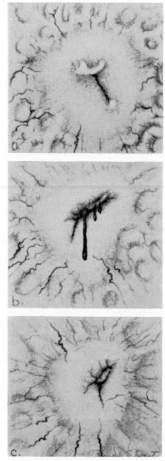

Figure 314.   Interstitial cystitis. The cystoscopic appearance of three separate areas of submucous fibrosis in a man. *a*, the gray line of necrosis on the apex of the ridge is connected by the line of submucous hemorrhage. *b*, the type showing submucous bleeding with distention from another line of submucous fibrosis. *c*, an earlier stage of submucous change. During the course of treatment these three apparently separate areas were found to connect (Hinman).

intractable than vesical cancer or tuberculosis. There is inflammatory infiltration and sclerosis of the submucosa and adjacent muscular coats of the bladder resulting in small superficial mucosal ulcerations with intense peripheral congestion as cystoscopically observed (Figs. 314 and 315). Lesions heal in one place while new ones appear elsewhere. There is a striking disproportion between the intensity of the vesical symptoms which simulate continuous acute cystitis and the comparative meagerness of the cystoscopic findings. Eventually there is inflammatory involvement of the entire bladder wall which thickens with leukocytic, lymphocytic and plasma cell infiltration, edema and muscular hypertrophy. The overlying peritoneum may be thickened and the vesical mucosa locally ulcerated.

Distention of the contracted bladder wall causes the appearance of numerous freely bleeding cracks in the mucosa and which may heal and totally disappear within two weeks; the cystoscopic diagnosis rests upon

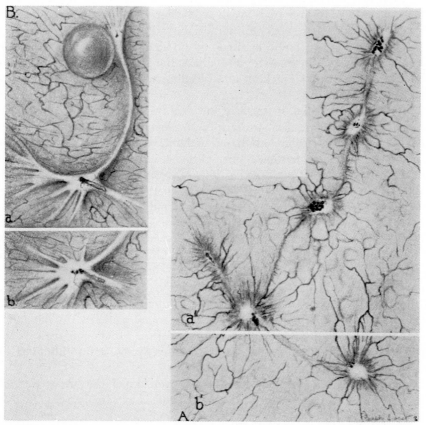

FIGURE 315. Composite drawing of cystoscopic pictures of submucous fibrosis showing the irregular arcuate character of the lesions, the upper area being near the air bubble and the lower at the right 2 cm. about the ureteral orifice. *A*, the general appearance before fulguration; the history indicated a duration of four or five years. *B*, the scarred appearance six months after treatment by fulguration; the lesions are almost healed. *a* and *a'* and *b* and *b'* are corresponding areas (Hinman).

this observation (Fig. 314). These lesions first appear over the bladder vertex but are later seen elsewhere as the disease progresses, and then become cystoscopically recognized as single or multiple brownish-red patches of various size and shape, surrounded by a radiating network of engorged blood vessels (Fig. 315). Large portions of the contracted bladder wall often appear normal. The inflamed areas ulcerate superficially, and later heal with whitish irregular or linear but extremely sensitive scarring which, if distended, splits and bleeds. Sometimes with healing, the local lesion completely disappears. As bladder wall contraction progresses, its capacity may be reduced to only two or three ounces so that the patient may have a physiologic or working capacity of only 20 or 30 cc. before having to void and yet there is no residual urine.

Symptoms. The striking clinical feature of interstitial cystitis is the clocklike regularity of the urinary frequency, increasing as the bladder contracts with diminishing capacity. Frequency often becomes every thirty minutes day and night with a bladder capacity of perhaps 40 to 60 cc., which of itself suggests interstitial cystitis or tuberculosis. Yet the cystoscopic diagnosis should be made by an alert urologist. When there is doubt, anesthetize the patient and dilate the bladder while performing the cystoscopic study; cracking and bleeding will appear in the areas of induration or scarring.

Treatment. None is certain; surgical resection has no place. At present the treatment most uniformly employed by urologists is electro-coagulation of the lesions with or without repeated hydraulic vesical distention. Vesical distention alone with the instillation of silver nitrate in strengths of 0.5 to 2 per cent has given favorable results in many hands and is the method I use chiefly. Education of the bladder and encouragement are essential collaterals in the therapeutic regimen. It is remarkable to see how many of these patients with an initial bladder capacity of only 2 or 3 oz. for example, will by periodic progressive hydraulic dilation under local anesthesia of the bladder lining or intravenous sodium pentathol anesthesia, achieve an increasing bladder capacity, ultimately to as much as 12 to 15 oz. or more and with complete symptomatic relief. Unfortunately vesical recontraction and symptoms recur after a variable period and require further treatment and many patients do not enjoy even this fortuitous progress. Yet with patience, satisfactory results are usually obtained and ureterosigmoidostomy, previously employed in many cases, is rendered unnecessary.

Prolapse of the bladder occurs as an eversion of the viscus through the urethral meatus and only in females, and is extremely rare. Relaxation of the vesical outlet and urethra is a predisposing cause and usually there is an antecedent history of urinary incontinence. Straining to cough, urinate or defecate is usually the immediate factor; dysentery has been reported in some cases and physical trauma in others. In vesical prolapse the trigone and ureteral orifice can usually be identified and serve to distinguish it from the less serious urethral prolapse, prolapse of a ureterocele, or polypoid tumor. With strangulation of the prolapsed vesical segment, gangrene may appear.

Treatment is reduction of the bladder which can usually be accomplished by pushing the organ back in place with the beak of a small cystoscope or a straight sound. Preferably this should be done under anesthesia and gently. With the bladder reduced, a small balloon catheter is anchored indwelling for a week to permit the vesical outlet and urethra to recontract. With recurrent vesical prolapse, the organ must be surgically suspended to the anterior abdominal wall and if permanent incontinence results from the stretching it may be necessary to correct this by sphincteroplasty (Kelly plication) or, in severe cases, in the manner employed in surgical treatment of advanced epispadias (q.v.).

Cystocele. Most cystoceles have their origin during pregnancy and labor. As a result of stretching and compression of the vaginal walls, and of the subvesical pelvic fascia including broad ligament layers attached to the pelvic wall (supporting the cervix, bladder and urethra), the support of these structures is weakened. The organs sag with progressive herniation into the vaginal cavity of the posterior bladder floor and anterior vaginal wall. With greater and wider sagging, the entire bladder floor, trigone and vesical outlet and sometimes even the posterior urethra bulge into the introitus. The ligamentous and fascial (broad and uterosacral ligaments, perivesical fasciae, levator ani muscles, pelvic floor, rectovaginal septum, etc.) stretching and damage may be much greater than in simple cystocele as just described, with variable prolapse of the bladder and uterus, and rectal herniation into the vagina.

The urologic importance of cystocele is concerned with the resulting urinary stasis and vesical residuum which not only offers a fertile field for the development of urinary infection, but perpetuates an established infection which may always be considered to involve the kidneys as well. Lower ureteral obstruction by angulation or compression, regularly occurs with cystocele and/or prolapse and causes upper urinary tract stasis, back pressure injury, and favors infection (see Chapters 5 and 7). Yet in mild cystocele with vesical irritability, treatment other than wide dilation of the urethra and sterilization of the urine is seldom necessary despite the zeal of the gynecologist and more particularly of the general surgeon to operate upon the condition. Pronounced cystocele and especially with rectocele requires major surgical repair.

INJURIES OF THE URINARY TRACT

The usual injuries of the urinary tract are discussed in Chapter 10.

Irradiation injuries have become an increasing problem as x-rays, radium, cobalt[60] and other ionizing agents are more widely used in the treatment of a variety of gynecologic conditions and cervical cancer in particular. Amenorrhea, bladder damage (ulceration, incrustation, scarring, telangectasia, necrosis, fistulization or contracture), proctitis and, frequently, intractable stricturization of the lower ureters are common late results. The management and treatment of these complications of irradiation, too often improperly or injudiciously used initially or even contraindicated, should be entrusted to one experienced in these problems. In some instances the only hope for relief lies in transplantation of the ureters to the rectum or, if the rectum has been badly injured by the irradiation, to the skin. One must be sure that new carcinoma has not developed in the irradiation injured structures!

FISTULA

The various urinary fistulas—vesicovaginal, urethrovaginal, ureterovaginal, or even vesicovaginorectal—which may result from trauma (surgical, obstetric, gynecologic or irradiation) are readily recognized. Their treatment is surgical, often highly complicated, and should be carried out by an expert urologist or urogynecologist.

URINARY INCONTINENCE

The many causes of urinary incontinence have been considered in Chapter 2 and elsewhere in this book. The more frequent are congenital (vesical extrophy, patent urachus, complete epispadias, ectopic ureter, absence of vesical sphincter); neuromuscular vesical disease, the various fistulas, congenital or acquired; overflow from vesical overdistention consequent to obstruction or neurogenic or due to acute urethrovesical irritation from inflammation, stone, foreign bodies, tumor or obstruction.

Stress incontinence is the commonest variety of lack of urinary control in women and occurs as a painless leakage of a few drops or even an ounce or more with abdominal exertion of laughing, coughing, sneezing, straining or even rising from a chair. It is to be sharply distinguished from the urinary leakage of urgency due to urethrovesical inflammation in which the patient wets herself before she can get to the toilet. Stress incontinence rarely appears before middle age and most often in stout or obese women who have borne children. Yet it occurs occasionally in virgins—especially older ones—with weak sphincters and no previous local injury.

Urethroscopy shows a relaxed, sluggish vesical outlet, often irregular and distorted by scar, and feebly closing on conscious effort of the patient. Vaginal palpation of the urethra against the urethroscope may disclose unsuspected localized, generalized or nodular peri-urethritis.

Fortunately many of these patients can be improved or even cured by nonoperative treatment consisting chiefly in (1) getting rid of obesity, (2) eradication of any irritable lesions in the urethra or bladder and including sterilization of the urine, (3) avoiding physical strain such as lifting, straining at constipated stools, chronic coughing, (4) general and vesical sedation (barbiturates, hyoscyamus), and (5) muscular exercises with or without the *perineometer* to strengthen the sphincter mechanism.

The perineometer is a rubber bulb device which is inserted into the vagina and is connected with a mercury manometer which records the contractile strength of the vaginal walls and vesical supports including the levator ani muscles. Although it may require diligent exercise daily or twice daily for several months before relief is achieved, excellent results have been obtained. The patient is continually encouraged as she becomes progressively able to squeeze the bulb harder in her vagina. Some women find the mechanism inconvenient or distasteful and in some of these satisfactory results have been obtained simply by the conscious practice of the vaginal squeezing exercise alone.

When the conservative treatment just outlined is unsatisfactory, surgery must be employed, the procedure used more than any other being the Kelly plication stitch of the vesical sphincter which in trained hands has cured nine-tenths of these women. Other procedures include fascial suspension of the urethra and bladder neck (Stoeckel, Miller, Aldridge, Millin, Marshall-Marchetti) and reconstruction of the periurethral fascia (Kennedy).

THE URETER

"He who knows ureteral obstruction (in the female) knows not only urology but also gynecology and has a faint idea of some of the problems of obstetrics" (Wharton). Ureteral disease such as stricture, calculi or extra-ureteral inflammation or compression may simulate appendicitis, salpingitis, or incite reflex urinary disturbances (too frequently called "cystitis"). It may cause innumerable needless appendectomies, salpingectomies, uterine suspensions, ureteral dilations and so forth to be performed as well as the endless administration of needless medicinal treatment. The reproduction of the pain complained of by ureteral distention with normal saline solution should give the diagnostic clue although the ureteral lesions(s) may result from adjacent disease.

Ureteral obstruction may result from stricture, stone, tumor, kinking, irradiation, trauma, infection or tuberculosis, precisely as it does in the male. Yet more often in women, lower abdominal or pelvic extra-ureteral masses or other lesions may cause ureteral compression. These include uterine fibroids or cancer, ovarian cysts, adenomas or cancer, uterine prolapse, or there may be hormonal influences causing relaxation, dilatation and urinary stasis as normally occurs in 95 per cent of pregnancies. In carcinoma of the cervix, the bilateral ureteral blockage from the tumor spread to the broad ligaments and pelvis, destroys the kidneys by urinary back pressure and makes uremia the commonest cause of death under such circumstances (Fig. 316). Ureteral obstruction may also result from angulation consequent to uterine prolapse, irradiation scarring, and surgical injuries especially during hysterectomy and even when performed with catheters in the ureters.

Upper tract obstruction and infection alone may account for the slight fever, malaise, headache, nausea and apathy which occurs so commonly in pregnant women but also in nonpregnant women with comparable obstruction and infection. The obstruction may cause only mild ureterectasis and pain in the loin or renal areas. To repeat, by passing the ureteral catheter and injecting the ureter and pelvis with saline solution, the pain complained of may be reproduced to localize it to the ureter.

Ureterospasm, localized and due to inflammation or disease of an adjacent organ or structure (appendix, ovary, tube, endometriosis or over-irradiation, for example) is a real clinical entity, often causes severe, sharp, dull or colicky pain and, unless stricture forms secondarily, may be expected to disappear following removal of its local cause. In the urogram of localized ureteral spasm, the spastic constriction is always at the same spot and in studies made at different times in the same series and on different days.

UROLOGIC CONDITIONS COMMON TO PREGNANCY

Pregnancy has no exemptions from the usual urologic diseases; I have uneventfully removed completely obstructing ureteral stones from a half dozen women between the sixth and eighth month of gestation. Pre-existing urethral stricture may close completely shut or nearly so and require dilation, or if term is not too distant, require indwelling catheterization. Urinary infection, commonly and inadequately diagnosed as "pyelitis of pregnancy" has been the usual urologic complication. Formerly occurring with an incidence of 12 to 15 per cent of all pregnant women, by virtue of greater urologic-mindedness of the obstetricians and modern antimicrobial therapy, not more than 1 to 2 per cent of pregnant women in enlightened areas today develop "pregnancy pyelitis." Yet true renal infection—suppurative pyelonephritis, infected hydronephrosis or even pyonephrosis—and usually with completely obstructed ureteral drainage, is still a serious complication as it may gravely jeopardize the mother, impair her future health, and increase infant mortality threefold.

The immediate danger of acute urinary infection and the injury it may cause to the mother and fetus is generally recognized but, if the infection is promptly eradicated, there is scant likelihood of permanent damage. Too commonly sight is lost of the potential late after effects when the infection is allowed to persist: chronic urinary stasis, urethral and/or ureteral stricture, hydronephrosis, calculous disease, chronic pyelonephritis, chronic nephritis, reduced renal function and, not infrequently, hypertension. Symptoms of urethrovesical irritation often persist or the mother simply feels "dragged out" all the time from the urinary toxemia. Pronounced anemia is common and may require whole blood transfusions. In any event, a complete urologic study is indicated and appropriate treatment administered (see Chapter 7).

The history indicates that in most women who develop urinary infection during pregnancy, there was pre-existing urologic disease such as ureteral stricture, hydronephrosis, chronic pyelonephritis and the like, and which should have been eliminated from the picture before the patient was permitted to become pregnant, or, if severe enough, to continue with the pregnancy. In many of these patients the initial urinary infection occurred in childhood, persisting, smoldering, low grade and usually unrecognized until the pregnancy or some other momentous or stasis-producing, debilitating condition occurs to engender an acute and often critical flareup of the renal infection.

Urinary Stasis in Pregnancy. In addition to the usual causes of urinary obstruction in people as a whole as described in Chapter 5, in pregnancy there is an important added factor—the hormonal—which largely accounts for the ureteral and general renal pelvic dilatation peculiar to this period. The hormone is *progestin* which has a relaxing effect on the ureteral smooth muscle and is present in increasing amounts as pregnancy progresses.

Upper urinary tract dilatation is seen in over 95 per cent of all pregnant women, is right sided in this same proportion and occurs on the left also but slightly less often (Figs. 317, 318). The progestin induces ureteral dilatation and atony with diminished peristalsis which results in urinary stasis and a fertile soil for infection. Other factors are the pressure of the gravid uterus on the ureter(s) and variable congestive swelling of the terminal ureters. Antecedent disease may play its part also.

Usually present by the end of the third month, ureteral dilatation increases up to the seventh month when it may variably recede. Following delivery the upper tract gradually returns to normal morphology in a month in three fourths of these women, but occasionally some dilatation remains permanently and even with variable hydronephrosis. The

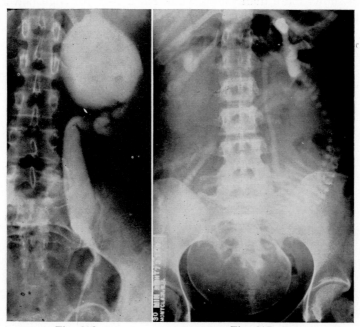

Fig. 316   Fig. 317

FIGURE 316. Advanced left ureteropelvic dilatation above blockage by pelvic extension of cervical carcinoma.
FIGURE 317. Dilatation of the upper urinary tract in pregnancy.

ureteral tonus and peristalsis is inverse to the degree of dilatation, i.e., the greater the dilatation, the greater the urinary stasis and favorable opportunity for infection to develop or persist.

Obstetric trauma of the bladder and urethra, the last crushed between the infant's head and the under side of the mother's pubis (Fig. 319), not only induces pronounced congestive and inflammatory changes with edema and even hematuria but may also engender acute urinary obstruction which, if not recognized and treated promptly by aseptic indwelling catheterization for at least twenty-four hours, is almost certain to invite important infection. Even though complete retention does not occur, a variably large residuum—urinary stasis—may persist for several days after delivery and encourage infection. In short, inadequate care of the postpuerperal bladder permits urinary retention and stasis as it does in other postoperative conditions and resulting infection may seriously increase the morbidity.

The symptoms of "pyelitis of pregnancy" are those of the usual urinary infection as outlined in Chapter 7 and the diagnosis is similarly made as described there.

Treatment. During pregnancy special attention must be devoted to (1) avoidance of complications, (2) maintenance of adequate fluid intake, (3) prevention of anemia, by transfusion if necessary, and (4) repeated urinalysis, at least once a month, preferably by catheterization (Chapter 3), and always by this method if the freshly voided and shaken urine specimen shows more than 6 to 8 white blood cells per high power field. Under this circumstance, obtain a urine culture examination of a cathe-

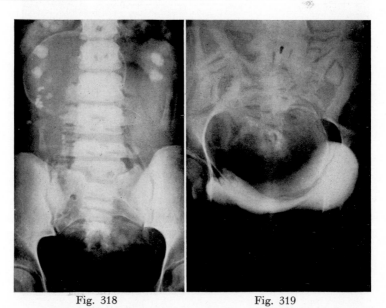

Fig. 318   Fig. 319

FIGURE 318.   Dilatation of the upper urinary tract in pregnancy. Breech.
FIGURE 319.   Vesical compression by the oncoming fetal head (see text).

terized specimen as well as urinalysis to learn precisely what the bacterial invader is, and the laboratory evidence of the severity of the infection.

Intelligently forearmed by appropriate antimicrobial prophylaxis and/or therapy many incipient infections can be aborted and the established ones kept under control. In antepartum management, the astute physician is ever on the alert for earliest evidence of complicating urinary infection that it may be intensively combated at once.

Without attempting to maintain such close antepartum attention of the patient, many obstetricians by rote have these pregnant women take a urinary antiseptic such as Gantrisin 1.0 gm. three times a day the first five or six days of each month. Whether this sterilizes the urine is problematic but such precautionary antisepsis has alone reduced the incidence of acute urinary infections in pregnancy by half (cf. Trout).

If the patient has had urinary infection or other urologic disease prior to becoming pregnant, the status of the urinary tract should be learned at once by (1) urine culture, (2) tests of renal function (phenol-sulfonphthalein excretion; nonprotein nitrogen determination of the blood), (3) an excretory urographic study, and, if this is not sharply definitive, cystoscopy, divided renal function studies and even retrograde pyelography. In addition, a careful checkup medical examination is indicated, especially of the heart and lungs, blood pressure, study of the eye grounds, observation of edema, and so forth.

With the onset of acute urinary infection during pregnancy, the treatment is that given in Chapter 7. If there is not prompt and satisfactory response to intensive antimicrobial treatment given according to bacteriologic indication and drug sensitivity tests, ureteral catheters (7 or 8 F., whistle tip and not stiff) should be inserted well up the ureters (25–30 cm.). These are anchored indwelling, irrigated with normal saline solution once or twice a day, and left in place until the temperature has been normal for at least twenty-four hours. Usually this will do the trick but when the infection persists hyperacute, make sure there is not renal abscess or perinephric abscess requiring nephrostomy, drainage or nephrectomy; the mother's condition may demand therapeutic abortion. Fortunately today few pregnant women with complicating urinary infection reach this stage.

Ectopic Kidney in Pregnancy. The multiplicity and coexistence of anomalies of the urinary and genital tracts is similar in both sexes; this has been discussed in Chapter 6. Yet of these anomalies one—congenital pelvic renal ectopia—is of great importance in pregnancy and delivery as a potential juxta-uterine obstructing mass. This congenital ectopia is to be distinguished from the more usual renal ptosis; in the congenital pelvic ectopia, the ureter is shorter than normal, the renal blood supply is from the adjacent lower aorta, iliac or hypogastric arteries, and, being anomalous, the organ is more prone to disease than the normally placed and formed kidney, especially to hydronephrosis and infection. The pelvic kidney may seriously interfere with delivery and while by good obstetrics there may be no maternal death under these conditions, one in ten viable infants will die at birth and with an average general fetal mortality of one in six. Yet, there have been maternal deaths, especially when the obstetrician, unaware of the pelvic kidney, has mistaken it for the fetus and tried to deliver it!

Although the ectopic kidney should be discovered before labor, it was overlooked in three fourths (74 per cent) of 209 cases collected by Anderson, was discovered during labor in 18 per cent, after pregnancy in 25 per cent and at autopsy in 7 per cent. Yet many of these kidneys are externally palpable in the abdomen (Fig. 75), and especially by bimanual vagino-abdominal examination, and good excretory urography should demonstrate nearly all of them. Therefore, for the best interest of the pregnant patient, routine satisfactory intravenous pyelographic studies will greatly broaden the obstetrician's knowledge of his patient and the status of her all-important urinary tract, painlessly, effectively and without jeopardy to the fetus.

Bibliography

GENERAL

Albright, F. and Reifenstein, E. C. Jr.: The Parathyroid Glands and Metabolic Bone Disease. Baltimore, Williams & Wilkins Co., 1948.

Allen, A. C.: The Kidney: Medical and Surgical Diseases. New York, Grune and Stratton, 1951.

Anson, B. J.: An Atlas of Human Anatomy. Philadelphia, W. B. Saunders Co., 1950.

Arey, L. B.: Developmental Anatomy. Ed. 6. Philadelphia, W. B. Saunders Co., 1954.

Bell, E. T.: Renal Diseases. Philadelphia, Lea & Febiger, 1946.

Best, C. H. and Taylor, N. B.: The Physiologic Basis of Medical Practice. Ed. 6. Baltimore, Williams & Wilkins Co., 1955.

Braasch, W. F. and Emmett, J. M.: Clinical Urography. Philadelphia, W. B. Saunders Co., 1951.

Campbell, M. F.: Editor: Urology. 3 Vol., Philadelphia, W. B. Saunders Co., 1954.

Campbell, M. F.: Clinical Pediatric Urology. Philadelphia, W. B. Saunders Co., 1951.

Davis, David M.: Mechanisms of Urologic Disease. Philadelphia, W. B. Saunders Co., 1953.

Everett, H. S.: Gynecological and Obstetrical Urology. Ed. 2. Baltimore, Williams & Wilkins Co., 1947.

Fulton, John F.: Textbook of Physiology. Ed. 17. Philadelphia, W. B. Saunders Co., 1955.

Goldblatt, H.: The Renal Origin of Hypertension. American Lectures in Pathology. Springfield, Ill., Charles C Thomas, 1948.

Gross, R. M.: The Surgery of Infancy and Childhood. Philadelphia, W. B. Saunders Co., 1953.

Higgins, C. C.: Renal Lithiasis. Springfield, Ill., Charles C Thomas, 1943.

Hinman, Frank: The Principles and Practice of Urology. Philadelphia, W. B. Saunders Co., 1936.

Hotchkiss, R. S.: Fertility in Men. Philadelphia, J. B. Lippincott Co., 1944.

Langworthy, O. R., Kolb, L. C. and Lewis, L. G.: Physiology of Micturition; Experimental and Clinical Studies with Suggestions as to Diagnosis and Treatment. Baltimore, Williams & Wilkins Co., 1940.

Moore, R. A.: A Textbook of Pathology. Ed. 2. Philadelphia, W. B. Saunders Co., 1951.

Moyer, C. A.: Fluid Balance. Chicago, The Year Book Publishers Inc., 1952.

Murphy, D. P.: Congenital Malformations. A Study of Parental Characteristics with Special Reference to the Reproduction Process. Ed. 2. Philadelphia, University of Pennsylvania Press, 1947.

Narath, Peter: The Renal Pelvis and Ureter. New York, Grune and Stratton, 1951.

Nelson, W. E.: Textbook of Pediatrics. Ed. 6. Philadelphia, W. B. Saunders Co., 1954.

Nesbit, R. M.: Transurethral Prostatectomy. Springfield, Ill., Charles C Thomas, 1943.

Patten, Bradley, M.: Human Embryology. Philadelphia, Blakiston and Co., 1946.

Prather, G. C.: Urological Aspects of Spinal Cord Injuries. Springfield, Ill., Charles C Thomas, 1949.

Smith, Homer, W.: The Kidney. Structure and Function in Health and Disease. New York, Oxford University Press, 1951.

Todd, J. C., Sanford, A. H. and Wells, B. B.: Clinical Diagnosis by Laboratory Methods. Ed. 12. Philadelphia, W. B. Saunders Co., 1953.

Wharton, L. R.: Gynecology with a Section on Female Urology. Ed. 2. Philadelphia, W. B. Saunders Co., 1942.

Wilkins, Lawson: The Diagnosis and Treatment of Endocrine Disorders in Childhood and Adolescence. Springfield, Ill., Charles C Thomas, 1950.

Young, H. H.: Genital Abnormalities, Hermaphroditism and Related Adrenal Diseases. Baltimore, Williams & Wilkins Co., 1937.

CHAPTER 1

Dorland: The American Illustrated Medical Dictionary. Ed. 23. Philadelphia, W. B. Saunders Co., 1957.

Fishbein, Morris: Medical Writing: The Technic and the Art. Philadelphia, The Blakiston Co., 1950.

Moore, T. D.: Urologic Diction and Usage. Urologists' Correspondence Club Letter (Dec. 27) 1955.

Style Manual: United States Government Printing Office. Washington, D. C.

CHAPTER 2

Campbell, M. F.: Viscerosensory phenomena in acute obstruction of the upper urinary tract. J.A.M.A., *92*:1327, 1929.

Olson, W. H. and Necheles, H.: Studies on anuria: Effect of infusion fluids and diuretics in the anuria resulting from severe burns. Surg., Gynec., & Obst., *84*:283, 1947.

Pitts, R. F.: Acid-base regulation by the kidneys. Am. J. Med., *9*:356, 1950.

CHAPTER 3

Bunge, R. G.: Delayed cystograms in children. J. Urol., *70*:729, 1953.

Hutchins, S. P. R.: A new catheter for pediatric use. J. Urol., *71*:767, 1954.

Matthei, L. P.: Excretory urography in children. J. Urol., *64*:417, 1950.

Smith, P. G., Rush, T. W. and Evans, A. T.: Evaluation of translumbar arteriography. J. Urol., *65*:911, 1951.

Stewart, C. M.: Delayed cystograms in children. J. Urol., *70*:588, 1953.

CHAPTER 4

Gruber, C. M.: Function of ureterovesical valve and experimental production of hydroureters without obstruction. J. Urol., *23*:161, 1930.

Richards, A. R.: Beaumont Foundation Lectures. Baltimore, Williams & Wilkins Co., 1929, 2.

CHAPTER 5

Creevy, C. D.: Distention of the urinary bladder. Arch. Surg., *25*:356, 1932.

Darrow, D. C.: Body fluid physiology: The role of potassium in clinical disturbances of body water and electrolytes. New England J. Med., *242*:978 and 1014, 1940.

CHAPTER 6

Anson, B.: Atlas of Human Anatomy. Philadelphia, W. B. Saunders Co., 1950.

Begg, R. C.: The urachus: its anatomy, histology and development. J. Anat., *64*:170, 1930.

Campbell, M. F.: Ureterocele: A study of ninety-four instances in eighty infants and children. Surg., Gynec. & Obst., *93*:705, 1951.

————: Urethrorectal fistula. J. Urol., *76:*411, 1956.

Carroll, W. A.: Malignancy in cryptorchidism. J. Urol., *61:*396, 1949.

Dean, A. L.: Cancers of the genito-urinary organs in children. J. Pediat., *15:*340, 1939.

Deming, C.: The evaluation of hormone therapy in cryptorchidism. J. Urol., *68:*354, 1952.

Engle, T.: Experimentally induced descent of the testis in the macacus monkey by hormones from the anterior pituitary and pregnancy urine. J. Endocrinol., *16:*513, 1932.

Gilbert, J. N.: Studies in malignant testis tumors: V. Tumors developing after orchidopexy: Report of two cases and review of 63. J. Urol., *46:*740, 1941.

Goldblatt, H.: Studies in experimental hypertension. Am. J. Clin. Path., *10:*40, 1940.

Gross, R. E.: Surgical experiences from 1222 operations for undescended testes. J.A.M.A., *160:*634, 1956.

Hildebrandt, A.: Weiterer Beitrag zur pathologischen Anatomie der Nierengeschwülste. Arch. f. klin. Chir., *48:*343, 1894.

Kampmeier, O. F.: A hitherto unrecognized mode of origin of congenital renal cysts. Surg., Gynec. & Obst., *32:*208, 1923.

Lewis, L. A.: Cryptorchidism. J. Urol., *60:*345, 1948.

McCollum, P. W.: Clinical study of spermatogenesis in undescended testicles. Arch. Surg., *31:*29, 1935.

McKenna, C. M. and Kampmeier, O. F.: Consideration of development of polycystic kidney. Tr. Am. Assn. Genito-urin. Surg., *26:*377, 1933; J. Urol., *32:*37, 1934.

Moore, C. R. and Quick, W. J.: The scrotum as a temperature regulator for the testes. Am. J. Physiol., *68:*70, 1924.

Moore, K. L., Graham, M. R. and Barr, M. L.: The detection of chromosomal sex in hermaphrodites from a skin biopsy. Surg., Gynec. & Obst., *96:*641, 1953.

Nordmark, B.: Double formations of the pelvis of the kidneys and the ureters. Acta Radiol., Stockholm, *30:*267, 1948.

Norris, R. F. and Herman, L.: Pathogenesis of polycystic kidneys: reconstruction of cystic elements in four cases. J. Urol., *46:*147, 1941.

Robinson, J. N. and Engle, E. T.: Some observations on the cryptorchid testes. J. Urol., *71:*726, 1954.

————: Cryptorchism: Pathogenesis and Treatment. Philadelphia. Pediatric Clinics. W. B. Saunders Co., pp. 729–736 (Aug.) 1955.

Sohval, A. R.: Histopathology of cryptorchidism: Study based upon comparative histology of retained and scrotal testes from birth to maturity. Am. J. Med., *16:*346, 1954.

Swenson, O., MacMahon, H. E., Jaques, W. E. and Campbell, J. S.: A new concept of the pathology of megaloureter. Bull. New England M. Center, *13:*157, 1951.

Wells, L. J. and State, D.: Misconception of the gubernaculum testis. Surgery, *22:*502, 1947.

White, R. R. and Wyatt, G. M.: Surgical importance of aberrant renal vessels in infants and children. Am. J. Surg., *58:*48, 1942.

Yarmudian, K. Y. and Ackerman, M. A.: Congenital polycystic kidneys. Urol. and Cut. Rev., *47:*147, 1943.

CHAPTER 7

Emmett, J. L., Alvarez-Ierena, J. J. and MacDonald, John R.: Atrophic pyelonephritis versus congenital renal hypoplasia. J.A.M.A., *148:*1470, 1952.

Hunner, G. L.: A rare type of bladder ulcer in women, with report of eight cases. Tr. South. Surg. & Gynec. A., *27:*1914; also Boston Medical and Surg. J., *172:*660, 1915.

Koppisch, E.: Manson's schistosomiasis. J.A.M.A., *121:*936–952, 1943.

Medlar, E. M., Spain, D. M. and Holliday, R. W.: Postmortem compared with clinical diagnosis of genito-urinary tuberculosis in adults. J. Urol., *61:*1078, 1949.

Spink, W. W., McCullough, N. B., Hutchings, L. M. and Mingle, C. K.: Diagnostic criteria for human brucellosis. J.A.M.A., *149:*805, 1952.

Sprunt, D. H. and McBride, A.: Morbid anatomic changes in cases of Brucella infection in man. Arch. Path., *21:*217, 1926.

CHAPTER 8

Allen, L. and Rinker, J. R.: The lymphatics of the tunica vaginalis with special reference to hernia and hydrocele. Anat. Rec., *94:*446, 1946.

Barr, M. L.: An interim note on the application of the skin biopsy test of chromosomal sex to hermaphrodites. Surg., Gynec. & Obst., *99:*184, 1954.

Bruskewitz, H. and Ewell, G. H.: The end results of the injection treatment of hydrocele. J. Urol., *59:*67–71, 1948.

Heckel, N. J., Rosso, W. A. and Kestel, L.: Spermatogenic rebound after testosterone therapy. J. Clin. Endocrinol., *2:*235, 1951.

✗ Kinsey, A. C., Pomeroy, W. B. and Martin, C. E.: Sexual Behavior in the Human Male. Philadelphia, W. B. Saunders Co., 1948.

Klinefelter, H. F., Jr., Reifenstein, E. C. Jr. and Albright, F.: Syndrome characterized by gynecomastia, aspermatogenesis, without aleydigism, and increased excretion of follicle-stimulating hormone. J. Clin. Endocrinol., *2:*615, 1942.

✗ McLeod, J.: The male factor in fertility and infertility. Fertil. & Steril., *1:*347, 1950.

McLeod, J. and Gold, R. Z.: Semen quality and certain other factors in relation to the case of conception. Fertil. & Steril., *4:*10–33, 1953.

MacLeod, J. and Hotchkiss, R. S.: The effect of hyperpyrexia upon spermatozoa count in men. Endocrinology, *28:*780, 1941.

Medlar, E. M., Spain, D. M. and Holliday, R. W.: Post mortem compared with clinical diagnosis in genito-urinary tuberculosis in adult males. J. Urol., *61:*1078, 1949.

Nelson, W. O. and Heller, C. G.: Hyalinization of the seminiferous tubules associated with normal or failing Leydig-cell function. J. Clin. Endocrinol., *5:*13, 1945.

Risman, G. C.: Effect of cortisone in orchitis of epidemic parotitis (mumps). J.A.M.A., *162:*875, 1956.

Turner, H. H.: Syndrome of infantilism, congenital webbed neck, and cubitus valgus. Endocrinology, *23:*566, 1938.

CHAPTER 9

Campbell, M. F.: A pharmacological study of the normal urinary tract in children. J. Urol., *43:*356, 1940.

Denny-Brown, D. E.: Nervous disturbances of the vesical sphincter. New England J. Med., *215:*647, 1936.

Emmett, J. L. and Helmholz, H. F.: Transurethral resection of the vesical neck in infants and children. J. Urol., *60:*463, 1948.

Swenson, O., MacMahon, H. E., Jaques, W. E. and Campbell, J. S.: A new concept of etiology in megaloureters. New England J. Med., *246:*41, 1952.

CHAPTER 10

Jewett, H. J.: A simple method for removing a constricting ring from the base of the penis. Urologists' Letter Club, July 29, 1949.

Prather, G. C. and Kaiser, T. F.: The bladder in fracture of the bony pelvis; the significance of the "tear drop bladder" as shown by cystogram. J. Urol., *63:*1019, 1950.

Trueta, J. et al.: Studies of the Renal Circulation. Chas. C Thomas. Springfield, Ill., 1947.

CHAPTER 11

Campbell, M. F.: Viscerosensory phenomena in acute obstruction of the upper urinary tract. J.A.M.A., *92:*1327, 1929.

Higgins, C. C.: Experimental production of urinary calculi. J. Urol., *29:*157, 1933.

————: Etiology and management of renal lithiasis. J. Urol., *62:*403, 1949.

McCarrison, R.: Experimental production of stone in the bladder. Brit. M. J., *1:*717, 1927; Causation of stone in India. ibid., *1:*1009, 1931.

Osborne, T. B., Mendel, L. B. and Perry, E. L.: Incidence of phosphatic urinary calculi in rats fed on experimental rations. J.A.M.A., *69:*32, 1917.

Prien, E. L. and Walker, B. S.: Salicylamide and acetylsalicylic acid in recurrent urolithiasis. J.A.M.A., *160:*355, 1956.

Randall, A.: The role of papillary pathology in renal calculus formation. Pennsylvania M. J., *44:*838, 1941.

Schorr, E.: Possible usefulness of estrogens and aluminum hydroxide gels in management of renal stone. J. Urol., *53:*507, 1945.

Suby, H. L., Suby, R. M. and Albright, F.: Properties of organic solutions which determine their irritability to the bladder mucous membrane. J. Urol., *48:*549, 1942.

CHAPTER 12

Broders, A. C.: Epithelioma of the genito-urinary organs. Am. Surg., *75:*574, 1922.

Busse, O.: Ueber Bau, Entwickelung und Eintheilung der Nierengeschwülste. Virchows Arch., *175:*346, 372, 1899.

Dean, A. L.: Diagnosis and treatment of testis tumors. New York State J. Med., *51:*485, 1951.

Dean, A. L. and Pack, G.: Treatment of malignant tumors of the kidney in children. J.A.M.A., *112:*408, 1939.

Deming, C. L.: Schwannoma. in Campbell's Urology (loc. cit.), Vol. II.

Dixon, F. J. and Moore, R. A.: Tumors of the Male Sex Organs. Washington, D. C., Armed X Forces Institute of Pathology, Section VIII, Fascicles 31b and 32, 1952.

Friedman, N. B. and Moore, R. A.: Tumors of the testis. Mil. Surgeon, *99:*573, 1946.

Geschickter, C. F. and Widenhorn, H.: Nephrogenic tumors (Wilms's tumors, cysto-denoma, and hypernephroma). Am. J. Cancer, *22:*620, 1934.

Grawitz, P.: Die sogenannten Lipome der Niere. Virchows Arch., *93:*39, 1883.

Huggins, C.: Effect of orchiectomy and irradiation on cancer of the prostate. Am. Surg., *115:*1192, 1942.

Jewett, H. J.: Significance of the palpable prostatic nodule. J.A.M.A., *160:*838–839, 1956.

Jewett, H. J.: Carcinoma of the bladder, J. Urol., *67:*672, 1952. Infiltrating carcinoma of the bladder; application of pathologic observations to clinical diagnosis and prognosis. J.A.M.A., *134:*496, 1947.

Muus, N. R.: Ueber die embryonalen Mischgeschwülste der Nieren. Virchows Arch. *155:* 401, 1899.

Nesbit, R. M. and Baum, W. C.: Serum phosphatase determination in diagnosis of prostatic cancer. A review of 1,150 cases. J.A.M.A., *145:*1321, 1951.

Nesbit, R. M. and Plumb, R. T.: Prostatic carcinoma: Follow-up in 795 patients treated prior to endocrine era and comparison of survival rates between these and patients treated by endocrine therapy. Surgery, *20:*263, 1946.

Papanicolaou, G. N.: Cytology of the urine sediment in neoplasms of the urinary tract. J. Urol., *57:*375, 1947.

Ribbert, W.: Üker ein Mego-sarkoma striocellulare des Nierenbeckens und des Ureters. Virchows Arch. f. Path. Anat., *106:*282, 1886.

Wilms, M.: Die Mischgeschwülste der Nieren. Leipzig, Arthur Georgi, 1899, p. 1–9.

CHAPTER 13

Addison, T.: On the Constitutional and Local Effects of Disease of the Suprarenal Capsules. London, D. Highley, 1855.

Bruce, G. M.: Ocular fundus in pheochromocytoma of adrenal gland; report of three cases. Trans. Am. Ophthal. Soc., *45:*201, 1947.

Cahill, G. F.: Adrenalectomy for adrenal tumors. Trans. Am. Assoc. of Genito-Urin. Surgeons, *44:*105, 1952.

Campbell, M. F.: Pediatric Urology, 2 Vol. New York, The Macmillan Co., 1937.

Chambers, W. L.: Adrenal cortical carcinoma in a male with excess gonadotropin in urine. J. Clin. Endocrinol., *9:*451, 1949.

Crooke, A. C.: Change in the basophile cells of pituitary glands common to conditions which exhibit syndrome attributed to basophile adenoma. J. Path. and Bact., *41:* 339, 1935.

Cushing, H.: The basophile adenomas of the pituitary body and their clinical manifestations (pituitary basophilism). Bull. Johns Hopkins Hosp., *50:*137, 1932.

Emlet, J. R., Grimson, K. S., Bell, D. M. and Orgain, E. S.: Use of piperoxan and regitine as routine tests in patients with hypertension. J.A.M.A., *146:*1383, 1951.

Fraser, R. W., Albright, F. and Smith, P. H.: The value of the glucose tolerance test, and glucose insulin tolerance test in the diagnosis of endocrinologic disorders of glucose metabolism. J. Clin. Endocrinol., *1:*297, 1941.

Fridericksen, C.: Nebennierenapoplexie bei kleinen Kindern. Jahrbuch f. Kinderh., *87:* 109, 1918.

Goldenberg, M., and Aranow, H., Jr.: Diagnosis of pheochromocytoma by the adrenergic blocking action of benzodioxane. J.A.M.A., *154:*1139, 1950.

Guarneri, V. and Evans, J. A.: Pheochromocytoma. Am. J. Med., *4:*806, 1948.

La Due, J. F., Murison, P. J. and Pack, G. T.: The use of tetra-ethyl ammonium bromide as a diagnostic test for pheochromocytoma. Am. Int. Med., *29:*914, 1948.

Marchand, F.: Ueber accessorische Nebennieren in Ligamentum latum. Virchows Arch., *92:*11, 1883.

Priestley, J. T., Randall, G. S., Walters, W. and Salassa, R. M.: Subtotal adrenalectomy for Cushing's disease. Am. Surg., *134:*464, 1951.

Robinson, F. J., Power, M. H. and Kepler, E. J.: Two new procedures to assist in the recognition and exclusion of Addison's disease: preliminary report. Proc. Staff Meet. Mayo Clin., *16:*577, 1941.

Roth, G. M. and Kvale, W. F.: A tentative test for pheochromocytoma. Am. J. Med. Sci., *210:*653, 1945.

Selye, H.: General adaptation syndrome and diseases of adaptation. J. Clin. Endocrinol., *6:*117, 1946: also Textbook of Endocrinology, University of Montreal Press, Montreal, Canada, 1947.

Spear, C., and Griswold, D.: The use of dibenamine in pheochromocytoma. New England J. Med., *239:*7366, 1948.

Thannhauser, S. J.: Hypoglycemia in the early phase of adrenocortical carcinoma. J. Clin. Endocrin., *9:*791, 1949.

Thorn, G. W. et al.: A test for adrenal cortical insufficiency. J.A.M.A., *137:*1005, 1948.

Thorn, G. W. et al.: Clinical studies in Addison's disease. Annals New York Acad. Med., 1949.

Thorn, G. W. et al.: Eosinophile fall as index of adrenal activity. New England J. Med., *241:*529, 1949.

Waterhouse, R.: A case of suprarenal apoplexy. Lancet, *1:*576, 1911.

Wilkins, L., et al.: The suppression of androgen secretion by cortisone in a case of congenital adrenal hyperplasia. Bull. Johns Hopkins Hosp., *86:*249, 1950.

Wittenborg, M. H.: Roentgen therapy in neuroblastoma. Radiol., *54:*679, 1950.

CHAPTER 14

Crabtree, E. G.: Urologic Diseases of Pregnancy. Boston, Little, Brown & Co., 1942.

Kegel, A. H.: Progressive resistance exercise in the functional restoration of the perineal muscles. Am. J. Gynec. & Obst., *56:*238, 1948.

Questions

CHAPTER 3

CHAPTER 14

Index